GYNECOLOGIC DERMATOLOGY

SYMPTOMS, SIGNS AND CLINICAL MANAGEMENT

GYNECOLOGIC DERMATOLOGY

SYMPTOMS, SIGNS AND CLINICAL MANAGEMENT

GUDULA KIRTSCHIG, MD, PhD
Consultant Dermatologist
University of Tübingen
Tübingen
Germany

SUSAN M COOPER, MD, FRCP
Consultant Dermatologist
Department of Dermatology
Oxford University Hospitals NHS Foundation Trust
Honorary Senior Clinical Lecturer
University of Oxford
Oxford
UK

JP medical publishers

London • Philadelphia • Panama City • New Delhi

Published by JP Medical Ltd, 83 Victoria Street, London, SW1H 0HW, UK
Tel: +44 (0)20 3170 8910 Fax: +44 (0)20 3008 6180
Email: info@jpmedpub.com Web: www.jpmedpub.com

ISBN: 978-1-909836-01-3

British Library Cataloguing in Publication Data
A catalogue record for this book is available from the British Library

Library of Congress Cataloging in Publication Data
A catalog record for this book is available from the Library of Congress

Publisher: Richard Furn
Associate Publisher: Sue Hodgson
Development Editor: Gavin Smith
Editorial Assistant: Katie Pattullo
Design: Designers Collective Ltd

Preface

Vulvar medicine spans the disciplines of dermatology, gynecology and sexual health. Many conditions affecting the vulva also affect the skin elsewhere, but their appearance may be modified by the vulvar environment, which is prone to heat, friction and occlusion. However, some conditions are unique to the vulvar site, influenced by hormonal and microbiological factors. Vulvar disorders may present, for example, as infections, inflammatory rashes or pigmented lesions, or simply cause pain. Time spent taking a careful history and carrying out a full examination is time well spent, increasing the chance of the correct diagnosis being made. The subsequent management of some vulvar conditions is complex and a multidisciplinary approach is often required.

Vulvar dermatology is still a developing discipline, and training and expertise is very variable amongst physicians. It is often difficult for practitioners to obtain practical help to deal with some of the problems they encounter in the clinic. There is a paucity of practical texts, with enough depth to satisfy the specialist but also be an aid to the generalist.

Gynecologic Dermatology: Symptoms, Signs and Clinical Management has been written to serve the specialist but also lead the generalist in a stepwise manner, offering basic knowledge about important vulvar conditions. The book has been written from a clinical perspective, and aims to assist the reader by providing a practical symptom- and sign-based approach. Features of the normal vulva are discussed in section one; section two covers diseases by symptoms such as itch and pain as well as by physical signs such as redness and white skin. In section three, individual diseases are each discussed in separate chapters written by experts in the field. Many tables and illustrations have been included to illuminate the text, highlight key points, and help the reader retain important information.

Many women still suffer in silence from irritating and often distressing vulvar symptoms, either because of embarrassment or because they believe that nothing can be done to help them. It is vital women receive the correct diagnosis and management when they seek professional help. The editors hope that *Gynecologic Dermatology: Symptoms, Signs and Clinical Management* supports the delivery of high quality care for patients with vulvar conditions and that, for some patients, it may help to change their lives for the better.

Gudula Kirtschig
Susan M Cooper
February 2016

Acknowledgements

We would like firstly to acknowledge our debt to Professor Fenella Wojnarowska who led the Oxford vulvar service for many years. She inspired both of us to work in vulvar dermatology and we are grateful for her enthusiastic support.

We are grateful to the colleagues who made this book possible by contributing chapters. Many more of our colleagues were also helpful during the preparation of *Gynecologic Dermatology*. We would particularly like to mention Professor Dr Theo M Starink and Dr Remco van Doorn of Leiden University Medical Center, and Dr Juliette Hoefnagel of Sint Lucas Andreas Ziekenhuis, Amsterdam, the Netherlands for their reviews and constructive criticism throughout the development of the book.

Dr Yves Bogaerts from Blankenberge in Belgium kindly provided the drawing of a 'normal vulva' (Figure 5.2) – a piece of artwork that is intended to serve as a master copy when taking notes in clinics and which may be copied freely.

Finally, we owe an enormous debt to our families for their understanding.

GK
SMC

Contents

Contributors

Ruth Asher, MB, ChB, FRCPath, DipRCPath(Derm)
Consultant Dermatopathologist
Department of Cellular Pathology
John Radcliffe Hospital
Oxford
UK

Tanja Gizela Bohl, MBBS, Dip RACOG, FACD
Jean Hailes Medical Centre for Women
Monash
Melbourne
Australia

Jan Brockie, SRN, NMP
Advanced Nurse Practitioner
Menopause Service
Women's Centre
John Radcliffe Hospital
Oxford
UK

Katherine Brown, MBBS, Dip RACOG, Dip Venereology, MSc M Forensic Medicine, FAChSHM, FFCFM
Medical Director, Ambulatory and Primary Health Care
Illawarra Shoalhaven Local Health District
Sydney Medical School
University of Sydney
Graduate School of Medicine
University of Wollongong
NSW
Australia

Fanny Camus, MD
Dermatologist and Venerologist
Department of Dermatology Venerology
Université Libre de Bruxelles (ULB)
Brussels
Belgium

Iskander H Chaudhry, MBChB, FRCPath
Consultant Pathologist
Department of Histopathology
St James's University Hospital
Leeds
UK

Susan M Cooper, MD, FRCP
Consultant Dermatologist
Department of Dermatology
Oxford University Hospitals NHS Foundation Trust
Honorary Senior Clinical Lecturer
University of Oxford
Oxford
UK

Christa De Cuyper, MD
Dermatologist
Department of Dermatology
AZ Sint-Jan Brugge-Oostende AV
Belgium

Joanne de Hullu, MD, PhD
Associate Professor
Gynecologic Oncologist
Radboud University Nijmegen Medical Centre
Nijmegen
The Netherlands

Marianne GR De Maeseneer, MD, PhD
Vascular Surgeon
Department of Dermatology, Phlebology Section
Erasmus University Medical Center
Rotterdam
The Netherlands

Barbara Eberz, MD
Specialist in Gynaecology and Obstetrics
Reference Center for Vulvar Diseases
Vice President, Interdisciplinary Interest Group for Vulvar Diseases
Mürzzuschlag
Austria

Sylvie M Franken, MD
Dermatologist
Department of Dermatology
VU Medical Centre
Amsterdam
The Netherlands

Karen L Gibbon, MB ChB, FRCP
Consultant Dermatologist
Department of Dermatology
Whipps Cross University Hospital
Barts Health NHS Trust
London
UK

Andreas R Günthert, MD
Professor of Gynecology and Obstetrics
Department of Gynecology and Obstetrics
Cantonal Hospital of Lucerne
Lucerne
Switzerland

Michael A Hambardzumyan, MD
Research Associate
Medical Scientific Centre of Dermatology and STI
Yerevan State Medical University
Armenia

Anne Lise Ording Helgesen, MD
Senior Consultant
Norwegian National Advisory Unit on Women's Health
Department of Dermatology and Faculty of Medicine
University of Oslo
Oslo
Norway

Aysha Javed, MBChB, MRCP(UK)
Consultant Dermatologist
Department of Dermatology
Lancashire Teaching Hospitals NHS Trust
Warrington
UK

Gregor B E Jemec, MD, DMedSc
Professor of Dermatology
Chairman, Department of Dermatology
Roskilde Hospital
Roskilde
Health Sciences Faculty
University of Copenhagen
Copenhagen
Denmark

Gudula Kirtschig, MD, PhD
Consultant Dermatologist
University of Tübingen
Tübingen
Germany

Claudia E Marchitelli, MD
Chief of Vulvar Disease and Surgery
President, International Society for the Study of
Vulvovaginal Diseases
Department of Gynecology
Hospital Italiano de Buenos Aires
Buenos Aires
Argentina

Janet McLelland, BSc, MBBS(Hons), MD, FRCP
Consultant Dermatologist
Dermatology Department
Newcastle upon Tyne Hospitals NHS Foundation Trust
Newcastle upon Tyne
UK

George Meligonis, MBBCh, FCPath(SA)
Consultant Histopathologist
Department of Histopathology
Addenbrooke's Hospital
Cambridge
UK

William James Merchant, MD, ChB, FRCPath
Consultant Histopathologist
St James's Hospital
Leeds
UK

Maja Mockenhaupt, MD, PhD
Senior Dermatologist; Head of German Registry
on Severe Skin Reactions (dZh); Coordinator of the
International RegiSCAR-Study Group
Medical Center, University of Freiburg
Department of Dermatology
Documentation Center for Severe Skin Reactions
Freiburg
Germany

Ruth Murphy, MbChB, MMEdSci (Med Ed), PhD, FRCP
Consultant in Paediatiric and Adult Dermatology
Sheffield University Teaching Hospitals
Sheffield Childrens' Hospital
Sheffield
Honorary Associate Clinical Professor
Nottingham University
Nottingham
UK

David Nunns, MD, FRCOG
Consultant Gynaecological Oncologist
Department of Gynaecological Oncology
Nottingham University Hospitals NHS Trust
Nottingham
UK

Dominique Parent, MD, PhD
Professor of Dermatology and Venerology
School of Medicine and Dentistry
School of Pharmacy
Université Libre de Bruxelles (ULB)
Brussels
Belgium

Mariola Pawlaczyk, MD, PhD
Assistant Professor of Dermatology and Venereology
Department of Skin Diseases Prophylaxis
Poznan University of Medical Sciences
Poznan
Poland

Michał Pawlaczyk, MD, PhD
Assistant Professor of Gynaecology and Obstetrics
Department of Gynaecology and Obstetrics
Szamotuły District Hospital
Szamotuły
Poland

Christiane Pfeiffer, MD, PhD
Department of Dermatology and Allergology
Ulm University
Ulm
Germany

Marjo J Ramakers, MD
Registered Sexologist NVVS/Fellow ECSM
CenSeRe (Center for Psychological, Relational and Sexual Health)
Voorschoten
The Netherlands

Sigrid Regauer, MD
Professor of Pathology
Institute of Pathology
Medical University Graz
Graz
Austria

Thomas Rustemeyer, MD, PhD
Professor of Dermato-Allergology and Occupational Dermatology
VU University Medical Centre
Amsterdam
The Netherlands

Ditte M Saunte, MD, PhD
Associate Professor and Consultant
Department of Dermatology
Roskilde Hospital
Roskilde
Denmark

Mirte Siemerink, MD
Dermatologist
Department of Dermatology
Erasmus University Medical Center
Rotterdam
The Netherlands

Michael Sticherling, MD
Professor of Dermatology
Skin Clinic, University Hospital Erlangen
Erlangen
Germany

Tom J Stoof, MD, PhD
Dermatologist
Department of Obstetrics and Gynaecology
VU Medical Centre
Amsterdam
The Netherlands

Kathy Taghipour, MD(Res), MRCP
Consultant Dermatologist
Department of Dermatology
Whittington Health
London
UK

Ad A van Bodegraven, MD, PhD
Departments of Gastroenterology, Geriatrics, Intensive Care Medicine, and Internal Medicine
Zuyderland Medical Centre
Heerlen-Sittard-Geleen
Department of Gastroenterology and Hepatology
VU University Medical Centre
Amsterdam
The Netherlands

Hedwig van de Nieuwenhof, MD, PhD
Resident in Obstetrics and Gynaecology
Radboud University Nijmegen Medical Centre
Nijmegen
The Netherlands

Irene A M van der Avoort, MD, PhD
Gynaecologist
Department of Obstetrics and Gynaecology
Ikazia Hospital
Rotterdam
The Netherlands

Laura T H Wang, MD
Assistant Professor of Clinical Obstetrics and Gynecology
University of South Carolina School of Medicine – Greenville
Department of Obstetrics and Gynecology
Greenville Health System
Greenville, South Carolina
USA

Jennifer Anne Yell, MBChB, FRCP, MD
Consultant Dermatologist
Central Manchester University Hospitals NHS Foundation Trust
Manchester
UK

Mirjana Ziemer, MD, PD Dr. Med. Habil.
University of Leipzig
Department of Dermatology, Venereology and Allergology
Leipzig
Germany

Martin Zikeli, MD
Consultant Dermatologist
Department of Dermatology
State Hospital Wiener Neustadt
Wiener Neustadt
Austria

Section 1

GENERAL CONSIDERATIONS

Chapter 1 Normal vulva

Andreas R Günthert

ETYMOLOGY

The Latin word vulva, earlier volva, from volvere 'to turn, twist, roll, revolve,' Sanskrit ulvam, was first used in the 14th century for the external genital organ. In common speech, the word vulva is rarely used, so many colloquialisms abound. Some authors prefer the Sanskrit word yoni. Furthermore, in the English language 'vagina' is often used synonymously with 'vulva,' which may lead to confusion as these are two distinct anatomical sites.

DEFINITION AND ANATOMY

There is great variability in the appearance of the normal vulva with differences in size, shape, and length of each individual structure. There is particular variation in the size of the labia majora and labia minora and the insertion of the labia minora. In addition, there are differences due to racial origin of skin pigment, hair color and distribution.

Vulva

The vulva consists of the external genital organs of the female mammal (**Figure 1.1**):

- Mons pubis
- Labia majora
- Labia minora
- Clitoris
- Bulb of vestibule (a mass of erectile tissue on either side of the vulva)
- Introitus vaginae (vaginal opening)
- Vulvar vestibule (part between labia minora)
- Bartholin glands
- Paraurethral Skene glands
- Sebaceous glands on labia minora and majora
- Orifice urethra (urethral opening)
- Frenulum labiorum pudendi (posterior fourchette)
- Perineum
- Ventral part of the anus

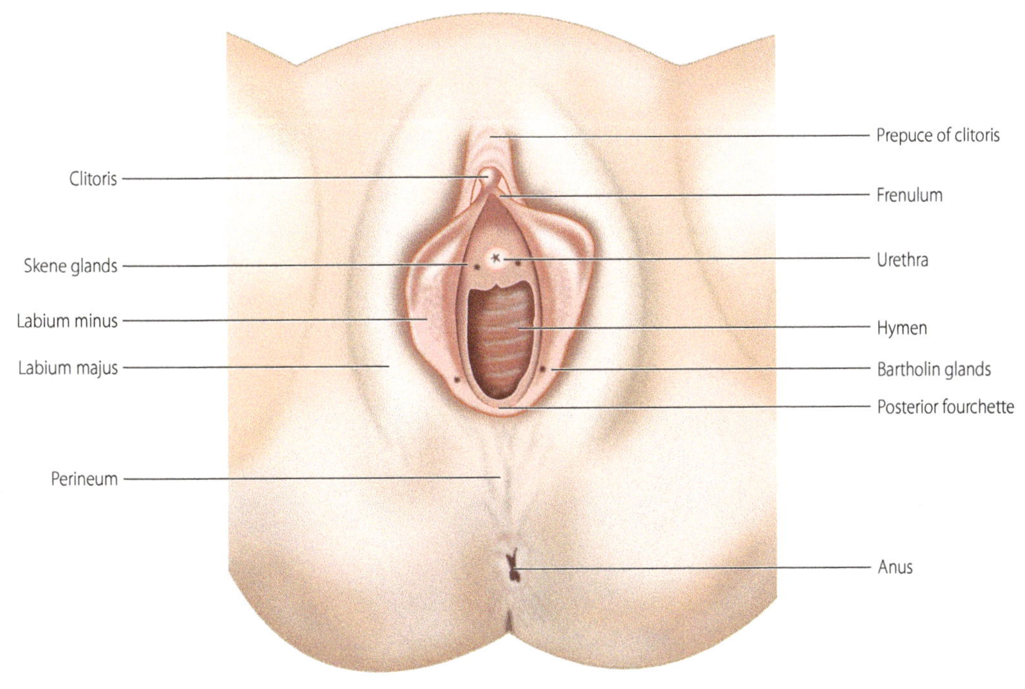

Figure 1.1 Anatomy of the adult vulva. Note: in a healthy nullipara, the vagina is not visible without manually parting the labia, which is often modified in anatomical drawings such as here.

The vulva is separated from the vagina by the hymen (O'Connell et al. 2008). Once the hymen is ruptured, the small skin elevations, which tend to occur in a circumferential pattern, are referred to as hymenal remnants.

A more recent anatomical classification involves classification of Muellerian parts of the vulva defined according to their ontogenetic origin (ontogenesis is defined as the development of structures from embryo to adulthood). This reflects and explains the development of some pathologic changes such as local cancer spread. Malignant solid tumors are confined to their ontogenetic compartment for a considerable time before spread occurs to other compartments. This may have important implications for surgical treatment of genital tumors (**Figure 1.2**) (Höckel et al. 2010, van der Putte 2005).

Clitoris

The clitoris was first described by Realdo Colombo, a student of Andreas Vesalius in the 16th century as a hidden part of the external genital, the amor veneris. The only visible part of the bulbo-clitoral organ is the glans clitoridis, which protrudes through the vestibulum through a channel. The transverse diameter of the glans is 3–10 mm, and it increases during sexual arousal. The prepuce partly covers the glans, which should be easily retractable.

Structures of the bulbo-clitoral organ (di Marino & Lepidi 2014)

- Cavernous structure parts (crura clitoridis) at the bottom of the labia minora
- Spongy structure parts (vestibular bulbs, commissure of the bulbs and glans)
- The junction of these parts
- Dense vascularization
- Dorsal clitoral nerve

The clitoris has double innervation, cerebrospinal via the pudendal nerve, and the autonomic nervous system via the inferior hypogastric plexus. Although the clitoris is a female's most erogenous zone, many women and gynecologists know little about its anatomy.

HORMONE RECEPTOR EXPRESSION

The growth of the vulva is predominantly regulated by androgens. During embryological development, the *SRY* gene of the Y-chromosome triggers the development of the external male organs, which can be inhibited by estrogens. The vulva as part of the genital tubercle remains androgen sensitive. The transition from vagina to vulva is marked by an increase in androgen and a decrease in estrogen and progesterone receptors (Hodgins 1998). Estrogens and progesterone regulate the hormonal changes during the menstrual cycle, and there is no effect of the menstrual cycle on measurements of vulvar structures (Morotti et al. 2013). In contrast, deprivation of androgens by antiandrogenic oral contraceptives may cause vulnerability to vulvar disease such as lichen sclerosus (Günthert et al. 2008).

DEVELOPMENT

Fetal period, neonate and childhood

In male and female embryos, the external genitalia start to differentiate after the 8th week when the fetus starts to produce its own hormones.

Dihydrotestosterone does not increase in females in contrast to males, resulting in differences in the male and female genitals (**Table 1.1**, Carlson 2014). In the neonate female, external genitals often look swollen and the clitoris enlarged which is an effect of the maternal hormones during pregnancy. During the 1st week after birth, the vulva will shrink in size and until the onset of puberty it does not undergo any change in appearance other than growing in proportion with the rest of the body (**Figure 1.3**). To avoid a hematocolpos in the menarche, it

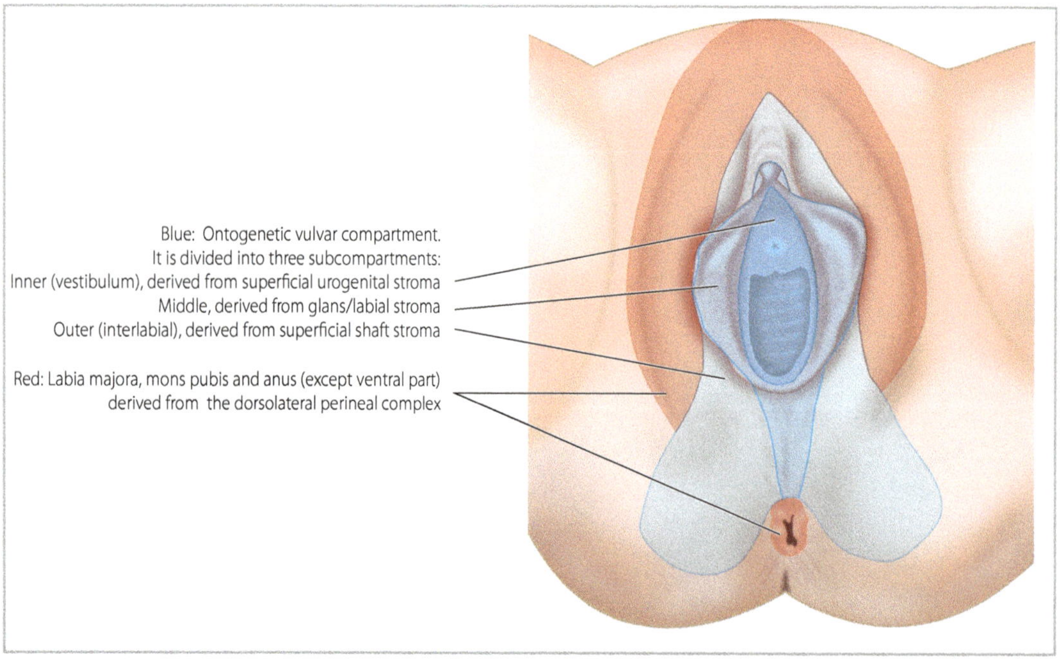

Figure 1.2 Ontogenetic compartments of the vulva (Höckel et al. 2010, van der Putte 2005). These compartments are anatomically separated regarding origin, sensomotor innervation, and vascularization.

Table 1.1 Differences in male and female genitals

	Females	Males
The genital tubercle forms the	clitoris	phallus
The genital folds form the	labia minora	penile urethra
The genital swellings form the	labia majora	scrotum

is very important to exclude an atresia hymenalis (imperforate hymen) at the first check-up of the neonate, because it is unlikely that the vulva will be examined in routine care during childhood.

Puberty

Stages I–V of pubertal development (Marshall & Tanner 1969)

- At the age of 10 years, short and downy hair starts to grow on the labia majora (II)
- During the next 3 years, hair becomes more coarse and curly and begins to extend laterally (III)
- Between 13 and 15 years, it extends across the mons pubis but spares medial thighs; its quality becomes those of adults (IV)
- After the age of 15, it extends to the lateral thighs but spares the linea alba, and finally it shows its typical upside down triangle (V)

Simultaneously, the mons pubis enlarges and increasingly separates the labia and the clitoris from the pubic bone, which varies according to body fat levels. The labia minora grow faster than other external genital structures and may protrude beyond the labia majora. Much of the variation in appearance of vulvas lies in the significant differences in size, shape, and color of the labia minora. On the inner side of the labia minora, multiple papillae develop, which vary in prominence. This is a normal finding but may sometimes be erroneously interpreted as human papilloma virus-related change. The skin of the vulva, excepting the labia majora, remains as hairless, moist, squamous epithelium.

Adults and childbirth

In adults, there is an enormous variety in size and shape of vulvar structures that are rarely defined by studies. Information on vulvar morphology is scanty and inaccurate in medical textbooks and publications (Andrikopoulou et al. 2013). By contrast, male genital measurements are widely available and were published as early as 1899. A cross-sectional study of 50 premenopausal women with no underlying pathologic vulvar condition was carried out in the United Kingdom to evaluate the measurements of the vulvar structures (Lloyd et al. 2005). Unsurprisingly, the women's outer genitals varied widely in size (**Table 1.2**, **Figure 1.4**).

During childbirth, the vulva and the distal part of the vagina might suffer from tears or be injured by an episiotomy. This can have a per-

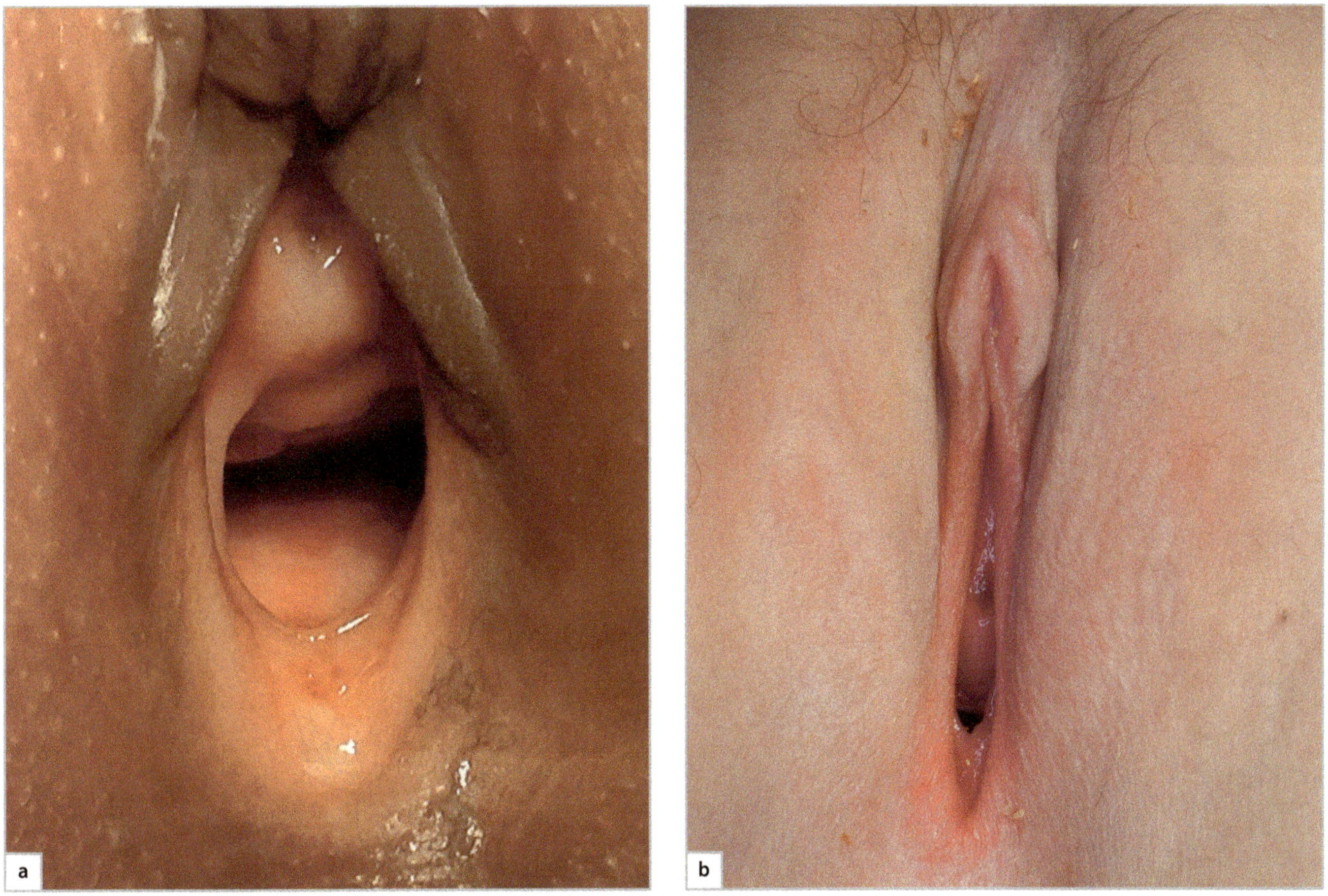

Figure 1.3 Prepubertal vulva. (a) The vulva of a 6-year-old girl lacks pubic hair and has small labia minora and an intact hymen with an open foramen. (b) In a 12-year-old girl, sparse pubic hair, labia minora, and the prepuce are starting to enlarge.

Table 1.2 Measurements of genitalia (data from Lloyd et al. 2005)

Measurement		Mean ± SD	Range
Clitoris	Length	19.1 ± 8.7	5–35 mm
	Width of glans	5.5 ± 1.7	3–10 mm
	Clitoris to urethra	28.5 ± 7.1	16–45 mm
Labia majora	Length	9.3 ± 1.3	7–12 cm
Labia minora	Length	60.6 ± 17.2	20–100 mm
	Width	21.8 ± 9.4	7–50 mm
Perineum	Length	31.3 ± 8.5	15–55 mm
Vagina	Length	9.6 ± 1.5	6.5–12.5 mm

manent impact on the width of the introitus and the condition of the pelvic floor. Although not confirmed by studies, the introitus and the distal part of the vagina in women after vaginal childbirth are often wider and sometimes require refashioning although this is usually for cosmetic rather than functional reasons.

Postmenopause

Concerns about postmenopausal vulvovaginal atrophy have created a market for hormone replacement therapy, although no large study has confirmed that age-related vulvar atrophy exists. With the postmenopausal reduction in estrogens and a bit later also androgens, the vascularization of the female vagina and vulva is reduced and sexual arousal and lubrication may decrease. However, based on the increased incidence of vulvar skin disorders such as lichen sclerosus after the menopause, there seems to be a protective effect of sex hormones. However, it is not known if hormone replacement therapy can protect a woman from lichen sclerosus. In fact, there is no evidence for a serious shrinkage of the external genitalia after menopause, irrespective of the age-related loss of elasticity of the skin as such. One cohort study from Turkey described a significant smaller vaginal length (8 mm) and width of labia minora (2.5 mm) in postmenopausal compared with premenopausal women, but the differences were small (Basaran et al. 2008). Interestingly, the mean labia minora width in the premenopausal cohort was much smaller compared with the UK group (Lloyd et al. 2005), suggesting a population-based and/or observer-based bias on the measurements of the 'normal' labia. Thus, the frequently postulated 'postmenopausal vulva atrophy' still needs to be confirmed.

PHYSIOLOGIC DISCHARGE

Lubrication is regulated by the autonomic nerve system and involves sweat, the Bartholin glands, the vaginal wall secretions, and the female

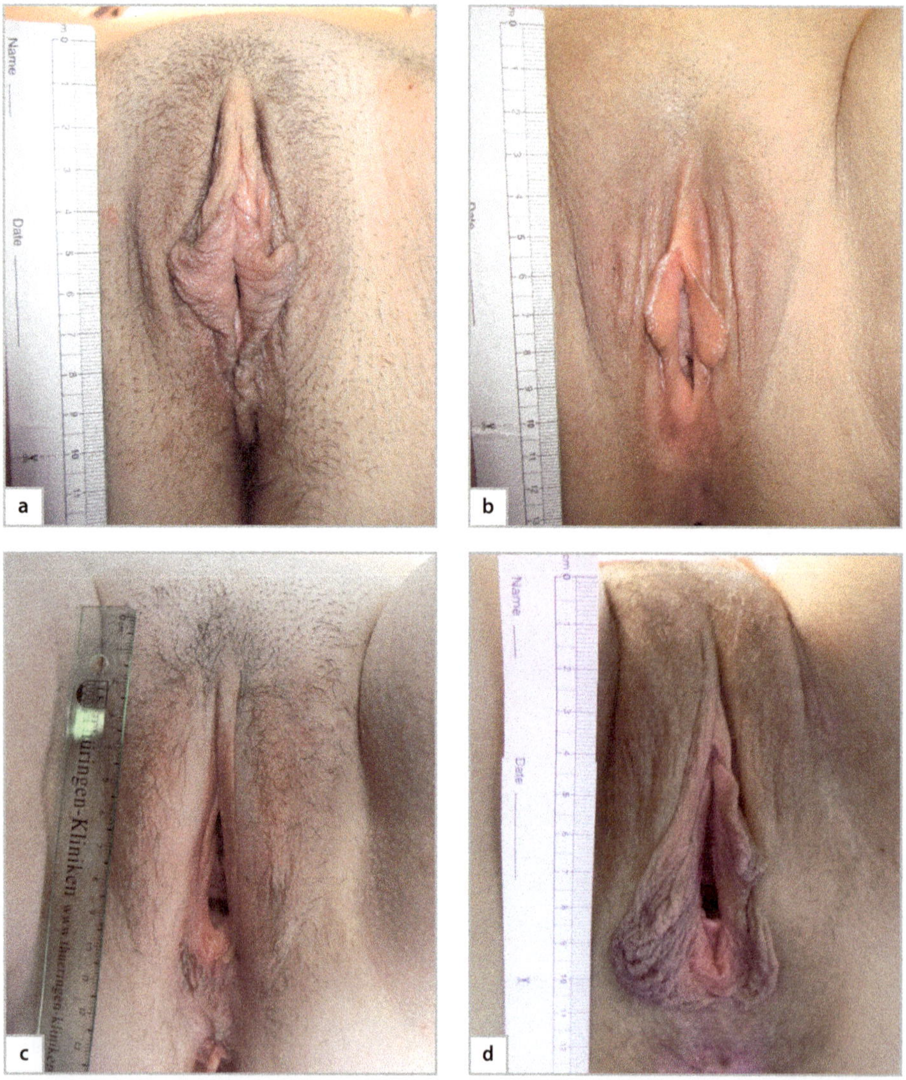

Figure 1.4 (a–d) Adult vulva. In adults, there is an enormous variety in the size and shape of vulvar structures. The normal vulva has not yet been defined. Considerable variability of the labia minora is noted including size and insertion.

prostate analog, the Skene glands. Smegma is a mixture of dead cells, sebum, and bacteria and can occur around the clitoris and in the interlabial sulci. Some women have physiologic skin bacteria that produce olfactory-stimulating aliphatic acids, and the concentration of these substances is affected by the menstrual cycle. Some authors described them as human pheromones, although there is no evidence that an olfactory relationship to pheromones exists in human comparable with those in rodents.

NORMALITY VERSUS 'SOCIETY'S IDEAL'

Currently, the practice of cosmetic genital surgery is increasing, driven by advertising, pornography showing 'idealized' external genitals, and mistaken understanding as to what is 'normal.' An increasing number of women and also girls with no underlying condition affecting their genital development seek surgery to alter their genital appearance. In particular, reduction in the labia minora or augmentation of the labia majora seems very popular. Since there is no definition of a normal vulva, it is surprising that some surgeons feel confident to achieve a 'normal' female genital appearance. One study has defined the labia minora as hypertrophic and thus deserving corrective surgery if the maximum distance from the base to edge exceeds 4 cm (Rouzier et al. 2000). A more recent study has demonstrated that the size of labia minora shows great variation far beyond the 4 cm claimed as being the maximum of 'normal' (Lloyd et al. 2005). Exposure to images of modified vulvas can change women's perception of what is normal and desirable (Moran & Lee 2014). In a large multicenter outcome, study of female genital plastic surgery, including 258 patients with different procedures, 91.6% of the patients were satisfied with their surgery (Goodman et al. 2010). It is likely that the number of women who seek plastic surgery to achieve 'society's ideal' for body and sexual well-being will increase in the next years. Thus, for physicians, it is important to understand these issues, and further studies are required to define the range of the normal vulval anatomy.

REFERENCES

Andrikopoulou M, Michala L, Creighton SM, Liao LM. The normal vulva in medical textbooks. J Obstet Gynaecol 2013; 33:648–650.

Basaran M, Kosif R, Bayar U, Civelek B. Characteristics of external genitalia in pre- and postmenopausal women. Climacteric 2008; 11:416–421.

Carlson BM. Human embryology and developmental biology, 5th edn. Philadelphia, PA: Elsevier, 2014:pp 376–399.

di Marino V, Lepidi H. Anatomic study of the clitoris and the bulbo-clitoral organ. Heidelberg: Springer, 2014.

Goodman MP, Placik OJ, Benson RH, et al. A large multicenter outcome study of female genital plastic surgery. J Sex Med 2010; 7:1565–1577.

Günthert AR, Faber M, Knappe G, Hellriegel S, Emons G. Early onset vulvar lichen sclerosus in premenopausal women and oral contraceptives. Eur J Obstet Gynecol Reprod Biol 2008; 137:56–60.

Höckel M, Schmidt K, Bornmann K, Horn LC, Dornhöfer N. Vulvar field resection: novel approach to the surgical treatment of vulvar cancer on ontogenetic anatomy. Gynecol Oncol 2010; 119:106–113.

Hodgins MB, Spike RC, Mackie RM, MacLean AB. An immunohistochemical study of androgen, oestrogen and progesterone receptors in the vulva and vagina. Br J Obstet Gynaecol 1998; 105:216–222.

Lloyd J, Crouch NS, Minto CL, Liao LM, Creighton SM. Female genital appearance: "normality" unfolds. BJOG 2005; 112:643–646.

Marshall WA, Tanner JM. Variations in pattern of pubertal changes in girls. Arch Dis Chil 1969; 44:291–303.

Moran C, Lee C. What's normal? Influencing women's perceptions of normal genitalia: an experiment involving exposure to modified and nonmodified images. BJOG 2014; 121:761–766.

Morotti E, Battaglia B, Persico N, et al. Clitoral changes, sexuality, and body image during the menstrual cycle: a pilot study. J Sex Med 2013; 10:1320–1307.

O'Connell HE, Eizenbern N, Rahman M, Cleeve J. The anatomy of the distal vagina: towards unity. J Sex Med 2008; 5:1883–1891.

Rouzier R, Louis-Sylvestre C, Paniel BJ, Haddad B. Hypertrophy of the labia minora: experience with 163 reductions. Am J Obstet Gynecol 2000; 182:35–40.

van der Putte SC. The development of the perineum in the human. A comprehensive histological study with a special reference to the role of the stromal components. Adv Anat Embryol Cell Biol 2005; 177:1–131.

Chapter 2 Normal histology of the vulva and anogenital area

Sigrid Regauer

The complex vulvar anatomy is reflected by the transition of hair-bearing skin in mons pubis and labia majora to glycogenated mucosa of the vestibulum featuring three different types of skin/mucosa and numerous glands. The vulva merges posteriorly with the perianal skin.

Key features of normal vulvar histology

- The vulva is composed of three types of epithelium/mucosa:
  - Hair-bearing skin
  - Non-hairy modified mucosa with cornified squamous epithelium
  - Glycogenated squamous mucosa
- There are three types of specialized glands:
  - Mammary-like glands
  - Skene glands
  - Bartholin glands
- The transition of modified to glycogenated mucosa is recognized as Hart line
- Melanocytes are evenly distributed within basal keratinocytes
- Subepithelial tissue (dermis) shows dense vascularization and sensory innervation

THE VULVA IN POSTPUBERTAL AND PREMENOPAUSAL WOMEN

Hair-bearing skin of mons pubis, labia majora (Table 2.1)

Hair-bearing skin consists of epidermis, the delicate papillary and collagen rich reticular dermis, and subcutaneous adipose tissue (**Figures 2.1a** and **2.2**). Epidermis and papillary dermis are connected by interdigitating epithelial and dermal ridges, which are separated by the basement membrane zone (junction zone). The epidermis is divided into basal and suprabasal keratinocyte layers (1), a continuous uniform granular cell layer (2), and a basket weave-stratum corneum (3) without nuclei (**Figure 2.1b**). A compact stratum corneum, retention of nuclei (parakeratosis), and discontinuous, wedge shaped or absent granular layer are features of various diseases.

Pubic/genital hair is thicker and longer than in an extragenital location. The superficial infundibular portion of the hair shaft within the epidermis contains a stem-cell population believed to be the origin of trichoepithelial tumors, basal cell carcinomas, and extramammary Paget disease. The isthmic portion is located within the dermis. Hair bulbs/roots extend into subcutaneous adipose tissue at a depth of 4–5 mm, an important distance for treatment decisions (e.g. laser versus surgical excision) when malignant disease extends along hair appendages [e.g. high-grade squamous intraepithelial lesions (HSIL) of the vulva and differentiated vulvar intraepithelial neoplasia (dVIN) in the infundibular portions] extramammary Paget cells can be found within the hair bulb (Regauer 2006). Sebaceous glands are located in the superficial reticular dermis, the secretory portions of eccrine and apocrine sweat glands in the deep reticular dermis. Apocrine and sebaceous glands terminate in the infundibulum of the hair shaft draining their secretions into the follicular lumen. Apocrine glands are lined by tall columnar cells with dense cytoplasm and luminal apocrine snouts resting on basal myoepithelial cells. Eccrine glands are lined by cuboidal cells sitting on a prominent basement membrane and terminate directly in the epidermis independently of hair shafts. A superficial and deep vascular plexus of blood vessels and lymphatic vessels supplies the dermis and adipose tissue, while the epidermis is devoid of blood and lymphatic vessels and supplied by diffusion. Androgen receptors are seen in epidermal keratinocytes, sebaceous glands, sweat glands, hair follicles, and dermal fibroblasts of vulvar skin, but no progesterone receptors are present. Estrogen receptors are restricted to basal keratinocytes (Hodgins et al. 1998) (**Table 2.2**).

'Modified mucosa' of interlabial sulci, labia minora, clitoris, clitoral prepuce

Modified mucosa lacks hair and is covered by a cornified squamous epithelium. It contains sebaceous glands that extend about 2 mm into the subepithelial tissue (**Figure 2.1c**). The density and amount of sebaceous glands vary considerably among individuals.

Table 2.1 Histological features of three types of skin/mucosa found at the anogenital site

	Hair-bearing skin	Modified mucosa	Glycogenated squamous mucosa
Location	Mons pubis and labia majora	Inner side of labia majora, interlabial sulci, outer side labia minora, clitoral hood, perineum	Vestibulum, including periclitoral and periurethral mucosa, introitus vaginae, and vagina
Stratum corneum	Present	Present	Absent
Granular cell layer	Present	Present	Absent
Skin appendages	Hair and adnexal structures	No hair, but sebaceous glands and specialized glands	Absent

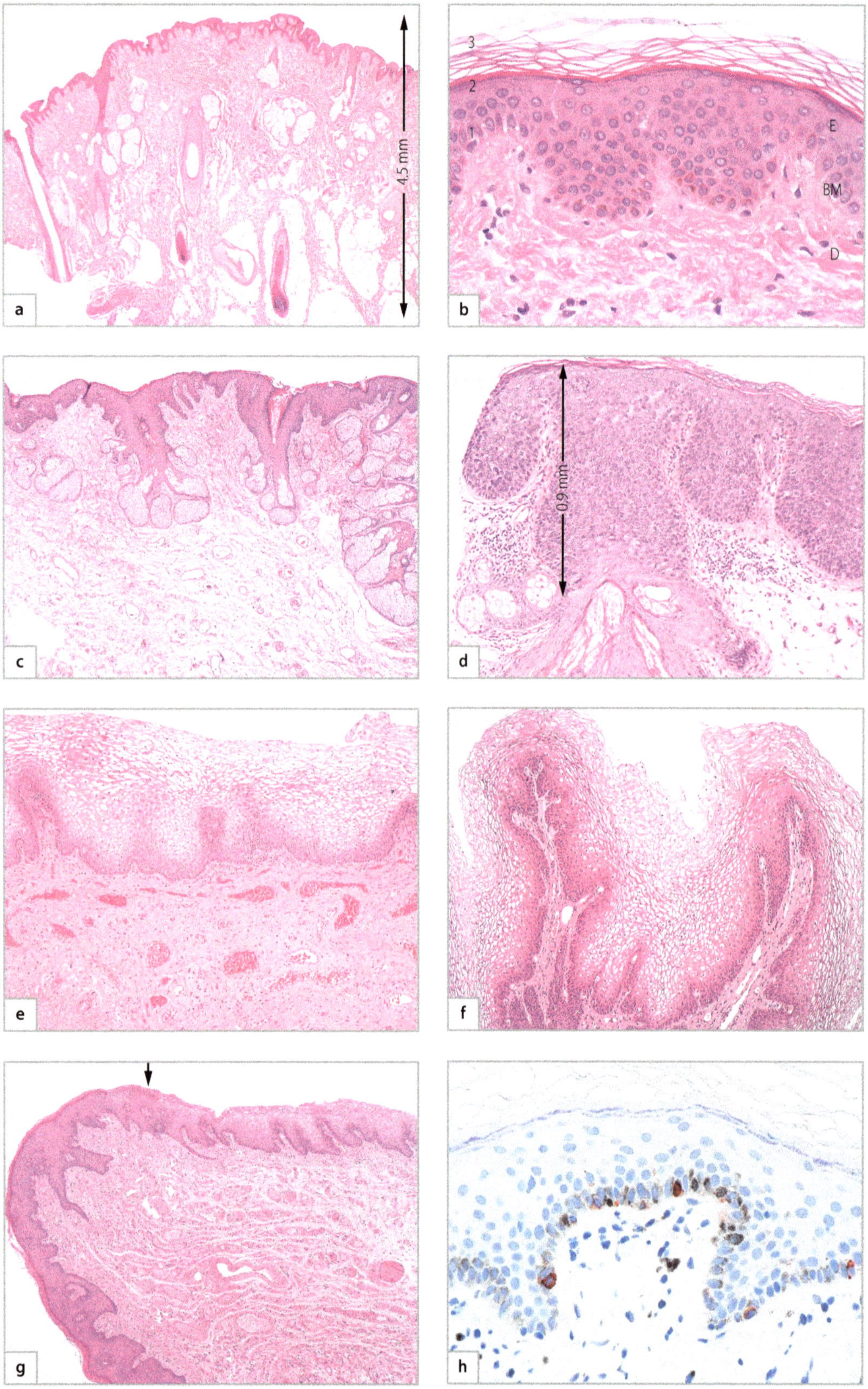

Figure 2.1 Histology of 'normal' vulva. (a) Hair-bearing skin with extension of hair bulb in subcutaneous fat at a distance of 4.5 mm. (b) The epidermis (E) is connected with the dermis (D) via the basement membrane (BM; barely visible in hematoxylin and eosin stain) and consists of a basal keratinocyte layer (1) resting on the BM and a suprabasal cell layer (synonym: spinous cell layer), a granular cell layer (2) and basket weave stratum corneum (3). (c) Modified mucosa with cornified squamous epithelium with sebaceous glands terminating directly in the epidermis. (d) Human papillomavirus (HPV)-induced high-grade squamous intraepithelial lesion) involving the infundibulum of a sebaceous gland with a vertical extension of almost 1 mm. (e) Stratified glycogenated mucosa of vestibulum devoid of skin appendages. (f) Vestibular papillomatosis. Note regular glycogenated epithelium without HPV-associated cell changes. (g) Cross section through the tip of a labium minus with the transition of cornified modified mucosa to glycogenated mucosa (arrow; Hart line). (h) Regular distribution of melanocytes (in red, immunohistochemistry with antibody to Mel-A) within basal keratinocyte layer.

They may be clinically recognized as yellow nodules or cysts with punctate openings (Fordyce spots). The infundibulum of sebaceous glands can be involved by HSIL (**Figure 2.1d**). The dermis is thinner, more delicate, and less collagenous than that of hair-bearing skin and contains numerous smooth muscle fibers, in particular in the labia minora. Subcutaneous adipose tissue is absent or scant. The vascular supply of the labia minora as part of the erectile tissues is more prominent than in hair-bearing skin and characterized by

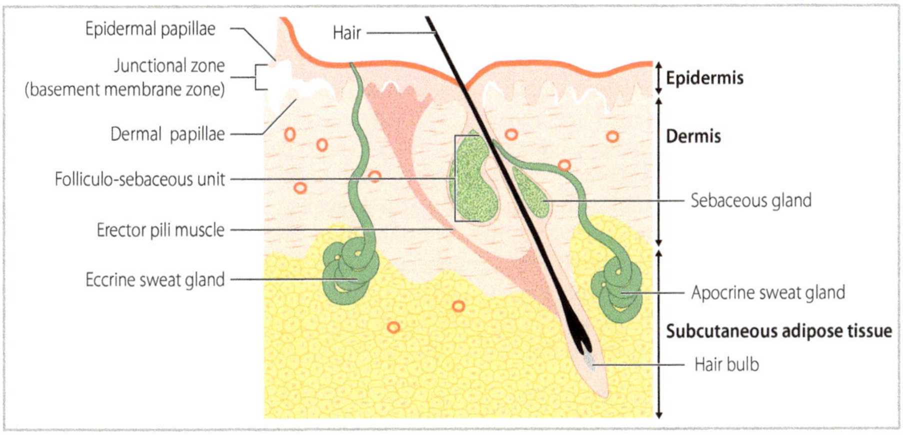

Figure 2.2 Sketch of normal skin showing the three layers of the skin with its appendages.

Table 2.2 Hormone receptors in vulvar epithelium

Receptor	Hair-bearing skin of labia majora	Modified mucosa of labia minora	Glycogenated mucosa of vestibulum
Estrogen	(+)	+	+++
Androgen	++	++	-

numerous thin, wide vascular channels, and thin-walled venous blood vessels. The erectile tissue of clitoris is composed of corpus cavernosum and spongiosum similar to that of penis with large irregular-shaped endothelial lined venous sinuses with longitudinal smooth muscle layers. Modified mucosa of the perineum and anoderm occasionally contains thin small hair. Hormone receptors for estrogens and androgens can be found. Androgen receptor expression is lower in modified mucosa of labia minora. Estrogen receptors are present in basal and suprabasal keratinocytes of the labia minora. Progesterone receptors are not present.

Glycogenated squamous mucosa of vestibulum including periurethral mucosa and introitus vagina

Glycogenated squamous mucosa is devoid of skin appendages and thin (**Figure 2.1e**), although it can assume a papillary configuration around the hymen (so-called vestibular papillomatosis) (**Figure 2.1f**), which is clinically often confused with human papillomavirus-induced condylomata. Glycogen content and epithelial thickness depend on estrogenization, e.g. receptors of estrogen α and β, but not of progesterone and androgen are expressed on basal and suprabasal keratinocytes. The highly vascularized subepithelial tissue lacks separation in papillary and reticular dermis and contains numerous smooth muscle fibers. The transition of modified to glycogenated mucosa (**Figure 2.1g**) is clinically often recognized as Hart line. The urethra is lined by urothelium, and the urethral orifice is covered by squamous epithelium.

Specialized vestibular glands

Glandular structures in the vulva are numerous. Mammary-like anogenital glands are found mainly in the interlabial sulcus between labium majus and labium minus (van der Putte 1994). They resemble mammary glands with tall columnar epithelium resting on a myoepithelial cell layer and express estrogen and progesterone receptors. They give rise to adenomas, hidradenoma papilliferum, adenocarcinomas, and the rare vulvar phyllodes tumors or invasive adenocarcinomas with overlying Paget disease (Kazakov et al. 2012). The small (about 1 mm) paired periurethral Skene glands resemble prostatic glands, express prostatic specific antigen, and are the origin of the extremely rare adenocarcinoma of Skene glands (Crum et al. 2014). The paired Bartholin glands (about 1 cm) in the deep posterolateral vestibule reveal tall columnar epithelium. The ductal portions with orifices lateral to the hymen show transitional epithelium. Minor vestibular glands in the posterior vestibulum are shallow tubular invaginations lined by tall columnar mucinous epithelium.

Normal pigmentation

Vulvar pigmentation shows wide constitutional (racial and genetic) variations. Melanocytes are of neuroectodermal origin and migrate from the neural crest into the respective organs, e.g. to vulvar skin. Melanocytes are regularly distributed among the basal keratinocytes, and their density is slightly higher in vulvar skin than in extragenital skin (1 melanocyte/15–25 keratinocytes, **Figure 2.1h**). Pigmentation depends on the type of melanin pigment (dark eumelanin, reddish pheomelanin) and melanosome maturation. Based on enzymatic activity and pigment content, melanosomes can be divided into stage I melanosomes (immature, no melanin granules) typical for mucosal sites to stage IV melanosomes (mature and pigmented) in skin and modified mucosa. Melanocytes transfer melanosomes via dendrites to adjacent basal keratinocytes in Caucasian or all keratinocytes layers in dark-skinned individuals.

Innervation

There is a network of myelinated and unmyelinated nerve fibers in the subepithelial tissues of hair-bearing skin and modified mucosa. Demonstration of sensory innervation is not possible on hematoxylin and eosin-stained sections but requires immunohistochemical staining with antibody to PGP9.5 (please note: S-100 antibody does not recognize sensory nerves). Various types of mechanoreceptors are identified in vulvar skin. Merkel cells are particularly common in modified mucosa of labia minora and the periclitoral mucosa. They are located either within the basal keratinocyte layer and/or immediately below the basement membrane. Meissner bodies are frequently found in hair-bearing skin and modified mucosa. Pacinian corpuscles are frequent near the clitoris.

Inflammatory infiltrate

As vulvar mucosal surfaces are constantly challenged by exogenous and endogenous antigens under physiologic conditions, small numbers of circulating lymphocytes, but no plasma cells, eosinophilic and neutrophilic granulocytes, or macrophages, are considered normal. Other cells involved in physiologic immune responses are submucosal mast cells and intraepithelial Langerhans cells, both of which require special stains for visualization.

THE VULVA IN PREPUBERTAL GIRLS AND POSTMENOPAUSAL WOMEN

In prepubertal girls, the major differences are observed in skin of mons pubis, labia majora, and perineum. They appear hairless, but histologically minute hair bulbs can be identified. Although the presence and distribution of hormone receptors show no difference in prepubertal girls and pre- and postmenopausal women, hormone-dependent growth of hair and increase of adipose tissue in children has not commenced. Sebaceous and apocrine glands are minute and 'atrophic' without secretion, and the amount of adipose tissue is scant. After menopause, atrophy as a result of lower levels of estrogen can be identified as thinner epithelium and decreased glycogen content and mildly atrophic sebaceous glands. In severe atrophy, degenerative atypia may be significant and raise the histological differential diagnosis of dysplasia. All other postmenopausal changes have no histological correlate.

REFERENCES

Crum C, Herrington S, McCluggage WG, Regauer S, Wilkinson E. Tumours of the vulva. Epithelial tumours. In: Kurman RJ, Carcangiu ML, Herrington CS, Young RH (eds), World Health Organisation classification of tumours of the female genital tract. Lyon: IARC, 2014:232–242.

Hodgins MB, Spike RC, Mackie RM, MacLean AB. An immunohistochemical study of androgen, oestrogen and progesterone receptors in the vulva and vagina. Br J Obstet Gynaecol 1998; 105:216–222.

Kazakov DV, Spagnolo DV, Kacerovska D, Michal M. Lesions of anogenital mammary-like glands: an update. Adv Anat Pathol 2012; 18:1–28.

Regauer S. Extramammary Paget's disease—a proliferation of adnexal origin? Histopathology 2006; 48:723–729.

van der Putte SC. Mammary-like glands of the vulva and their disorders. Int J Gynecol Pathol 1994; 13:150–160.

Chapter 3 Vulvovaginal care

Jan Brockie

This chapter covers general care of the vulva and care of the aging/postmenopausal vulva and vagina.

GENERAL CARE

Key points

- A woman should be encouraged to regularly self-examine her vulva to detect and report any changes
- All women should be aware of general vulvar skin care as vulvar disease is often caused or worsened by personal hygiene and self-treatments
- Women with vulvar disease need evidence based and relevant information about their condition and treatment
- Women should be encouraged to be involved in and take control of their own care
- Support groups and networks can help women with long-term treatment compliance

Vulvar skin is sensitive to irritants, and self-care and hygiene behavior can cause or contribute to vulvar disease. Likewise, good care may help prevent problems and enhance treatment effects (Marin et al. 2000). In addition, proximity of the vulva to the rectum, urethra, and vagina with irritant effects of urine and faeces and the mechanical effects of sanitary or incontinence protection may increase susceptibility to vulvar disorders.

Patient history

Women generally will not provide information about their vulvar hygiene unless specifically asked, as they mistakenly believe that their hygiene practices and self-treatments are safe. Often, 'special' products are used for vulvar care in the belief that normal skin care products are not suitable. Over 60% of women unknowingly use irritants and allergens (Marin et al. 2000). Possible irritants are numerous and sometimes allergies to products may develop after many years of use. Therefore, specific questioning is required to elucidate adverse hygiene or self-treatment practices. Women should be specifically asked about urinary and fecal incontinence. Symptoms are reported to be exacerbated by stress.

Information and support

Ideally, all women should be informed about appropriate general vulvar care, to promote safe hygiene and avoidance of irritants (**Table 3.1**). However, patients with vulvar disease should be provided with detailed information on their condition (**Table 3.2**) (UK National Guideline 2014). This encourages women to take control and manage their condition more effectively in the long term.

In addition to information, follow-up care and access to a support network can be helpful (BSSVD 2013). Patient support groups offer practical, emotional support and reduce feelings of isolation. Social media can also give easy access to mutual support while reinforcing information, treatment advice, and raising public awareness generally of vulvar disease.

Table 3.1 General advice for all vulvar conditions

Washing the vulva
• Wash the vulvar area with plain water. If water only causes dry skin or itching use a soap substitute as suggested by your health-care provider. Shower rather than bath. Do not wash the vagina • Do not wash the vulva too often as this may cause irritation, once daily is usually enough • Avoid products that cause irritation of your vulva such as soaps, shower gel, scrubs, shampoo, bubble baths, deodorants, baby wipes, antiseptics, fabric conditioners, biological washing powders, essential oils, and talcum powder. Thrush treatments and herbal products may contain possible allergens and irritants • Shampoo your hair over a basin if possible to avoid contact with affected skin • Avoid using sponges or flannels to wash the vulva, instead use your hand. Dry thoroughly, gently dab the vulvar area with a soft towel and do not rub
Clothing
• Avoid close-fitting occlusive clothing that trap sweat, promote candidosis or chafe the skin such as tights, G-strings, or tight jeans. Wear loose-fitting silk or 100% cotton underwear, change daily and sleep without underwear. Wash new underwear before wearing • Consider wearing a skirt with no underwear at home • Wash your underwear separately using a non-biological washing product. Wear white or light colored underwear as dark fabric dyes are more likely to cause allergies
Sanitary protection
• If possible use tampons not sanitary towels during periods. If necessary use sanitary pads with natural cotton, hypoallergenic and not those with plasticized 'one-way' top sheets that can cause sweating. Change sanitary products regularly. Avoid wearing panty liners or sanitary towels on a regular basis • Avoid colored or scented toilet paper and pat the vulva, do not rub
Other advice
• If you tend to scratch your skin, avoid wearing nail varnish and keep nails short • Shaving pubic hair and vulvar hair removal products may damage the vulvar skin • When, e.g. swimming (or going to the toilet/urinating), protect the vulva with a moisturizer such as soft paraffin before and again after contact with water • If the vagina feels dry or intercourse is uncomfortable use a simple vaginal lubricant around the vulva and vagina that is formulated for vaginal use. Oil-based vaginal lubricants cause deterioration in condoms and condoms with spermicides can be sensitizing to vulvar skin so may need to be avoided

Table 3.2 Care provision for women with vulvar problems

• A detailed explanation of the condition should be given, and this should include the long-term implications for both the patient and her partner. This needs to be reinforced with clear written information • Specific advice on care and treatments related to the condition should be provided by a healthcare provider; this may include other specific practical advice to aid comfort • Patients must receive education on the importance of avoiding potential skin irritants and possible comfort measures, using only vulvar products suggested by the healthcare provider • Patients should be given contact details of the healthcare provider if they notice a change or are concerned about their condition • Clear information about follow-up arrangements should be given, and these should be in line with current guidelines (e.g. 2014 UK National Guideline)

Self-examination

Regular self-examination of the vulva is crucial for early recognition of malignant change, enabling prompt diagnosis and treatment. It is recommended for all women aged > 18 years and those who are sexually active. Monthly self-examinations should be encouraged between periods. With the help of a hand mirror, the mons pubis, clitoris, labia majora, labia minora, perineum, and anus should be closely inspected in turn for notable changes, such as skin color (both whitening and increased pigmentation) or any new lumps, warts, skin tags, ulcers, or blisters. Any soreness, swelling, irritation, or pain that continues for more than a few weeks should be reported to a physician rather than self-treated (UK National Guideline 2014). Patient leaflets to guide women are available in some countries.

Sexual problems

A thorough history will reveal if disorders are contributing to sexual problems and also if adverse sexual behavior is contributing to vulvar disorders (see Chapter 39). Advice about the use of simple vaginal lubricants can help reduce pain and trauma during intercourse.

CARE OF THE AGING VULVA/VAGINA

Key points

- Vulvovaginal problems due to hormonal deficiency are common among postmenopausal women, and a detailed history, with specific questioning on vulvar, sexual, and continence problems, will aid diagnosis and effective management
- Treatment should be individualized depending on patient medical and menstrual history and personal preferences
- Both systemic and topical estrogen therapy may take several months to effectively reverse atrophic vaginal changes
- Vaginal atrophy will return if estrogen therapy is stopped, and its treatment may need to be continued in the long term
- Vaginal moisturizers and lubricants provide symptom relief but do not reverse the postmenopausal atrophic changes
- There is no proven benefit for the topical treatment of the vulva itself

Estrogen receptors are present in the vagina, lower urinary tract, and pelvic floor musculature, and low postmenopausal estrogen levels lead to atrophic changes in these areas. These changes may result in distressing vaginal and urinary symptoms (Sturdee 2014) (**Table 3.3**) in about 40% of women. Older women are reluctant to seek help (Kingston 2010). Urogenital atrophy should be considered alongside other causes of vaginal or vulvar discomfort in postmenopausal women. Also, as women age, the skin and hormonal changes increase the risk of vulvar and vaginal infection and slow the healing process (Kingston 2010). There is no evidence that vulvar atrophy due to hormonal decrease exists, since the majority of vulvar skin is not estrogen dependent, but decrease in androgens in postmenopausal situation might also contribute to vulvar changes.

All women should be encouraged to continue following general advice on vulvar care. In addition, as the incidence of urinary and fecal incontinence increases with age, if incontinence products are necessary, women should be encouraged to use products that contain a hydrophobic layer. This layer draws urine away from the surface of the pad keeping the skin dry, unlike some sanitary products.

Estrogen hormone therapy

Hormone therapy (HT) can be given either systemically or topically. HT has been available for decades, and recent evidence, global consensus, and national recommendations support appropriate use of HT, clarifying years of confusion over its safety (de Villiers et al. 2013). The global consensus states that local low-dose estrogen is preferred if menopause symptoms are limited to urogenital atrophy and dyspareunia and that the dose and duration should be consistent with the individual's treatment goals and safety issues. HT reverses the postmenopausal urogenital changes, but improvement can take several months. In severe cases of urogenital atrophy, a combination of systemic and local treatment may be needed. However, until now there is no proven advantage for local application of topical estrogens or any other hormonal creams or ointments on the vulva to prevent or reverse atrophy.

There are many systemic HT preparations, containing estrogen or combined estrogen and progestogen, and it is prescribed according to a woman's history and menopause status. Systemic estrogen preparations differ worldwide and include tablets, patches, gels, vaginal rings, and sprays. There are some relative contraindications to systemic estrogen therapy including a history of endometrial cancer, porphyria,

Table 3.3 Postmenopausal vulvar and vaginal atrophy symptoms and changes

Symptoms • Vaginal or vulvar dryness • Vaginal or vulvar itching • Vaginal burning • Dyspareunia • Skin fissuring around the introitus and fourchette • Dysuria • Urinary urgency • Urinary frequency • Urinary incontinence • Increased number of urinary infections
Changes • The vulva becomes paler • The labia are thinner and smaller • The clitoral hood is less obvious • The vaginal epithelium becomes thinner and loses its rugae • The vagina looks pale and dry or erythematous with fine petechial hemorrhages • Reduced vaginal and cervical secretions • Evidence of trauma such as skin splitting

severe active liver disease, thromboembolic disorders, undiagnosed abnormal vaginal bleeding, and breast cancer.

Topical vaginal estrogen therapy

Low-dose topical estrogen options vary around the world and contain different types of low-dose estrogen, given as cream, pessaries, ovules, vaginal tablets, or ring (**Table 3.4**). Systemic absorption is low with vaginal estrogen products, the extent depending on dose and formulation. Absorption is greatest initially but as the atrophy is reversed, systemic absorption drops. There is no evidence that these topical preparations cause endometrial stimulation, and the addition of progestogen is not necessary. Conjugated equine estrogen cream has greater systemic absorption and is now little used.

All topical estrogen preparations have a significant effect compared with placebo or non-hormonal products, reversing postmenopausal atrophy, improving vaginal comfort and dryness, restoring vaginal wall cells and elasticity, lowering vaginal pH so reducing risk of vaginal and urinary infections and improving sexual function. Atrophy will reoccur when treatment is stopped, and although there are no studies of use of vaginal estrogen beyond 12 months duration, it can be used in the long term (Sturdee 2014), and annual review is recommended (Sanchez-Borrego et al. 2014). Vaginal estrogen use is associated with minimal side effects, although local irritation or sensitization to their ingredients may occur.

If there is an inadequate treatment response after 3 months to a usual topical estrogen regime, changing the vaginal preparation, increasing the treatment frequency or dose, or using combination therapy may be considered. The global consensus advice recognizes that dose should be tailored to meet treatment goals (de Villiers et al. 2013). New lower dose vaginal estrogen products are now available, but improvements with these are not so great (Rees et al. 2012). So if deep vaginal atrophy continues, a vaginal cream rather than tablet or use of two vaginal estrogen tablets inserted simultaneously (one delivered to the posterior fornix and the second to the lower vagina) may treat the total length of the vagina more effectively. If areas of atrophy continue in the lower vagina or vulva, additional topical estrogen cream could be used and applied directly to problematic areas using a fingertip.

Use of topical vaginal estrogens, including promestriene, is usually discouraged in women with a history of breast cancer or other hormone-responsive cancer due to insufficient data. Local guidelines may exist or advice from an oncologist should be sought.

Table 3.4 Low-dose local vaginal estrogen therapies

Vaginal tablets
• Estradiol hemihydrate: 10 µg tablet vaginally for 2 weeks, then one tablet 2–3 times weekly
Vaginal cream
• 17β-estradiol: 2–4 g/day for 1–2 weeks, then 1 g for 1–3 times weekly
Vaginal ovules/pessaries/cream
• Estriol: 1 applicatorful daily for 2 weeks, then twice weekly 0.01% or 0.1%
• Promestriene: 1 application 2–3 times/day, then one application daily diethyl-ether of estradiol
Vaginal ring
• 17β estradiol: one ring with 2 mg estradiol replaced every 90 days

Ospemifene

This oral/systemic selective estrogen receptor modulator is licensed in some countries for the treatment of urogenital atrophy. Ospemifene acts as estrogen agonist in the vagina, reducing dyspareunia, but it is not licensed for women with a history of breast cancer. As an oral therapy, it can offer a useful alternative to vaginal products for women with limited dexterity to cope with topical application.

Non-hormonal vaginal moisturizers

Non-hormonal vaginal moisturizers are alternatives if estrogen preparations are to be avoided. Applications can offer effective symptom relief for 2-4 days and reduce the vaginal pH; however, they do not reverse the postmenopausal changes. Various products are available, and the active component, either hyaluronic acid or polycarbophil, contains many times their own weight in water that is gradually released over a number of days to provide a moisturizing effect.

Vaginal lubricants

Non-hormonal vaginal lubricants are primarily used to aid comfort during intercourse, and they can be used alongside topical vaginal estrogen therapy or moisturizers. Used daily, they too can help with atrophic symptoms. Lubricants specifically formulated for vaginal use should be encouraged, as they are designed to replicate the natural vaginal secretions. If a preparation causes stinging (mainly water-based products), advise using another product. Both water- and oil-based products are available; any oil-based product may affect the integrity and therefore safety of condoms; however, they are often better tolerated. Traditionally, many natural products have been used to help with vaginal comfort, but evidence on effectiveness is limited. Like moisturizers, lubricants do not reverse the postmenopausal changes; however, regular sexual intercourse will help maintain vaginal health.

REFERENCES

British Association for Sexual Health and HIV. 2014 UK national guideline on the management of vulval conditions. 2014. http://www.bashh.org/documents/UK national guideline for the management of vulval conditions 2014.pdf (accessed 22 Oct 2015).

British Society for the Study of Vulval Disease BSSVD 2013. Standards of care for women with vulval conditions. https://www.pcc-cic.org.uk/sites/default/files/articles/attachments/standards_of_care_vulval_conditions_report.pdf (accessed 22 Oct 2015).

de Villiers TJ, Gass MLS, Haines CJ, et al. Global consensus statement on menopausal hormone therapy. Maturitas 2013; 74:391–392.

Kingston A. Vulval disease in the postmenopausal patient: a guide to current management. Menopause Int 2010; 16:117–120.

Marin MG, King R, Sfameni S, Dennerstein GJ. Adverse behavioural and sexual factors in chronic vulval disease. Am J Obstet Gynecol 2000; 183:34–38.

Rees M, Perez-Lopez FR, Ceasu I, et al. EMAS clinical guide: Low-dose vaginal estrogens for postmenopausal vaginal atrophy. Maturitas 2012; 73:171–174.

http://www.rcog.org.uk/files/rcog-corp/GTG58Vulval22022011.pdf

Sanchez-Borrego R, Manubens M, Navarro MC, et al. Position of the Spanish Menopause Society regarding vaginal health care in postmenopausal women. Maturitas 2014; 7:146–150.

Sturdee D. Urogenital atrophy. Post Reprod Health 2014; 20:73–75.

Chapter 4 Taking a vulvar history and examination of the vulva

Barbara Eberz

HISTORY

A detailed history is the most important step to accurate diagnosis. It should be performed carefully using a structured approach before examination and, if necessary, be completed afterward. A questionnaire may be helpful. However, it is vital to remain vigilant to the patient's cues as patients are often embarrassed or reluctant to divulge some information, and if there is too much focus on a structured history, these clues may be missed. Basic elements include a description of vulvar symptoms, previous vulvar treatments, and diagnoses, followed by a gynecological, general, and sexual history when appropriate. It is essential to allow sufficient time for patients with vulvar complaints.

Key points

- A thorough history is vital for correct diagnosis
- Allow sufficient time when taking a vulvar history
- Follow a structured procedure for taking a vulvar history (e.g. questionnaire)
- Listen to patient´s symptoms and description of vulvar changes
- Ascertain prior treatments (prescribed and non-prescribed) and treatment effect
- Obtain dermatological, gynecological, and general medical history
- Address sexual difficulties and psychosexual issues when appropriate

Specific vulvar history

When a patient is referred, request a detailed letter of referral. The patient should be allowed to explain her symptoms in detail including the presence of itching, pain, soreness, and any vulvar changes seen or felt by self-examination or by a partner. This may be problematic because some patients lack correct expressions for 'vulva' and may use the term 'vagina.' It can be helpful to ask patients to describe the symptom of pain in more detail as it may be stabbing, sharp, burning, or a dull ache (the presence of sharp stabbing pains may indicate neuropathic pain, Chapter 38). Use the visual analog scale for patients with pain and inquire about other pain problems including painful micturition and defecation, pelvic- and bowel-associated pain, migraine, and muscle and joint aches.

The next step is an assessment of localization, intensity, duration, and trigger factors of symptoms including questions about the onset and course of symptoms. The presence and absence of concomitant vaginal symptoms should be documented. Knowledge of preceding local, systemic, surgical and also specific therapeutic procedures (e.g. laser therapy, pelvic floor re-education, psychosexual therapy), and treatment success or worsening effects of therapies is essential. All previous vulva-related diagnoses may be relevant for present complaints. Inquire about self-treatment and vulvar hygiene practices, e.g. the frequency of washing, use of soaps and disinfectants, and the use of sanitary towels. Ask if the patient has problems with holding urine or stool (incontinence will worsen or cause certain dermatoses). The most common conditions assigned to chronic/recurrent vulvar complaints are summarized in **Table 4.1**.

Gynecological history

A thorough gynecological history is often helpful. Information about menstruation including the age of menopause is important, as an early menopause may alert the physician to postmenopausal atrophic changes. A history of cervical intraepithelial neoplasia (CIN) or abnormal smears including the presence of human papillomavirus (HPV) may make one more alert to the possibility of vulvar intraepithelial neoplasia.

Table 4.1 Most common conditions assigned to chronical/recurrent vulvar symptoms

Pruritus	Pain	Soreness or tendency to fissuring
Lichen sclerosus	Vulvodynia	Lichen planus
Candida infection	Lichen planus	Lichen sclerosus
Lichen simplex chronicus Contact dermatitis	Herpes simplex virus infection	Incorrect vulvar care
Psoriasis inversa	Lichen sclerosus	Psoriasis
Lichen planus	Certain neoplasms	*Candida* infection

Key points

• Menstruation	Regular, any complaints, change of symptoms?
• Menopause	Age at onset?
• Hormone treatments	Present/past, local/systemic (contraception)?
• Obstetric history	Number of pregnancies, instrumental delivery, episiotomies, tears, terminations?
• Other conditions	Vaginal discharge, recurrent yeast infections, endometriosis?
• Sexually transmitted diseases	Pelvic inflammatory disease, herpes, chlamydia?
• Surgical	Hysterectomy, prolapse repair?
• Cervical screening	PAP-smear, human papilloma virus infection/cervical intraepithelial neoplasia? Any treatment for this?

Medical history

A comprehensive history includes medical conditions such as diabetes, hypertension, autoimmune diseases, or cancer. If a patient has diabetes, it is prudent to inquire about diabetic control as poor control is frequently associated with vulvar symptoms and Candida infection. Knowledge of all current medication is essential. Lichen planus (LP) may be induced by a number of medications for heart and kidney disease and estrogen depriving treatments for breast cancer may give rise to severe postmenopausal symptoms. A family history of autoimmune disease should be sought as the common vulvar conditions, lichen sclerosus (LS) and LP, are frequently associated with other autoimmune diseases (Cooper et al. 2008).

Key points

- Medical history especially diabetes, autoimmune, bowel disease
- Previous history of cancer particularly breast cancer
- Family history of conditions (autoimmune, bowel disease, etc.)
- Immunosuppression
- Medications
- Smoking
- Alcohol and drug abuse

Dermatological history

It is important to ask about other skin diseases, particularly eczema and psoriasis, and to inquire about signs and symptoms elsewhere in the body (Eberz et al. 2008). This may give a clue to diagnosis as patients with genital psoriasis and eczema frequently have disease elsewhere and patients with genital LP often have oral or nail involvement (see other chapters for details).

Key points

- Allergies: Type I (pollen, latex, etc.), type IV (metals in jewelry, creams, etc. Chapters 16 and 17)
- Atopy: Eczema (in childhood), allergic rhinitis or asthma; family history (Chapter 16)
- Psoriasis: (see Chapter 22)

Sexual history

This is an important aspect of history taking and most patients should be asked about whether there are any problems with intercourse. This is especially important in patients with vulvar pain, after surgical procedures or diseases with vulvar architectural changes. Patients with difficulty with intercourse may need a more detailed history including frequency, penetrative, or non-penetrative intercourse (Nunns et al. 2010). All doctors should be able to elicit the basics of a sexual history, but training in sexual medicine is advised for dealing with more complex problems (see Chapters 38 and 39). Remember that older women and women without regular partners may still be sexually active. It is worth establishing if her sex life was good before the onset of the vulvar pain and whether there has ever been any unwanted sexual attention. This needs to be asked sensitively.

Key points

- Current partner – any relationship problems?
- Intercourse possible?
- Pain on intercourse (superficial, at the introitus/deep in the vagina)?
- Is pain only on sexual activity?
- Problems with sexual arousal and orgasm?
- When did the sexual problem start?
- Dryness – use of lubricants?
- Description of sexual activity in patient's own words (what happens when you are sexually active?)
- What is the partner's response to the difficulty?

EXAMINATION

The examination of the vulva should be performed as a structured and careful procedure, bearing in mind the patient's history. Sometimes, especially in the early stages of disease, findings may be subtle and are easily missed. Offer a friend, partner, or chaperone to accompany the patient and put the patient at ease, although sometimes it may be inhibiting when talking about sexual problems to have another person in the room. It is very important to examine the patient's skin generally including an examination of the mouth, nails, scalp, eyes, and rest of the skin.

General examination of skin and mucous membranes

Examination of the skin frequently gives clues to diagnosis and ideally should be performed at the first visit. This can be performed quickly by doing a visual check of the nails; looking at the elbows, knees, and trunk; examining the scalp and external ears; pulling down the lower eyelids to observe the conjunctiva; and examining the mouth including the buccal and gingival mucosa and tongue.

Key points

• Nails	Observe, e.g. pitting and onycholysis in psoriasis, scarring in LP
• Scalp	Scaling in seborrheic dermatitis, psoriasis, alopecia in LP and lupus erythematosus
• Ears	Scaling in seborrheic dermatitis, psoriasis
• Mouth	Changes seen in LP and mucous membrane pemphigoid
• Elbows/knees	Scaling and plaques in psoriasis
• Eyes	Pallor of conjunctiva in anemia, scarring in mucous membrane pemphigoid, persistent tearing in lacrimal duct occlusion in LP
• General	For example, extragenital LS and LP, eczema, psoriasis, and vitiligo

Inspection of the vulva, perianal region and vagina

A complete examination includes inspection of vulva, perineum, perianal region, and vagina. In cases of pain or architectural/focal changes, this will be followed by palpation of the affected sites and, when appropriate by vulvoscopy, staining with acetic acid and special examinations like saline preparations, and microbiological and/or viral swabs.

Key features

- Visualization and examination of vulva using gynecological chair if available, otherwise the patient should lie on their back or on one side with their legs open
- Inform the patient about the examination step-by-step, do not touch the vulva unexpectedly; take particular care in very young patients, those who are anxious or have pain
- Examine the vagina and perianal region (and rest of skin/mucosa)
- Describe anatomical changes and lesions (Chapter 5)
- Take a photo if possible (and with the patient's consent)
- Use 3–5% acetic acid in evaluation of precancers (take a biopsy if suspicious)
- Take swabs or biopsy if necessary (consent)

A thorough evaluation of the vulva documents all findings including normal features. First, the gross anatomy is evaluated including whether structures are present, missing, or reduced (female genital mutilation, labial fusion, scarring, atrophy, or buried clitoris in LS and LP). For visualization of the clitoris, it is crucial to spread the labia minora and to retract the prepuce (**Figure 4.1a** and **b**). Simultaneous traction backward and lateral allows a good estimation of appearance and width of the entrance of the vagina. This also allows inspection of the perianal region (**Figure 4.2 a** and **b**). Careful digital examination starting with one finger can ascertain whether there is an involuntary vaginal muscle spasm known as vaginismus. Afterward, specific changes such as macules, papules, including color, dimension, texture, number, borders, and presence of scale, crust, or scars tissue defects, etc. are documented (see Chapter 5). Taking a photograph is helpful.

For inspection of the vagina, some training is usually required to handle the speculum. It is useful to have at least two or three sizes available. A sufficient vaginal inspection allows inspection of the entire vaginal walls, the fornices, and the cervix and the sampling of vaginal discharge for wet mount tests and microbiological cultures and viral tests like HPV.

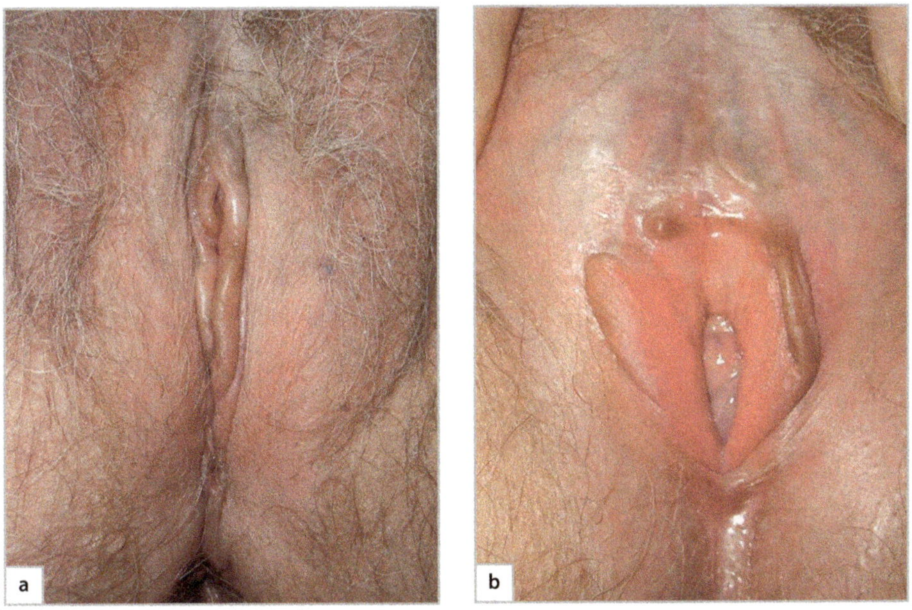

Figure 4.1 Advanced lichen sclerosus in a 63-year-old woman (a) with partial shrinkage of labia minora and severe (peri) clitoral synechiae seen only by spreading of the labia (b).

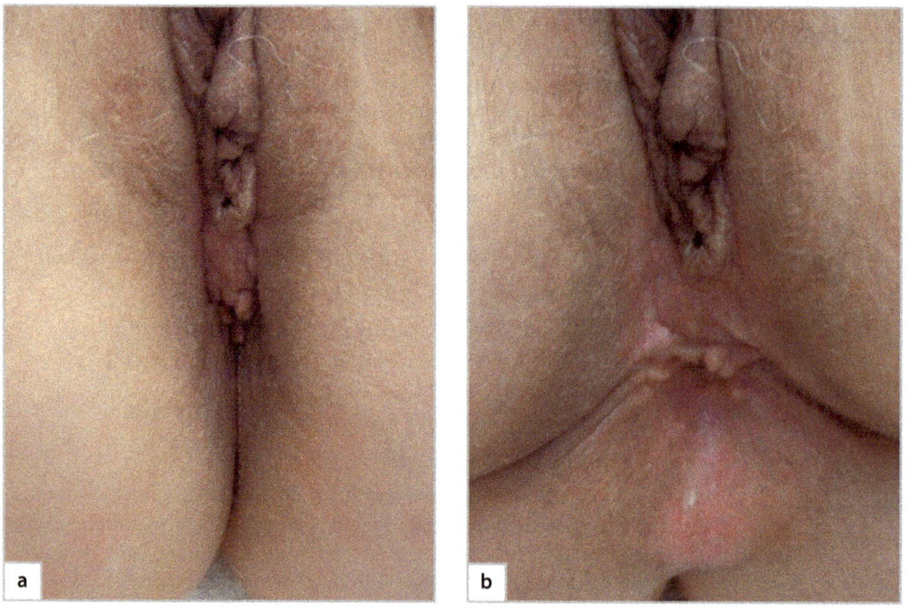

Figure 4.2 Perianal disease in a 50-year-old woman with advanced lichen sclerosus. The disease is not visible when examining only the vulva (a), but when the perianal area is examined and the skin parted, the changes are visible (b).

Evaluation of vulvar and vaginal pain

For patients with vulvar pain, it is vital to verify potential triggers of pain, to localize painful areas, and to evaluate the severity of pain. Applying pressure of varying intensity with a cotton stick ('Q-tip-test/cotton stick test') allows discrimination of areas with mild, moderate, or severe pain from painless areas. Findings should be documented on a pain mapping diagram (Haefner et al. 2005). Dynamic provoked pain can be assessed by gentle wiping. The patient should classify the level of pain by using a visual analog scale (1-10). Painful areas of the vagina can be examined also with a cotton stick (see also Chapter 38).

Equipment

The basic equipment consists ideally of a gynecological examination chair, a good flexible source of light, at least two sizes of specula, cotton swabs, plastic loops for sampling material for wet mount tests from vulva (and vagina), transport swabs for microbiological and viral tests, saline solution, glass slides, coverslips and a microscope, 3% and 5% acetic acid, and biopsy tools.

Additional examinations

Vulvoscopy

A colposcope is a good flexible light source with a 6-40-fold magnification. It allows demonstration of small lesions and evaluation of texture and depth of defects.

Saline preparations

Especially for persistent itching or burning complaints, it is essential to differentiate fungal or bacterial infections from other conditions with similar symptoms. Fungal elements, bacteria, and other infecting microorganisms like trichomonas vaginalis can be visualized in a wet mount preparation of vaginal discharge and abrasion material of the vulva. Evaluation of inflammatory cells and morphology of vaginal epithelial cells allows discrimination between infection and colonizing, and evaluation of estrogenization of vestibulum and vagina.

Staining with acetic acid

The application of 5%, in case of pain-sensitive patients 3%, acetic acid solution to the vulva for several minutes improves the detection of HPV-associated changes. HPV lesions appear as well-demarked white plaques or macules.

Microbiological scrapings, swabs for cultures, and viral tests

For precise classification of microorganisms (bacterial, fungal, viral) specimens can optionally be obtained from the groins, vulva, vagina, or cervix can be examined in clinics or sent to a microbiological laboratory for diagnosis, and it is occasionally necessary to obtain information about antibiotic sensitivities.

REFERENCES

Cooper S, Ali I, Baldo M, et al. The association of lichen sclerosus and erosive lichen planus of the vulva with autoimmune disease. Arch Dermatol 2008; 144;1432–1435.

Eberz B, Berghold A, Regauer S. High prevalence of concomitant anogenital lichen sclerosus and extragenital psoriasis in adult women. Obstet Gynecol 2008; 111:1143–1147.

Haefner HK, Collins ME, Davis GD, et al. The vulvodynia guideline. J Low Genit Tract Dis 2005; 9:40–51.

Nunns D, Mandal D, Byrne M, et al. Guidelines for the management of vulvodynia. Br J Dermatol 2010; 162:1180–1185.

Chapter 5 Scoring and recording of vulvar disease

Gudula Kirtschig, Susan M Cooper

Scoring of vulvar disease encompasses accurate recording of symptoms and signs requiring certain terminology (**Table 5.1**) and evaluation of their severity. It may include notes of the effect of the disease on the patient's quality of life including sexual functioning. Accurate and standardized documentation recording the severity, extent, and evolution of vulvar disease is important in daily practice to monitor disease progress and success of treatment. Furthermore, accurate assessment and quantification of disease symptoms and their evolution are important in research studies to accurately evaluate efficacy of therapies. For many diseases, e.g. psoriasis and eczema, standardized scoring systems are available; however, the scoring and documentation of the clinical features of inflammatory vulvar disease are not standardized (Simpson & Murphy 2012). Recently, a scoring system was published for lichen sclerosus, which needs further clinical evaluation (Günthert et al. 2012). There exist various pain scores, e.g. the visual analog scale also used in vulvar pain (Murina et al. 2008), a common

Table 5.1 Dermatological terminology.

	Definition	Clinical appearance	Examples of diseases
Primary lesions	**Characteristic first signs in diseases**		
Macule (macula)	A macule is a change in the color of the skin. It is flat, if you run your fingers over the surface of a purely macular lesion, you cannot detect it		Vitiligo, lentigo simplex
Papule (papula)	A papule is a circumscribed, solid elevation of skin with no visible fluid, varying in size from a pinhead to 1 cm	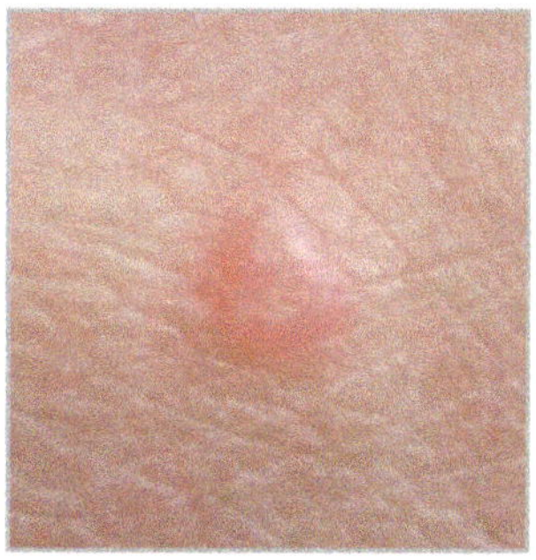	Intradermal naevus, papular lichen planus
Nodule (nodus)	A nodule is a localised swelling, bigger than a papule	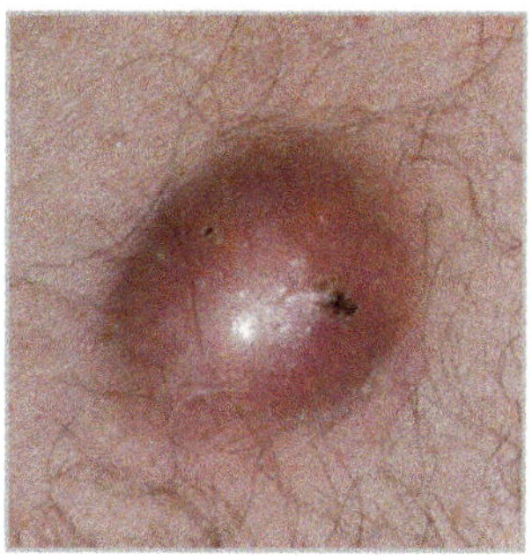	Big tumor, lipoma, cyst (shown here)

	Definition	Clinical appearance	Examples of diseases
Plaque	A plaque describes a palpable flat lesion greater than 1 cm in diameter or a confluence of papules	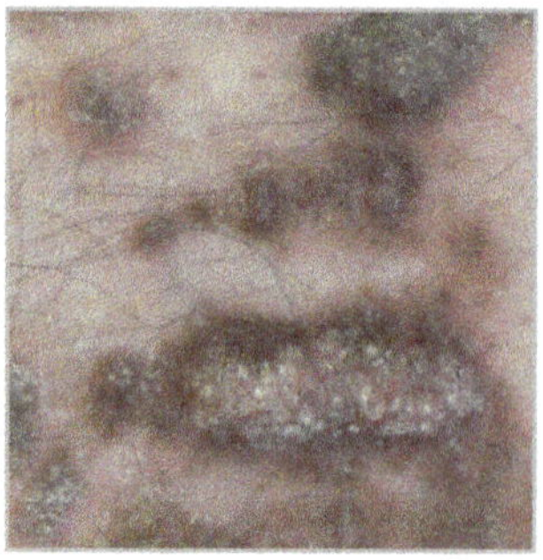	A plaque in psoriasis or confluent papules in lichen planus as shown
Wheal (urtica)	Wheals are raised areas surrounded by a red base, very itchy, they typically disappear quickly within 24 or 48 hours	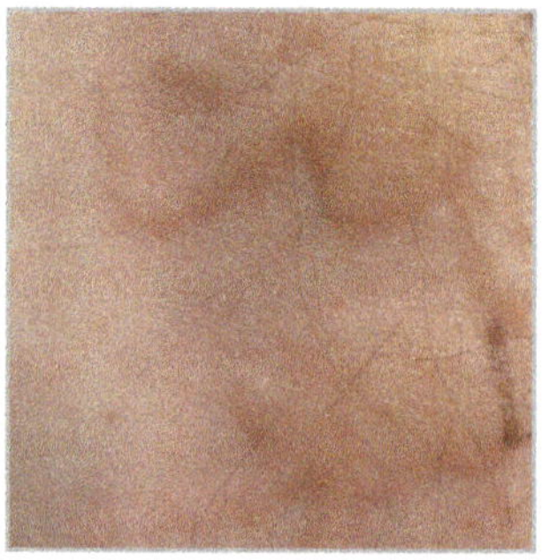	Dermographism or urticaria
Vesicle (vesicula)	A vesicle is a circumscribed, fluid-containing, epidermal elevation generally considered less than either 10 mm in diameter	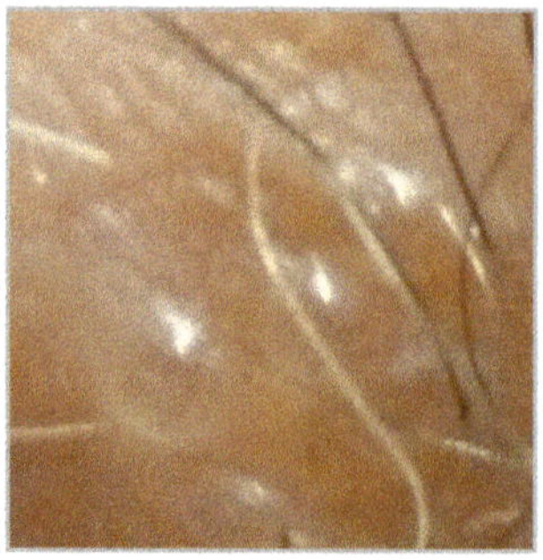	Herpes simplex, acute eczema
Blister (bulla)	A bulla is a large vesicle, a rounded or irregularly shaped blister containing (serous) fluid	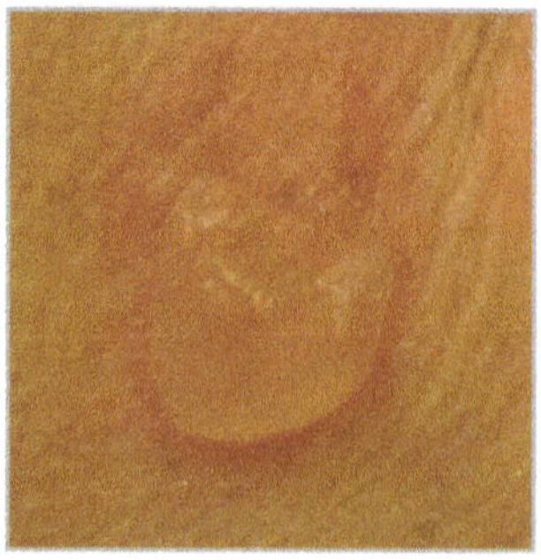	Bullous pemphigoid, bullous insect bite
Pustule (pustule)	A pustule is a small elevation of the skin containing pus	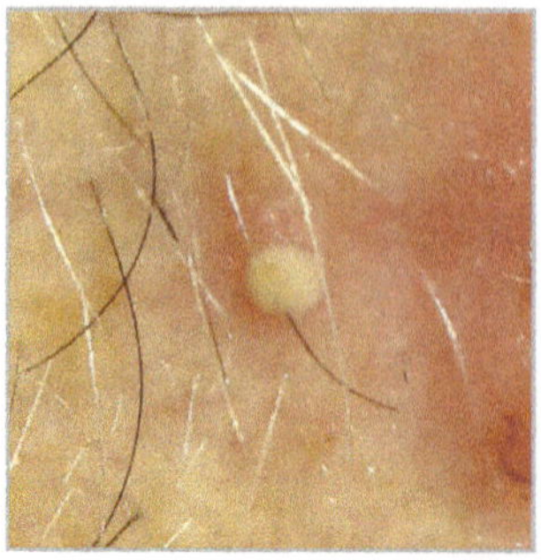	Pustule in staphylococcal infection

	Definition	Clinical appearance	Examples of diseases
Secondary lesions	**Lesions developing in the course of a disease**		
Scale (squama)	Scales are dry or greasy laminated masses of keratin that represent thickened stratum corneum	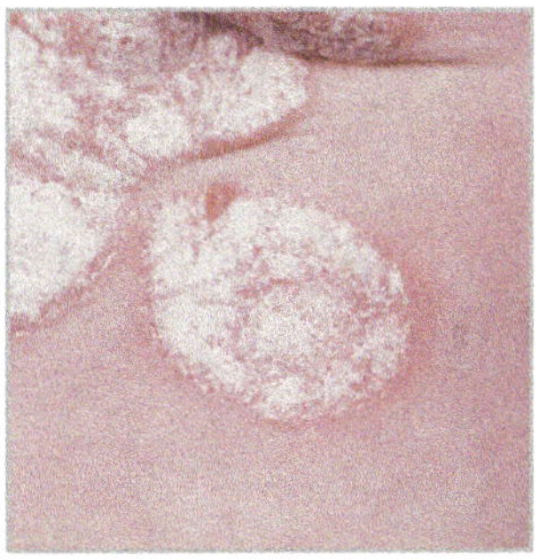 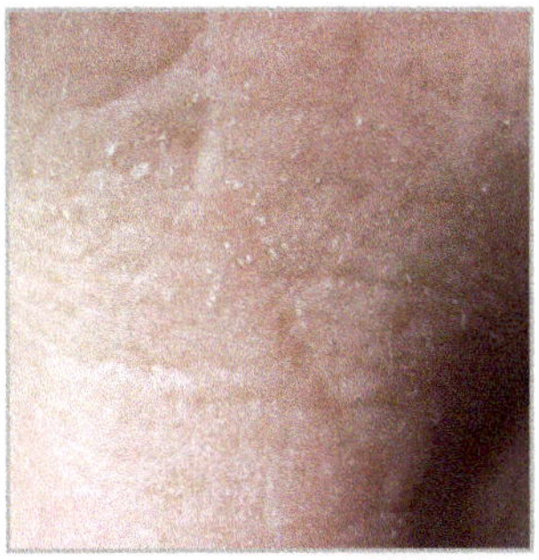	Scales in psoriasis or seborrheic dermatitis
Crust (crusta)	A crust is dried serum, pus, or blood usually mixed with epithelial and sometimes bacterial debris	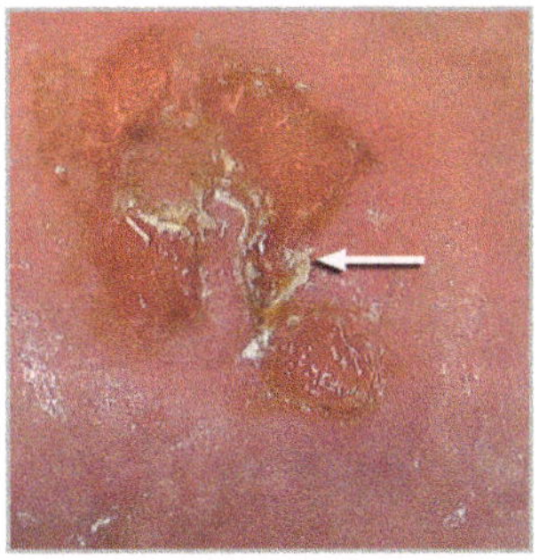	Crust on top of an ulcer
Erosion (exesa)	An erosion is a discontinuity of the skin or mucosa exhibiting incomplete loss of the epithelium, a superficial defect of the skin	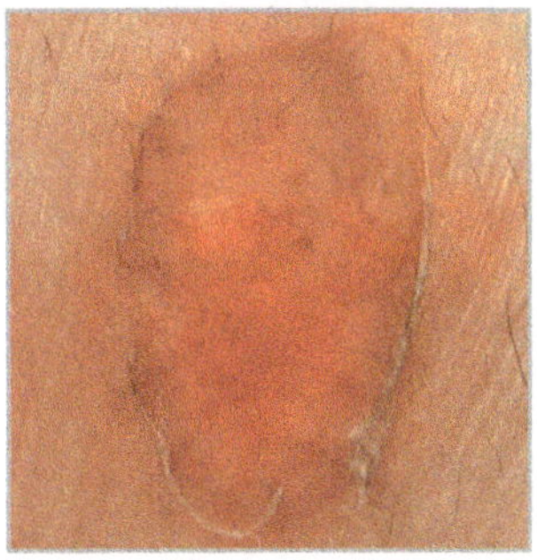	Erosion after a ruptured blister
Ulcer (ulcus)	An ulcer is a discontinuity of the skin or mucosa exhibiting complete loss of the epithelium and often portions of the dermis and even subcutaneous fat	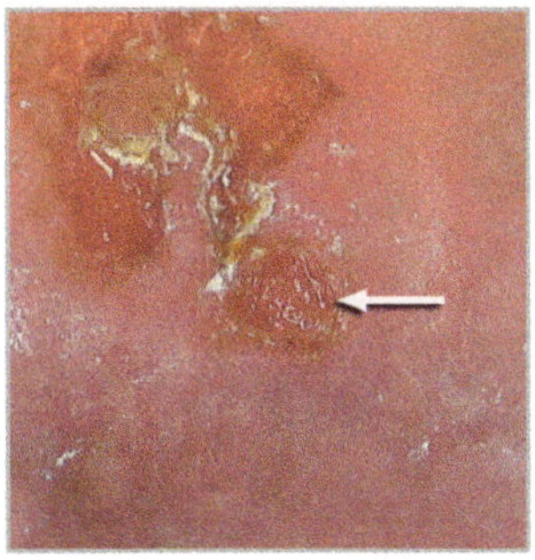	

	Definition	Example	Disease
Fissure (rima / fissura)	A fissure is a crack in the skin that is usually narrow but deep	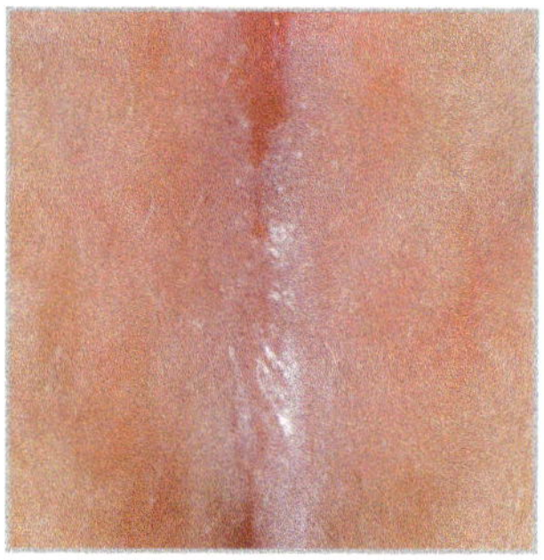	Lichen sclerosus, eczema
Atrophy (atrophia)	Atrophy is a loss of tissue, and can be epidermal, dermal, or subcutaneous. With epidermal atrophy, the skin appears thin, translucent, and wrinkled. Dermal or subcutaneous atrophy is represented by depression of the skin	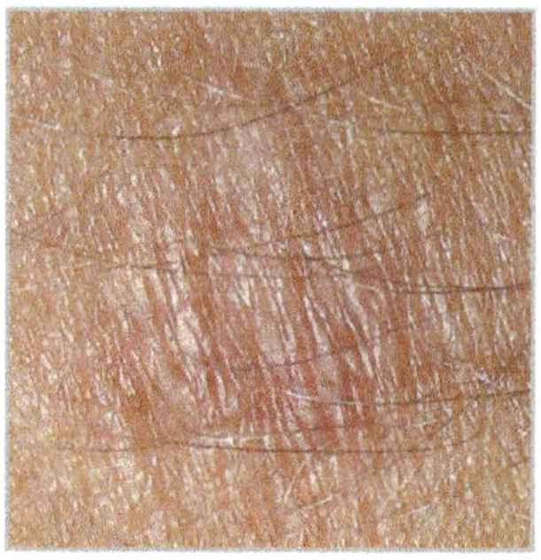	Atrophic scars in epidermolysis bullosa acquisita or striae distensae after pregnancy
Scar (cicatrix)	A scar is a replacement after a tissue defect; it replaces the original tissue and is usually visible and of less good quality	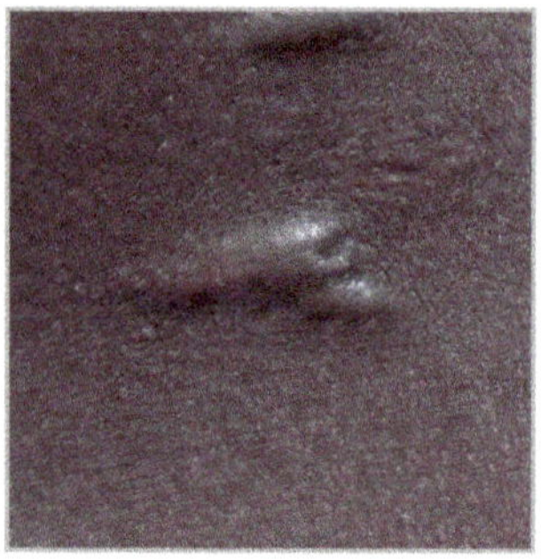	After an injury or surgery, they may appear spontaneously as keloids
Commonly used terms			
Erythema	Redness of the skin		After sunburn
Excoriation	A punctate or linear abrasion (erosion) produced by mechanical means (often scratching), usually involving only the epidermis, but commonly reaching the superficial dermis	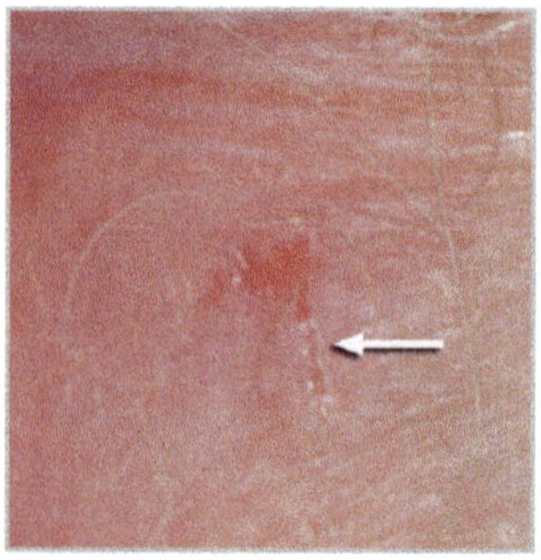	After scratching in eczema
Induration	Dermal thickening causing the cutaneous surface to feel thicker and firmer		In scleroderma

	Definition	Example	Disease
Lichenification	Epidermal thickening characterized by visible and palpable thickening of the skin with accentuated skin markings; elephant skin	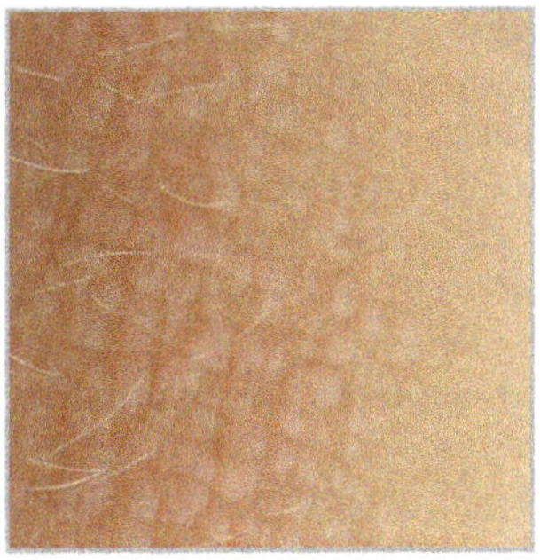	Lichenification is often caused by continuous scratching, finally leading to lichen simplex
Maceration	Softening and turning white of the skin due to being consistently wet	see Figure 29.2	Intertrigo
Histopathologic terminology			
Acanthosis	Acanthosis is diffuse epidermal hyperplasia (thickening of the skin)		Psoriasis
Hyperkeratosis	Hyperkeratosis is thickening of the stratum corneum (the outermost layer of the epidermis)		Psoriasis plaque or other scaly disorders
Parakeratosis	Parakeratosis is a mode of keratinization characterized by the retention of nuclei in the stratum corneum. In mucous membranes, parakeratosis is normal		Psoriasis
Dyskeratosis	Dyskeratosis is abnormal keratinization occurring prematurely within individual cells or groups of cells below the stratum granulosum		Darier disease
Papillomatosis	Papillomatosis is skin surface elevation caused by hyperplasia and enlargement of contiguous dermal papillae		Severe lymphedema
Spongiosis	Spongiosis is mainly intercellular edema (abnormal accumulation of fluid) in the epidermis, and is characteristic of eczematous dermatitis, manifested clinically by intraepidermal vesicles (fluid-containing spaces)		Eczema
Acantholysis	Acantholysis is the loss of intercellular connections, such as desmosomes, resulting in loss of cohesion between keratinocytes		Pemphigus

terminology and classification for vulvar pain/vulvodynia endorsed by the International Society for the Study of Vulvovaginal Disease in 2003 (see Chapters 9 and 38), scores for sexual functioning (Marinoff & Turner 1992), and grading systems for vulvar intraepithelial neoplasia (see Chapter 35). The impact of vulvar disease on quality of life may be measured by using a dermatology-specific tool 'Skindex-29' (Ponte et al. 2009) or Dermatology Life Quality Index (Finlay & Khan 1994) or a general utility measure, the 'Short Form 36' (Brazier et al. 1992).

Marinoff dyspareunia scale

0 – No dyspareunia

1 – Causes discomfort but does not interfere with frequency of intercourse

2 – Sometimes prevents intercourse

3 – Completely prevents intercourse

Accurate recording starts with a thorough inspection of vulvar and perianal area; knowledge of the normal features of the vulva in different age groups is mandatory (see Chapter 1). It is useful to do this in a systematic fashion inspecting the groins, outer and inner aspects of the labia majora, interlabial sulcus, outer and inner aspects of the labia minora, the clitoris, clitoral hood, the introitus vaginae, the vagina and cervix if possible, the perineum, and perianal region including the anus. It is good practice to thoroughly inspect the rest of the skin including the oral mucosa, nails, and scalp.

Skin color (red, white, brown/black), skin texture (lichenification, hyperkeratosis, scaling, atrophy, fissures, erosions, blisters, or tumors, etc.), the distribution, and extent of skin changes must be documented; it is important to record whether the architecture is normal or abnormal (scarring may lead to fusion or disappearance or structures) (physician-administered score). Symptoms such as discharge and subjective symptoms like pain and itch need to be assessed (patient-administered symptom score).

Günthert et al. (2012) evaluated a patient-administered symptom score in lichen sclerosus rating pruritus, burning, soreness, and dyspareunia using a numeric scale ranging from 0 (no complaints) to 10 (extreme complaints) for each symptom. A score ranging from a minimum of 0 and a maximum of 40 gave a total score for the patient. Six items were considered for the physician-administered clinical score namely erosions, hyperkeratosis, fissures, agglutination, stenosis, and atrophy. Each item was scored on a 3-point scale ranging from 0 to 2, with 0 representing normal findings, 1 moderate changes, and 2 severe changes (Günthert et al. 2012).

The schematic representations in **Figure 5.1** show features of a normal vulva (1) and architectural changes (2–6) that may be encountered in inflammatory diseases such as lichen sclerosus and lichen planus. Simple drawings during clinic may help record architectural changes. If photo documentation is available, it is a very useful tool for monitoring disease development. A photo taken, e.g. before treatment and then months or years later in the course of the disease allows patients and physicians to recognize changes.

The use of preprinted schematic representations may allow users to draw on them and accurately sketch the distribution of skin lesions (**Figure 5.2**).

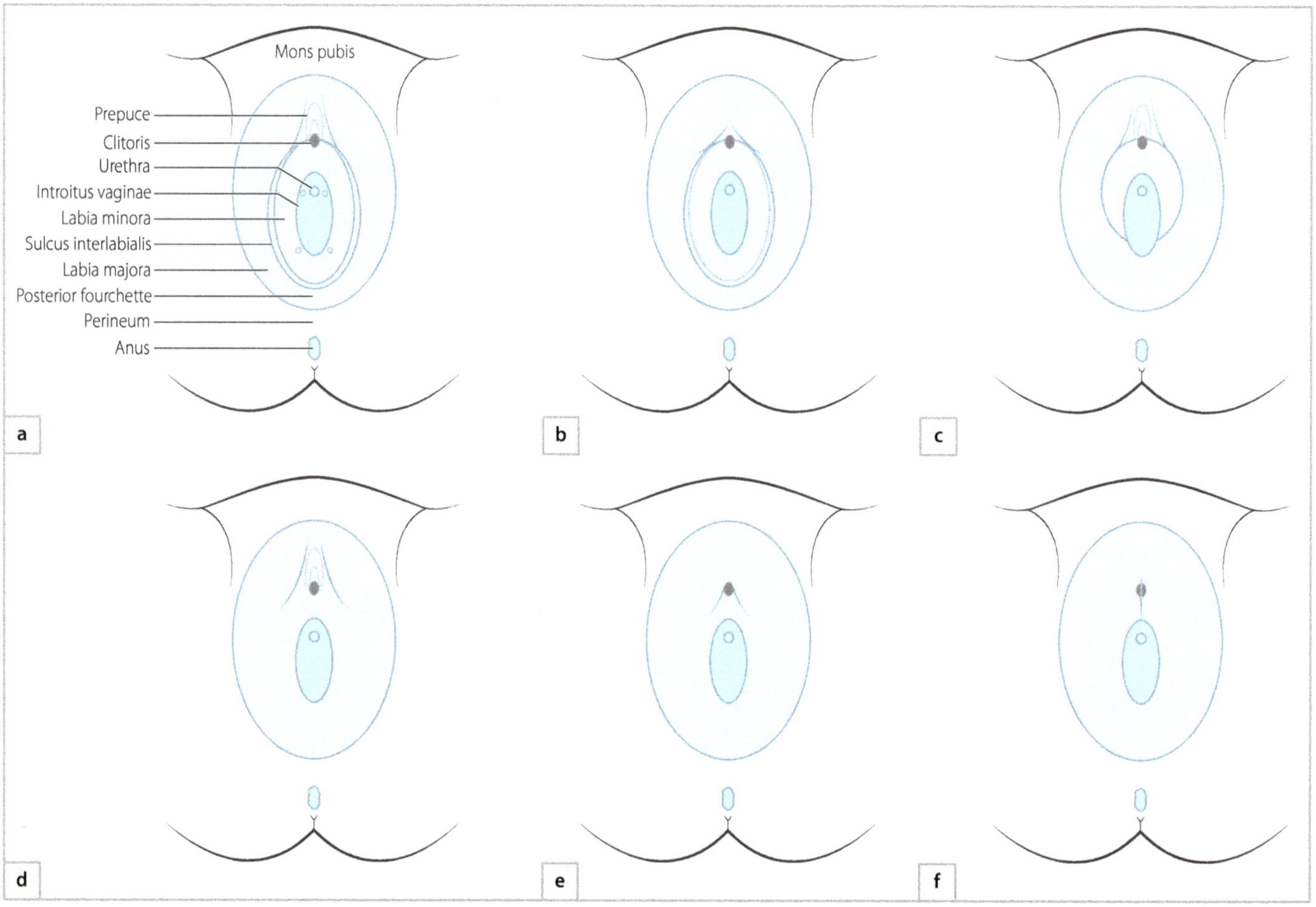

Figure 5.1 The normal vulva and changes due to disease. (a) Normal vulva. (b) Fusion of the clitoral hood. (c) Partial inferior labia minora absorption (posterior fourchette). (d) Completely absorbed labia minora. (e) Completely absorbed labia minora and fused clitoral hood. (f) Absorbed labia minora and completely fused clitoral hood.

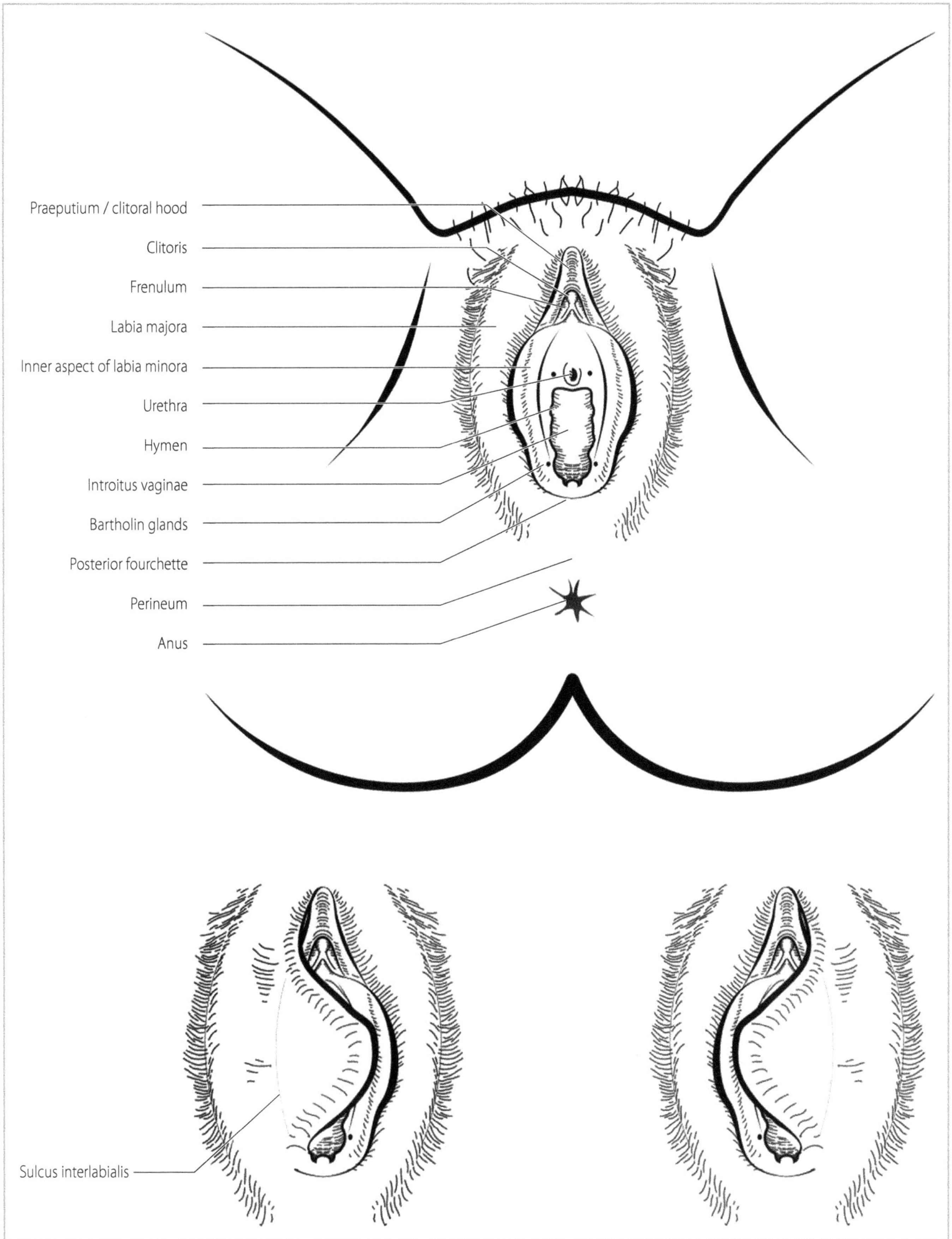

Figure 5.2 A normal vulva. (This can be copied for use in the clinic when recording distribution of lesions.)

REFERENCES

Brazier JE, Harper R, Jones NM, et al. Validating the SF-36 health survey questionnaire: new outcome measure for primary care. BMJ 1992; 305:160–164.

Finlay AY, Khan GK. Dermatology Life Quality Index (DLQI)—a simple practical measure for routine clinical use. Clin Exp Dermatol 1994; 19:210–216.

Günthert AR, Duclos K, Jahns BG, et al. Clinical scoring system for vulvar lichen sclerosus. J Sex Med 2012; 9:2342–2350.

Marinoff SC, Turner MLC. Vulvar vestibulitis syndrome. Dermatol Clin 1992; 10:435–444.

Murina F, Bianco V, Radici G, et al. Transcutaneous electrical nerve stimulation to treat vestibulodynia: a randomised controlled trial. BJOG: an International Journal of Obstetrics & Gynaecology 2008; 115:1165–1170.

Ponte M, Klemperer E, Sahay A, Chren MM. Effects of vulvodynia on quality of life. J Am Acad Dermatol 2009; 60:70–6.

Simpson RC, Murphy R. Considerations for disease impact and outcome measures in vulvar disease. J Low Genit Tract Dis 2012; 16:460–463.

Chapter 6 How to take a vulvar biopsy and what to expect from a histopathological examination

Barbara Eberz, Sigrid Regauer

HOW TO TAKE A VULVAR BIOPSY

Introduction

A vulvar biopsy is a simple and relatively painless method to obtain a histopathological evaluation of tissue. It helps to evaluate common clinical symptoms and signs such as itching or redness, which are a feature of many conditions but may show specific features when examined under the microscope. A biopsy is essential to diagnose differentiated vulvar intraepithelial neoplasia (dVIN), high-grade squamous intraepithelial lesions (HSIL) or other malignant change. Sometimes one biopsy will not lead to a (clinically suspected) diagnosis and repeated biopsies are needed. In case of discrepancy between the clinical and histopathological findings, e.g. if neoplastic changes mimic inflammatory diseases, repeated biopsies are advised.

Key points

- Medical history, informed written consent, and ideally photographic documentation should be taken prior to biopsy
- Local topical treatment, in particular potent topical steroids, should be stopped 2–4 weeks before biopsy
- Local anesthesia is usually sufficient except for clitoral biopsies
- Use 4 to 6-mm punch biopsies
- Biopsies must not be crushed or squeezed by instruments
- Take biopsies from the most typical and suspicious area and/or site of maximal complaints
- Never biopsy the ulcer bed, but the edge of a defect containing a portion of intact skin

Prebiopsy medical history, written consent and information for the pathologist

The reason for a biopsy must be explained, e.g. to help establish a diagnosis or rule out malignancy. It is helpful to provide written information as patients are frequently very anxious when told they need a biopsy. Potential complications such as bleeding, infection, and a scar must be documented and explained. Prior to biopsy, it is advisable to obtain written consent and to check patient identifiers.

Information needed

- Allergies (e.g. local anesthetics, latex, disinfectants, antibiotics)
- Infection risk (e.g. HIV, hepatitis)
- Anticoagulation (e.g. acetylic acid, non-steroidal anti-inflammatory drugs, warfarin)
- Pacemaker or implantable defibrillator
- Diseases or medication influencing the biopsy or wound healing such as immunosuppression

Photographic documentation before biopsy is useful as small lesions may be totally removed or lesions may change dramatically after therapy. Ideally, all local therapies should be stopped 2–4 weeks prior to biopsy for a primary diagnosis, or otherwise the type and duration of current treatments need to be provided to the pathologist. In particular, topical steroids, calcineurin inhibitors, imiquimod, and podophyllotoxin (O'Mahony et al. 2010) can affect histological features.

Information for pathologist

- General information about patient
- Location/duration of lesion
- Description of lesion
- Current treatment
- Suspected diagnosis
- Indicate if there was a previous biopsy

Local anesthesia

Local anesthesia is sufficient for vulvar biopsies except for clitoral biopsies or possibly vulvar biopsies in children. After cleaning the skin with a colorless skin and mucosa-compatible disinfectant, every biopsy site will be infiltrated with 0.5–1 mL of, e.g. lidocaine or mepivacaine 1% +/− adrenalin/epinephrine using a 25–30 gauge needle. Pain-sensitive areas can be pretreated with a 5% prilocaine/lidocaine cream or 2% lidocaine gel for 30 minutes as some patients experience an unpleasant burning sensation when injecting the local anesthesia. Lidocaine may be buffered with (8.4%) sodium bicarbonate, which appears to reduce the pain when injecting the lidocaine. The use of an anesthetic spray alone is insufficient for adequate anesthesia.

Biopsy technique

For evaluation of most inflammatory vulvar diseases, a punch biopsy is adequate; however, in some circumstances, e.g. in suspected malignancy, it may be more appropriate to perform an excision biopsy. A 4 mm punch is adequate in thick-hair-bearing skin. For thin glycogenated and modified mucosal areas, such as the inner aspects of the labia minora, 6 mm punches are preferred. Damaging the biopsy by grabbing it too hard or squeezing may cause artifacts that hinder histopathological evaluation. For some diseases, samples from at least two sites should be taken. In case of widespread or multifocal lesions, multiple areas must be biopsied (documented in a 'vulvar mapping' sketch) and submitted in separate containers. In erosive and ulcerated diseases, biopsies should be obtained from the edge of the defect, including intact skin, never from the ulcer bed. The biopsy punch is placed on top of the skin and inserted with screwing movements to a depth of 3–5 mm through the slightly stretched skin. The punch cylinder is cautiously fixed with a skin hook, small forceps, or an injection needle, while the base is cut with scissors, and transferred to 4% buffered formalin (**Figure 6.1a**). Bleeding after a 4 mm biopsy will stop after applying pressure with cotton gauze (**Figure 6.2a–c**). More intense bleeding can be stopped with potassium-silver nitrate sticks, aluminum- or iron chloride (**Figure 6.1b**). Sutures with atraumatic absorbable material are usually required in anticoagulated patients, potentially also after a 6 mm biopsy. It is important to document the exact site of the biopsy, e.g. labia minora or majora, perineum. Biopsying the clitoris should be avoided (unless cancerous growth is suspected) as this may lead to a loss of sensation and is very painful.

Aftercare

It is helpful to provide information on aftercare. It is important to keep the area clean, but it is not necessary to keep the area dry. The vulvar area is very vascularized, and therefore it is important to explain how to apply pressure in the event of bleeding (pressing for 15 minutes with a clean towel). It is usually not possible to apply a dressing but instead gauze can be put in the patient's underwear; sanitary towels/panty liners may be provided in clinics after a biopsy. Most stitches dissolve but can be removed in 1 week if they have not dissolved.

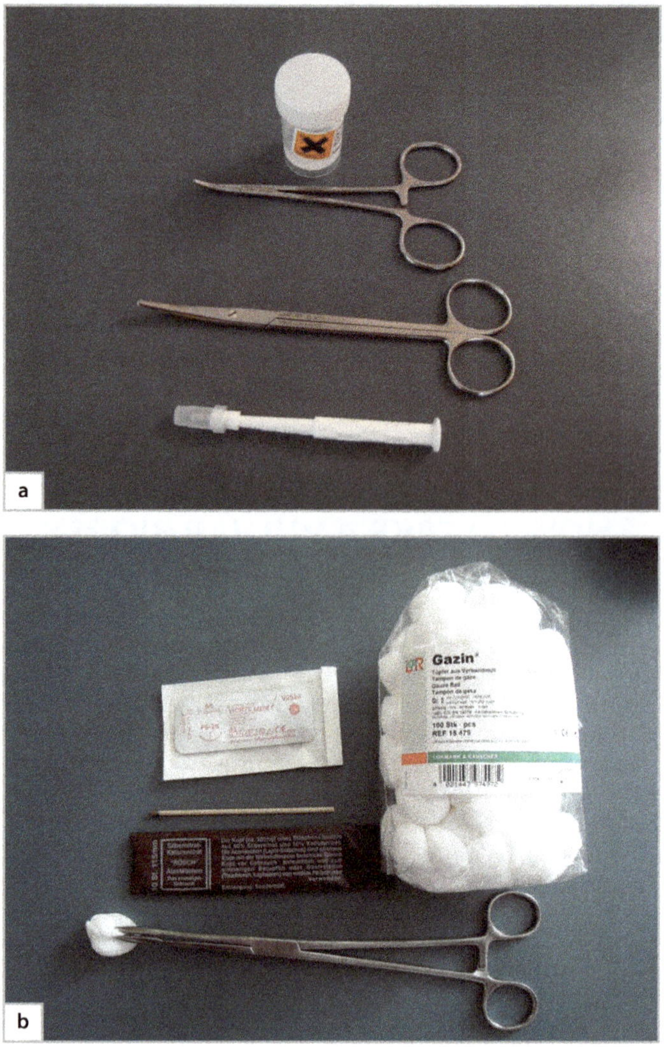

Figure 6.1 (a) Biopsy instruments: Biopsy punches between 3 and 6 mm, a small mosquito clamp, a small curved dissecting scissors, and 4% buffered formalin-filled specimen bottle. (b) Equipment for hemostasis including cotton balls, potassium-silver nitrate sticks, and an atraumatic absorbable suture.

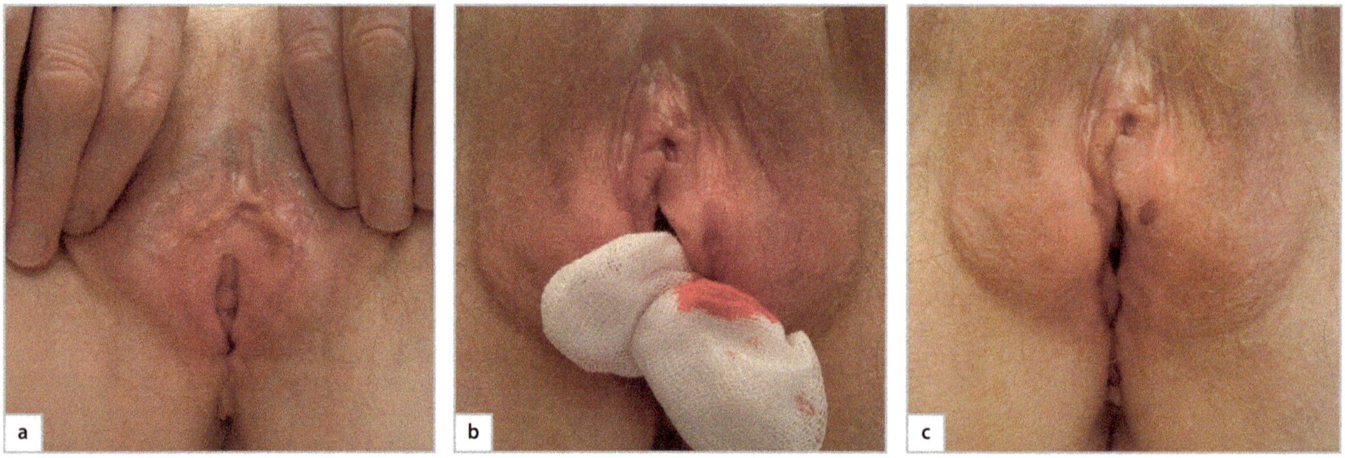

Figure 6.2 Vulvar site before and after performing a biopsy. (a) A 71-year-old woman with early stage of lichen sclerosus in remission. (b) Punch cylinder after inserting the biopsy punch in the left interlabial fold. (c) Small defect after cutting the base of the cylinder.

WHAT TO EXPECT FROM A HISTOLOGICAL EXAMINATION

Introduction

Close cooperation between clinician and (dermato)pathologist ensures optimal histopathological evaluation of diseases. Clinicians expect confirmation or exclusion of a suspected condition and/or assistance in therapeutic decisions. A detailed description of lesions (optimally by photodocumentation) preceding topical treatments and differential diagnoses will support the pathologist in interpreting the histological features. Sometimes the clinical diagnosis does not fit with the histopathological interpretation and conclusion of a biopsy; in these cases, it is advisable to discuss the results with the pathologist and re-biopsy if needed.

Key points

- Close cooperation between clinician and pathologist is crucial
- Gold standard is a definitive and unequivocal diagnosis, not only a histological description
- In case of precancerous lesions, distinction between human papillomavirus (HPV)-induced and HPV-negative lesions is important for adequate patient management
- Additional information from immunofluorescence tests may be needed in suspected autoimmune diseases

Biopsy report and diagnosis

A biopsy report consists of three integral parts:

1. A macroscopic description for larger and complex specimens, not necessarily biopsies
2. A histological description
3. A diagnosis

For the most common vulvar conditions (e.g. lichen sclerosus, lichen planus, psoriasis, eczema, invasive cancers, malignant melanoma), a work-up with hematoxylin and eosin (HE) stains and periodic acid-Schiff (PAS) reaction is sufficient. Depending on the clinical differential diagnoses, additional special stains and immunohistochemical analysis may be necessary.

WHAT TO EXPECT FROM A BIOPSY

1. The gold standard is an unequivocal and definitive diagnosis. The aim should be the diagnosis of a specific condition such as lichen sclerosus, lichen planus, psoriasis, or precancerous lesions, not merely a description of histopathological findings.

   For chronic inflammatory dermatoses, a histopathological report should comment on certain features, including the presence and quantity of inflammatory cells, the type of infiltrate (e.g. lymphocytes, mast cells), and the presence of vasculitis (Regauer et al. 2004). Since lichen planus and lichen sclerosus carry a cancer risk (Crum et al. 2014, Regauer et al. 2014), the presence of mitotic activity and/or dysplasia should be noted.

   The etiology of an epithelial precancerous lesion (e.g. HPV-induced or HPV negative) influences treatment decisions. The most recent WHO classification (Crum et al. 2014) lists HPV-induced precancerous lesions as high-grade squamous intraepithelial lesions (synonymously VIN, basaloid VIN, usual VIN, Bowen disease, bowenoid papulosis) with $p16^{ink4a}$ overexpression and with slow progression to invasion. In contrast, the HPV-negative and $p16^{ink4a}$-negative precancerous lesion differentiated VIN (synonym: simplex carcinoma in situ), often associated with lichen sclerosus and lichen planus, is rapidly progressing to invasive cancer (Regauer 2011, Regauer et al. 2014) and needs urgent treatment. An unequivocal distinction is possible with HE histology and immunohistochemistry with antibody to $p16^{ink4a}$, an indirect marker for a transforming infection with HPV-high-risk genotypes (Reuschenbach et al. 2011).
2. In the absence of unequivocal diagnostic criteria, or when a non-specific histological reaction pattern is present, e.g. psoriasiform hyperplasia, the report should list differential diagnoses to be correlated with the clinical information provided.
3. A PAS stain should be performed, particularly in patients with unclear symptoms and non-diagnostic histopathological features to exclude fungal infections. Cells of extramammary Paget disease are also PAS positive.
4. In potentially HPV-related malignant changes [squamous cell carcinoma (SCC), HSIL, giant condylomata] or certain infectious diseases (herpes simplex/zoster), polymerase chain reaction (PCR) and immunohistochemistry investigations may be needed to determine if and which type of viruses are present that may cause the disease. These tests need to be discussed with the patient and the pathologist, e.g. if and how (biopsies or swabs) these tests can be done in the pathology laboratories.
5. A direct immunofluorescence test is required in suspected autoimmune bullous disorders. A biopsy of uninvolved skin is taken, about 2 cm away from the lesion and transported either frozen in liquid nitrogen or in physiological saline to a specialized laboratory (see also Chapter 26 and talk to the pathologist).
6. In vulvar pain patients, a biopsy may be obtained to exclude or demonstrate an underlying disease causing the pain and to allow an immunohistochemical workup possibly demonstrating sensory hyperinnervation (antibody to PGP9.5) and increased mast cells (antibody to mast cell tryptase) seen in some patients with neuropathic pain, e.g. vulvodynia (Regauer & Eberz 2010, Regauer & Beham-Schmid 2014, Regauer et al. 2015). Note that antibody to S-100 does not recognize sensory nerves.

REFERENCES

Crum C, Herrington S, McCluggage WG, Regauer S, Wilkinson E. Tumours of the Vulva. Epithelial tumours. In: Kurman RJ, Carcangiu ML, Herrington CS, Young RH (eds.),World Health Organisation, Classification of Tumours of the Female Genital Tract. Lyon: IARC, 2014:232–242.

O'Mahony C, Yesudian PD, Stanley M. Imiquimod use in the genital area and development of lichen sclerosus and lichen planus. Int J STD AIDS 2010; 21:219–221.

Regauer S. Residual anogenital lichen sclerosus after cancer surgery has a high risk for recurrence: a clinicopathological study of 75 women. Gynecol Oncol 2011; 123:289–294.

Regauer S, Beham-Schmid C. Benign mast cell hyperplasia and atypical mast cell infiltrates in penile lichen planus in adult men. Histol Histopathol 2014; 29:1017–1025.

Regauer S, Eberz B. Diagnosis and management of vulvodynia should include biopsy and histological examination. Br J Dermatol 2010; 163:663–665; author reply 665–666.

Regauer S, Eberz B, Beham-Schmid C. Mast cell infiltrates in vulvodynia: benign reactive mastocytosis or neoplastic disease? APMIS 2015; 123:452–456.

Regauer S, Liegl B, Reich O, Beham-Schmid C. Vasculitis in lichen sclerosus—an under recognized feature? Histopathology 2004; 45:237–244.

Regauer S, Reich O, Eberz B. Vulvar cancers in women with vulvar lichen planus: a clinicopathological study. J Am Acad Dermatol 2014; 71:698–707.

Reuschenbach M, Seiz M, von Knebel Doeberitz C, et al. Evaluation of cervical cone biopsies for coexpression of p16INK4a and Ki-67 in epithelial cells. Int J Cancer. 2011; 130:388–394.

Section 2

SYMPTOMS AND SIGNS OF DISEASE

Chapter 7 General treatment considerations

Susan M Cooper, Gudula Kirtschig

Many women erroneously believe that 'special' products such as deodorants, feminine washes, and wipes are necessary for daily care; however, they may harm the vulvovaginal environment by disturbing the skin barrier, normal vaginal bacterial flora and pH increasing susceptibility to irritation or infections. If used for prolonged periods, they may cause allergies. The proximity of the genital, urinary and gastrointestinal systems means that diseases of these organs may affect the anogenital skin so it is wise to inquire about the function of the urinary and gastrointestinal tracts.

Main principles of management

- Avoidance of frequent cleansing with water (and soap)
- Soap substitutes
- Emollients
- Inquiry about potential irritants and allergens
- Written advice and information on relevant patient support groups
- Specific advice on how and where to apply treatments
- Copy patient in to any correspondence with primary care physician wherever possible

Avoidance of irritants and allergens

Women with vulvar disease benefit from advice on avoidance of potential irritants such as shower gels and soaps (**Table 7.1**). Moist toilet wipes and feminine wet wipes should be specifically be inquired for as they can cause contact dermatitis, typically containing preservatives and fragrances. Underwear made from soft natural fiber such as cotton or silk is less irritant and occlusive than synthetic fiber; G-strings, tight jeans, and hard saddles may cause friction; white underwear is preferred as textile dyes in dark clothing may rarely induce allergies (D'Antuono et al. 2011).

Table 7.1 Possible irritants of anogenital skin

- Soaps and bubble baths
- Shower gels
- Talcum powder
- Wet cleansing wipes
- Intimate cleansing
- Deodorants
- Antiseptics
- Sanitary towels and tampons
- Shaving procedures
- Urine
- Feces
- Spermicidal gels
- Tight clothing

Soap substitutes and emollients (Table 7.2)

Many medical emollients can be used as soap substitutes for washing. If the skin is open, emollients should be applied at least twice a day to keep skin hydrated and act as a barrier. To protect the skin from fluids, it may be useful to apply greasy emollients before exposure to urine or water such as when swimming or showering. It is helpful to offer a choice of emollients with samples as patients' preferences vary. Lighter cream emollients are more pleasant to use than greasy ointments but may sting the skin if skin is very inflamed. Greasier ointments may be better tolerated if skin is very sore. Although allergy to the constituents of emollients is unusual, some women may develop allergy to excipients such as parabens, chlorocresol, cetostearyl alcohol, or lanolin (Nardelli et al. 2004). Emollients may help maintain remission in lichen sclerosus (Simonart et al. 2008).

Special situations

In recurrent skin infection, antimicrobial emollients/soap substitutes containing benzalkonium chloride or chlorhexidine may be useful. Benzalkonium may result in irritant contact dermatitis if used very frequently so it is normally advised not to use more frequently than twice daily. When skin is fissured or ulcerated as in erosive lichen planus (see Chapter 20), urination is painful thus protection with, for example, petroleum jelly prior to urination is helpful. Spray emollients containing soft paraffin can be prescribed if the skin is too sore to touch.

Topical corticosteroids

Many women are anxious about applying topical steroids so it is best to anticipate this by discussing package inserts that may warn against application on genital skin. This may be compounded by well meaning pharmaceutical advice to apply sparingly. Give advice specifically on and where to put the ointment and how much to use (a large pea-sized application is generally sufficient to cover the anogenital area). Emollients should be applied first leaving 30 minutes before applying steroid. In general, steroid ointments instead of creams are preferred because they have fewer excipients than creams reducing the risk of allergic contact dermatitis and are less likely to sting.

Table 7.2 Soap substitutes and emollients

- Very greasy ointments with high lipid to water content such as 50% white vaseline and 50% liquid paraffin
- Less greasy cream emollients usually containing cetostearyl alcohol or lanolin as a base
- Lotions have the lowest lipid to water content and are therefore lighter, being more suitable for use as soap substitutes
- Shower preparations, usually lotions or oils
- Bath oils

INFORMATION ON THE DIAGNOSIS AND TREATMENT

Written patient information such as that available on the website of the International Society for the Study of Vulvovaginal Disease is helpful. Patient support groups are valuable for some patients and are available in many countries.

TREATING VULVAR DISEASE AROUND OR AFTER THE MENOPAUSE

Some women develop soreness after their primary skin disease has been adequately treated, which may be due to postmenopausal atrophic changes. This is not always recognized and treatment of the original disease may be escalated without good effect. In conjunction with disease-specific treatment, topical vaginal estrogen may relieve these symptoms (see Chapter 3).

PSYCHOLOGICAL SUPPORT

This may be required in some cases including counseling and psychosexual counseling (see Chapter 39).

REFERENCES

D'Antuono A, Bellavista S, Gaspari V, Filippini A, Patrizi A. Dermasilk briefs in vulvar lichen sclerosus: an adjuvant tool. J Low Genit Tract Dis 2011; 15:287–291.

Nardelli A, Degreef H, Goosens A. Contact allergic reactions of the vulva: a 14 year review. Dermatitis 2004; 15:131–136.

Simonart T, Lahaye M, Simonart J-M. Vulvar lichen sclerosus: effect of maintenance treatment with a moisturizer on the course of the disease. Menopause 2008; 15:74–77.

Chapter 8 Pruritus

Tanja Gizela Bohl

INTRODUCTION

Pruritus or itch (these terms are used synonymously throughout the chapter) is the commonest symptom experienced by females of all ages with vulvar disorders. It can be caused and modulated by systemic factors as well as by skin conditions arising in the anogenital area. Despite the common nature of this complaint and the significant morbidity and disturbance of quality of life that it causes, there is no specific tool for measuring the severity and quality of vulvar itch (Simpson et al. 2013).

The lengths to which a woman will go to gain relief provides a useful indication on how distressing she finds her pruritus and also a potential tool with which to measure improvement. Many will volunteer that they find the sensation of soreness or pain more bearable than pruritus and may scratch with their fingernails, a cloth, hairbrush, or apply cold water or caustic solutions to gain some relief. This can lead to excoriations, erosions, ulceration, and exudate increasing the risk of secondary infection. Many women will wear sanitary napkins to 'protect' their vulva. It is important to listen to such information with empathy, not judgment. These additional features may make the diagnosis more challenging. All contributing factors will require attention (**Figure 8.1**).

Vulvar pruritus may be caused by the primary condition such as dermographism (**Figure 8.2**) or arise as a consequence of efforts to achieve relief. This can include the use of multiple over the counter topical preparations that can act as irritants and/or allergens, making clinical assessment all the more difficult. Once established, the itch-scratch cycle can be difficult to break even after resolution of the initiating condition. The exact pathogenesis remains unknown; however, recent studies into the pathogenesis of pruritus suggest that this may be a combination of permanent tissue damage, small fiber neuropathy, and possibly altered central processing of this sensation. Clinically, these more chronic developments equate to thickening of the skin and exaggerated skin markings known as lichenification (**Figure 8.3**).

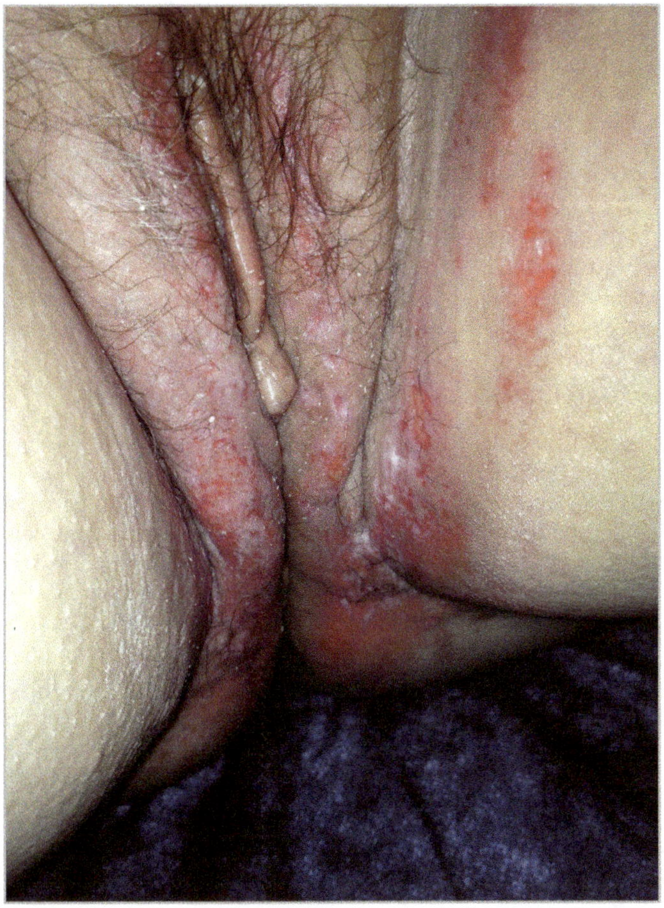

Figure 8.1 Extensive excoriations of the vulva and inner thighs due to irritant contact dermatitis. The cause was identified as chafing from pads and urinary incontinence.

PATHOPHYSIOLOGY OF PRURITUS

As early as 1660, itch was defined as an unpleasant sensation provoking the desire to scratch. Although it is a useful description, patients will also describe itch as irritation, crawling, pins and needles, general discomfort, and abnormal vulvar awareness. It is important to allow the patient to use her own words to describe what she is feeling. Many patients use the words scratch and itch interchangeably. A useful distinction between pruritus and pain is that pruritus is a 'hands-on sensation' where the patient has a desire to touch to gain relief, whereas pain is a 'hands-off' sensation as touch usually makes it worse.

Our understanding of the pathogenesis of pruritus is increasing (Davidson et al. 2014). Although the current classification for pruritus

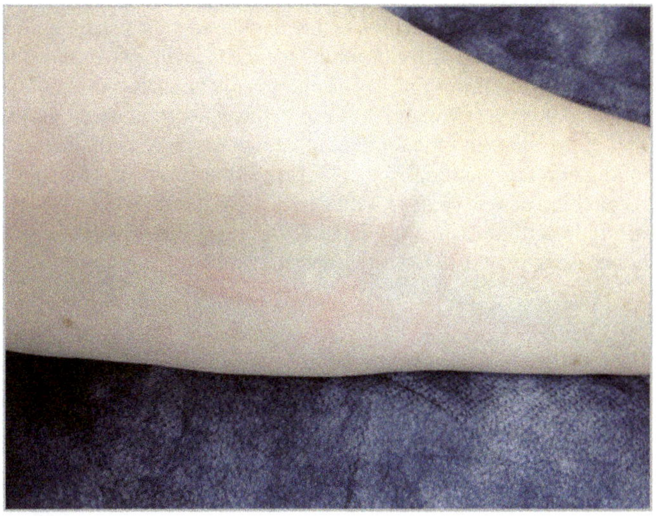

Figure 8.2 A typical raised weal following scratching typical of dermographism.

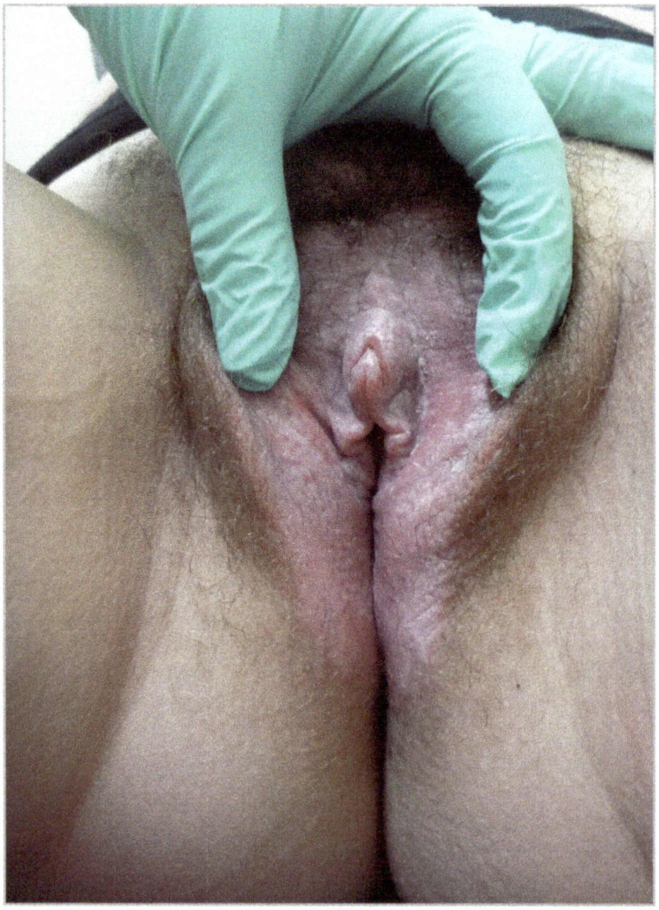

Figure 8.3 Intense pruritus and chronic scratching leading to lichenification in a 21-year-old diabetic. *Candida albicans* infection was missed initially as a periodic acid–Schiff stain was not performed on the histologic specimen.

uses the origin of the injury or underlying disease as the basis, there is increasing evidence that dedicated itch-transmitting neurones exist in both peripheral and central afferent pathways (Metz & Ständer 2010). The sensation of pruritus is transmitted by polymodal, small (0.2–1.5 μm), nociceptive, unmyelinated C fibers. These fibers end at the dermo-epidermal junction and to date no specific itch receptors have been identified. Itch can only be evoked in intact skin or mucous membranes like the vagina or oral mucosa but not if the epidermis is removed. Keratinocytes are involved in the generation of the sensation of pruritus, and the number of known pruritus mediators and modulators is expanding. Hopefully, in the future this will result in the recognition of new targets for therapy such as interleukin-31 (IL-31) in atopic dermatitis, new modalities of therapy, and overall improve our management of this most distressing problem.

Pruritus mediators and modulators (Darsow et al. 2011)

- Histamine
- Prostaglandin E2
- Acetylcholine
- Serotonin
- Substance P
- Mast cell chymase
- Endogenous opioid neuropeptides
- Proteinases
- Calcitonin gene-related peptide
- Cytokines, e.g. IL-31 in atopic dermatitis

Current classification of pruritus (Twycross et al. 2003)

- Pruritogenic pruritus originating in the skin due to inflammation, dryness, or other skin damage
- Neuropathic pruritus occurs as a result of pathology located at any point along the afferent pathways
- Neurogenic pruritus originating centrally but without evidence of neural pathology
- Psychogenic pruritus is associated with psychological abnormalities

Vulvar pruritus is complex and can involve more than one type of itch. Pruritogenic itch is not homogenous and pruritic skin stimuli can induce two distinct responses, although it is not known if they are transmitted via the same neural pathways. First, itch that persists only briefly once the stimulus is removed is known as spontaneous itch, and second, there may be a poorly localized area surrounding the original area affected by the stimulus, that does not itch spontaneously but itches intensely when subjected to light touch or other minor stimuli, which is known as 'alloknesis' and is also referred to as generally 'itchy skin.'

The phenomenon of 'itchy skin' is a common complaint in atopic individuals who complain of 'sensitive skin' that requires very little to set off intense itch. Known factors that evoke itch include heat, perspiration, and clothing brushing against the skin during dressing or undressing.

CAUSES OF VULVAR PRURITUS

The 'normal' vulva changes in appearance throughout life secondary to endocrine and reproductive influences. Unsurprisingly, conditions that may cause vulvar pruritus vary through life. The causes of vulvar pruritus are summarized in **Table 8.1** organized according to condition and patient's age, neonate/infant, prepubertal, reproductive years, and postmenopause. Common conditions and important other considerations have been included, and therefore, it is not entirely limited to conditions of the vulva.

Table 8.1 Causes of vulvar pruritus

Conditions/dermatoses	Neonate/infant	Prepubertal	Reproductive years	Postmenopause
Lichen sclerosus (Chapter 19)	No	Yes	Yes	Yes
Lichen simplex chronicus (Chapter 16) (Figure 8.3)	No	Yes	Yes	Yes
Atopic dermatitis (Chapter 16)	Yes	Yes	Yes	Yes

Continued opposite...

Table 8.1 Causes of vulvar pruritus. *Continued*

Conditions/dermatoses	Neonate/infant	Prepubertal	Reproductive years	Postmenopause
Urticaria	Uncommon	Yes	Yes	Yes
Dermographism (Figure 8.2)	Uncommon	Yes	Yes	Yes
Contact dermatitis (Chapter 17) • Irritant contact dermatitis (Figure 8.1) • Allergic contact dermatitis	 Yes Uncommon	 Yes Uncommon	 Yes Yes	 Yes Yes
Seborrheic dermatitis (Chapter 16)	Yes	No	No	No
Lichen planus (Chapter 20)	No	Uncommon	Yes: usually pain	Yes: usually pain
Intertrigo	Yes	Yes	Yes	Yes
Fox–Fordyce disease	No	No	Yes	No: usually resolves
Darier disease (Chapter 27)	No	Yes	Yes	Yes
Hailey–Hailey disease (Chapter 27)	No	Uncommon	Yes	Yes
Infection/infestation				
Candidosis (Chapters 39 and 42)	Yes	No	Yes	Yes: under certain situations*
Molluscum contagiosum (Chapter 30)	Usually No	Yes	Yes	Yes
Pinworms/threadworms (Chapter 42)	Usually No	Yes	Yes	Unlikely
Scabies	Yes	Yes	Yes	Yes
Perianal/perineal streptococcal disease (Olson & Edmonson 2011)	Possibly	Yes: most common	Yes	No
Congenital syphilis (Chapter 31)	Yes	No	No	No
Herpes simplex (Chapter 30)	Unlikely	Unlikely	Yes	Yes
Dermatophytosis (tinea) (Chapter 29)	No	No	Yes	Yes
Pediculosis pubis (Chapter 31)	No	No	Yes	Yes
Trichomoniasis (Chapter 31)	No	No	Yes	No
Tumors				
Syringomata (benign) (Chapter 33)	No	No	Yes	No
Lymphangioma circumsripta	No	Yes	Yes	Yes
Vulvar intraepithelial neoplasia (premalignant) (Chapter 35)	No	No	Yes: • HPV associated • LS associated	Yes: • LS associated
Basal cell carcinoma (Chapter 35)	No	No	Yes	Yes
Paget disease (malignant) (Chapter 36)	No	No	Uncommon	Yes
Langerhans histiocytosis (malignant) (Chapter 36)	Yes	Yes: very unlikely	Yes: very unlikely	Yes
Granular cell tumor (malignant and benign) (Chapter 35)	Yes	Yes	Yes: peak 30s and 40s	Unlikely
Cloacogenic carcinoma (malignant)	No	No	Yes: rare	Yes: rare
Anal and lower bowel disorders				
Hemorrhoids	No	No	Yes	Yes

Continued overleaf...

Table 8.1 Causes of vulvar pruritus. *Continued*

Conditions/dermatoses	Neonate/infant	Prepubertal	Reproductive years	Postmenopause
Anal fissures	No	Yes	Yes	Yes
Fistulas	No	No	Yes	Yes
Inflammatory bowel disease	No	Very rare	Yes	Yes
Proctitis	No	No	Yes	Yes
Adenomatous polyps	No	No	Yes: increase with age	Yes
Anal intraepithelial neoplasia	No	No	Yes: • HPV associated • LS associated	Yes: • LS associated
Anal, rectal malignancy	No	No	Yes	Yes
Neurogenic/musculoskeletal disorders				
Pudendal nerve entrapment	No	No	Yes	Yes
Radiculopathy	No	No	Yes	Yes
Lumbar facet joint disease	No	No	Yes	Yes
Endocrine/other disorders				
Estrogen deficiency (atrophic vulvovaginitis)	No	Yes	No Yes: • postpartum • breast feeding • medroxyprogesterone injection • etonogestrel implant • aromatase inhibitors • estrogen receptor blockers	Yes: normal No: HRT
Diabetes	Unlikely	Possible	Yes: increased candidosis	Possibly increased candidosis
Immunosuppression				
HIV†	Yes	Yes	Yes	Yes
Medication‡	Yes	Yes	Yes	Yes

*Diabetes, hormonal replacement therapy (HRT)
†Clinical picture will depend on age of patient, seborrheic dermatitis, candidosis, sexually transmitted diseases must be considered
‡The increased incidence of organ transplantation and use of immunosuppressant therapy for varied conditions means that pruritus vulvae may occur as a consequence of infections such as candidosis or drug eruptions
HPV, human papillomavirus; LS, lichen sclerosus

Most causes of vulvar pruritus may be elucidated following a careful history and examination that includes examination of the skin generally. It is especially important to determine whether there is any inflammatory skin disease of the vulvar skin. It is useful to observe whether there is any architectural change of the vulva since the scarring disorderssuch as lichen sclerosus and lichen planus are more likely. Investigations including biopsy, swabs, and blood tests may be required as there are a number of systemic conditions such as anemia and hypothyroidism that may contribute to itch (**Table 8.2**). If the vulvar pruritus is part of generalized itch, it can be useful to look for other causes of itch.

Urticaria is a common condition and may also involve the vulva. Dermographism (**Figure 8.2**) may be itchy and is caused by scratching or other mechanical triggers like pressure in some individuals. Taking a careful history of potential triggers and the duration of symptoms is essential to discover this condition that may show no signs at presentation. Scratching the skin of the forearm with a blunt tool may be useful to provoke dermographism (raised red streaks after scratching).

Investigations to consider in pruritus

- Hemoglobin (anemia, polycythemia)
- Ferritin or iron studies (low iron can cause itch even if hemoglobin is normal)
- Thyroid function tests (hypothyroidism)
- Blood glucose (diabetes mellitus)
- Renal and hepatic function (renal failure and liver disorders especially primary biliary cirrhosis)
- Chest radiography in selected cases only (lymphoma)
- Protein electrophoresis (elderly patient with unexplained itch, myeloma)

Table 8.2 Systemic causes of pruritus and vulvar pruritus

Metabolic: • Uremic/kidney disease • Hepatic disease: – Primary biliary cirrhosis – Intrahepatic biliary obstruction – Extrahepatic biliary cirrhosis
Endocrine: • Hyperthyroidism • Hypothyroidism • Diabetes
Infections: • Human immunodeficiency virus
Malignancy related: • Polycythemia vera • Lymphoma: Hodgkin disease (mainly) and other including mycosis fungoides • Carcinoid syndrome • Leukemia • Multiple myeloma • Solid tumors (breast, gastric, lung), (possibly as part of paraneoplastic syndrome)
Other: • Atopic manifestations other than eczema: asthma, allergic rhinitis, dermographism • Iron deficiency anemia • Multiple sclerosis • Brain abscess • Stroke • Psychogenic/factitial

REFERENCES

Darsow U, Pfab F, Valet M, et al. Pruritus and atopic dermatitis. Clin Rev Allergy Immunol 2011; 41:237–244.

Davidson S, Moser H, Giesler G. Ascending pathways for itch. In: Carstens E, Akiyama T (eds), Itch: mechanisms and treatment (Chapter 22). Boca Raton, FL: CRC Press, 2014.

Metz M, Ständer S. Chronic pruritus–pathogenesis, clinical aspects and treatment. J Eur Acad Dermatol Venereol 2010; 24:1249–1260.

Olson D, Edmonson MB. Outcomes in children treated for perineal group A beta-haemolytic streptococcal dermatitis. Pediatr Infect Dis J 2011; 30:933–936.

Simpson RC, Thomas KS, Murphy R. Outcome measures for vulval skin conditions: a systematic review of randomized controlled trials. Br J Dermatol 2013; 169:494–501.

Twycross R, Greaves MW, Handwerker H, et al. Itching: scratching more than the surface. Q J Med 2003; 96:7–26.

Chapter 9 Pain

Susan M Cooper, Gudula Kirtschig

Pain may vary in character and be described in many ways including discomfort, soreness, burning, sharp, or stabbing; it may be experienced as persistent genital arousal (Markos & Dinsmore 2013). Vulvar pain may involve the outer aspect of the genitals, the vulva ('superficial pain'), or the deeper parts or inner organs including the vagina ('deep pain'). If a woman has pain during penetration, we call it dyspareunia; this is divided into superficial, affecting the outer aspect of the vulva or deep dyspareunia, affecting the vagina or other inner organs; superficial and deep dyspareunia may occur together.

Most pain is caused by inflammation or infection or trauma/injury; however, there may be no obvious visible reason (**Table 9.1**).

Vulvar pain may have many different causes:

- Inflammation – e.g. lichen sclerosus, (Chapter 19), lichen planus (Chapter 20), bullous disease (Chapter 26/27)
- Infection – e.g. *Candida* (Chapter 29), herpes simplex/zoster (Chapter 30)
- Trauma/injury – e.g. after surgery or damage of nerves for other reasons, e.g. herpes neuralgia, spinal nerve compression
- Neoplasms – benign neoplasms are not usually painful, in contrast to squamous cell carcinomas which are usually painful
- Pain syndromes – e.g. vulvodynia (Chapter 38)

Table 9.1 Causes of pain and particular sensation

Clinical correlate	Sensation	Chapter
Fissures		
In eczema, lichen sclerosus, psoriasis, candida, and bacterial infection	Localized pain, possibly induced after putting tension on the skin (after cleansing/rubbing the skin, during defecation)	11
Erosions		
Lichen planus	Pain, soreness, superficial and possibly deep vaginal dyspareunia	20
Lichen sclerosus	Pain, soreness, superficial dyspareunia, and itch	19
Bullous diseases	Pain, soreness, superficial dyspareunia	27
Ulcers		
Herpes simplex/zoster	Burning pain, often prodromal burning before skin changes	30
Possibly other STDs	Ulcers in syphilis are not painful	31
Aphthous ulcers	Pain	28
Pyoderma gangrenosum	Pain	28
Local trauma		
Various causes	Acute/chronic pain	40, 41
Tumors		
Squamous cell carcinoma	Localized pain and soreness	35
Vulvar intraepithelial neoplasia	Localized pain and soreness	35
Paget disease	Localized pain and soreness	36
Hormonal changes		
Postmenopausal atrophic changes	Generalized soreness, dryness, dyspareunia	3
Breast feeding	Generalized soreness, dryness, dyspareunia	3
Pain syndromes		
Vulvodynia	No visible morphological change: sharp, burning, stabbing pains, often superficial dyspareunia	38

The International Society for the Study of Vulvovaginal Disease (ISSVD) re-established 'vulvodynia' as the preferred term for 'idiopathic vulvar pain,' vulvar pain in the absence of a recognizable condition (Moyal-Barracco & Lynch 2004, Haefner 2007). The terminology and classification of vulvodynia continue to evolve, much remains to be understood about this distressing condition, and worldwide consensus has not been reached. However, the current consensus classification for vulvar pain is a useful approach to enable the communication among various specialties.

Consensus classification and terminology of persistent vulvar pain (2015)

1. Vulvar pain related to a specific disorder
   a. Infectious
   b. Inflammatory
   c. Neoplastic
   d. Neurologic
   e. Trauma
   f. Iatrogenic
   g. Hormonal deficiencies
2. Vulvodynia (vulval pain of at least 3 months duration), without clear identifiable cause)
   a. Descriptors
      i. Localized (e.g. vestibulodynia, clitorodynia, generalized or mixed
      ii. Provoked (e.g. insertional, contact), spontaneous or mixed
      iii. Onset (primary or secondary)
      iv. Temporal pattern (intermittent, persistent, constant, immediate, delayed)
   b. Generalized
      i. Provoked (sexual, non-sexual, or both)
      iii. Unprovoked
      iii. Mixed (provoked and unprovoked)
3. Localized (vestibulodynia, clitorodynia, hemivulvodynia)
   a. Provoked (sexual, non-sexual, or both)
   b. Unprovoked

When faced with a patient with vulvar pain, it is helpful to answer a few questions:

IS THE PAIN ACUTE OR CHRONIC?

Acute pain is usually due to infection, inflammation, or injury, and the cause is usually obvious on examination. Chronic pain may be due to an underlying chronic inflammatory disorder such as lichen sclerosus but may also be a feature of vulvodynia.

IS THERE ANY VISIBLE CAUSE FOR PAIN?

Vulvar examination will usually help determine, if there is any inflammatory or infectious cause of the pain. If there is no obvious visible cause for pain, vulvodynia may be suspected.

WHAT IS THE QUALITY OF THE PAIN?

Pain in vulvodynia is usually described as burning, sharp, or stabbing. Allodynia (pain due to stimuli that do not normally cause pain such as light touch) may also be a feature. These types of pain may sometimes occur in inflammatory disease but are less common except in herpes neuralgia. Pain due to nerve entrapment, e.g. pudendal nerve compression causes burning pains similar to those seen in vulvodynia and herpes zoster neuralgia. Generalized soreness, dryness and dyspareunia are typical in postmenopausal atrophic changes.

CAN THE PAIN BE LOCALIZED?

Pain is usually localized to the area of fissuring, ulceration or inflammation. In vulvodynia, pain may be localized to one part of the vulva, e.g. the clitoris in 'clitorodynia' or at the vestibule in 'vestibulodynia.'

ARE THERE ANY PROVOKING FACTORS?

Inserting tampons or having intercourse often provokes pain, which is called 'provoked vestibulodynia.'

REFERENCES

Haefner HK. Report of the International Society for the Study of Vulvovaginal Disease terminology and classification of vulvodynia. J Low Genit Tract Dis 2007; 11:48–49.

Markos AR, Dinsmore W. Persistent genital arousal and restless genitalia: sexual dysfunction or subtype of vulvodynia? Int J STD AIDS 2013; 24:852–858.

Moyal-Barracco M, Lynch PJ. 2003 ISSVD terminology and classification of vulvodynia: a historical perspective. J Reprod Med 2004; 49:772–777.

Chapter 10 Red skin

Gudula Kirtschig, Susan M Cooper

INTRODUCTION

Many skin diseases will show some degree of redness. There are three main causes of 'red changes' of the skin with variable etiology:

Causes of redness

Hyperemia (temporary vascular dilatation)	Seen as erythema due to inflammation
Vascular changes (permanent)	Seen as telangiectasia/varices/ hemangioma
Erythrocyte extravasation	Seen as purpura/ecchymoses/ hematoma

Inflammation is a stereotypical reaction of the skin seen in a variety of diseases (**Table 10.1**). In addition to erythema, other clinical signs including swelling, scaling, blistering, or ulceration may accompany the process; pain and itch may be accompanying symptoms. Inflammation of the skin is a response to any stimuli. Sometimes, it is difficult to appreciate erythema, in particular in skin of color, as there is variable normal 'redness' of the vulva especially at the vaginal introitus, which can be confusing even for the experienced observer. Over interpretation of erythema may occur although appearances are physiological, e.g. in vestibulodynia (previously vestibulitis).

Pathogenetic factors

- Auto-inflammatory processes
- Autoimmune processes
- Allergies
- Irritancy
- Pathogens (bacteria, viruses, fungi)
- Tumor cells

Sometimes, the typical clinical appearances (**Table 10.1**) will reveal the cause of inflammation; however, as the anogenital site is occluded and exposed to friction, typical features of disease seen at other body sites; e.g. scaling in psoriasis or blisters in autoimmune blistering diseases may not be observed. Examination of the skin elsewhere may give clues. Often, the underlying cause may not be obvious and histopathological or microbiological investigations are needed. Clinical appearances can vary according to the stage of disease; e.g., in the early stages of lichen sclerosus, there may be erythema indistinguishable from eczema before the typical pallor develops. Secondary infection may complicate established disease, e.g. candidosis in lichen sclerosus. Overuse of topical steroids may lead to diffuse erythema; this will resolve when the steroids are stopped (**Figure 10.1**).

Malignant diseases such as differentiated vulval intraepithelial neoplasia (dVIN), high-grade squamous intraepithelial lesions (HSIL),

Table 10.1 Clinical features differentiating the most common inflammatory vulvar diseases

	Candida	Dermatitis/eczema	Lichen sclerosus (LS)	Psoriasis	Lichen planus (LP)
Anatomy	No changes	Usually no changes	Loss of labia minora and labial fusion possible	Usually no changes	Loss of labia minora and labial fusion possible
Site	Vulva and perianal; vaginal	Vulva and perianal; not vaginal; anywhere else on the skin	Vulvar and perianal 'Figure of 8'; no vaginal changes	Vulva and perianal; not vaginal; anywhere else on the skin	Vulva (and vagina and oral)
Sign	Diffuse erythema; satellite lesions outside main erythema; possibly fissures, white curds	Diffuse erythema; possibly scaling, papulovesicular, lichenification, fissures	Hypopigmentation, hyperkeratosis, sclerosis, erythema, fissures, atrophy, ecchymoses	Sharply demarcated symmetrical erythema; possibly fissures and some scaling	Sharply demarcated glazed erythema/erosions, Wickham striae
Symptom	Itch, discharge	Itch	Itch > pain or asymptomatic in some	Soreness, itch or asymptomatic	Pain > itch
Extragenital	Extragenital unlikely	Commonly extragenital	Extragenital LS is rare	Possibly extragenital	Possibly extragenital LP
Nail	No nail changes	No nail changes	No nail changes	Nail changes such as pitting frequent	Possibly typical nail changes
Oral	Usually no oral symptoms	Usually no oral symptoms	Usually no oral disease	Oral symptoms not typical	Often oral disease

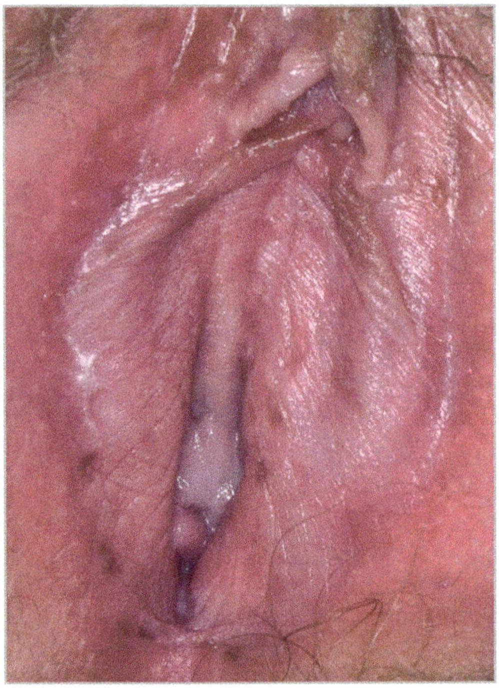

Figure 10.1 Diffuse erythema in a patient with lichen sclerosus who applied too much topical steroid for several years.

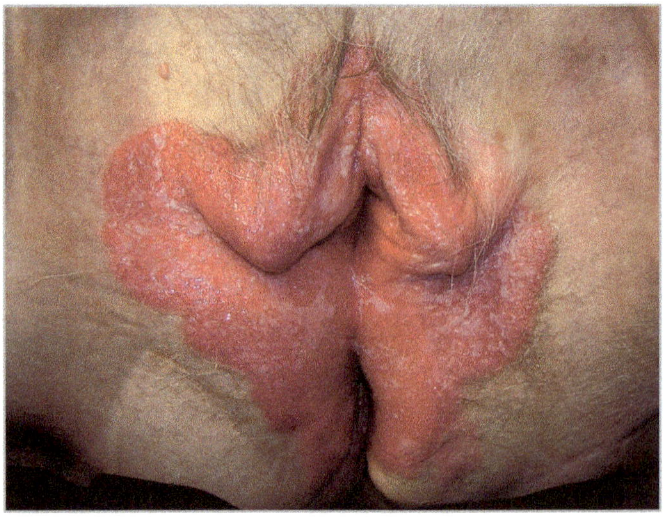

Figure 10.2 Paget disease showing erythema with erosions and hyperkeratosis.

squamous cell carcinomas, or Paget disease (**Figure 10.2**) will show some redness due to inflammation and neovascularization (see Chapters 35 and 36) (**Table 10.2**).

Table 10.2 Examples of diseases causing vulvar redness listed according to frequency of occurrence

Disease	Clinical features	Chapter
Candida infection	Red/white islands, discharge, itch	29
Dermatitis (atopic/irritant/allergic)	Fine scales, diffuse margins, fissures, vesicles	16, 17
Lichen sclerosus	White hyperkeratosis, fissures, ecchymoses	19
Lichen simplex	Lichenification/thickened skin, intense itch	16
Psoriasis	Possibly scales, fissures, sharp margins	22
Bacterial infection (streptococci)	Intense spreading erythema, fissures, perianal, often in children	29, 42
Lichen planus	Papules with white striae or erythema, scars	20
HSIL & dVIN	Variable; additional flat papules or erosions	35

VASCULAR CHANGES

The redness in vascular changes (see Chapter 37 for further reading) is usually well circumscribed (e.g. nevus flammeus). There may be additional papules or nodules (e.g. hemangioma). Dilation of vessels is observed as telangiectasia/spider nevi (small vessels; not usually seen at the vulva) or vulvar hemorrhoids and varices (larger vessels), sometimes seen after pregnancy. There is well defined redness or, if deeper skin layers are involved, bluish discolorations. They are often not troublesome; however, if larger vessels are involved, swelling may be a problem.

Angiomata or hemangiomata are proliferations of vessels that may present shortly after birth, like cavernous hemangioma in children or may be acquired later in life. Spontaneous remission in children is likely. In adults, cherry angiomata or angiokeratomata (multiple small papules with some scale) may occur and may be seen in lichen sclerosus (**Figure 10.3**). Newly developing single red nodules may be benign, e.g. pyogenic granuloma but should be excised as the differential diagnosis includes amelanotic malignant melanoma and bleeding may be troublesome.

ERYTHROCYTE EXTRAVASATION

If vessel walls are damaged, erythrocytes leak from the vessels and are deposited in the surrounding tissue, seen as petechiae or purpura. This may be very subtle and is not usually observed in the vulva. Larger areas seen as purple, red flat macules (ecchymoses) are, e.g. a feature of lichen sclerosus (**Figure 10.4**), secondary to vascular fragility. These changes do not require special treatment but will resolve when the underlying skin disease is treated. A hematoma is usually a result of trauma or intraoperative bleeding. Blood may expand rapidly into the loose tissue and swelling may be troublesome. A typical yellowish discoloration will occur but resolve with time.

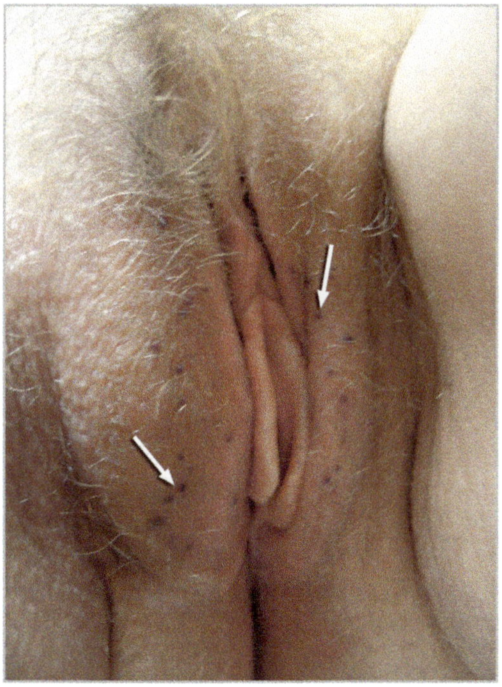

Figure 10.3 Angiokeratomata in lichen sclerosus.

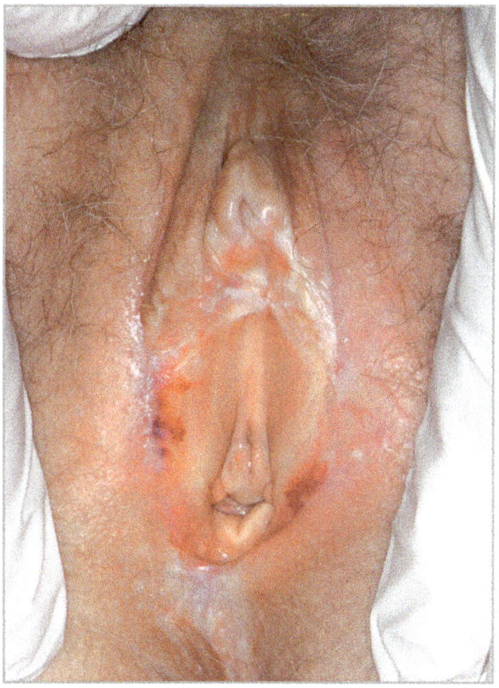

Figure 10.4 Red macules, ecchymoses, a feature of lichen sclerosus secondary to vascular fragility.

Chapter 11 Broken skin

Gudula Kirtschig, Susan M Cooper

There are many causes of 'broken skin.' Broken skin is usually painful with some exceptions, most notably the chancre of syphilis. Clinically, we distinguish between superficial defects that only affect epidermal layers, which usually heal without scarring and deep defects that involve dermal layers, which will usually heal with scars (Chapter 14). However, any chronic inflammatory process at the vulva, with or without skin defect, may lead in time to changes of skin structure and architecture.

Features of broken skin

- Fissure: fine, linear, superficial breaks
- Erosion: shallow, well-defined breaks with intact dermal tissue
- Ulcer: complete loss of the epidermis, extending to the dermis and sometimes the fat layer

The skin may be broken in only fine lines, usually termed as fissures. They most often occur at the perineum or in the interlabial sulci between the labia majora and minora (**Figure 11.1**). In the special situation of fissuring at the fourchette, this can be aggravated by an anatomical band of tissue caused by scarring secondary to inflammatory disease, e.g. lichen sclerosus, postmenopausal atrophy, due to surgery or birth trauma or sometimes due to a presumed anatomical variant.

Erosions refer to well-demarcated superficial breaks in the skin, whereas ulcers are deeper. Erosions and ulcers may be primary features of disease like ulcers in Behçet disease or pyoderma gangrenosum and erosions in erosive lichen planus or high-grade squamous intraepithelial lesions of the vulva (**Figure 11.2**) or develop secondary to disease as seen in the blistering diseases, which will lead to a skin defect once the blister has ruptured (**Figure 11.3**).

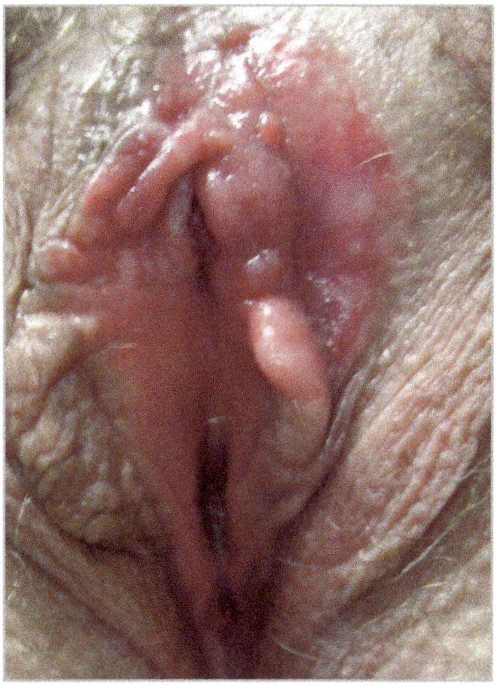

Figure 11.2 More generalized erosions in high-grade squamous intraepithelial lesions of the vulva.

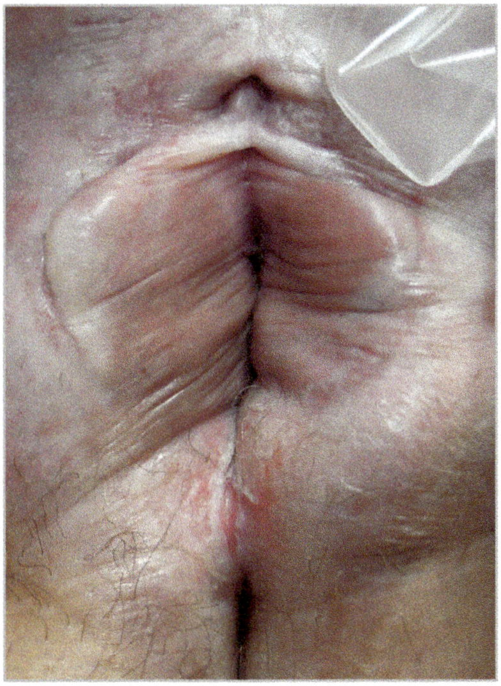

Figure 11.1 Fissure at the perineum in lichen sclerosus showing typical linear conformation.

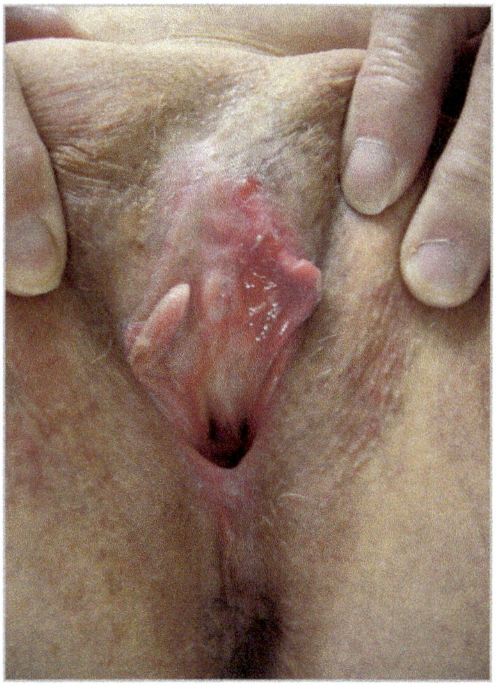

Figure 11.3 Well-circumscribed erosions after the rupture of blisters in mucous membrane pemphigoid.

CARE OF BROKEN SKIN

Broken skin is usually painful, and even small defects may lead to severe interference with daily life. The skin should be protected with greasy topicals like vaseline or a mixture of white vaseline and liquid paraffin (1:1). It is helpful to apply the topical several times daily and in particular before the skin is exposed to liquids like water (showering or bathing) or urine. Small fissures may be protected with paste containing zinc oxide or 'drying lotions' also suitable for superficial erosions. Cleaning the broken skin may cause problems and again, greasy topicals such as unperfumed baby oil or petrolatum-based emollients instead of water may help (Chapter 7). Fissures may cause severe pain when stretched. This may be a particular problem after defecation in lichen sclerosus affecting the perianal site; soft stool diminishes the problem and a diet containing lots of fibers, e.g. in cereals, fruit, and vegetables, is recommended.

Table 11.1 Examples of vulvar diseases accompanied by broken skin

Kind of defect	Skin diseases	Diagnostic test	Chapter
FISSURES			
	Candida infection	Swab	29
	Streptococcal infection	Swab	29
	Eczema, atopic/irritant/allergic	History and biopsy	16, 17
	Psoriasis (inversa)	History and biopsy	22
	Lichen sclerosus	History and biopsy	19
	Lichen planus	History and biopsy	20
	Postmenopausal	History and evidence of atrophy	2
	Sexual abuse	History	39
EROSION			
	Lichen planus	Biopsy at edge of defect	20
	Lichen sclerosus	Biopsy at edge of defect	19
	HSIL, dVIN, Paget disease	Biopsy	35, 36
	Reactions to drugs (TEN, EEM)	History	18
	Graft versus Host Disease	History, biopsy	18
	Lupus erythematosus	Biopsy, serology	25
	Zinc deficiency syndrome	History, blood tests	
	Scratch artifacts, dermatitis artefacta, tight clothing	Patient's history	
Secondary to blisters	Mucous membrane pemphigoid, Hailey–Hailey disease and others autoimmune, and inherited blistering diseases	Biopsy of blister and extralesional for immunofluorescence test	26, 27
	Glucagonoma	Blood tests, etc.	
	Herpes/Epstein–Barr virus infections	Swab, serology	30
Secondary to pustules	Fungal and bacterial infections	Swab, skin scrapings	29
ULCERS			
Non-infectious	Aphthous ulcers	History	28
	Lipschütz disease	History, swab	28
	Behçet disease	Other sites?	28
	Crohn disease (long knife–cut ulcers pathognomic)	Biopsy, intestine?	24
	Pyoderma gangrenosum	No specific test	28
	Langerhans cell histiocytosis	Biopsy	28
	Malignancies	Biopsy	35
Infectious	Sexually transmitted diseases	Swab, serology	31

dVIN, differentiated vulvar intraepithelial neoplasia; EEM, erythema multiforme; HSIL, high-grade squamous intraepithelial lesions; TEN, toxic epidermal necrolysis

FURTHER READING

Cebesoy FB, Balat O, Inaloz S. Premenarchal vulvar ulceration: is chronic irritation a causative factor? Pediatr Dermatol 2009; 26:514–518.

Deitch HR, Huppert J, Adams Hillard PJ. Unusual vulvar ulcerations in young adolescent females. J Pediatr Adolesc Gynecol 2004; 17:13–16.

Mirowski GW, Schlosser BJ, Stika CS. Cutaneous vulvar streptococcal infection. J Low Genit Tract Dis 2012; 16:281–284.

Pipkin C. Erosive diseases of the vulva. Dermatol Clin 2010; 28:737–751.

Wong CS, Andrew S, Yell J. Isolated vulval splitting—is this normal or pathological? J Obstet Gynaecol 2004; 24:899–902.

Chapter 12 White skin

Susan M Cooper, Ruth Asher, Gudula Kirtschig

Many vulvar skin conditions show some pallor or whitening of the skin. Racial differences in skin color may affect the appearance of the skin disease.

Reasons for the appearance of white skin (see Tables 12.1 and 12.2)

- Reduced melanocytes or melanin with or without change of skin texture
- Scarring or sclerosis
- Thickened epidermis due to hyperkeratosis or acanthosis
- Reduced skin blood flow

When approaching the differential diagnosis of white skin in the vulva, it is helpful to start with answering the following questions:

IS THE SKIN TEXTURE NORMAL OR ABNORMAL?

In lichen sclerosus (LS) pallor is typically crinkly with loss of normal skin markings (**Figure 12.1**), but in vitiligo and postinflammatory hypopigmentation, texture is normal. In postmenopausal atrophy skin is dry and in lichen simplex very thickened with lichenification (**Figure 12.2**). In high-grade squamous intraepithelial lesions (HSIL) skin may be warty and thickened.

IS THE PALLOR SYMMETRICAL OR ASYMMETRICAL?

LS and vitiligo are usually symmetrical skin diseases, whereas dVIN or HSIL are usually asymmetrical.

ARE THE PALLOR LESIONS NUMEROUS AND WIDELY DISTRIBUTED OR LOCALIZED IN ONE PATCH?

Early LS can start as a pale patch, but established disease usually shows diffuse pallor as also seen in postinflammatory hypopigmentation of eczema. HSIL or dVIN may be one patch or multiple; condylomata are usually multiple.

Table 12.1 Diseases causing vulvar whitening

Skin disease	Clinical features	Chapter
Loss or reduction of melanin or melanocytes without change of skin texture		
Vitiligo	Sharply demarcated, symmetrical	
Postinflammatory hypopigmentation, e.g. in eczema	Partial depigmentation, history of previous inflammation poorly demarcated, usually symmetrical	16, 17
Nevus depigmentosus (achromic nevus)	Usually solitary, hypopigmentation rather than complete depigmentation, normal skin texture	
Hypopigmentation in connection with epidermal atrophy, scarring, or sclerosis with change of skin texture		
Postmenopausal atrophy/age-related	Subtle generalized pallor usually symmetrical, skin feels dry	1, 3
Scarring	History of surgery or episiotomy, often linear	14
Lichen sclerosus	Crinkly pallor, hyperkeratosis, fissures, ecchymoses, 'figure of 8,' usually symmetrical	19
Thickened epidermis due to hyperkeratosis or acanthosis (change of skin texture)		
Lichen simplex	Thickened skin, lichenification, intense itch	16
Lichen sclerosus	Crinkly pallor, hyperkeratosis, fissures, ecchymoses, 'figure of 8,' usually symmetrical	19
Lichen planus (Figure 12.4)	White plaques, may be other signs of lichen planus such as violaceous papules with striae	20
Condylomata acuminata/lata	Flat plaques or papules with whitish surface	30, 31
Vulvar intraepithelial neoplasia	Variable, white plaques, red erosions	35
Hypopigmented mycosis fungoides	White macules widespread, usually part of more generalized skin condition	
Reduced skin blood flow (no change of skin texture)		
Nevus anemicus	Congenital vascular anomaly. Skin changes undetectable on diascopy (pressing skin with glass slide). Wood lamp examination is normal	

Table 12.2 Differential diagnoses of common conditions causing pale skin in the vulva

Disease/features	Vitiligo	Lichen sclerosus	Postinflammatory change in eczema	Postmenopausal/age-related changes
Clinical description	Sharply demarcated symmetrical depigmentation	Hypopigmentation, possibly accompanied by hyperkeratosis, sclerosis, erythema, fissures, excoriations, ecchymoses in later disease	Hypopigmentation, possibly accompanied by erythema and fine scales	General subtle pallor, dryness
Architecture	No architectural change	Architectural changes	Usually no architectural change (exception children)	Minor architectural change possible
Sites involved	Vulva and perianal; extragenital lesions likely	Vulvar and perianal; extragenital LS is rare	Vulvar and perianal, extragenital lesions possible	Age-related skin, vulvar, and vaginal changes
Symptoms	Asymptomatic	Itch > pain, may be asymptomatic	Itch > pain	Soreness and dryness
Medical history	Personal or family history of autoimmune disease	Personal or family history of autoimmune disease	History of eczema, allergies	Menopausal symptoms

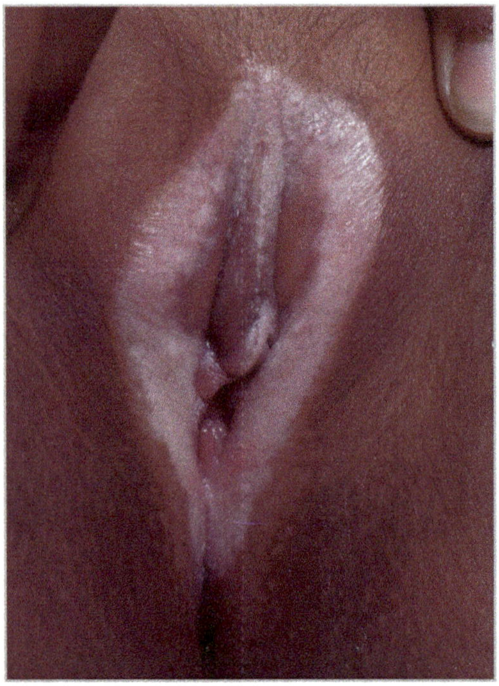

Figure 12.1 Typical well-demarcated pallor of lichen sclerosus with shiny, crinkly changes.

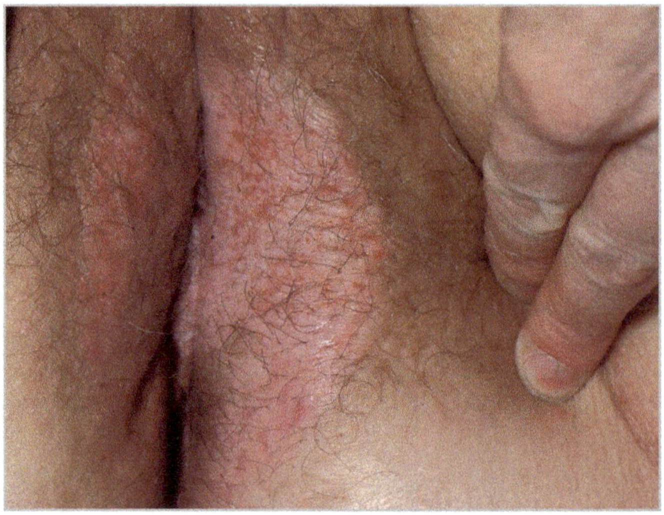

Figure 12.2 Thickened, excoriated plaque typical of lichen simplex. The outer surface of the labia majora is the most common site.

IS PALLOR WELL DEMARCATED OR HAS IT DIFFUSE MARGINS?

Pallor in vitiligo (**Figure 12.3**) and LS has well-demarcated borders, whereas postinflammatory hypopigmentation often has diffuse margins.

Diagnostic tools

- A biopsy is often needed to make a diagnosis
- Use of the Wood lamp can be helpful in vitiligo but is most helpful in Fitzpatrick phototypes (II–VI)

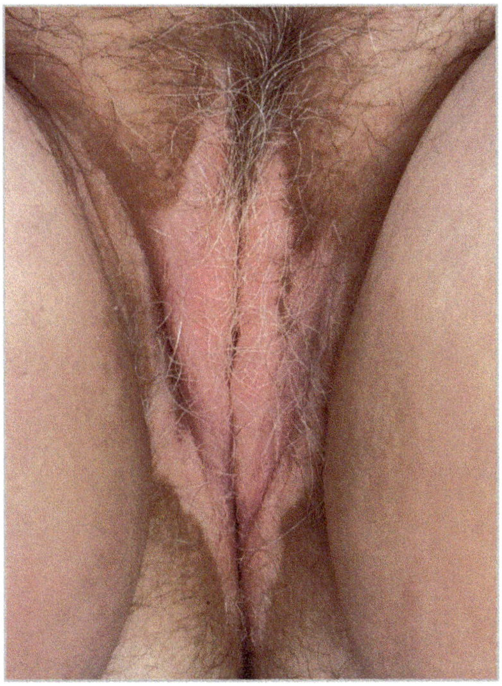

Figure 12.3 Well-demarcated pallor of vitiligo; the skin has a normal texture.

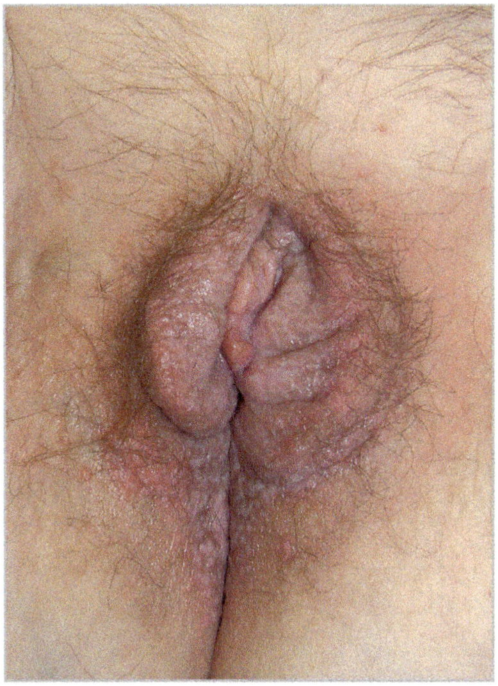

Figure 12.4 Hypertrophic asymmetrical white plaque typical of lichen planus; however, a biopsy is necessary to exclude vulvar intraepithelial neoplasia/high-grade squamous intraepithelial lesions or squamous cell carcinoma.

Chapter 13 Pigmented skin

Susan M Cooper, Ruth Asher, Gudula Kirtschig

Pigmentation of the skin may be due to melanin (see Chapter 34), increased vascularization (varices, angioma) (see Chapter 37), erythrocyte deposition (petechiae, hematoma), hemosiderin (later stage of petechiae and hematoma), or artificial pigment such as tattoos (see Chapter 41). This chapter will concentrate on pigmentation induced by melanin. There is considerable variation in normal skin color reflected in the skin of the vulva varying from skin of no color to black skin (Fitzpatrick skin types I–VI). The labia minora vary in color often being darker in women with skin of color and become darker during pregnancy.

It is helpful to divide pigmentation of the vulva into localized or diffuse pigmentation (**Table 13.1**). Causes of localized pigmentation include postinflammatory hyperpigmentation (e.g. following inflammation of lichen planus or lichen sclerosus) (**Figure 13.1a** and **b**), lentigines, melanosis (**Figure 13.2a** and **b**), nevi (**Figure 13.3**), and melanoma (**Figure 13.4**) (Chapter 34). A history of change in a melanocytic lesion, which may indicate malignancy, is rarely obtained for a pigmented lesion in the vulva. Vulvar dermoscopy may give more information particularly when assessing vascular vulvar lesions such as angiokeratoma, but a biopsy is required if the diagnosis is uncertain to rule out melanoma. Diffuse pigmentation may occur in some genodermatoses such as Dowling–Degos and Galli–Galli disease and systemic endocrine conditions such as Addison disease or acanthosis nigricans benigna (**Figure 13.5**) or maligna. There are several syndromes associated with anogenital hyperpigmentation including multiple lentigines in Peutz–Jeghers, the Carney complex, or Bannayan–Riley–Ruvalcaba syndrome (**Table 13.2**).

Table 13.1 Spectrum of brown pigmented lesions of the vulva

Lesion	Vulvar findings	Other skin findings	Histology	Disease associations	Chapter
Melanocytic vulvar pigmented lesions					
Lentigo	<4-mm macule, single or multiple	Possibly, if occurring in a syndrome	Increased number of basal melanocytes, hyperpigmented basal cell layer, and elongated rete ridges	Nil or seen in syndromes (Table 13.2)	34
Benign nevus	Discrete pigmented lesions, even in color and outline	Nil	Variable depending on type, nests of melanocytes, no atypia	Nil	34
Melanoma and melanoma in situ	Asymmetrical, irregular border with variable pigmentation	Nil	Confluent proliferation and expansile nodules of melanocytes with severe atypia	Nil	34
Non-melanocytic vulvar pigmented lesions					
Postinflammatory hyperpigmentation	Normal skin markings, normal texture	Nil	Normal or increased melanin pigment in the basal cell layer, dermal melanin pigment in macrophages (melanophages)	Frequently follows inflammatory diseases including lichen sclerosus, lichen planus or in scars, e.g. after tears, episiotomy or bruising	19 and 20
Seborrheic keratosis	Warty, greasy plaque, usually outer surface of labia majora	Nil	Acanthosis, hyperkeratosis, horn cysts	Rarely in combination with neoplasms, Leser–Trélat sign	33
Genital wart (condyloma)	Warty or smooth papules or plaques, may be numerous	Nil	Acanthotic epidermis with papillomatosis, hyperkeratosis, focal parakeratosis, and some koilocytes	HPV	30
Vulvar intraepithelial neoplasia	Flat plaques anywhere on the vulva, single or multiple	Nil	Full thickness dysplasia	HPV, cervical, anal, and vaginal disease	35
Pigmented basal cell carcinoma	Isolated nodule	Nil	Basaloid islands of cells with peripheral palisading with surrounding retraction artifact. Increased melanin in lesional cells	Nil	35

Continued overleaf...

Continued...

	Vulvar findings	Other skin findings	Histology	Disease associations	Chapter
Diffuse melanocytic vulvar pigmentation					
Vulvar melanosis (benign vulvar melanosis)	Large macules often asymmetrical labia minora and majora. Uniform in color, well demarcated but borders may be irregular	Nil	Increased basal cell pigmentation, a slight increase in the number of basal melanocytes but no melanocyte atypia	None	34
Diffuse non-melanocytic vulvar pigmentation					
Lichen simplex chronicus	Lichenification, usually outer surfaces of labia majora	Not necessarily	Hyperkeratosis, acanthosis, there may be some spongiosis and patchy parakeratosis	Anemia, hypothyroid state	16
Acanthosis nigricans benigna or maligna (as a paraneoplastic syndrome)	Velvety pigmentation (gray/black) labia majora, inguinal folds	Flexural areas, e.g. axillae, groins, neck	Hyperkeratosis, mild acanthosis, papillomatosis, no increase in melanocytes but may be increased melanin deposition in basal layer	Multiple including insulin resistance, obesity, familial, malignancy	
Dowling–Degos disease (pigmented reticulate anomaly of the flexures)	Dappled or reticulate pigmentation of vulva and/or inguinal region	Flexural involvement	Epidermis shows elongated branched rete ridges with increased melanin pigmentation at the tips, no increase in melanocyte number	None	
Addison disease	Darkening of mucous membranes including vagina	Darkening of buccal mucosa and generalized skin pigmentation	Increased melanin in basal keratinocytes and often in keratinocytes in the upper spinous layer. The number of melanocytes is normal. Variable melanophages in the papillary dermis	Adrenal insufficiency leading to weakness, fatigue , hypoglycemia, etc.	

HPV, human papillomavirus.

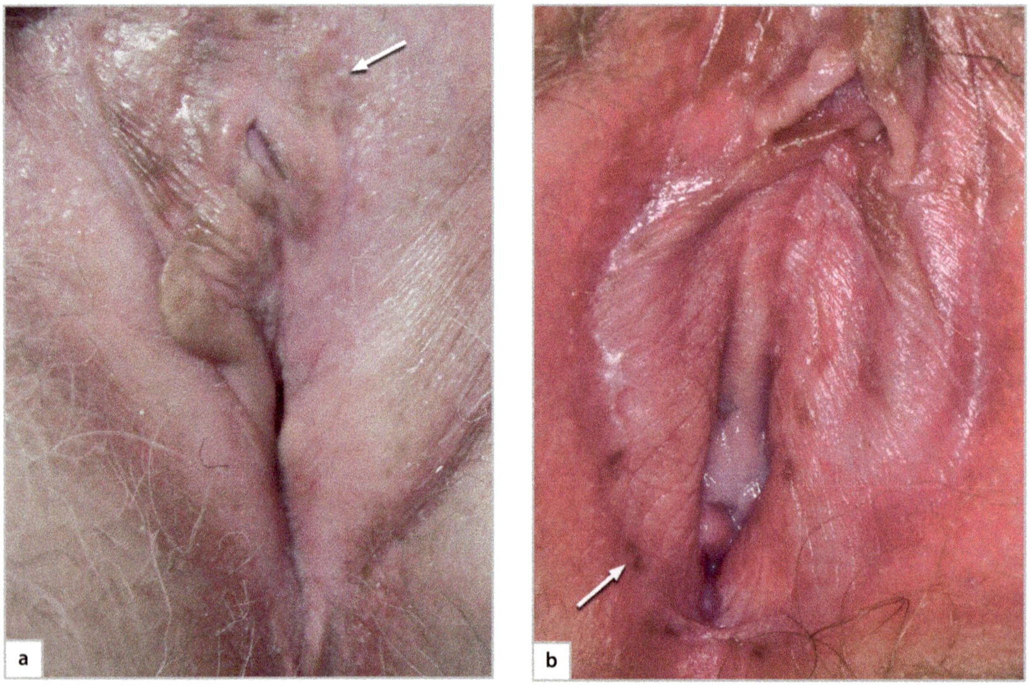

Figure 13.1 Postinflammatory pigmentation in lichen sclerosus (a) Subtle, diffuse hyperpigmentation. (b) Darker, discrete pigmentation.

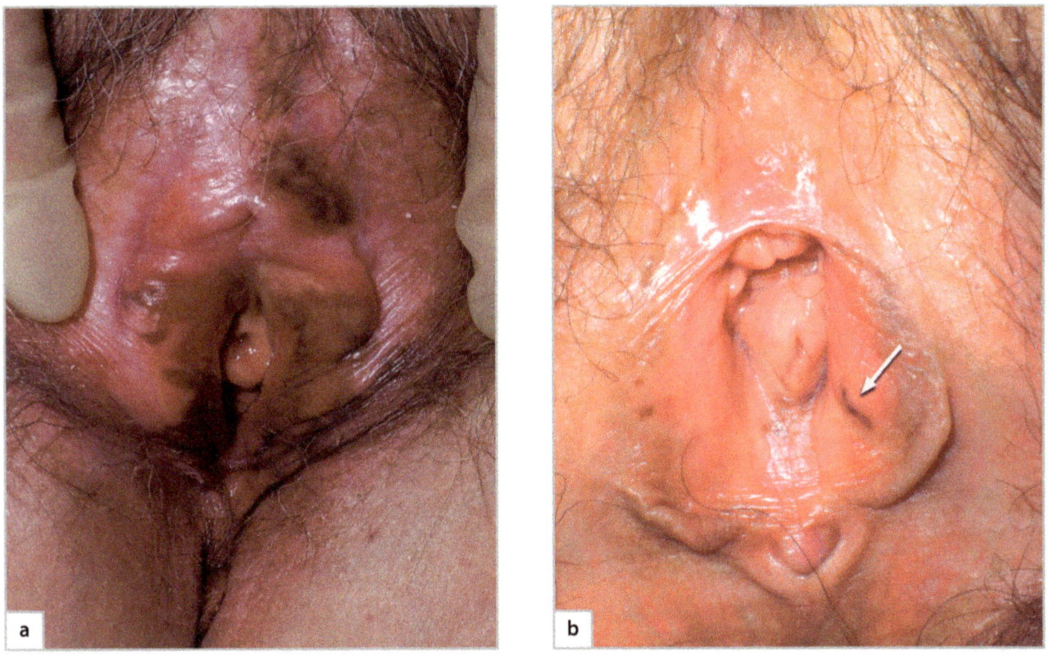

Figure 13.2 Benign vulvar melanosis. (a) Large, dark macules: some are sharply demarcated and angular. (b) Subtle linear pigmentation. By courtesy of Dr Vanessa Venning, Oxford, UK.

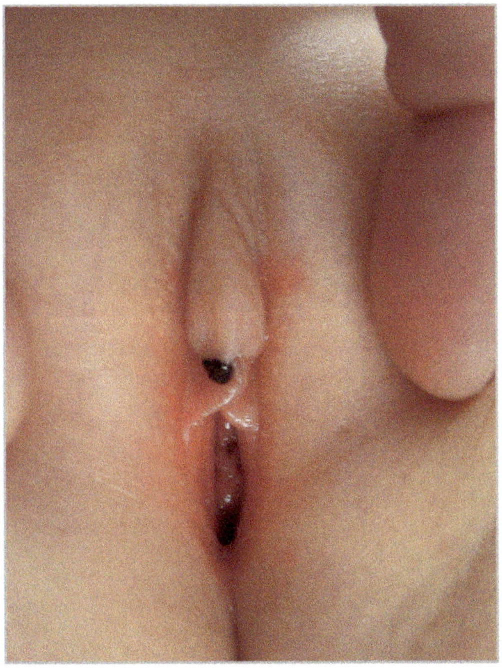

Figure 13.3 Spitz nevus in a child.

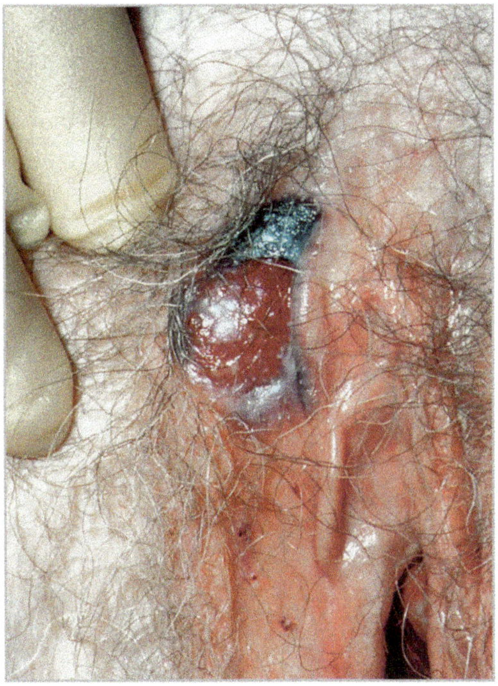

Figure 13.4 Melanoma.

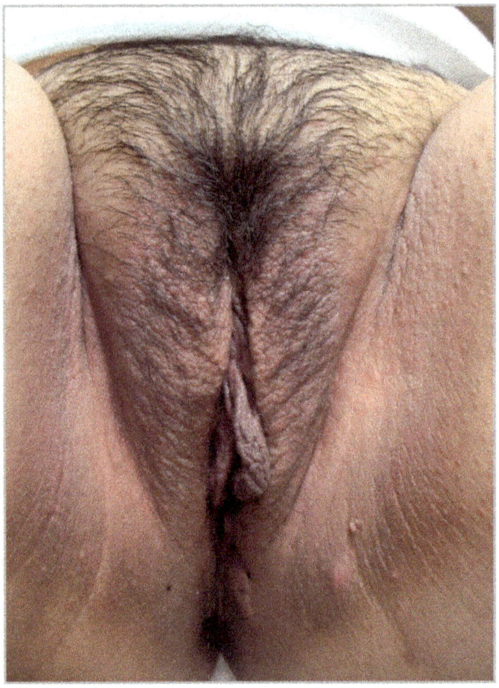

Figure 13.5 Acanthosis nigricans benigna displaying typical velvety skin.

Table 13.2 Syndromes associated with multiple lentigines

Syndrome	Vulvar findings	Other skin findings	Disease associations
Peutz–Jeghers	Multiple lentigines (<4 mm) mucous membranes and skin of vulva	Buccal mucosa, perioral, and skin	Hamartomatous gastrointestinal polyps, increased risk of cancer
Laugier–Hunziker	Multiple lentigines in genital and perianal area	Longitudinal melanonychia, lentigines of oral mucosa including hard and soft palate	No systemic associations
Carney complex (also known as LAMB, NAME)	Brown, black lentigines	Widespread lentigines, blue nevi	Multiple including atrial myxomas and endocrine disease
LEOPARD syndrome	Multiple lentigines	Multiple cutaneous	Multiple including cardiac and genitourinary, short stature
Bannayan–Riley–Ruvalcaba syndrome	Multiple lentigines in the genital area	Lipomas, vascular malformations	Hamartomatous gastointestinal polyps, increased risk of cancer especially thyroid, macrocephaly

Chapter 14 Scarring

Gudula Kirtschig, Susan M Cooper

Scars are areas of fibrous or atrophic tissue that replace normal skin after injury or disease. Scar tissue is less elastic and may be more easily injured after trauma: fissures or ulcerations in scars will heal slowly. There are a number of possible causes of scarring:

- Trauma including episiotomies, sexual abuse, or female circumcision/mutilation may cause variable scarring. There are different types of circumcision that will lead to more or less mutilation, scars, and other complications (Hearst & Molnar 2013, Strickland 2001)
- Radiotherapy possibly followed by radio dermatitis (**Figure 14.1**) may cause scars and difficult-to-heal ulcerations
- Inflammatory diseases including lichen sclerosus, lichen planus, and certain infectious diseases cause various forms of scarring. Fused labia minora, small or completely lost labia minora, clitoral pseudocysts, and atrophic or sclerotic changes of, e.g. the posterior fourchette are often observed (**Figures 14.2** and **14.3**). Scarring is unusual in vulvar psoriasis or eczema; however, eczema in young children may cause labial fusion

Scarring in inflammatory diseases may be diffuse involving the entire vulva as seen in lichen sclerosus, lichen planus, Graft versus Host Disease, or radiotherapy or circumscribed, e.g. after ulcers in Crohn or Lipschütz disease.

PREVENTION OF SCARRING

There is evidence that early treatment of inflammatory diseases will prevent scar formation (Kirtschig et al. 2015, Lee et al. 2015). The prophylactic application of topical corticosteroid in patients undergoing radiotherapy may significantly reduce the incidence of acute radio dermatitis and possibly scar formation (Meghrajani et al. 2013). Early treatment of disease is prudent as scarring is irreversible.

TREATMENT OF SCARRING

Established scars are difficult to treat. Massage using various techniques (simple emollients, topicals containing silicone or corticosteroids, ultrasonography) steroid injections, surgical procedures, and systemic treatments are tried with variable success. Re-adhesion after surgical release of vulvar or vaginal adhesion may be prevented by manual massage, the use of dilators, or sexual intercourse. If there is underlying inflammatory disease such as lichen planus or lichen sclerosus, the early use of topical corticosteroids is also beneficial in preventing re-adhesion; see Chapters 20 and 40 for more information.

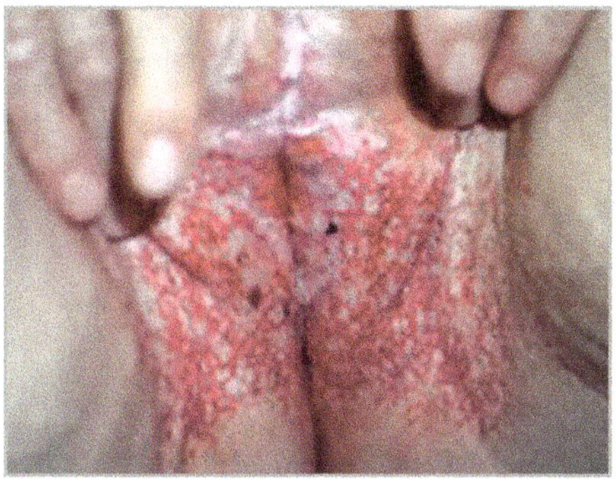

Figure 14.1 Radiodermatitis showing erythema and atrophy of the vulvar skin.

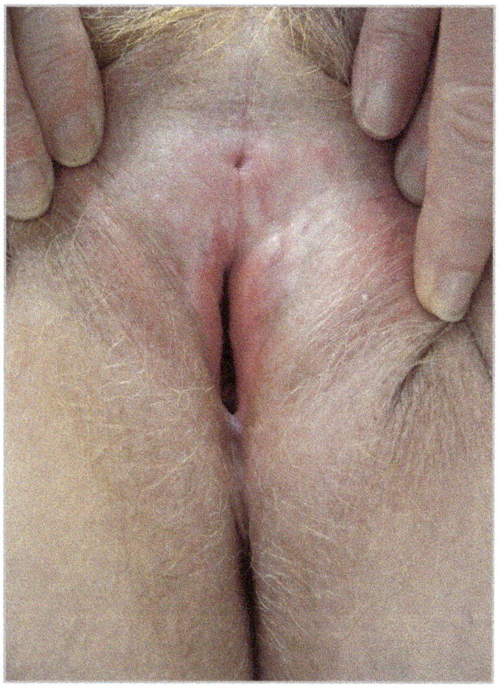

Figure 14.2 Advanced scarring due to longstanding lichen sclerosus. There is extensive midline fusion, burying of the clitoris and complete loss of the labia minora. Note the featureless vulva.

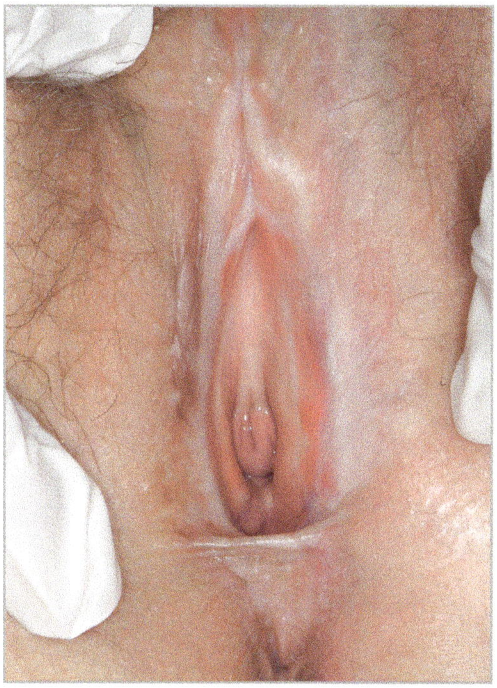

Figure 14.3 Fusion of the clitoral hood due to lichen sclerosus with only a very small part of the right labium minus still visible. There is a bridge of skin at the fourchette which may be vulnerable to splitting.

Table 14.1 Examples of conditions that may be accompanied by scar formation

Kind of scarring	Clinical signs of early disease	Chapter
'Superficial' atrophic scars usually diffuse, often with architectural change		
Lichen planus/Graft versus Host Disease	Pain, erythema, and erosions, later absorption of tissue with change of architecture	20, 18
Lichen sclerosus	Itch, pain, erythema, white changes, and fissures, later absorption of tissue with change of architecture	19
Eczema	Erythema and itching, not usually scarring, but labial fusion and absorption of labia minora may be seen	16
'Superficial' atrophic scars usually circumscribed, without architectural change		
Mucous membrane pemphigoid	Erosions and blisters result in atrophic scars; not usually change of architecture	26
Behçet disease, pyoderma gangrenosum	Painful ulcers leading to single or multiple atrophic scars	28
Severe aphthous and Lipschütz ulcers	Painful ulcers that may lead to scars	28
Fibrotic, keloid like scars		
Hidradenitis suppurativa	Abscesses and fistulas, linear cord-like scars, grouped comedones	23
Crohn disease	Variable, erythematous swellings, deep knife-cut ulcers	24
Langerhans cell histiocytosis	Itch, burning, puffy skin, ulcerated and papillomatous lesions, inguinal lymphadenopathy	
Infections (STD)	Variable, erythema, ulcers, possibly edema and inguinal lymphadenopathy	29, 31
Scarring after trauma		
Surgery	Usually small firm scars, often linear	40
Radiotherapy	Atrophic skin; acute RD may be treated with topical steroids to prevent further damage	
Accidents/self-induced		41

REFERENCES

Hearst AA, Molnar AM. Female genital cutting: an evidence-based approach to clinical management for the primary care physician. Mayo Clin Proc 2013; 88:618–629.

Kirtschig G, Becker K, Günthert A, et al. Evidence-based (S3) guideline on lichen sclerosus. J Eur Acad Dermatol Venereol 2015; 29:e1–e43.

Lee A, Bradford J, Fischer G. Long-term management of adult vulvar lichen sclerosus: a prospective cohort study of 507 women. JAMA Dermatol 2015;151:1061–1067.

Meghrajani CF, Co HC, Ang-Tiu CM, Roa FC. Topical corticosteroid therapy for the prevention of acute radiation dermatitis: a systematic review of randomized controlled trials. Expert Rev Clin Pharmacol 2013; 6:641–649.

Strickland JL. Female circumcision/female genital mutilation. J Pediatr Adolesc Gynecol 2001; 14:109–112.

Chapter 15 Swollen vulva

Susan M Cooper, Gudula Kirtschig

Vulvar swelling can be localized or generalized. This chapter concentrates on generalized swellings (**Table 15.1**) as localized swelling may be caused by a wide variety of cysts, benign, and malignant lesions covered in Chapters 32–35.

Orthostasis and the lax tissue of the vulva make this area vulnerable to fluid accumulation. Most swelling is secondary to edema. When assessing the patient, it is helpful to answer the following questions:

IS THE SWELLING ACUTE OR CHRONIC?

Acute swelling associated with erythema and pain is usually due to infection (**Figure 15.1**). Angioedema may be idiopathic or secondary to type I immediate hypersensitivity reactions, e.g. to latex or seminal fluid (**Figure 15.2**). Chronic swelling may be seen in lymphedema, Crohn disease and Melkersson–Rosenthal syndrome.

ARE THERE ANY ASSOCIATED SYMPTOMS?

There may be fever and pain with infection, a history of bowel problems in Crohn disease (**Figure 15.3**) (but not always as vulvar Crohn disease may present before bowel symptoms become apparent, Chapter 24). In the rare inherited C1-esterase-inhibitor-deficiency, there may be associated abdominal pain and a family history of angioedema. Vascular lesions may vary in size depending on the degree of vascular filling, which is influenced by a variety of factors including tension, stasis and temperature (Chapter 37).

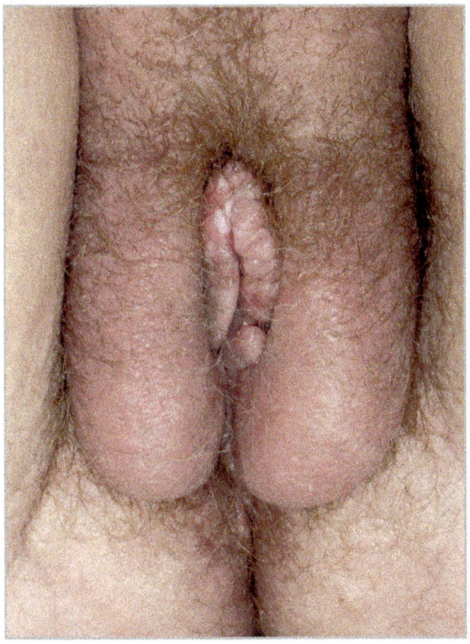

Figure 15.1 Acute swelling due to recurrent erysipelas of the vulva.

DOES THE UNDERLYING SKIN APPEAR ABNORMAL?

In the presence of infection, skin is red, warm to touch, and painful. In lymphedema, skin will be firm and dimpled. In Crohn disease, skin may initially look normal but knife-cut ulcers, swellings, tags, and sinuses will develop. In angioedema, there is swelling but skin is of normal color.

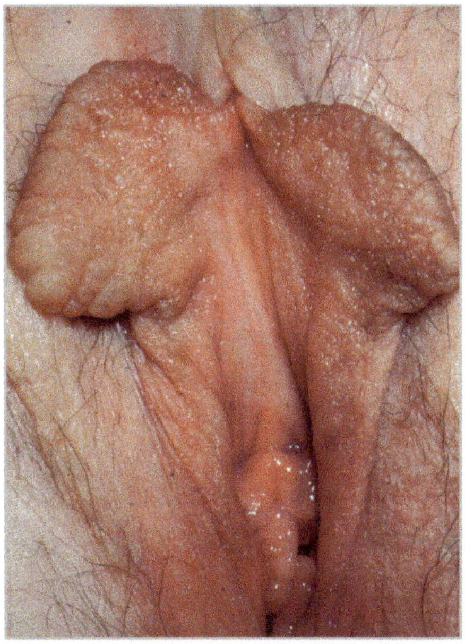

Figure 15.2 Swelling due to angioedema, skin texture is normal.

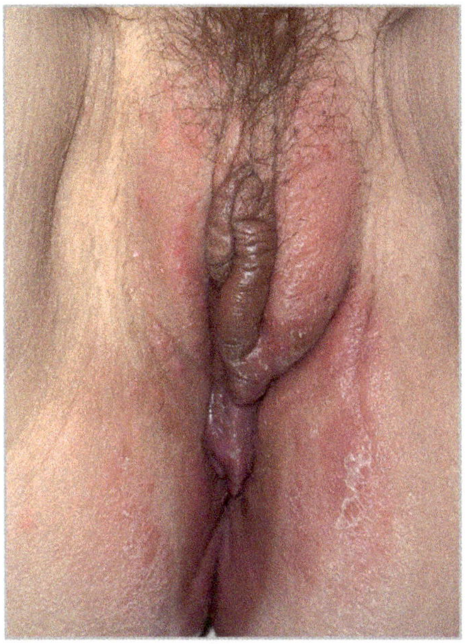

Figure 15.3 Crohn disease with asymmetrical swelling and erythema of labia majora (see Chapter 24).

Table 15.1 Diseases causing general vulvar swelling

Skin disease	Clinical features	Chapter
Acute swelling normal skin texture and color		
Idiopathic angioedema	Swelling with no immediate cause. Check for aspirin and NSAID and ACE inhibitor use	
Pressure urticaria	Often associated with dermographism, but there is a delayed form that can present with swelling a few hours rather then immediately after intercourse	17
Seminal fluid allergy	Type I immediate hypersensitivity reaction. Acute swelling usually within an hour of unprotected sexual intercourse. May be systemic symptoms, anaphylaxis in very severe cases. Confirmed by specific IgE or skin prick testing	17
Latex allergy	Type I immediate hypersensitivity reaction. Acute swelling usually within an hour of exposure to, e.g. condoms or after examination with latex gloves. May be systemic symptoms, anaphylaxis in very severe cases. History of reaction to latex at other body sites. Confirmed by specific IgE or skin prick testing	
C1-esterase-inhibitor-deficiency	Very rare cause of angioedema without urticaria. Usually, a positive family history. Inquire about abdominal cramps. Tested by assaying C1 esterase inhibitor with low C4	
Acute swelling with erythema and pain		
Infection	Diffuse erythema, pain, warm to touch, sometimes with systemic symptoms. Usually *Candida* or streptococcal infections	29, 30, 31
Chronic swelling		
Lymphedema	Fixed swelling although initially intermittent. Skin firm and woody. Skin dimpled and may be verrucous in long-standing problem. May be due to congenital lymphatic problem when there would be associated swelling of lower legs or secondary, e.g. due to filariasis in developing countries, other infections, or pelvic surgery	37
Hidradenitis suppurativa	Sinuses, linear cords of scarring, grouped comedones	23
Crohn	Variable presentation, e.g. with fissures, ulcers, red nodules, tags, and sinuses	24
Melkersson–Rosenthal syndrome	Recurrent swelling of, e.g. the tongue, eye lids, or vulva; it may become permanent, granulomas on histology	24
Sarcoidosis	Nodules and plaques, widespread usually part of more generalized skin condition	24
Vascular anomalies	Long-standing, variable in size. Often bluish/purple in color. May have a bruit	37
ACE, angiotensin-converting enzyme; IgE, immunoglobulin E; NSAID, non-steroidal anti-inflammatory drug		

ARE THERE ANY TRIGGERS?

Unprotected sexual intercourse will provoke swelling in seminal fluid allergy and the use of condoms if latex allergic. Inquire about aspirin, non-steroidal anti-inflammatory drugs (NSAID) and angiotensin-converting enzyme (ACE) inhibitor usage; all of these can precipitate angioedema. Multiple previous episodes of cellulitis in the vulvar area predispose to lymphedema as does vulvar surgery especially with lymph node dissection and a history of pelvic cancer or radiotherapy.

Pressure urticaria may occur after mechanical triggers such as sexual intercourse or riding a bike. Prolonged cycling in elite athletes can cause fixed swelling called 'cyclist edema' (Coutant-Foulc et al. 2014, Trofaier et al. 2015).

REFERENCES

Coutant-Foulc P, Lewis FM, Berville S, et al. Unilateral vulval swelling in cyclists: a report of 8 cases. J Low Genit Tract Dis 2014; 18:e84–89.

Trofaier ML, Schneidinger C, Marschalek J, et al. Pelvic floor symptoms in female cyclists and possible remedies: a narrative review. Int Urogynecol J 2015 Aug 4. [Epub ahead of print]

Section 3

VULVAR DISEASES

Chapter 16 Atopic eczema, lichen simplex, seborrheic dermatitis

Karen L Gibbon

There are several different types of eczema that may affect the vulvar area, including atopic, seborrheic, lichen simplex chronicus (LSC), and contact dermatitis (allergic and/or irritant). Different types of eczema may coexist, and atopic eczema in childhood may be replaced with other types of eczema in adulthood. Pointers as to the type of eczema may be gleaned from a careful personal and family history. A full examination of the rest of the skin will frequently give clues; e.g. a scaly scalp and nasolabial folds may alert the clinician to the possibility of seborrheic dermatitis. Clinical signs of these types of eczema can fluctuate quite quickly and taking time to carefully examine the whole of the anogenital tract in good lighting is essential to make the correct diagnosis.

ATOPIC ECZEMA

Synonyms

Endogenous dermatitis, atopic dermatitis (AD), flexural eczema, 'neurodermatitis' in German-speaking literature.

Key features

- Vulvar atopic eczema is characterized by intense pruritus
- Common in prepubertal girls and often disrupts sleeping
- Frequently accompanied by either irritant or allergic contact dermatitis
- Vulvar architecture is preserved – in keeping with other forms of dermatitis below

Introduction

Atopic dermatitis affects approximately 10–20% of children and 2–5% of adults. It is an inflammatory disease presenting with characteristic itchy skin lesions, immune dysregulation, disrupted epidermal barrier function, and immunoglobulin E (IgE)-mediated hypersensitivity reactions to food and environmental allergens. AD solely affecting the vulva, however, is rare and more frequently affects girls than adult women (Fischer & Rogers 2000). Diagnostic guidelines for the diagnosis of atopic eczema are not very sensitive for the vulva. A personal or family history of atopy may therefore be more useful for making a diagnosis (Crone et al. 2000).

Epidemiology

Atopic eczema affects all ethnic groups and is increasing in frequency across the world.

Pathogenesis

Atopic dermatitis is a multifactorial disease that is increasing in prevalence. The exact cause of AD is unknown. However, it is generally agreed that AD results from a combination of genetic and environmental factors. Twin studies support a high rate of concordance; identical twins have a sevenfold increased risk for AD, and fraternal twins have a threefold increased risk (Wolter & Price 2014).

Immunology

Immunological events in atopic individuals include activation of the T-helper 2 (Th2) immune response with synthesis of cytokines interleukin (IL)-4, IL-5, IL-10, and IL-13. IL-4 and IL-5 produce elevated IgE levels and eosinophilia. Recently, a new cytokine IL-33 has been shown to be a promoter of Th2 inflammation. It is released from mechanically injured or barrier-disrupted skin (Tamagawa-Mineoka et al. 2014).

Genetics

Familial clustering of the disease along with asthma and allergic rhinitis supports a significant heritable component. Loss-of-function mutations in the filaggrin gene, whose product is a key structural protein in the stratum corneum, provide an explanation for disease initiation in many patients. Once barrier function disruption is established other environmental and immunological sequelae perpetuate epidermal inflammation (O Regan & Irvine 2010).

Environmental factors/triggers

More than 90% of chronic eczema lesions contain *Staphylococcus aureus*, often in large numbers. Even in the absence of overt superinfection, *S. aureus* is thought to serve as a superantigen, acting as a significant driver of disease, and may be correlated with more severe skin disease. An impaired IL-17 immune response partially explains why patients with AD fail to clear *S. aureus* from their skin (Kilian et al. 2009).

Clinical presentation

Atopic eczema presents in one of the three clinical patterns. Acute atopic eczema presents with a vesicular, weeping, crusting eruption. Subacute atopic eczema presents with dry, scaly, erythematous papules, and plaques. Chronic atopic eczema shows lichenification from repeated scratching characteristically over the labia majora or buttocks (**Figures 16.1** and **16.2**). Mild redness and desquamation may also be seen in the labia minora. Characteristic plaques of non-genital AD usually coexist (**Figure 16.3**) (Rimoin et al. 2013).

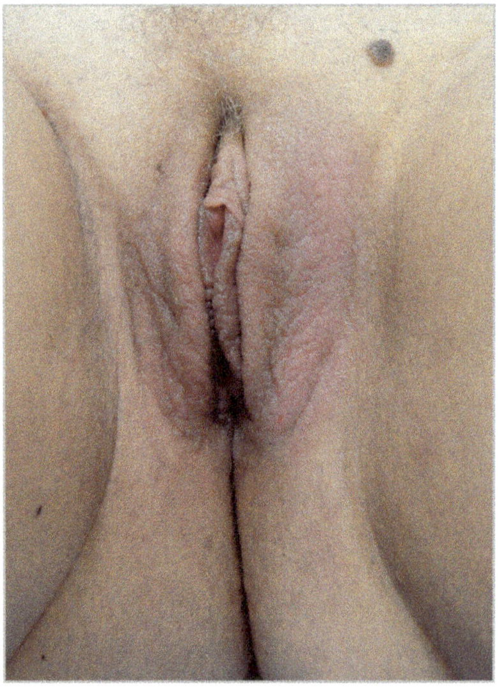

Figure 16.1 Chronic atopic eczema affecting the labia majora.

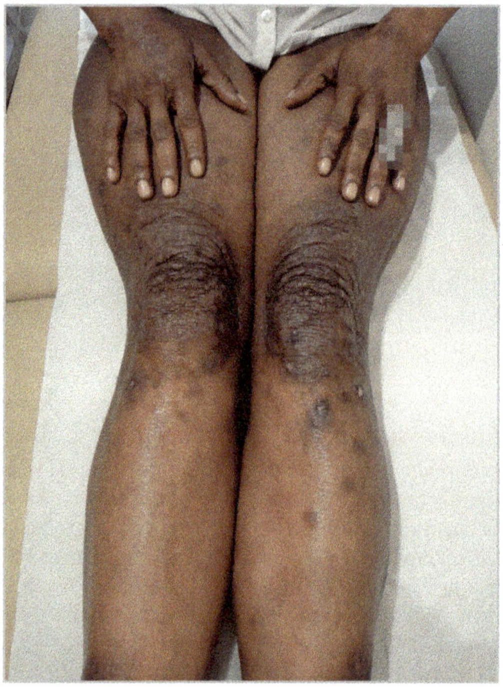

Figure 16.3 Typical lichenified plaques of atopic eczema on non-genital skin.

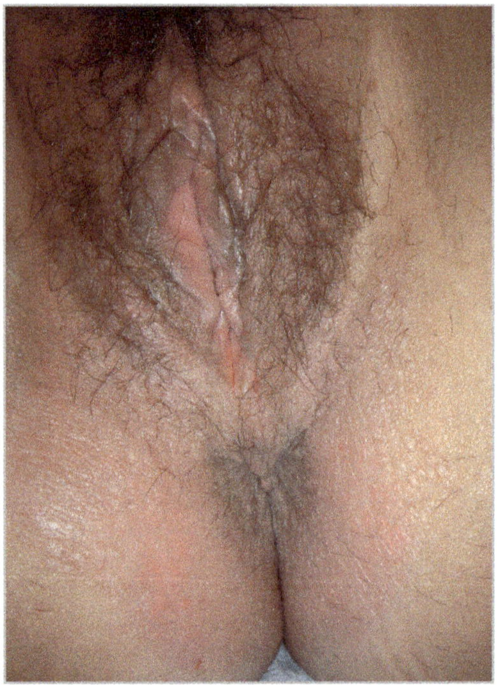

Figure 16.2 Chronic atopic eczema affecting medial buttocks and lower labia majora.

Histopathology

- Scale crusts in stratum corneum
- Spongiosis, microvesicles
- Irregular epidermal hyperplasia
- Exocytosis of inflammatory cells (mainly lymphocytes)
- Superficial perivascular infiltrate of lymphocytes and eosinophils

Differential diagnoses

Vulvar and vaginal swabs should be taken to exclude candidosis or bacterial infection. Candidosis in prepubertal children is rare. Psoriasis usually has more demarcation of scaly plaques over the labia majora. Irritant or allergic contact dermatitis may require patch testing to confirm. In the early stages of lichen sclerosus, the genital skin may be red and be confused with eczema.

Principles of management

These are common to all types of dermatitis and include avoiding all irritants including soap, bubble baths, moist tissue wipes, and shampoo. Wearing loose clothing and cotton underwear is important.

Treatment

An emollient of the patient's choice should be used as a soap substitute and reapplied at least twice daily. A mild-to-moderate topical steroid, e.g. clobetasone butyrate 0.05% should be used nightly for 2 weeks to gain control of the eczema. Maintenance treatment with 1% hydrocortisone or 0.05% clobetasone butyrate used twice weekly may prevent subsequent flares. Alternative steroid sparing agents such as pimecrolimus 1% or tacrolimus 0.1% may be tried, but some patients report a burning or hot sensation when used on the vulva.

Course and prognosis

Atopic dermatitis frequently relapses and remits even with appropriate treatment. Psychological support for their eczema in general may be helpful, e.g. habit reversal therapy to reduce scratching behavior. Childhood AD usually improves and is rarely a problem in isolation in adult women.

LICHEN SIMPLEX

Synonyms

Lichen simplex chronicus–LSC; 'neurodermatitis' (this term is used in the English-speaking literature for LSC but in the German-speaking literature instead describes atopic eczema)

Key features

- 'Itch-scratch-itch' cycles of behavior
- Paroxysms of scratching that interfere with sleeping
- Associated psychological issues are common
- Triggers include heat, sweating, menstruation, friction
- Polypharmacy and complaints about ineffective therapies are common
- It may be primary or secondary to other vulvar dermatoses

Introduction

Lichen simplex of the anogenital area is an eczema characterized by cycles of unremitting itching and scratching. It frequently occurs in individuals with a personal or family history of atopy. Psychological distress, anxiety, or depression is frequently either causal or contributing factors to its perpetuation.

Epidemiology

The LSC is a very common condition thought to affect up to 0.5% of the population in Western Europe and America.

Pathogenesis

Environmental factors stimulate histamine releasing, type C, non-myelinated sensory nerve endings. These include heat, sweat retention, friction from clothing, excessive use of cleansers or irritating topical products, and irritation from menstrual products and panty liners. LSC can also arise secondary to other pruritic vulvar disease, e.g. lichen sclerosus or chronic vulvovaginal candidosis.

Environmental factors/triggers

Coexisting conditions, e.g. poorly controlled diabetes mellitus, hypothyroidism, or iron deficiency will aggravate LSC and require separate treatment. Obesity causes increased frictional/shearing forces on the skin aggravated by sweating and tight clothing.

Clinical presentation

Patients characteristically describe intense bouts of scratching for around 5–15 minutes often shortly after getting into bed. The scratching that can be initially pleasurable is followed by a burning pain accompanied by bleeding or weeping of the skin secondary to mechanical disruption of the epidermis. The dominant hand and finger nails may be used, but other objects, e.g. hairbrush or clothing may be used to violently rub the skin.

Common sites include the labia majora, perineum, or perianal skin. Erythematous plaques of LSC may be bilateral, unilateral, or generalized and are lichenified with exaggerated skin markings, induration, and edema (**Figures 16.4** and **16.5**). The surface of the lesions may be rough and the thickened stratum corneum appears white or gray/black in pigmented skin (**Figures 16.6** and **16.7**). Excoriations, fissures, erosions, or ulcers may be seen within the plaques or surrounding skin (Thorstensen & Birenbaum 2012).

Patients frequently report that medication is ineffective or the response is very short lived. A wide variety of other topical preparations will often have been used, e.g. aloe vera, T-tree oil, moist tissue wipes, antiseptics, or hemorrhoid preparations raising the possibility of a coexisting allergic or irritant intact dermatitis.

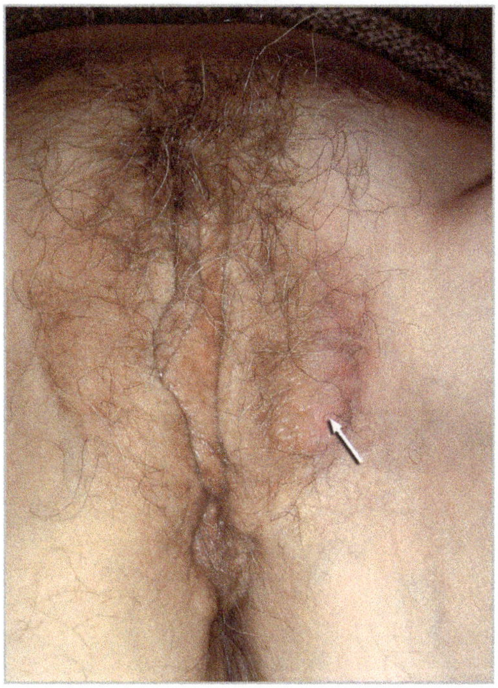

Figure 16.4 Unilateral plaque of lichen simplex chronicus.

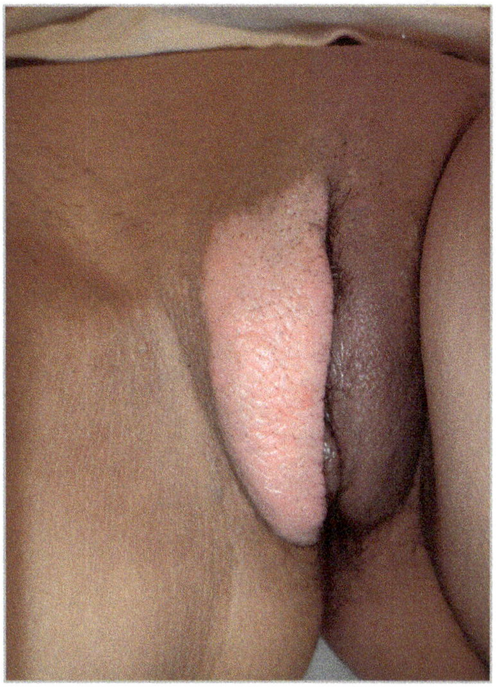

Figure 16.5 Edema and striking hypopigmentation with lichenification affecting right labium majus.

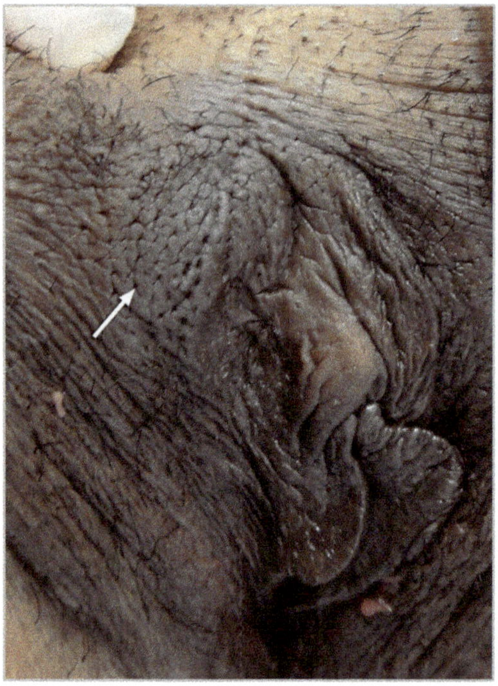

Figure 16.6 Lichen simplex chronicus affecting right labium majus.

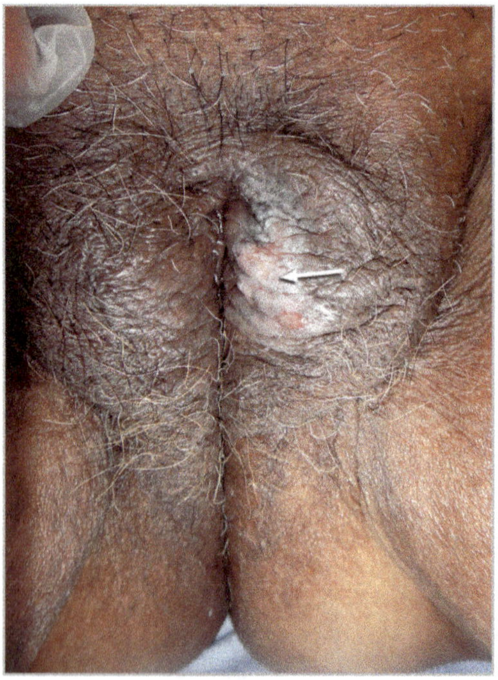

Figure 16.7 Lichenification, edema, and erosions secondary to scratching.

Histopathology

- Orthohyperkeratosis
- Acanthosis
- Psoriasiform elongation of rete ridges
- Broad dermal papillae with vertically oriented collagen bundles and blood vessels
- Perivascular and interstitial infiltrate of mononuclear cells

Differential diagnoses

It is important to establish whether LSC is primary or secondary, i.e. superimposed on some other underlying disease (**Table 16.1**).

Principles of management

Four important steps need to be put in place to resolve LSC (Lynch 2004).

Treatment

The principles of treatment are the same as for all types of vulvar dermatitis (**Table 16.2**).

Topical treatments

Potent or super potent topical steroids, e.g. beclomethasone valerate 0.1% or clobetasol propionate 0.05% daily for 4–8 weeks initially. Maintenance treatment with twice weekly application for a few weeks or a few months will reduce risk of epidermal atrophy and rebound flares. The potent topical steroids can and should be stopped once

Table 16.1 Differential diagnoses of lichen simplex

Differential diagnosis	Clinical or investigative features
Lichen sclerosus	Architectural change, violaceous color, epidermal atrophy
Psoriasis	Beefy red plaques with silvery scale, other affected sites, e.g. scalp, nails
Vulvar intraepithelial neoplasia/HSIL (**Figure 16.8**)	Previous history of cervical intraepithelial neoplasia (CIN), history of genital warts, biopsy
Extramammary Paget disease	Erythematous poorly demarcated moist eroded plaques, biopsy
Tinea (**Figure 16.9**), bacterial infection, or candidosis	Scrapings for mycology, swabs for microscopy and culture, sexual health referral
Contact dermatitis	Treatment stops working, condition worsens, patch testing
Atrophic vulvovaginitis	Elevated vaginal pH, pale atrophic vagina with punctate erythema, swabs
Seborrheic dermatitis	Fissuring common, less pruritus, other affected sites, e.g. scalp, axillae, natal fold

Table 16.2 Management of lichen simplex

Principles of management	Treatment
Identify underlying disease/ infection	Treat/optimize management of all correctable conditions. Sexual health screening, e.g. persistent candidosis
Repair barrier function	Soap substitute for bathing. Avoid all irritants and allergens, e.g. moist tissue wipes, fragrance products. Use occlusive emollients regularly. Avoid urea or lactic acid containing emollients as they sting if applied to fissured skin
Reduce inflammation	Potent or superpotent topical steroids
Break the 'itch-scratch-itch' cycle	Oral sedating antihistamine or antidepressant/anxiolytic medication

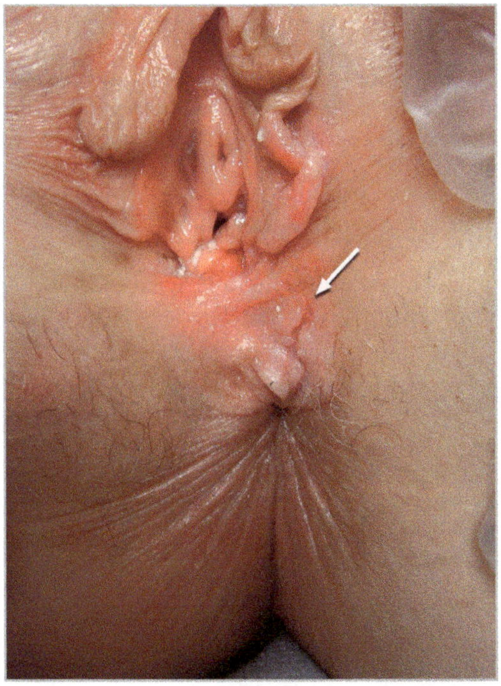

Figure 16.8 Lichenification within plaques of vulvar intraepithelial neoplasia over perineum.

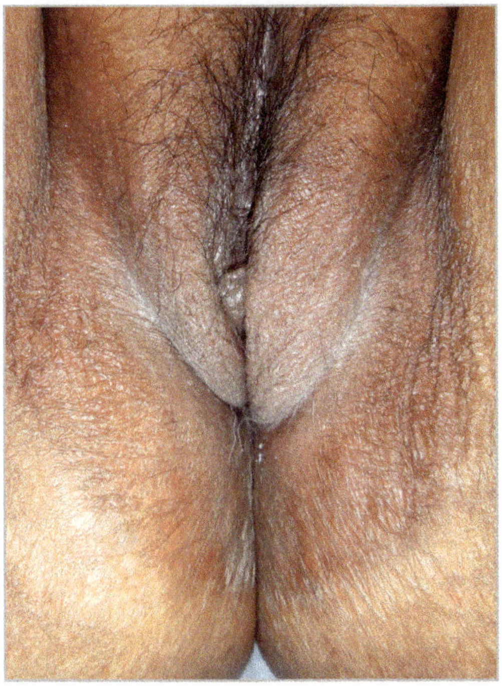

Figure 16.9 Lichen simplex chronicus secondary to tinea (dermatophyte infection).

the skin is recovered; however, this may take months. Patients have to be instructed that relapses may be possible and treatment should be re-introduced if necessary.

Systemic treatments

Sedating antihistamine taken 2 hours before bedtime, e.g. hydroxyzine initially 10–25 mg up to 75 mg. Alternative treatment includes the tricyclic (sedative) antidepressant doxepin 10–25 mg nocte. Obsessive compulsive disorders (OCD) or other psychiatric symptoms, e.g. anxiety or depression may require a selective serotonin reuptake inhibitor, e.g. fluoxetine or sertraline. Referral to a psychologist for 'habit reversal' may help.

Surgical intervention

Intralesional triamcinolone 10–20 mg into very thick plaques may be beneficial. Particularly, recalcitrant areas may benefit from surgical excision, e.g. if LSC accompanies lesions of hidradenitis suppurativa.

Course and prognosis

LSC is stubborn and frequently relapses, so any treatment plan needs to anticipate this. Written information and appropriate guidance from patient information leaflets may be beneficial. Addressing any accompanying psychosexual issues will encourage women to recognize that they may need additional help to maintain any improvement. Time should be set aside to explain the nature of the condition and the various steps that need to remain in place. Frequent follow-up is needed initially as the patient learns to regain control of her life and medication adjustments can be undertaken.

SEBORRHEIC DERMATITIS (SEBORRHEIC ECZEMA)

Key features

- Pruritus more variable and soreness more predominant
- Frequent fissuring of interlabial sulci, posterior fourchette, or natal fold
- Symptoms can be disproportionate to signs
- Often accompanied by vestibulodynia in type I skinned women
- If very severe or widespread consider HIV testing or investigations for immunosuppression

Introduction

Seborrheic dermatitis is a very common condition affecting around 5–10% of the population. It usually starts around puberty, peaks in incidence around 40 years, and is commoner in males. It is a chronic inflammatory disease affecting the scalp, eyebrows, eyelids, nasolabial creases, lips, ears, sternal area, submammary folds, umbilicus, groins, vulva, and natal fold. Scaling, which is faintly orange/yellow and greasy, appears on an erythematous base (Gupta & Bluhm 2004). Genital involvement is highly variable and poorly reported. At this site, it is frequently misdiagnosed and treated as chronic or recurrent 'thrush.'

Pathogenesis

In adults seborrheic dermatitis is dependent on the presence on the skin of the yeast *Malassezia furfur*. This is a commensal, lipophilic yeast found in the acroinfundibulum of hair follicles. After puberty colonization increases and *M. furfur* activates complement through an alternative lipase-producing pathway. The role of seborrhea especially in anogenital skin is debatable in accounting for flares of dermatitis. The pathogenesis of infantile seborrheic dermatitis is not clear, and many authors regard this as a separate condition (Ooi & Tidman 2014).

Genetics

A family history of seborrheic dermatitis is very common. It can, however, appear to 'skip' a generation so asking about grandparent's skin history can be very helpful. No candidate genes have been identified for seborrheic dermatitis.

Environmental factors/triggers

Overcolonization of the skin with *M. furfur* may trigger flares as may over-tiredness and stress. Alcohol can flare facial seborrheic dermatitis and some patients report worsening anogenital dermatitis too. *Demodex folliculorum* a saprophytic mite of human pilosebaceous units is found within the terminal hair of the mons pubis; however, its role in contributing to lesions of seborrheic dermatitis is unclear.

Clinical presentation

Vulvar seborrheic dermatitis may present in infancy as napkin dermatitis accompanied by scalp involvement or 'cradle cap.' The condition often disappears in a few months only to re-appear in teenage years and early adulthood. Soreness and pruritus are often disproportionate to clinical signs. These include recurrent linear fissuring of the interlabial sulci, mons pubis (**Figures 16.10 and 16.11**), perineum, perianal skin, and natal fold (**Figure 16.12**). Smaller areas of pruritic fissuring occur in the midline skin above the clitoris where it meets the fold of the mons pubis. Scaling may be noted over the mons pubis, but it is often absent in the interlabial sulci or around the introitus (McKay 1991). Seborrheic dermatitis affects all ethnic groups, but women with type I skin are more likely to develop a secondary vestibulodynia with a burning dysesthesia around the vestibule. This typically presents with superficial dyspareunia and difficulty inserting tampons or riding a bike. These patients have often used repeated courses of intravaginal anticandida preparations with short lived or no benefit.

Histopathology

- Scale-crust formation surrounding the follicular ostia within the stratum corneum
- Spongiosis at the edges of the follicular openings
- Neutrophils present within the scale-crust and spongiotic foci
- Slight hyperplasia of interfollicular epidermis with parakeratosis

Differential diagnoses

Vulvar seborrheic dermatitis and flexural or inverse psoriasis can look very similar (both clinically and histologically), and some authors prefer the unifying term sebopsoriasis. Other differential diagnoses are shown in **Table 16.3.**

Principles of management

These are broadly similar to those for LSC and include identifying and treating any underlying disease, e.g. checking HIV status if

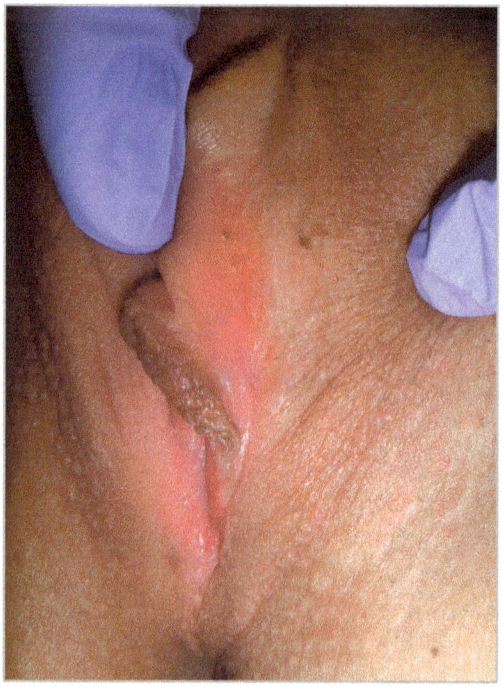

Figure 16.11 Fissuring of left interlabial sulcus.

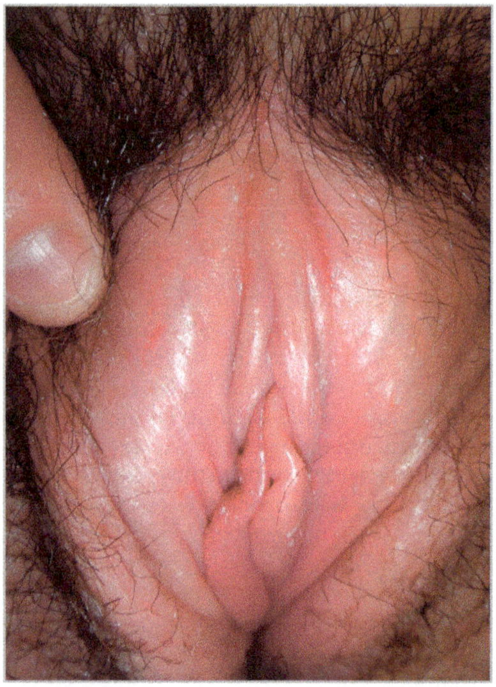

Figure 16.10 Fissuring of anterior vestibule and midline mons.

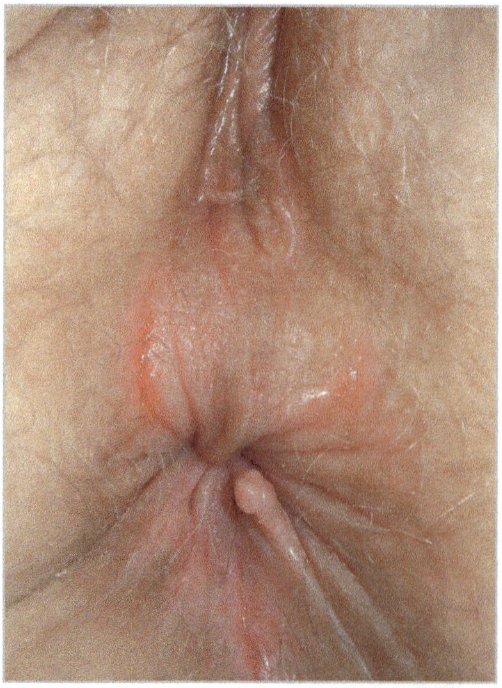

Figure 16.12 Perianal fissuring in seborrheic dermatitis.

Table 16.3 Differential diagnoses of seborrheic dermatitis

Differential diagnosis	Clinical features, diagnostic test
Atopic or allergic contact dermatitis	More pruritic patches or plaques, patch testing required
Pediculosis or tinea	Scabetic burrows present elsewhere, tinea cruris uncommon in women. Skin scrapings to confirm
Benign familial pemphigus, pemphigus foliaceus	Axillae, face, and interscapular areas may be affected. Biopsy and immunofluorescence studies
Acrodermatitis enteropathica	Failure to thrive, irritability, alopecia, and diarrhea
Langerhans cell histiocytosis	Similar rash but with systemic upset, hepatosplenomegaly, lymphadenopathy, and bone involvement
Vestibulodynia	Pain and burning on touching the introitus. Responds to 5% lidocaine or amitriptyline

seborrheic dermatitis is particularly severe or more widespread. Repairing skin barrier function and reducing inflammation is best achieved with regular emollients and topical steroid therapy. Patients generally prefer creams rather than ointments for their dermatitis, although type I skinned women may complain that they 'sting' when applied.

Topical treatments

An emollient cream should be prescribed and the patient instructed to use it when washing and re-apply it afterward, twice daily. A moderately potent topical combination preparation such as clobetasone butyrate 0.05%, oxytetracycline 3%, nystatin 100,000 units/g, may be used initially for 2–4 weeks to gain control of the dermatitis. After this it can be reduced to once or twice weekly. Alternatively, the strength of the steroid can be reduced to a 0.5% or 1% hydrocortisone combination preparation, e.g. hydrocortisone 0.5%, nystatin 100,000 units/g, benzalkonium chloride solution 0.2%, dimethicone '350' 10%, or hydrocortisone 1%, miconazole nitrate 2% and used alternate days as needed. Topical lithium succinate 8% or topical ketoconazole 2% cream are also useful therapies.

Five percent lidocaine may be needed to help with superficial dyspareunia if fissuring and burning dysesthesia (vestibulodynia) continue to be problematic. Shampoo containing 2.5% selenium sulfide or 2% ketoconazole can be used on anogenital hair-bearing sites monthly to reduce the burden of *Malassezia* yeast. Tar or lithium containing preparations for seborrheic dermatitis are not well tolerated on genital skin.

Systemic treatments

Patients with recurrent flares of seborrheic dermatitis may benefit from a short course of oral itraconazole 100 mg daily for 15 days.

Surgical intervention

Persistent fissuring of the posterior fourchette interfering with sexual intercourse may be helped with a modified Fenton procedure when all other contributing factors such as recurrent *Candida* infection have been excluded.

Course and prognosis

Management of the patient's expectations is very important. They need to understand that this condition has idiopathic and environmental triggers, which mean the condition may wax and wane in a rather unpredictable but not indefinite fashion. Patients should be given written information and a treatment plan that allows them to adjust their treatment quickly and not wait for days in misery before they can get to see a health-care professional. Other psychological conditions in addition to vestibulodynia, e.g. obsessive compulsive disorder or eating disorders may coexist with anogenital seborrheic dermatitis and patients may appreciate time to discuss these or be referred for further psychological assessment.

REFERENCES

Crone A, Stewart E, Wojnarowska F, et al. Aetiological factors in vulvar dermatitis. J Eur Acad Dermatol Venereol 2000; 14:181–186.
Fischer G, Rogers M. Vulvar disease in children: a clinical audit of 130 cases. Ped Dermatol. 2000; 17:1–6.
Gupta A, Bluhm R. Seborrheic dermatitis. J Eur Acad Dermatol Venereol 2004; 18:13–26.
Kilian E, Pennino D, Scarponi C, et al. IL-17 in atopic eczema: linking allergen-specific adaptive and microbial-triggered innate immune response. J Allergy Clin Immunol 2009; 123:59–66.
Lynch P. Lichen simplex chronicus (atopic/neurodermatitis) of the anogenital region. Dermatol Ther 2004; 17:8–19.
McKAY M. Vulvar dermatoses. Clin Obs Gynecol 1991; 34(3): 614–629.
Ooi E, Tidman M. Improving the management of seborrhoeic dermatitis. Practitioner 2014; 258:23–6.
O'Regan G, Irvine A. The role of filaggrin in the atopic diathesis. Clin Exp Allergy 2010; 40:965–972.
Rimoin L, Kwatra S, Yosipovitch G. Female-specific pruritus from childhood to postmenopause: clinical features, hormonal factors, and treatment considerations. Dermatol Ther 2013; 26:157–167.
Tamagawa-Mineoka R, Okuzawa Y, Masuda K, et al. Increased serum levels of interleukin 33 in patients with atopic dermatitis. J Am Acad Dermatol 2014; 70:882–888.
Thorstensen K, Birenbaum D. Recognition and management of vulvar dermatologic conditions: lichen sclerosus, lichen planus, and lichen simplex chronicus. J Midwifery Women's Health 2012; 57:260–275.
Wolter S, Price H. Atopic Dermatitis. Pediatr Clin North Am 2014; 61:241–260.

Chapter 17 Contact dermatitis (irritant and allergic), fixed drug eruption and immediate hypersensitivity reactions

Martin Zikeli, Sylvie M Franken, Thomas Rustemeyer

CONTACT DERMATITIS OF THE VULVA

Synonyms

Contact eczema

Key features

- Contact dermatitis may be either allergic or, more frequently, irritant
- Primary or associated with other vulvar disorders
- Common on vulvar skin due to particular susceptibility
- Clinical signs may be indistinguishable from other types of eczema
- Allergic contact dermatitis (type IV cell-mediated allergy) is confirmed by patch testing

Introduction

Contact dermatitis is an inflammatory skin condition characterized by erythema, scaling, and vesicles occurring after contact with an external trigger. Contact dermatitis is difficult to distinguish from other types of dermatitis occurring in the vulvar area by clinical signs alone. There are two forms of contact dermatitis: irritant and allergic (Farage 2005). Irritant contact dermatitis is caused by a non-immunologic skin reaction. Allergic contact dermatitis is based on a T-cell mediated delayed hypersensitivity reaction. A typical example of irritant dermatitis of the hands is by frequent contact with water and soaps or of allergic dermatitis by contact to nickel in costume jewelry.

The female anogenital area is a distinct anatomical location with sensitive skin prone to develop contact dermatitis. A number of exogenous and endogenous factors contribute to the development of irritant and allergic dermatitis, including friction, occlusion, urine and fecal residues, hygiene products, washing procedures, and administration of various topical agents.

Epidemiology

Contact dermatitis is a common disorder that affects all age groups with high prevalence and incidence. Contact dermatitis of the vulva also is common, with the majority having irritant dermatitis and only 20% allergic (Margesson 2004). The most relevant allergens of the vulva are fragrances, preservatives, local anesthetics, and neomycin.

Pathophysiology

Irritant contact dermatitis is caused by skin damage, direct cytotoxic effects, or cutaneous inflammation from contact with an irritant.

Allergic contact dermatitis is a type IV, T cell mediated, delayed hypersensitivity reaction in which an allergen is detected by dendritic cells in the epidermis. These Langerhans cells process the allergen and present the protein to T cells in regional lymph nodes, thus activating them. T cells differentiate into sensitized Th1 cells, return to affected sites, and initiate an inflammatory cascade.

The vulvar epithelium is thin with just a few layers of keratinocytes and an absent stratum corneum in the mucosal area. Many hair follicles, sweat glands, and sebaceous glands are present on the mons pubis and labia majora. The density of Langerhans cells in vulvar keratinized epithelium and non-keratinized mucosa is similar to other areas of body skin. Greater friction, occlusion, and hydration affect permeability in comparison with other sites (depending on the nature of the applied substance) leading to easier penetration of irritants and allergens. Hence, it is possible that weaker irritants or allergens unable to elicit a reaction on 'normal' skin cause problems in the vulvar area (Farage & Maibach 2004).

Immobility, obesity, incontinence, lack of estrogen, coexistent pathologies of the vulva, and atopic constitution with an impaired skin barrier are endogenous predisposing factors.

Factors influencing the susceptibility and severity of contact dermatitis (Brasch et al. 2014)

- Strength and amount of irritant/allergen applied
- Frequency of exposure
- Environmental factors, e.g. occlusion and humidity
- Skin susceptibility, e.g. atopic constitution
- Filaggrin loss-of-function mutations predispose to irritant and allergic contact dermatitis
- Body site

Etiology

Common substances that cause contact dermatitis of the vulva are as follows (Margesson 2004):

Irritants

Washing procedures

- Excessive washing, e.g. water, soaps, detergents, vaginal douches

Mechanical factors

- Tight clothes
- Friction from sanitary towels
- Scratching
- Sports, e.g. biking, riding
- Sexual intercourse

Body fluids

- Sweat, e.g. relevant in folds and obesity, excess vaginal discharge
- Incontinence (urine, feces)

Topical products

- Topical medications, e.g. tar, podophyllin, benzalkonium, calcipotriol
- Cosmetic preparations, e.g. wet wipes, deodorant sprays

Allergens

- Fragrances, e.g. balsam of Peru, eugenol, e.g. in moist toilet paper, peppermint in herbal teas
- Preservatives, e.g. methylchloroisothiazolinone/methylisothiazolinone (e.g. in moist toilet paper), methyldibromo glutaronitrile/phenoxyethanol, formaldehyde releasing preservatives, parabens
- Ointment bases/emulsifiers, e.g. lanolin, cetylstearyl alcohol in medicaments/creams
- Local anesthetics, e.g. benzocaine
- Topical antibiotics, e.g. neomycin
- Antimycotics, e.g. clotrimazole
- Antivirals, e.g. acyclovir
- Antiseptics, e.g. benzalkonium chloride
- Topical steroids, e.g. hydrocortisone, triamcinolone
- Rubber chemicals in condoms, sexual toys
- Colors, e.g. textile dyes in fabric of panties
- Self-administered 'natural' treatments like calendula, propolis, arnica
- Nail varnishes

The most frequent sensitizers in patients with anogenital complaints vary slightly in different studies:

Benzocaine, neomycin, and fragrance (Goldsmith et al. 1997), bufexamac, fragrance mix I and II, propolis and methyldibromo glutaronitrile (Bauer et al. 2011), methylisothiazolinone (Uter et al. 2013), and balsam of Peru, benzocaine, fragrance mix and quaternium-15 (O'Gorman & Torgerson 2013) are reported.

Preservatives, perfumes, and local therapeutics seem to be the most frequent sensitizers. Contact to these allergens is mostly through cosmetics, sanitary padding, intimate products, or iatrogenic. It is therefore wise to test the patient's own products.

Rarely, allergic contact dermatoses in the vulva may be caused by oral allergen exposure such as herbs (Vermaat et al. 2008).

Clinical presentation

Key clinical features

	Irritant	Allergic
	- Burning sensation - Well-demarcated margins - Reaction limited to site of contact	- Pruritus as dominant symptom - Diffuse margins - In certain situations lesions at distant sites (secondary generalization in very severe or prolonged cases)
Acute	Moist, intensive redness, edema	
	- Occurs minutes to hours after contact - Decreasing symptoms (decrescendo) - Monomorphic lesion: erythema, sometimes necrosis	- Manifests 1–2 days after contact - Increasing symptoms (crescendo) - Polymorphic lesion: erythema, papules, vesicles
Chronic	Dry, faint redness with slight scaling lichenification of the skin	
	- Slowly undulant course even if irritant is eliminated	- Heals more quickly after avoidance of allergen

Clinical features

Both irritant and allergic contact dermatitis present with an erythematous and slightly scaling lesion. During the acute stage, various features help distinguishing between irritant (**Figure 17.1**) and allergic (**Figure 17.2**) dermatitis, although chronic lesions look very similar. In general, allergic contact dermatitis rather provokes pruritus, whereas irritants cause burning, pruritus, and pain. Irritant lesions present with distinct borders especially in the acute stage, in contrast to blurred margins and sometimes generalized lesions of allergic contact dermatitis. Excoriations from scratching may be present.

Acute irritant contact dermatitis is easier to diagnose by clinical features and history because patients are often aware of the possible irritant or toxic agent. In contrast, the cause for chronic eczema and allergic reactions is rather difficult to identify without further examinations. Chronic lesions usually present with a slightly scaling erythema in the area of the outer labia minora and labia majora as well as in the perivulvar and perianal skin.

Constant scratching is an irritant factor itself, leading to further impairment of the skin barrier, which aggravates inflammation and

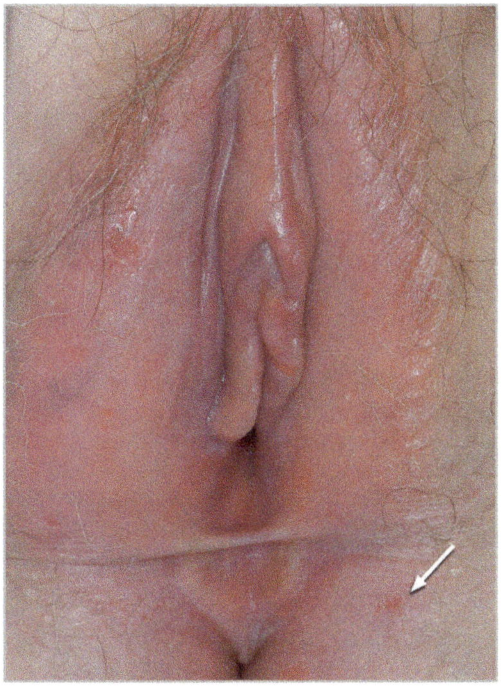

Figure 17.1 Irritant contact dermatitis after frequent washing of the vulva; notice the excoriation at the arrow. By courtesy of Gudula Kirtschig, Tübingen, Germany.

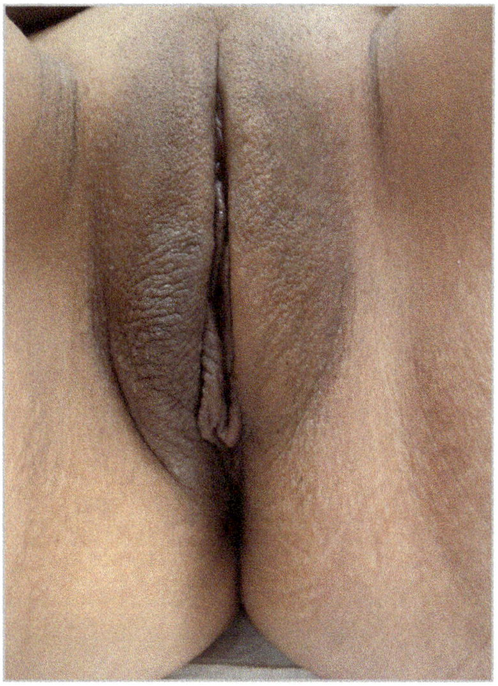

Figure 17.3 Lichen simplex chronicus showing lichenification (thickening of the vulvar skin by constant rubbing). By courtesy of Gudula Kirtschig, Tübingen, Germany.

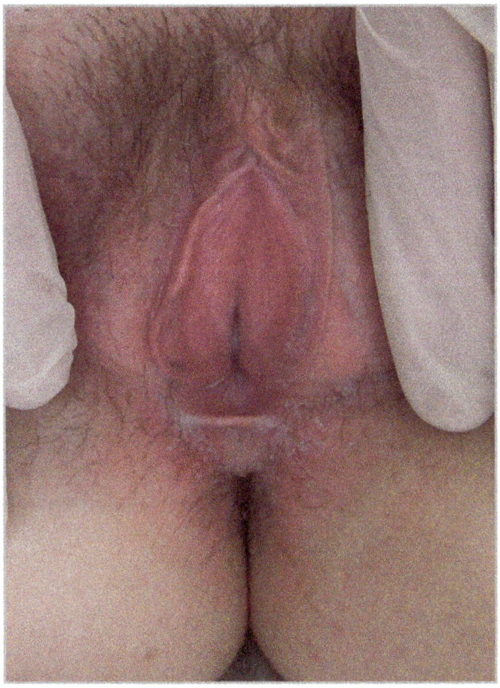

Figure 17.2 Allergic contact dermatitis in a patient with lichen sclerosus. Her symptoms were not well controlled despite adequate treatment for lichen sclerosus. The patient was allergic to methyldibromo glutaronitrile, disperse blue 106, sorbitan sesquioleate, fragrances and various spices, and her own shaving gel.

pruritus, which, in turn, enhances further scratching and rubbing. The vicious circle of scratching and itching leads to hypertrophy of the epidermis, resulting in a leathery appearance of the skin. This condition is called lichen simplex chronicus (**Figure 17.3**).

Investigations

Histopathology

Histopathology of both types of reactions shows spongiosis, parakeratosis, a superficial perivascular infiltrate with lymphocytes and irregular hyperplasia of the epidermis. In allergic contact dermatitis, eosinophils are more prominent than in irritant contact dermatitis. Acute toxic lesions present with hydrops or even necrosis of keratinocytes, neutrophils within the epidermis, and a superficial perivascular infiltrate with lymphocytes and neutrophils (Kerl et al. 2003).

Patch testing

Patch testing is usually required to exclude or prove type IV allergic reactions but cannot be used to diagnose irritant contact dermatitis (**Figure 17.4**).

Indications for patch testing for vulvar problems

- Eczema unresponsive to treatment or recurring frequently
- Otherwise unexplained eczema
- Poor response to treatment or deterioration of other vulvar dermatoses
- History of reaction to medicaments including emollients or corticosteroids

Patch testing depending on patient history

- Standard (European) battery
- Preservatives
- Ointment bases and emulsifiers
- Rubber additives
- Local therapeutics (e.g. corticosteroids and antimicrobials)
- Textile dyes and finishes
- Own products

In a typical patch test protocol, suspected haptens are applied to the skin of the back for 48 hours. Skin reactions are assessed at 48 and

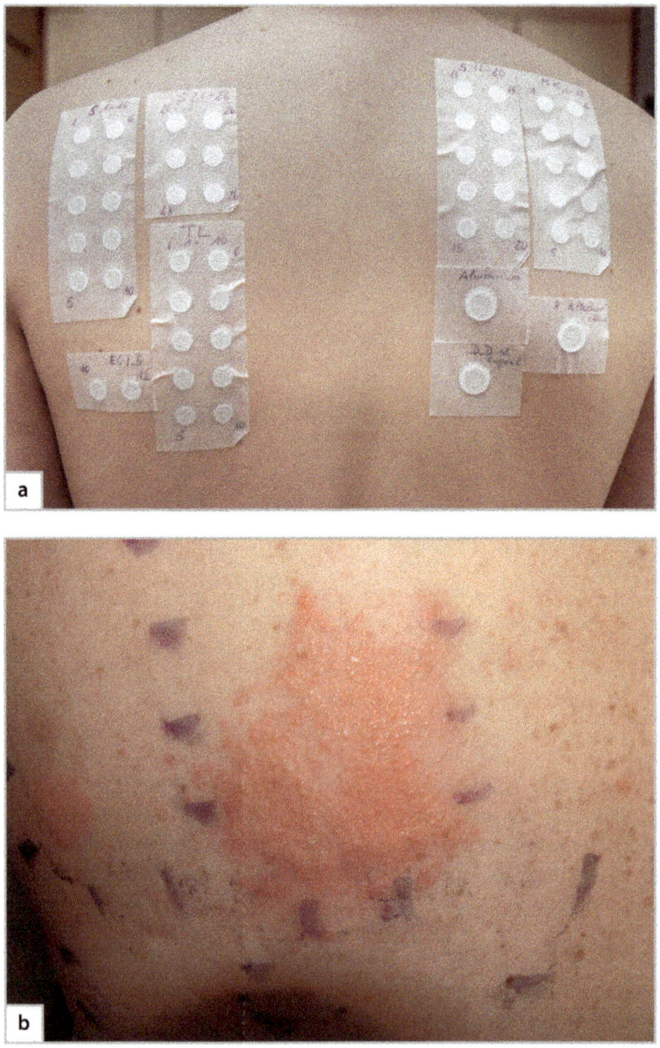

Figure 17.4 (a) Patch test on the back with allergens applied. (b) Reading after 72 hours having been applied for 48 hours with a positive reaction with palpable erythema and vesicles (2+ reaction). This was a relevant reaction as the patient was using fragranced products in the genital area.

72 hours, in case of corticosteroids additionally after 96 hours. Positive reactions show erythema and palpable infiltrate (+), in moderate cases vesicles (++) and in strong cases bullae (+++).

There are limitations to patch testing of potential vulvar contact allergens because sensitivity of the vulvar epithelium differs to the skin on the back and also the volar forearm. This may lead to false-negative results. Therefore, various modifications of patch testing have been developed. A feasible method is stripping the horny layer with adhesive tape before application of the patch test to increase its sensitivity. The repeated open application test (ROAT) is a 'use test,' which is helpful either in finally confirming contact hypersensitivity or in the assessment of clinical relevance of an equivocal result of a patch test. The ROAT is performed by applying a small amount of suspected substance twice daily onto the skin of the ulnar fossa over a period of 1–2 weeks or until dermatitis develops in the exposed site.

Patch testing should not be confused with other types of allergy testing including skin prick test or radioallergosorbent tests used for diagnosis of type I hypersensitivity, such as immediate type I reaction to latex, aeroallergens, and food allergies.

Diagnosis

Contact dermatitis shows typical features of eczema, but differentiation between irritant and allergic reactions is difficult and sometimes impossible.

A patient's history is crucial in making the diagnosis, since the potential causative agent must be elicited before tests are performed. When a possible cause is found, the first step in confirming the diagnosis is avoidance of the irritant or allergen to see if the eczema resolves.

If avoidance and empiric treatment fail (e.g. with potent topical steroid ointments), lesions recur and diagnoses or specific triggers remain unknown, patch testing should be performed to exclude or prove delayed hypersensitivity reaction.

A positive result of a patch test is not equal to the diagnosis of allergic contact dermatitis. The clinical relevance of a positive patch test must be established to answer the question 'does the positive patch test really explain the patient's symptoms?'.

Optionally, swabs and histopathology may be performed to rule out differential diagnoses.

Differential diagnoses

- Atopic dermatitis
- Seborrheic dermatitis
- Candidosis
- Inverse psoriasis
- Lichen sclerosus
- Lichen planus

Treatment

Management of irritant and allergic contact dermatitis requires identification and avoidance of causative factors. Patient education is fundamental. Patients are taught about skin care, intimate washing and shaving, vulvar hygiene during toilet and menses. Advice is given on clothing choices and hobbies. Positive patch test results are explained with written information and advice on avoidance of the specific allergens.

Contact dermatitis is usually successfully treated with mid- or high-potency topical steroids (preferably ointments) once or twice daily over a period of about 2 weeks. Subsequently, long-term skin care with non-irritating emollients, moisturizers, or barrier creams is necessary in irritant contact dermatitis to prevent recurrence.

FIXED DRUG ERUPTION

Introduction

A fixed drug eruption is a cutaneous adverse reaction (type IV allergy) to systemic medication that occurs at the same (fixed) site or sites each time the causative drug is ingested. The genital area is one of the sites of predilection (Ozkaya-Bayazit 2003, Revuz & Valeyrie-Allanore 2008).

Epidemiology

Fixed drug eruptions may account for as much as 16–21% of all cutaneous drug eruptions. The prevalence has been reported to range from 1% to 5%.

Pathophysiology

It is a dose-independent, immunologic type IV hypersensitivity reaction based on cytotoxic T cells. The offending drug functions as a hapten that binds to keratinocytes. Through liberation of cytokines, T cells are attracted and perpetuate tissue damage. CD8+ memory T cells play an important role in rapid reactivation of lesions with re-exposure of the drug.

Etiology

Most often, causative agents are medications taken episodically, mainly non-steroidal anti-inflammatory drugs, antibiotics, and, rarely, food ('fixed food eruption') such as quinine or cashew. The most common cause is trimethoprim–sulfamethoxazole.

Several cases of fixed drug eruption on the genitalia have been reported in patients who were not ingesting the drug but whose sexual partner was taking the offending drug and the patient was exposed to the drug through sexual contact (Zawar & Chuh 2006).

Clinical presentation

The initial lesion typically appears within 2 weeks of initial exposure of the drug. It is often solitary but may be multiple or very rarely generalized and frequently located on the lips or genitalia (Revuz & Valeyrie-Allanore 2008). Other common locations are the dorsum of the basal joint of the thumb, the lower trunk, and hip.

The characteristic lesion is a round or oval, sharply demarked, brownish-livid patch (**Figure 17.5**). The center may blister or become necrotic. Local symptoms include burning, pruritus, and pain. Vulvar involvement usually presents with acute swelling.

Lesions persist from days to weeks after discontinuation of the drug and fade to residual hyperpigmented patches. Subsequent re-exposure to the medication results in a flare-up at the initial site within 1–48 hours. Readministration of the causative agent poses the risk of increased pigmentation, size, and number of lesions, leading to a generalized bullous fixed drug eruption.

Differential diagnoses

A cutaneous drug reaction involving mucous membranes is indicative of a severe adverse event.

Differential diagnoses for cutaneous drug reaction involving mucous membranes

- Erythema multiforme
- Stevens–Johnson syndrome and toxic epidermal necrolysis
- Pemphigus vulgaris

Investigations

Histopathology

Histopathology shows vacuolar interface dermatitis with necrotic keratinocytes in every layer of the epidermis, spongiosis, acanthosis, and a superficial and deep dermal infiltrate with neutrophils, eosinophils, and melanophages (Kerl et al. 2003).

Patch testing

Patch testing with the suspected causative agent has to be performed in loco; this means at the site where the fixed drug reaction occurs (Andrade et al. 2011) as testing will be negative when applied on the back as with conventional patch testing. If there is a negative result, an oral provocation test should be considered.

Diagnosis

The history is crucial in making this diagnosis, and it is essential to specifically inquire about over-the-counter medication as well as prescribed medications. If the diagnosis is established but the causative agent remains unknown, patch testing in loco and, when indicated, drug challenge should be performed. A biopsy helps to rule out differential diagnoses.

Treatment

High-potency topical steroids have anti-inflammatory effect. Discontinuation of the offending drug is curative.

IMMEDIATE TYPE I REACTION

In contrast to the delayed type IV reactions described above, specific IgE-mediated immediate type I reactions may occur at the genital

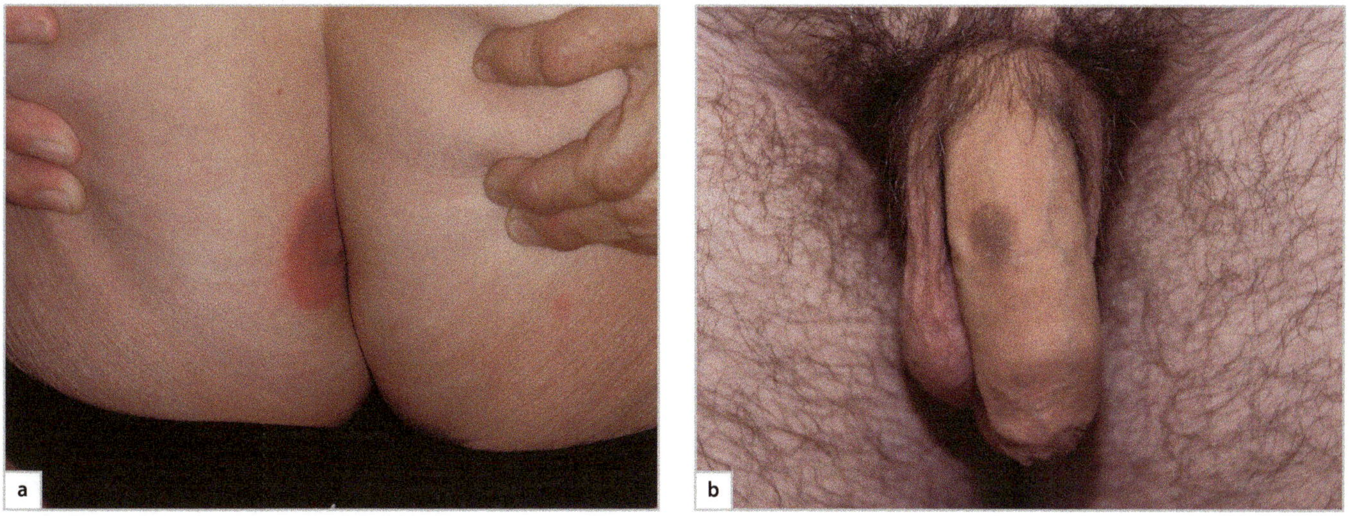

Figure 17.5 Fixed drug reaction at the anal fold presenting as an erythema (a) and on the penis as a hyperpigmented macule (b).

site. Type I allergies occur less frequently than type IV reactions. These reactions are characterized by their abrupt onset (typically within 30 minutes of exposure) and the possibility of very severe reactions including anaphylaxis.

Seminal fluid

Seminal fluid allergy is an underreported cause of vaginal and vulvar complaints (Bernstein 2011, Best et al. 1988). Infections/colonization, friction, or psychosocial components need to be differentiated.

Patients typically report of local pruritus and swelling within a few minutes after contact to seminal fluid (Lee-Wong et al. 2008, Weidinger et al. 2006). Generalized anaphylactic reactions presenting with urticaria, angioedema, bronchospasm, and hypotension may occur. The absence of symptoms when using a condom is characteristic. Patients often have an atopic constitution.

No one allergen has been identified with multiple allergenic proteins with molecular weights ranging from 12 to 75 kDa being identified; however, sperm proteins have only rarely been implicated. A protein with a similar molecular weight to prostate-specific antigen was identified in one case of anaphylaxis. Cross-reactivity between the allergen and dog epithelial allergen has been proposed, but this is not proven and many patients with seminal fluid allergy are not allergic to dogs. It is noteworthy that some allergens of, e.g. peanuts, tree nuts, crustaceans, or penicillin present in seminal fluid may lead to an immediate type I allergic reaction in a sensitized partner after unprotected intercourse (Eubel et al. 2014).

Desensitization

In seminal fluid allergy intravaginal desensitization with human seminal fluid may be conducted. However, to maintain tolerance contact to seminal fluid has to be achieved at least every 48 hours. This treatment is not widely available.

Latex

Use of condoms may cause the same symptoms described above in latex-allergic patients; this also needs to be considered when examining a patient with gloves (latex-free gloves are needed). The longer and more intensive the contact, the more severe may be the symptoms. Cross-reactions to banana, avocado, kiwi, and chestnut may be relevant. Latex-free condoms are provided by several manufacturers.

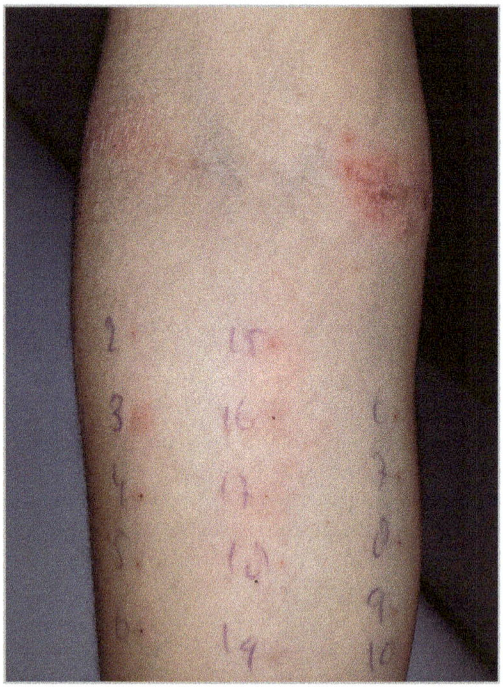

Figure 17.6 Prick testing showing reading at 15 minutes performed on the forearm in a patient with atopic eczema. A positive control, histamine (1) and a negative control, saline / 0.9% NaCl (2) is always done. There were positive tests to the positive control and spring trees (3).

Specific tests

- Skin prick test with relevant allergens, e.g. latex, seminal fluid, and seminal plasma (**Figure 17.6**)
- Specific IgE testing to allergens, e.g. latex, seminal fluid
- Prick to prick testing with latex/condoms

REFERENCES

Andrade P, Brinca A, Gonçalo M. Patch testing in fixed drug eruptions—a 20-year review. Contact Dermatitis 2011; 65:195–201.

Bauer A, Oehme S, Geier J. Contact sensitization in the anal and genital area. Curr Probl Dermatol 2011; 40:133–141.

Bernstein JA. Human seminal plasma hypersensitivity: an underrecognized women's health issue. Postgrad Med J 2011; 123:120–125.

Best CL, Walters C, Adelman DC. Fixed cutaneous eruptions to seminal-plasma challenge: a case report. Fertil Steril 1988; 50:532–534.

Brasch J, Becker D, Aberer W, et al. Guideline contact dermatitis. Allergo J Int 2014; 23:126–138.

Eubel J, Diepgen TL, Weisshaar E. Allergien im Genitalbereich. Hautarzt 2015; 66:45–52.

Farage MA. Vulvar susceptibility to contact irritants and allergens: a review. Arch Gynecol Obstet 2005; 272:167–172.

Farage M, Maibach HI. The vulvar epithelium differs from the skin: implications for cutaneous testing to address topical vulvar exposures. Contact Dermatitis 2004; 51:201–209.

Goldsmith PC, Rycroft RJ, White IR, et al. Contact sensitivity in women with anogenital dermatoses. Contact Dermatitis 1997; 36:174–175.

Kerl H, Garbe C, Cerroni L. Allergische und toxisch-irritative Kontaktdermatitis. In: Histopathologie der Haut. Berlin, Heidelberg: Springer, 2003:92–101.

Lee-Wong N, Collins JS, Nozad C, Resnick DJ. Diagnosis and treatment of human seminal plasma hypersensitivity. Obstet Gynecol 2008; 111:538–539.

Margesson LJ. Contact dermatitis of the vulva. Dermatol Ther 2004; 17:20–27.

O'Gorman SM, Torgerson RR. Allergic contact dermatitis of the vulva. Dermatitis 2013; 24:64–72.

Ozkaya-Bayazit E. Specific site involvement in fixed drug eruption. J Am Acad Dermatol 2003; 49:1003–1007.

Revuz J, Valeyrie-Allanore L. Drug reactions. In: Bolognia JL, Jorizzo JL, Rapini RP (eds), Dermatology. Maryland Heights, MO: Mosby, 2008:311.

Uter W, Geier J, Bauer A, Schnuch A. Risk factors associated with methylisothiazolinone contact sensitization. Contact Dermatitis 2013; 69:231–238.

Vermaat H, Smienk F, Rustemeyer T, Bruynzeel DP, Kirtschig G. Anogenital allergic contact dermatitis, the role of spices and flavour allergy. Contact Dermatitis 2008; 59:233–237.

Weidinger S, Mayerhofer A, Raemsch R, Ring J, Köhn FM. Prostate-specific antigen as allergen in human seminal plasma allergy. J Allerg Clin Immunol 2006; 117:213–215.

Zawar V, Chuh A. Fixed drug reaction may be sexually induced. Int J Dermatol. 2006; 45:1003–1004.

Chapter 18 Erythema multiforme majus, Stevens–Johnson syndrome/toxic epidermal necrolysis and Graft versus Host Disease

Maja Mockenhaupt, Mirjana Ziemer

ERYTHEMA MULTIFORME MAJUS, STEVENS–JOHNSON SYNDROME/ TOXIC EPIDERMAL NECROLYSIS

Synonyms

Erythema multiforme majus, Erythema (exsudativum) multiforme with mucosal involvement, Stevens–Johnson syndrome (SJS)/toxic epidermal necrolysis (TEN), Lyell syndrome

Key features

- Erythema multiforme majus (EMM), SJS/TEN are adverse reactions to drugs or infections
- Erythema multiforme majus and SJS/TEN are distinct entities
- Mucous membrane involvement occurs in >90% of the SJS/TEN-cases and 100% of EMM cases
- Mucous membrane involvement may lead to scarring, strictures, and long-lasting functional disability

Introduction

Erythema multiforme varies widely in severity. Erythema multiforme minus represents a localized eruption of the skin with minimal or no mucosal involvement: this is not outlined in this chapter. EMM and SJS or TEN, however, are more severe, and SJS/TEN are potentially life-threatening disorders with mucosal involvement including the vulva and vagina.

Erythema multiforme majus and SJS are often erroneously used interchangeably. However, large epidemiologic studies confirm that they are distinct conditions in terms of clinical pattern, demographics, and etiology (Auquier-Dunant et al. 2002). By definition, mucosa is always affected in EMM, whereas in SJS and TEN 'only' about 90% have mucosal lesions. SJS and TEN are considered a single disease entity of different severity with a common pathogenesis (Mockenhaupt 2011). These diseases are rare but genital involvement is very frequent.

Epidemiology

There are no reliable data on the incidence or prevalence of EMM. The combined incidence of SJS/TEN is estimated at 1-2 cases per one million per year (Mockenhaupt 2011, Ziemer & Mockenhaupt 2011). In a population-based registry, the average age of patients with SJS, SJS/TEN-overlap, and TEN was 53.4 years (1-94 years), but >80% of patients with EMM are <40 years. More men develop EMM (almost 70%), whereas for SJS/TEN the distribution of gender is almost equal (slightly more females) and a female preponderance of around 65% can be observed in SJS/TEN-overlap. Mortality in SJS is 9%, in SJS/TEN-overlap 29%, and in TEN 48% increasing with age (Mockenhaupt 2011). Risk factors for death in SJS/TEN are severity of the reaction (high percentage of skin detachment) and age of the patient (Sekula et al. 2013).

Pathogenesis

- Genetic predisposition (HLA and ethnic factors)
- Specific external trigger such as medication or infection
- Drug-specific lesional lymphocyte-derived cytotoxic proteins cause epidermal destruction
- Humoral autoimmunity to epithelial antigens is not established

Autoantibodies against epithelial proteins, e.g. plakin, desmoplakin I/II, envoplakin, and periplakin were not detectable in EMM ruling out humoral autoimmunity as a common denominator in its pathogenesis (Komorowski et al. 2013).

SJS/TEN occurs in genetically predisposed patients exposed to an external trigger such as medication. A very strong association has been observed between carbamazepine-induced SJS/TEN and HLA-B*1502 in Han-Chinese patients (Chung et al. 2004) and between allopurinol-induced SJS/TEN and HLA-B*5801 in Chinese (Hung et al. 2006); this strong association was not shown in Europeans (Lonjou et al. 2008, Phillips et al. 2011). Thus, a genetic predisposition to develop SJS/TEN is highly associated with specific drugs. T-cells, especially CD8 + lymphocytes play an important role in this process, mediated by cytokines (Pichler et al. 2011). The cytotoxic mitochondrial protein granulysin seems the most important factor for the epidermal destruction (Chung et al. 2008).

Etiology

EMM is mainly triggered by infectious agents

- Herpes simplex
- Mycoplasma pneumoniae
- Other infections of the upper respiratory tract ('flu and 'flu-like infections)

SJS/TEN is mainly triggered by drugs (75%)

High-risk drugs include:

- Allopurinol
- Sulfonamides including sulfasalazine
- Anti-epileptic drugs (carbamazepine, lamotrigine, phenobarbital, phenytoin)
- Nevirapine
- Non-steroidal anti-inflammatory drugs (NSAIDs) of the oxicam type

Moderate-risk drugs include:

- Antibiotics, e.g. cephalosporins, macrolides, quinolones, tetracyclines
- NSAIDs of the acetic acid type, e.g. diclofenac

Common drugs not associated with an increased risk:

- Beta-blockers, ACE-inhibitors, calcium channel blockers
- Sulfonamide-related diuretics and sulfonylurea antidiabetics, insulin, and propionic acid NSAIDs like ibuprofen
- In up to 25% of cases, infections may trigger SJS/TEN
  - Upper respiratory and mycoplasma pneumoniae infection
  - Influenza-like illness

Erythema multiforme majus and minus are mainly triggered by infectious agents and SJS/TEN is predominantly triggered by drugs (75%) with up to 25% attributed to infection (Mockenhaupt 2011, Mockenhaupt et al. 2008b). Medications taken 1-4 weeks before onset of disease are most likely triggers. Medications taken for years or those taken just around the time of onset are rather unlikely to be causative. It is important to take a very clear history of all medications (prescribed and non-prescribed). The possible interaction of infection and medication remains unclear. There is no reliable in vitro or in vivo test to determine the link between a specific drug and a cutaneous adverse reaction, and the detection of the culprit drug mainly relies on the time interval between beginning of drug use and onset of the adverse reaction.

Clinical presentation

EMM

Typical target lesions are well defined round lesions composed of three concentric zones with a central blister (**Figure 18.1**). If they are raised, palpable and less defined they are termed 'atypical.' They occur mainly on the limbs but sometimes over the face and trunk, especially in children. Involvement of the palms and soles is characteristic. Skin detachment in EMM is usually very limited [2-5% of the body surface area (BSA)].

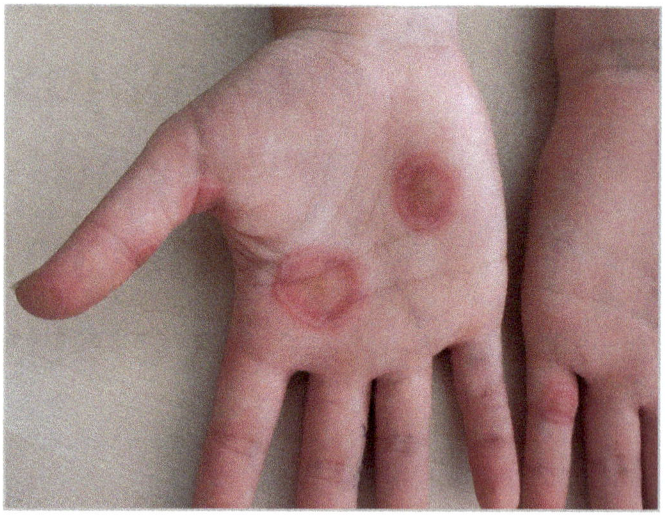

Figure 18.1 Typical target lesions in erythema exsudativum multiforme of the palm. By courtesy of Dr Gudula Kirtschig, Tübingen, Germany.

SJS/TEN

SJS and TEN are characterized by dusky erythema evolving into extensive blistering and detachment resembling a second-degree burn. Nikolsky sign is positive. SJS presents with a generalized dissemination of atypical target lesions and macules. Confluent blisters may merge. Detachment of the skin affects <10% of BSA in SJS. More than 30% skin detachment is seen in TEN with macules. In a very rare form of TEN with widespread erythema <10% of BSA detaches. SJS/TEN-overlap has been defined as blisters and erosions affecting 10–30% of BSA (Bastuji-Garin et al. 1993) (**Table 18.1, Figure 18.2**). The reactions are often accompanied by fever and malaise.

Mucosal involvement

Severe mucosal involvement may occur in EMM and SJS/TEN with hemorrhagic blisters and erosions affecting any mucosal site including eyes, nose, lips, mouth, pharynx, conjunctiva, vulva, vagina, and urethra (**Figures 18.3 to 18.8**), less frequently the trachea, bronchi, bronchioli, esophagus, and intestines. Cutaneous disease usually precedes genital involvement.

Scarring and long-term effects may result from mucosal involvement. Oral sequelae include impaired taste and adhesions of lips and oral mucosa. Eye involvement may result in dryness, damage to the lacrimal duct entropium, fibrosis, trichiasis, symblepharon, or blindness.

Vaginal scarring and adhesions, mucosal dryness, pruritus, and recurrent bleeding of the genital mucosa may occur in women after SJS/TEN with genital involvement (Mockenhaupt et al. 2008a). Introital adenosis and vaginal stenosis have also been observed (Bonafe et al. 1990).

Histopathology

EMM and SJS/TEN show a typical histological pattern and share many features, but histopathologic differentiation is impossible. The dermal infiltrate in early EMM and SJS/TEN is superficial and mostly perivascular. It decreases with the severity of the disease, being intermediate or even dense in the majority of cases of EM and rather sparse in TEN (Rzany et al. 1996, Ziemer & Mockenhaupt 2011).

Table 18.1 Consensus definition of SJS/TEN (data from Bastuji-Garin et al. 1993)

Criteria	EM majus	SJS	SJS/TEN overlap	TEN with macules	TEN on large erythema (without macules)
Skin detachment (%)	<10%	<10%	10–30%	>30%	>10%
Typical target lesions	+	-	-	-	-
Atypical target lesions	Raised	Flat	Flat	Flat	-
Macules	-	+	+	+	-
Distribution	Mainly limbs	Widespread	Widespread	Widespread	Widespread

EM, erythema multiforme; SJS, Stevens–Johnson syndrome; TEN, toxic epidermal necrolysis

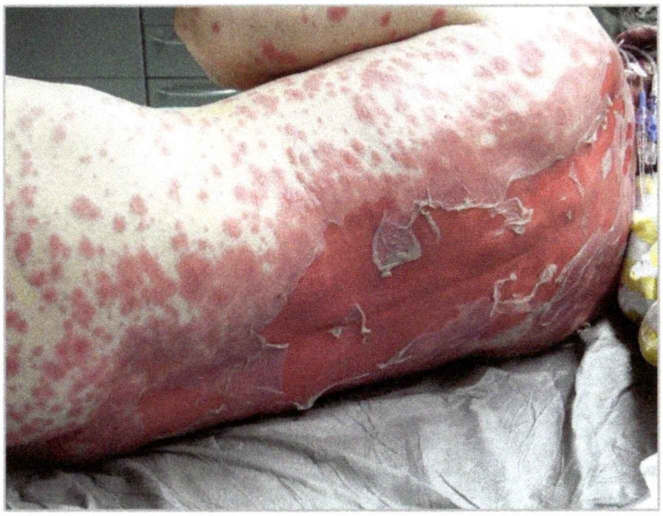

Figure 18.2 Stevens–Johnson syndrome/toxic epidermal necrolysis-overlap with loss of skin at the back and surrounding macular lesions.

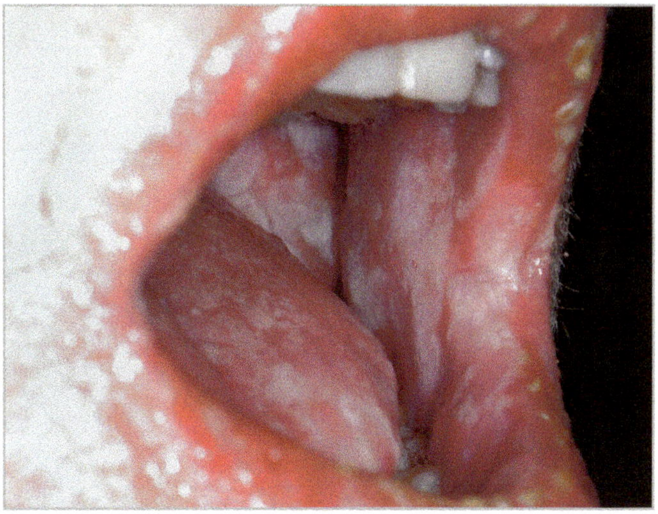

Figure 18.3 Oral erosions in erythema exsudativum multiforme majus or Stevens–Johnson syndrome/toxic epidermal necrolysis.

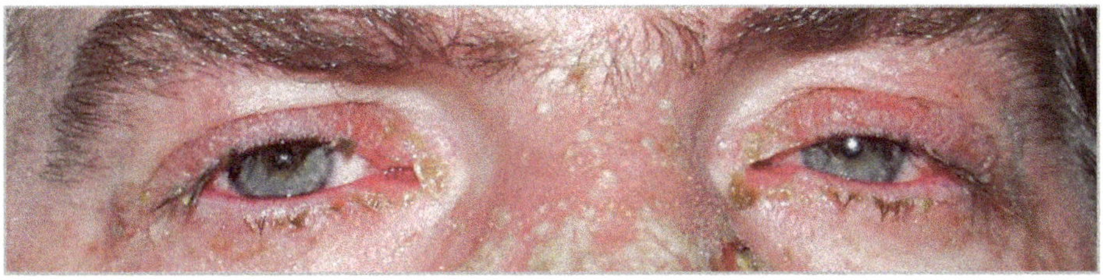

Figure 18.4 Ocular and periocular inflammation in Stevens–Johnson syndrome/toxic epidermal necrolysis.

Histopathology of early erythematous lesions

- Dermo-epidermal junction (DEJ):
  - Vacuolar alteration at the DEJ often in company with some lymphocytes (vacuolar interface dermatitis)
- Lower part of the epidermis:
  - Necrotic keratinocytes are scattered throughout
- Superficial dermis:
  - Sparse to moderate perivascular and interstitial infiltrate, occasionally eosinophils

Histopathology of fully developed lesions

- Subepidermal blistering and necrotic keratinocytes either in wide dissemination or full-thickness necrosis of the epidermis to extensive apoptosis (Figure 18.9)

Immunohistopathology

Predominance of CD4+ cells in the dermis and CD8+ cells in the epidermis similar to Graft versus Host Disease (GvHD).

Differential diagnosis

- Generalized bullous fixed drug eruption (GBFDE)
- Staphylococcal scalded skin syndrome (SSSS)
- Paraneoplastic pemphigus

Generalized bullous fixed drug eruption is characterized by brown/violaceous patches with flaccid blisters; however, bright erythematous patches may occur. Blistering usually affects only a small percentage of BSA, and sizable areas of intact skin are seen between large blisters.

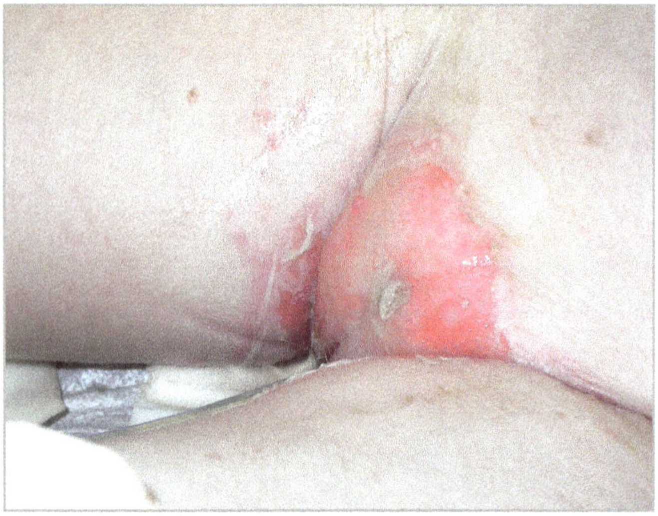

Figure 18.5 Erosions of the vulva in Stevens–Johnson syndrome/toxic epidermal necrolysis.

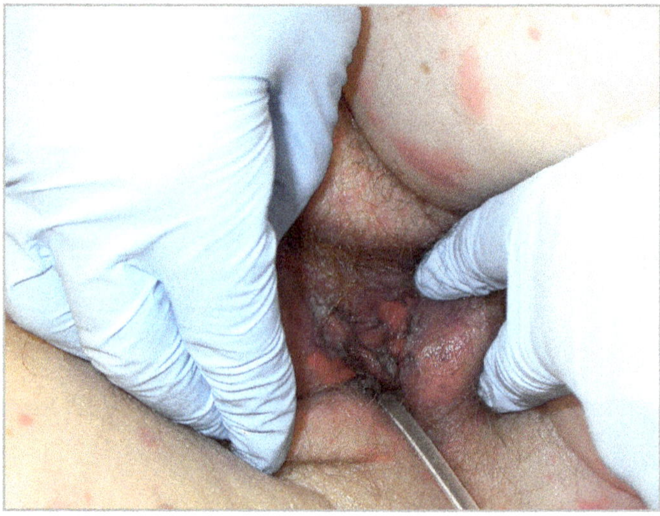

Figure 18.7 Erosions at the introitus in an acute phase of Stevens–Johnson syndrome/toxic epidermal necrolysis.

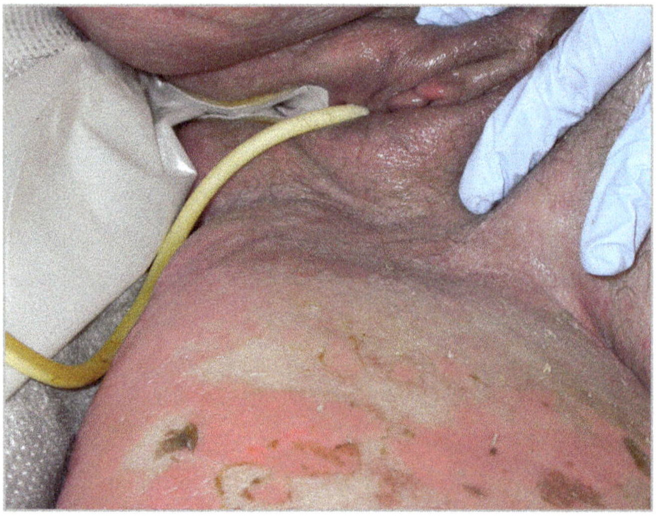

Figure 18.6 Erosions of the skin in Stevens–Johnson syndrome/toxic epidermal necrolysis, note the erosion of the clitoris.

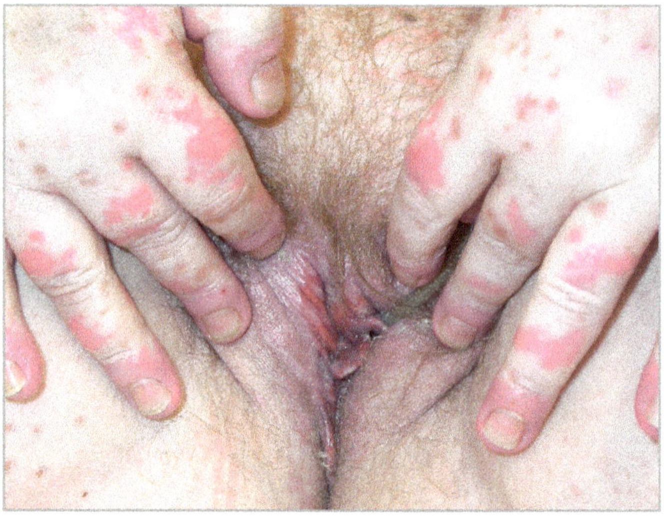

Figure 18.8 Erosions of introitus vaginae in healing phase in Stevens–Johnson syndrome/toxic epidermal necrolysis.

Erosive mucosal involvement is mild. However, in 77% of patients with GBFDE mucous membrane involvement, mainly affecting the genitals in men (58%) and women (48%), is reported (Mockenhaupt et al. 2010). Most patients report a history of a similar, often local reaction of fixed drug eruption; however, repeated exposure to the drug can lead to increasingly widespread detachment of the skin. Histopathological differentiation may be difficult, in particular in biopsies of early lesions, because there is overlap with features seen in EMM and SJS/TEN.

Staphylococcal scalded skin syndrome rarely affects mucous membranes and the macular confluent exanthema seen in SJS/TEN is absent. SSSS is less common in adults than SJS/TEN; it has a variable age distribution with peak incidences in early childhood and in immunocompromised adults. Skin detachment is very superficial and can be distinguished histopathologically.

Paraneoplastic pemphigus may present with mucosal erosions and skin detachment, but immunofluorescence tests will help to distinguish (see Chapter 26).

In the early stage of SJS/TEN, before blisters occur, the reaction may resemble a benign macular or maculopapular eruption, often caused by viral infections.

Management

In EMM, infections must be treated appropriately, e.g. with antibacterial or antiviral agents, and in SJS/TEN suspected drugs must be withdrawn. In many adults with erythema multiforme supportive topical treatment of skin and mucous membranes and pain relief will suffice expecting resolution within 2–3 weeks. In severe cases of EMM, especially in children, and in cases of SJS/TEN hospitalization is necessary. Patients of SJS/TEN-overlap and TEN often need access to intensive care facilities.

Treatment is usually symptomatic and supportive. Mucosal lesions do not respond well to immunomodulation; scars and strictures are observed in patients with and without immunomodulating therapy.

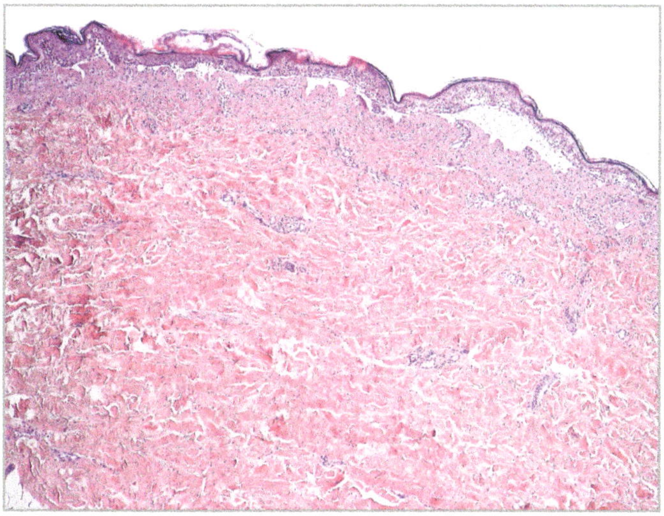

Figure 18.9 Histopathology of Stevens–Johnson syndrome/toxic epidermal necrolysis showing subepidermal blistering and necrotic blister roof.

A non-specific effect of systemic corticosteroids in a moderate dose (1–2 mg/kg body weight/day for 2–4 days) on mucous membranes is reported; this is probably due to reduction of swelling and pain.

- **General supportive care** for severe cases includes adjustment of ambient temperature, pressure relieving bedding, fluid replacement, nutrition, pain management using intensive care protocols. Erosions are treated with disinfectants such as chlorhexidine, octenidine hydrochloride or polyhexanide solutions and covered with non-adherent mesh gauze; spray emollients containing Vaseline are used too. Although blisters in SJS/TEN are fragile, they should be left in place and only punctured if they are a mechanical hindrance, since the blister roof serves as a natural cover.
- **Eye care.** Daily visit by ophthalmologist with eye drops and rodding with loosening of adhesions.
- **Genital erosions.** There are no standardized protocols for care; however, it is important to try and prevent scarring. Genital involvement is usually treated with appropriately placed wet dressings or vaginal dilators and sitz baths. Tampons (covered with, e.g. Vaseline) have been suggested with daily change to prevent adhesions of the vagina. Mild corticosteroid ointments may be soothing. Genital examination is recommended even in asymptomatic patients since genital involvement may develop in the course of the disease (Wilson & Malinak 1998).
- **Urethral care.** Catheter usually advised to prevent adhesions.
- **Systemic.** In severe cases, systemic therapy is considered but remains controversial including intravenous immunoglobulins (IVIGs), cyclosporine, and steroids.

Various immunomodulating treatments for SJS/TEN have been proposed, such as glucocorticosteroids, IVIGs, and cyclosporine, but their usefulness is still discussed controversially. Cyclosporine 3 mg per kg body weight for 10 days seems to be the therapy with the highest chance to halt the progression of skin detachment (Valeyrie-Allanore et al. 2010); however, the exact mechanism is not understood. Antibodies in pooled human IVIG are thought to block the Fas-mediated necrosis of keratinocytes in vitro. Interestingly, granulysin levels could not be reduced by IVIG, which might explain the lack of effect of IVIG on disease progression and treatment with IVIG is therefore questioned (Bachot et al. 2003, Chung et al. 2008). A large retrospective observational study revealed that treatment with corticosteroids in doses between 60 mg and 500 mg/day suggests a benefit for SJS/TEN-patients with a reduced mortality, whereas treatment with IVIG did not (Schneck et al. 2008). Plasmapheresis, hyperbaric oxygen, and cyclophosphamide have been reported as a successful treatment of TEN in case reports and small case series. Thalidomide, an effective TNF-α-inhibitor in vitro and successfully used in GvHD, caused a higher death rate in the only randomized controlled trial in TEN; therefore, treatment with TNF-α-inhibitors has to be used with caution (Mockenhaupt 2011).

GRAFT VERSUS HOST DISEASE

Key features

- Graft versus Host Disease is an inflammatory disease affecting many organs including skin and mucous membranes developing after allogeneic transplants
- In 25–35% mucous membranes of female genitalia are involved
- Mucous membrane involvement may lead to scarring and strictures and long-lasting functional disability

Introduction

GvHD is a multiorgan disease that occurs when donor alloreactive immunocompetent T cells identify foreign antigens on recipient cells and attack them. The dysfunction usually occurs after allogeneic hematopoietic stem cell transplantation (allo-HSCT) and donor lymphocyte infusions; it may also rarely occur after transplantation of solid organs.

Epidemiology

The survival rate for severe acute GvHD (aGvHD) in stage III (maculopapular rash affecting >50% body surface area) clinical disease is about 30% in the first year after transplantation; in stage IV (generalized erythema and bullous formation) clinical disease, it is < 10%. With an average prevalence of 50%, chronic GvHD (cGvHD) is the most serious long-term complication of HSCT with skin the most frequently affected organ. Female genital tract GvHD is a common complication of allo-HSCT and may involve the vulva, vagina, and perineal area. It is an under-recognized complication with a major impact on quality of life.

A retrospective analysis of the incidence of genital GvHD showed 35% at 1 year and 49% at 2 years, but late onset has been reported (Riera et al. 2010, Zantomio et al. 2006). The cGvHD of the genital tract is often associated with oral and ocular GvHD (Marks et al. 2011, Zantomio et al. 2006).

Pathogenesis

Epithelial cells are the main target in aGvHD, whereas cGvHD may affect various mucocutaneous compartments (epithelia/epidermis, dermis) as well as the subcutis. Although the functional mechanisms of aGvHD are increasingly well understood, the primary pathophysiological mechanisms underlying the development of cGvHD are not fully understood.

Etiology

The etiology of GvHD is usually related to allo-HSCT and donor lymphocyte infusions.

Clinical presentation

In acute GvHD skin and mucous membranes are most frequently affected. Patients with severe disease will have widespread epidermolysis and erosions of the adjacent mucosae (in particular stomatitis, vaginitis, vulvitis). Grade IV cutaneous aGvHD is a life-threatening disease.

The most common morphological types of chronic GvHD are lichenoid and sclerotic forms.

Genital GvHD presents with pain, burning, dyspareunia. There may be tenderness on cotton-tipped applicator palpation of vestibular gland openings and vulvar mucosa. Erosions and erythema with similar feature to those of erosive lichen planus, possibly scarring with labial fusion or clitoral hood agglutination, and narrowing of the introitus may be observed. Vaginal examination may show erythema, fibrinous vaginal adhesions, circumferential fibrous vaginal banding, vaginal shortening, synechiae, or complete vaginal stenosis (Lara et al. 2010, Mueller et al. 2013, Shanis et al. 2012, Smith Knutsson et al. 2014, Zantomio et al. 2006).

Lichenoid cGvHD

- Papules and plaques resembling lichen planus
- Pruritus, xerosis, and scaling are frequent (Figures 18.10 & 18.11)
- Persistent hyperpigmentation
- Mucosal changes resembling lichen planus:
  - White reticulated lines and patches of erythema
  - Painful erosions and sometimes ulcerations or fissures
  - After healing vaginal adhesions, strictures or obliteration of the introitus may occur
- Sicca symptoms

Sclerotic cGvHD

- Superficial sclerosis (resembling lichen sclerosus or superficial morphea)
- Deep sclerosis (resembling localized scleroderma or diffuse sclerosis)
- Erosions and stenosis due to scarring
- Burning, pruritus, pain, to touch
- Affecting vulva and vagina dyspareunia and complete obliteration of the vagina
- Affecting urethra and anus dysuria and impaired defecation may occur

Investigations

Repeated genital examination by dermatologists and gynecologists is recommended for GvHD even in asymptomatic patients. Genital involvement may develop, especially in patients with involvement of eyes and mouth.

Labia majora should be spread to inspect the vulva. Vestibular gland openings (Skene and Bartholin), labia minora and majora should gently be touched with a cotton stick. The vaginal wall is palpated with a single digit to detect bands, shortening, narrowing, or other signs of vaginal scarring.

Diagnostic features of genital cGvHD (based on the consensus recommendations of the GvHD working group of the US National Institute of Health) are shown in **Table 18.2**. If there is any uncertainty, a biopsy should be performed. Indurated areas or those that are abnormal on palpation may require further histopathological evaluation to rule out squamous cell carcinoma.

Differential diagnosis

Very early forms of aGvHD are indistinguishable from viral rashes showing a macular or maculopapular eruption. Histopathology may show very similar features; however, if vacuolar interface dermatitis

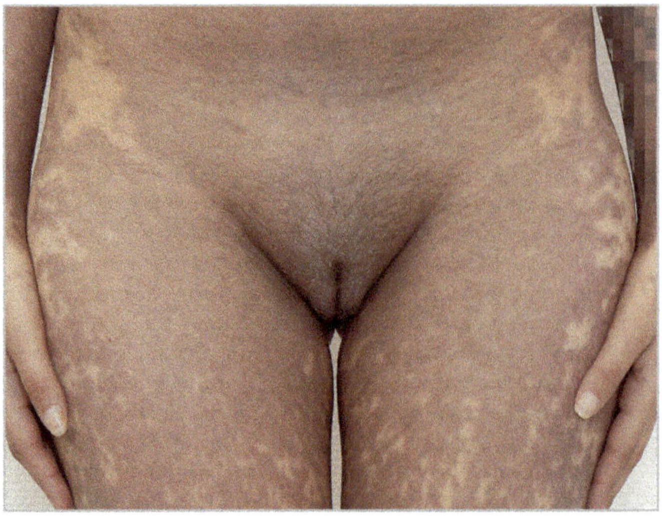

Figure 18.10 Chronic lichenoid Graft versus Host Disease with confluent brownish lichenoid papules and xerosis of the vulva.

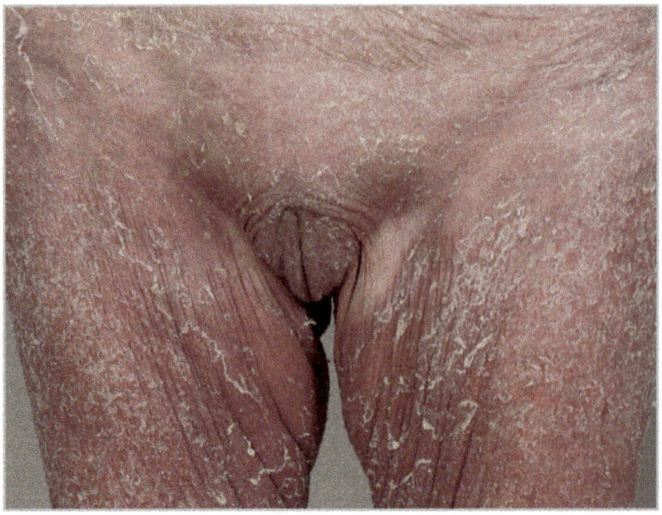

Figure 18.11 Chronic lichenoid Graft versus Host Disease with erythematous plaques and diffuse scaling.

Table 18.2 Clinical scoring of chronic Graft versus Host Disease for genital mucosa 11 (Filipovich et al. 2005)

	Score 0	Score 1	Score 2	Score 3
Genital tract	No signs	Mild signs and females may have symptoms* with discomfort on examination	Moderate signs and females may have symptoms† with discomfort on examination	Severe signs with or without symptoms‡

Severity of signs:

*Mild (any of the following); erythema on vulvar mucosal surfaces, vulvar lichen planus or vulvar lichen sclerosus
†Moderate (any of the following); erosive inflammatory changes of the vulvar mucosa, fissures in vulvar folds
‡Severe (any of the following); labial fusion, clitoral hood agglutination, fibrinous vaginal adhesions, circumferential fibrous vaginal banding, vaginal shortening, synechiae, dense sclerotic changes, and complete vaginal stenosis

and necrotic keratinocytes are found, a viral eruption is highly unlikely. In patients with more severe clinical symptoms of aGvHD SJS/TEN needs to be considered. Chronic lichenoid GvHD needs to be distinguished from idiopathic or drug-induced lichen planus and sclerotic cGvHD from scleroderma. The patient's history is important because histopathology may be the same in those diseases.

Histopathology

Key features of aGvHD

Early stage

- Vacuolar alteration at the DEJ of the epidermis and adnexal epithelia often in association with some lymphocytes (vacuolar interface dermatitis)
- Sparse, superficial, lymphocytic inflammatory infiltrate

With disease progression

- Necrotic keratinocytes, epidermal and adnexal

In severe disease

- Epidermal necrosis and areas of epidermolysis

In persisting skin lesions

- Hyperkeratosis and hypergranulosis
- Melanophages in papillary dermis as a sign of pigment release and subsequent phagocytosis

Histopathological grading is of little predictive use in aGvHD in terms of clinical severity. The extent of the lymphocytic inflammation and the numbers of apoptotic keratinocytes do not automatically correlate with the clinical severity of disease or its course.

cGvHD

This may be divided into a lichen-planus-like (epidermal) and a sclerotic (dermal) variant; however, often a combination of epidermal and dermal changes is seen. Sclerotic changes can extend into the fatty tissue and fascia.

Key features of cGvHD

Lichen-planus-like changes (Figure 18.12)

- Hyperkeratosis and hypergranulosis
- Vacuolar alteration at the DEJ (*vacuolar interface dermatitis*) necrotic keratinocytes in lower layers of the epidermis and adnexal epithelia
- Lymphocytic infiltrate is more pronounced and often band-like (*lichenoid interface dermatitis*)
- Melanophages in papillary dermis as a sign of pigment release and subsequent phagocytosis

Sclerotic changes

- Early stages:
  - Superficial and/or deep perivascular lymphocytic infiltrate sometimes with a few plasma cells
- Fully developed stages (Figure 18.13):
  - Homogenization and thickening of the collagen fibers
  - Simultaneous loss of adnexal structures and subcutaneous fat lobules
- Residual signs of interface dermatitis in the form of clusters of melanophages in the papillary dermis are often present

Management

Treatment of GvHD requires a multidisciplinary team. Early therapy with local corticosteroid application and dilator use to prevent fusion may reduce genital scarring in females (**Table 18.3**) (Riera et al. 2010, Zantomio et al. 2006).

Genital management

- Good genital care advice on the use of emollients and soap substitutes (see also Chapters 3 and 7).
- Vaginal dilators may be useful to maintain patency particularly if there is lack of penetrative intercourse.
- High-potency topical steroids (e.g. clobetasone dipropionate 0.05%) are the first choice. For short-term use, steroids may also

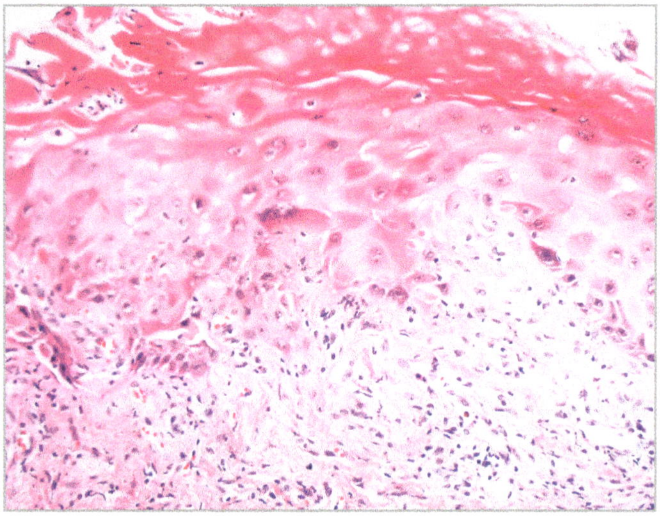

Figure 18.12 Chronic lichenoid Graft versus Host Disease with hyperkeratosis, vacuolar degeneration along the basal cell layer as well as keratinocyte apoptosis, especially in the lower layers of the epidermis and a sparse lichenoid lymphocytic infiltrate.

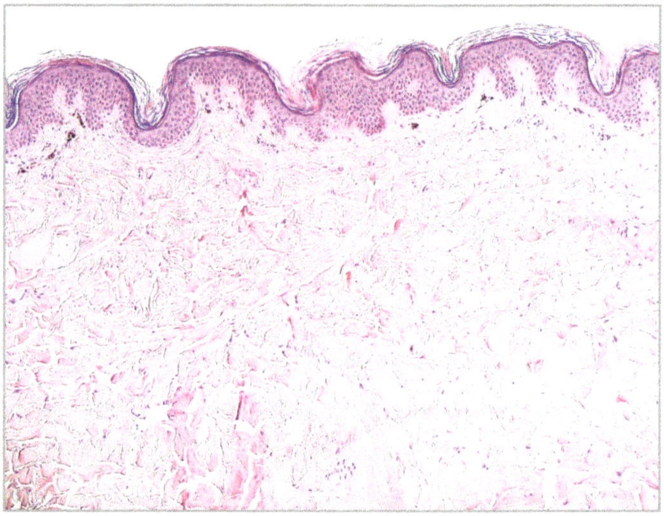

Figure 18.13 Histopathology of sclerotic chronic Graft versus Host Disease with homogenization of the collagen fibers, loss of adnexal structures, and melanophages in the papillary dermis.

Table 18.3 Topical treatment options for chronic Graft versus Host Disease of the skin (adapted from Marks et al. 2011 and Wolff et al. 2011)

	Medication	Recommendation	Evidence	Response rate	Side effect	Comment
Skin	Topical steroids	C-1	III-1	Unknown	Skin atrophy	Trunk and extremities: medium- and high-potency steroids Face: hydrocortisone Application twice daily
	Tacrolimus/ pimecrolimus	C-1	III-1	~70%	Potential long-term risk of skin cancer	Application twice daily
	UVA1 340–400 nm	C-1	III-1	~60–70%	Potential phototoxicity, potentially increased long-term risk of skin cancer	Medium to high dosage; max. single dose of 60 J/cm^2 is sufficient; Use in lichenoid and sclerotic forms of GvHD
	Oral PUVA 320–400 nm	C-1	III-1	~75%	Potential phototoxicity, potentially increased long-term risk of skin cancer	Preferably used in lichenoid forms UV protection needed after therapy
	UVB 311 nm and broadband UVB 280–320 nm	C-1	III-2	~60%	Potential phototoxicity, potentially increased long-term risk of skin cancer	Lacking effectiveness in sclerosis of the skin
Genital mucosa	Topical steroids	B	III-3	Unknown	Increased risk of local infections and atrophy	Application twice daily for short term use, than tapered
	Topical tacrolimus, pimecrolimus, cyclosporine	B	III-3	Unknown	Sometimes burning	Application twice daily

AE, adverse effects; B, general use; C-1, first-line therapy; C-2, second-line therapy (at most); cGvHD, chronic Graft versus Host Disease; III- 2, one retrospective uncontrolled study or retrospective evaluation; III-1, several case reports on retrospective evaluations or small uncontrolled clinical studies; III-3, case reports only.

be applied under occlusion. Depending on the clinical signs and symptoms they will be tapered.

- Topical cyclosporine inhibitors, such as pimecrolimus and tacrolimus, may be combined with topical steroids or used as monotherapy for cutaneous and mucosal lesions (Choi & Nghiem 2001).

Topical tacrolimus 0.1% is applied twice daily for 3 weeks. Depending on the response, the dose should be tapered to 0.03% once daily until a complete remission is achieved. If there is no response after 4 weeks other options should be considered. Pimecrolimus is preferably used in children.

Similar to positive experience with erosive mucosal changes in lichen planus, these preparations may also partly be used for the treatment of GvHD of the adjacent mucosae (Brown et al. 2013). The potentially increased long-term risk of skin cancer has to be taken into account, and close clinical checks and, if necessary, biopsies have to be performed.

- Topical cyclosporine is an alternative for use on the mucous membranes. Ready-to-use preparations are available as a 0.05% emulsion for ophthalmological use (Restasis, Allergan Inc., Irvine, CA, USA). However, in many countries, topical cyclosporine is only available as an individual prescription; it has to be taken into account that cyclosporine is a highly lipophilic peptide with very poor solubility in water.
- In cutaneous GvHD, phototherapy [ultraviolet (UV)-B, systemic PUVA, and UVA1 therapy] may be used. In some institutions topical PUVA is performed with a special device for body cavities.
- Extracorporeal photopheresis (ECP) is increasingly used and is considered the first choice among second-line therapies in steroid-refractory disease. ECP does not increase the risk of infection (Flowers et al. 2008, Knobler et al. 2014). In the largest retrospective study on 71 patients with steroid-refractory cGvHD, the response rate in cutaneous manifestations was 59% (Couriel et al. 2006). Of the 21 patients with sclerotic GvHD, 67% responded to treatment. The response rate among patients with involvement of the oral mucosa was 77%.
- Surgical intervention is sometimes required for adhesions and strictures of mucosal surfaces; complete obliteration of the vagina is described. Adhesiolysis of the entire vaginal length using either sharp or blunt dissection until the cervix is visible may need to be performed. Topical corticosteroid treatment is recommended to avoid recurrence after surgery.
- Oral hormonal replacement therapy does not prevent synechiae (Riera et al. 2010).

REFERENCES

Auquier-Dunant A, Mockenhaupt M, Naldi L, et al. for the SCAR Study Group. Correlations between clinical patterns and causes of erythema multiforme majus, Stevens-Johnson syndrome, and toxic epidermal necrolysis. Arch Dermatol 2002; 138:1019–1024.

Bachot N, Revuz J, Roujeau JC. Intravenous immunoglobulin treatment for Stevens-Johnson syndrome and toxic epidermal necrolysis. A prospective noncomparative study showing no benefit on mortality or progression. Arch Dermatol 2003; 139:33–36.

Bastuji-Garin S, Rzany B, Stern RS, et al. Clinical classification of cases of toxic epidermal necrolysis, Stevens-Johnson syndrome, and erythema multiforme. Arch Dermatol 1993; 129:92–96.

Bonafe JL, Thibaut I, Hoff J. Introital adenosis associated with Stevens-Johnson syndrome. Clin Exp Dermatol 1990; 15:356–357.

Brown RS, Edwards D, Walsh-Chocolaad T, et al. Topical tacrolimus with custom trays in the treatment of severe oral chronic graft-versus-host disease refractory to a potent topical steroid therapy: a case report. Oral Surg Oral Med Oral Pathol Oral Radiol 2013; 115:e26–30.

Choi CJ, Nghiem P. Tacrolimus ointment in the treatment of chronic cutaneous graft-vs-host disease: a case series of 18 patients. Arch Dermatol 2001; 137:1202–1206.

Chung WH, Hung SI, Hong HS, et al. A marker for Stevens-Johnson syndrome. Nature 2004; 428:486.

Chung WH, Hung SI, Yang JY, et al. Granulysin is a key mediator for disseminated keratinocyte death in Stevens-Johnson syndrome and toxic epidermal necrolysis. Nat Med 2008; 14:1343–1350.

Couriel D, Carpenter PA, Cutler C, et al. Ancillary therapy and supportive care of chronic graft-versus-host disease: national institutes of health consensus development project on criteria for clinical trials in chronic Graft-versus-host disease: V. Ancillary Therapy and Supportive Care Working Group Report. Biol Blood Marrow Transplant 2006; 12:375–396.

Filipovich AH, Weisdorf D, Pavletic S, et al. National Institutes of Health consensus development project on criteria for clinical trials in chronic graft-versus-host disease: I. Diagnosis and staging working group report. Biol Blood Marrow Transplant 2005; 11:945–956.

Flowers ME, Apperley JF, van Besien K, et al. A multicenter prospective phase 2 randomized study of extracorporeal photopheresis for treatment of chronic graft-versus-host disease. Blood 2008; 112:2667–2674.

Hung SI, Chung WH, Jee SH, et al. Genetic susceptibility to carbamazepine-induced cutaneous adverse drug reactions. Pharmacogenet Genomics 2006; 16:297–306.

Knobler R, Berlin G, Calzavara-Pinton P, et al. Guideline on the use of extracorporeal photopheresis. J Eur Acad Dermatol Venereol 2014;28(Suppl 1):1–37.

Komorowski L, Mockenhaupt M, Sekula P, et al. Lack of a specific humoral autoreactivity in sera from patients with early erythema exsudativum multiforme majus. J Invest Dermatol 2013; 133:2799–2802.

Lara LA, De Andrade JM, Mauad LM, et al. Genital manifestation of graft-vs.-host disease: a series of case reports. J Sex Med 2010; 7:3216–3225.

Lonjou C, Borot N, Sekula P, et al. A European study of HLA-B in Stevens-Johnson syndrome and toxic epidermal necrolysis related to five high-risk drugs. Pharmacogenet Genomics 2008; 18:99–107.

Marks C, Stadler M, Hausermann P, et al. German-Austrian-Swiss Consensus Conference on clinical practice in chronic graft-versus-host disease (GVHD): guidance for supportive therapy of chronic cutaneous and musculoskeletal GVHD. Br J Dermatol 2011; 165:18–29.

Mockenhaupt M. The current understanding of Stevens-Johnson syndrome and toxic epidermal necrolysis. Expert Rev Clin Immunol 2011; 7:803–815.

Mockenhaupt M, Herb T, Liß Y, Bork K, Haustein UF. Generalized bullous fixed drug eruption: analysis of 62 cases. Eur Ann Allergy Clin Immunol 2010; 42(2/2010):43.

Mockenhaupt M, Sekula P, Roujeau JC, et al. Mortality and long-lasting sequelae in patients with severe cutaneous adverse reactions. Pharmacoepidem Dr S 2008a; 17:115–116.

Mockenhaupt M, Viboud C, Dunant A, et al. Stevens-Johnson syndrome and toxic epidermal necrolysis: Assessment of medication risks with emphasis on recently marketed drugs. The EuroSCAR-study. J Invest Dermatol 2008b; 128:35–44.

Mueller SM, Haeusermann P, Rovo A, et al. Genital chronic GVHD in men after hematopoietic stem cell transplantation: a single-center cross-sectional analysis of 155 patients. Biol Blood Marrow Transplant. 2013; 19:1574–1580.

Phillips EJ, Chung WH, Mockenhaupt M, Roujeau JC, Mallal SA. Drug hypersensitivity: pharmacogenetics and clinical syndromes. J Allergy Clin Immunol 2011; 127(3 Suppl):S60–S66.

Pichler WJ, Naisbitt DJ, Park BK. Immune pathomechanism of drug hypersensitivity reactions. J Allergy Clin Immunol 2011;127(3 Suppl):74–81.

Riera C, Deroover Y, Marechal M. Severe vaginal chronic graft-versus-host disease (GVHD): two cases with late onset and literature review. Eur J Gynaecol Oncol 2010; 31:703–704.

Rzany B, Hering O, Mockenhaupt M, et al. Histopathological and epidemiological characteristics of patients with erythema exsudativum multiforme majus (EEMM), Stevens-Johnson syndrome (SJS) and toxic epidermal necrolysis (TEN). Br J Dermatol 1996; 135:6–11.

Schneck J, Fagot JP, Sekula P, et al. Effects of treatments on the mortality of Stevens-Johnson syndrome and toxic epidermal necrolysis: a retrospective study on patients included in the prospective EuroSCAR Study. J Am Acad Dermatol 2008; 58:33–40.

Sekula P, Dunant A, Mockenhaupt M, et al. Comprehensive survival analysis of a cohort of patients with Stevens-Johnson syndrome and toxic epidermal necrolysis. J Invest Dermatol 2013; 133:1197–1204.

Shanis D, Merideth M, Pulanic TK, et al. Female long-term survivors after allogeneic hematopoietic stem cell transplantation: evaluation and management. Semin Hematol 2012; 49: 83–93.

Smith Knutsson E, Bjork Y, Broman AK, et al. Genital chronic graft-versus-host disease in females: a cross-sectional study. Biol Blood Marrow Transplant 2014; 20:806–811.

Valeyrie-Allanore L, Wolkenstein P, Brochard L, et al. Open trial of ciclosporin treatment for Stevens-Johnson syndrome and toxic epidermal necrolysis. Br J Dermatol 2010; 163:847–853.

Wilson EE, Malinak LR. Vulvovaginal sequelae of Stevens-Johnson syndrome and their management. Obstet Gynecol 1998; 71:478–479.

Wolff D, Gerbitz A, Ayuk F, et al. Consensus conference on clinical practice in chronic graft-versus-host disease (GVHD): first-line and topical treatment of chronic GVHD. Biol Blood Marrow Transplant 2011; 16:1611–1628.

Zantomio D, Grigg AP, MacGregor L, et al. Female genital tract graft-versus-host disease: incidence, risk factors and recommendations for management. Bone Marrow Transplant 2006; 38:567–572.

Ziemer M, Mockenhaupt M. Severe drug-induced skin reactions: clinical pattern, diagnostics and therapy. In: Khopkar U (ed.) Skin biopsy. Rijeka, Croatia: InTech, 2011. www.intechopen.com/articles/show/title/severe-drug-induced-skin-reactions-clinical-pattern-diagnostics-and-therapy (accessed 25 November 2015).

Chapter 19 Lichen sclerosus

Janet McLelland, Susan M Cooper, Gudula Kirtschig

Synonyms

Lichen sclerosus et atrophicus, kraurosis vulvae, lichen albus, hypoplastic dystrophy

Key features

- Inflammatory disease of the skin
- Propensity to sclerosis and scarring
- Mainly affects anogenital site
- Can occur at any age including childhood but most frequently presents in adult women
- Responds well to potent topical corticosteroids
- Usually persists indefinitely
- Increased risk of developing squamous cell carcinoma (SCC) in genital but not extragenital lesions

INTRODUCTION

Lichen sclerosus (LS) is a chronic inflammatory dermatosis that has a predilection for the genital skin of both sexes. It may be asymptomatic but frequently causes itching or discomfort in women. LS often leads to architectural change that may affect urinary and sexual function.

EPIDEMIOLOGY

LS may occur at any age, although the incidence increases with age. There are peaks of incidence in the prepubertal child and in women after the menopause. The suspected prevalence varies between 0.1% and 3% for children and older women, respectively; however, the exact prevalence of LS is unknown (Goldstein et al. 2005, Leibovitz et al. 2000, Wallace 1971). Some women may be asymptomatic or do not seek medical advice.

PATHOGENESIS

LS is thought to be a T-cell-mediated disorder, but the cause is unknown.

Immunology

T cells/Autoimmune

LS is characterized by increased levels of Th1-specific cytokines, a dense T cell infiltrate, and enhanced BIC/miR-155 expression, a microRNA involved in regulation of the immune response (Terlou et al. 2012). Women with LS may have higher frequencies of autoantibodies compared with controls particularly to thyroid and gastric parietal cells (Cooper et al. 2008, Goolamali et al. 1974). Circulating autoantibodies to extracellular matrix protein and bullous pemphigoid antigen BP180 are also more prevalent, although their significance is unknown (Baldo et al. 2010, Oyama et al. 2003).

Disease associations

Most studies show that autoimmune diseases such as thyroid disease, alopecia areata, pernicious anemia, morphea are more frequent in patients with LS (Cooper et al. 2008, Meyrick Thomas et al. 1996), although a recent case-control study found no association with autoantibodies or autoimmune disease other than diabetes (Higgins & Cruickshank 2012, Hofer et al. 2014). There is also an association with increased body mass index, and smoking in men (Hofer et al. 2014). Consideration should be given to screening for autoimmune disorders, including full blood count, thyroid function tests, and B12 for active disease or autoantibodies for potential disease.

Genetics

Familial

A familial incidence is recognized in women (Higgins & Cruickshank 2012, Kirtschig & Kuik 2014, Sherman et al. 2010).

HLA

Inherited genotype seems to have a significant effect on whether a person develops LS. There is a significant association with the human leukocyte antigen (HLA) class II antigen DQ7 and DRB1*12 (Marren et al. 1995) and DRB1*12 (DR12) and the haplotype DRB1*12/DQB1*0301/04/09/010 (Gao et al. 2005). There is a lower frequency of DRB1*0301/04 (DR17) and haplotype DRB1*03/DQB1*02DRB1*0301/DQB1*0201/02/03 in LS patients compared with controls. HLA-DR and DQ antigens or their haplotypes appear to be involved in both susceptibility to and protection from LS.

Epigenetics

Epigenetics refers to functionally relevant changes, other than those of DNA sequence, in the genome that lead to changes in gene expression or cellular phenotype. Vulvar LS is associated with altered expression of isocitrate dehydrogenase enzymes and aberrant hydroxymethylation indicating an epigenetic background for the pathogenesis of vulvar LS (Gambichler et al. 2014). There are reported increases in extracellular matrix proteins and connective tissue growth factor compared to normal controls (Gambichler et al. 2012).

Cell kinetics

Tan et al. showed an altered p53 expression and epidermal cell proliferation in vulvar LS compared with normal vulvar skin and extragenital LS (Tan et al. 1994).

Environmental factors/triggers

Mechanical

The Köbner phenomenon where disease occurs in sites subject to trauma is seen in extragenital LS and may be a factor in genital LS. Mechanical factors like friction due to tight clothing, occlusion, surgical trauma, trauma after sexual abuse, urinary incontinence, radiotherapy, sunburn, and scars are thought to play an important role in triggering and maintaining LS. Higgins & Cruickshank 2012 did not find any association with number or type of vaginal deliveries, perineal suturing, or a history of pelvic radiotherapy; however, the risk of LS may be greater in parous women than in nulliparous women (Higgins & Cruickshank 2012).

Infectious triggers

There is no clear evidence for an infective etiology with either *Borrelia burgdorferi* or human papilloma virus infection.

Hormonal

The prepubertal and postmenopausal peaks in incidence and reported increased incidence in women with Turner syndrome (who have low estrogen levels) support a possible role for hormones in the pathogenesis of LS. In a case-control study, after adjustment for age, menopausal status was not associated with LS (Higgins & Cruickshank 2012), but use of hormone replacement therapy was associated with a reduced risk. Antiandrogenic oral contraceptives have been associated with LS and may trigger early onset LS in a subgroup of susceptible women (Günthert et al. 2008). Progesterone-only contraceptives (Higgins & Cruickshank 2012) may protect from LS, but there is no consistent benefit from estrogen or testosterone treatment.

Drugs

There are very few reports of an association of LS with drugs. The use of beta-blockers, angiotensin-converting-enzyme inhibitors, hormone replacement therapy, and progesterone only methods for contraception may be protective (Baldo et al. 2014, Higgins & Cruickshank 2012).

CLINICAL PRESENTATION

Key clinical symptoms

- Pruritus
- Pain, soreness
- Fragility of genital skin
- Dyspareunia or apareunia
- Poor urinary stream
- Constipation (children)

Key clinical signs

- Pallor, ivory white with wrinkled appearance
- Figure of eight distribution around vulvar and perianal area
- Fissures
- Purpura/ecchymoses
- Hyperkeratosis
- Variable degree of scarring
- Ulceration/erosions
- Bullae (rare)
- Follicular plugging (extragenital)

Skin affected by LS is very itchy and sore, although some women with LS are asymptomatic. If skin fissures, it will be painful. Women may experience pain on intercourse. In children, painful defecation due to perianal disease may lead to constipation (see Chapter 42 for LS in children).

The skin may change appearance becoming ivory white, shiny, and wrinkled and in some cases hyperkeratotic. LS usually affects the clitoral area, labia minora, sulcus interlabialis and/or outer surfaces of the labia majora (**Figures 19.1** and **19.2**), it may present perianally in a figure-of-eight distribution (**Figure 19.3**). If the skin is inflamed the vulva may be erythematous and the classical white appearance may not be seen initially (**Figure 19.4**). Scarring occurs in 80% of women and 30% of girls (Cooper et al. 2004) and may lead to resorption of the labia minora, fusion in the midline (**Figure 19.5**) with burying of the clitoris (**Figure 19.6**). Erosions and fissures will produce pain. Narrowing and fissuring of the vaginal introitus may cause problems with sexual intercourse. Purpura and ecchymoses (**Figure 19.7**) may be a feature, which may raise the concern of sexual abuse particularly in childhood. Sometimes LS lesions may be bullous or eroded.

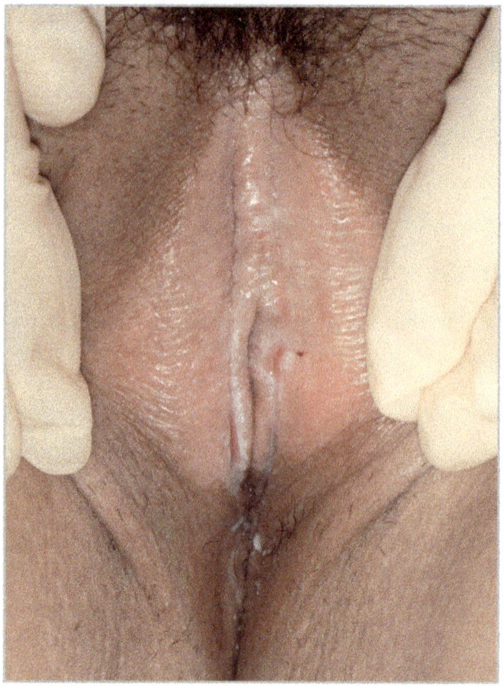

Figure 19.1 White symmetrical plaques of lichen sclerosus.

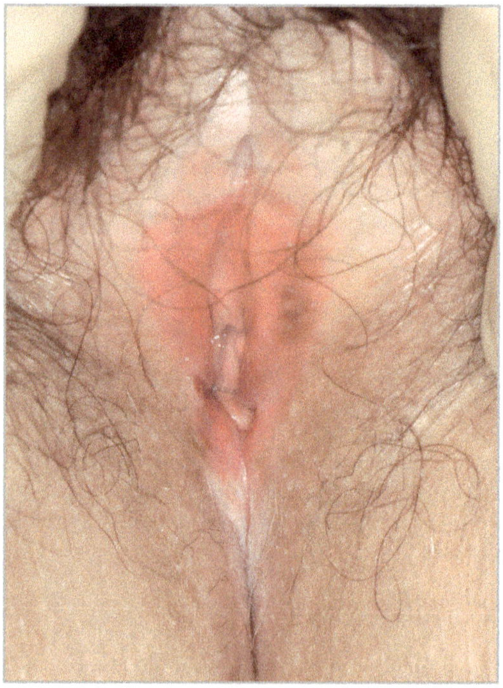

Figure 19.2 Erythema and pallor.

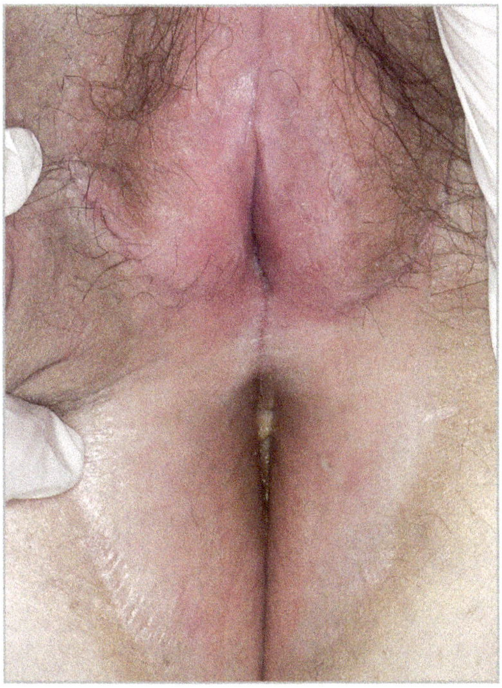

Figure 19.3 Typical 'figure-of-eight' distribution involving the vulvar and perianal skin.

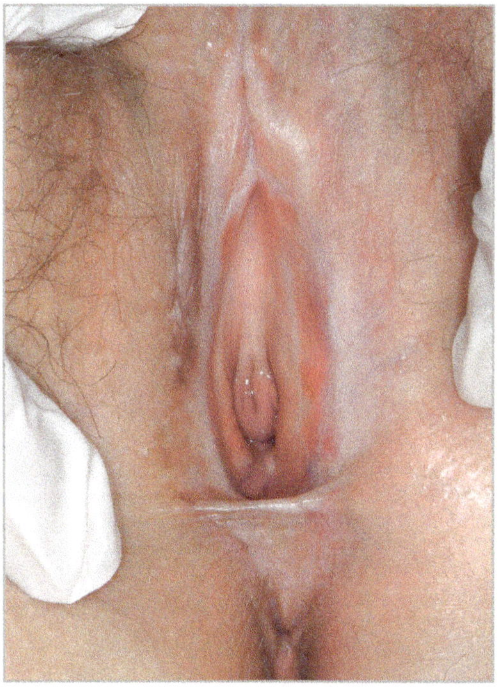

Figure 19.5 Loss of the labia minora.

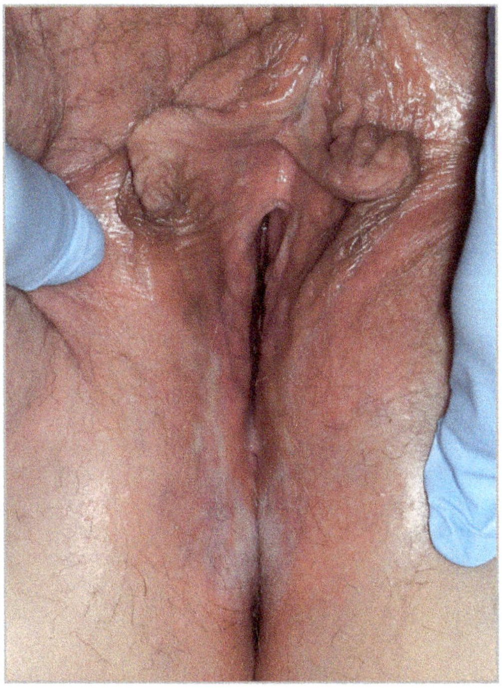

Figure 19.4 Subtle pallor of early lichen sclerosus affecting the perineum. This is a common site for the first skin changes.

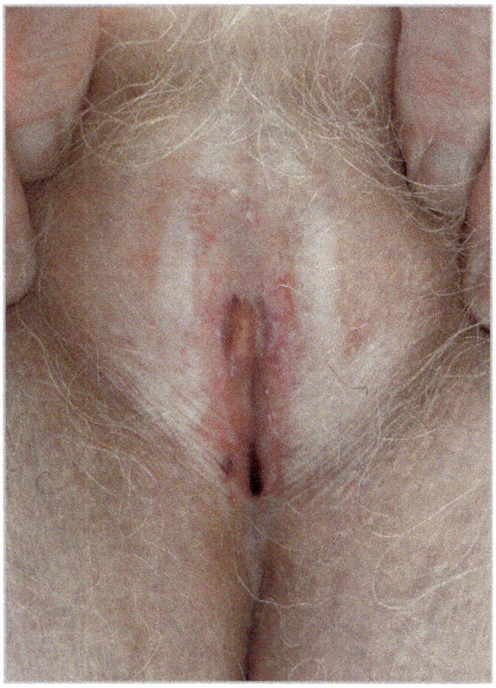

Figure 19.6 Extensive midline fusion with burying of the clitoris.

Extragenital LS (**Figure 19.8**) occurs in about 6% (Wallace 1971) to 11% (Meyrick et al. 1996) of women. Plaques often occur on the upper trunk, neck, axillae, and flexor surface of the wrists. They are often asymptomatic or cause itching and may have hemorrhage or erosions in the lesions. The Köbner phenomenon, where lesions occur after minor trauma, e.g. scratching, is well recognized. Lesions typically do not involve the vagina or mouth, although occasional cases have been reported.

Pregnancy and delivery are unlikely to be significantly affected by LS (Dalziel 1995) and Higgins and Cruickshank reported no problems with healing after delivery (Higgins & Cruickshank 2012).

In typical cases a biopsy with histopathological confirmation may not be needed.

A biopsy should be performed:

- If the clinical diagnosis is uncertain
- If dysplasia is suspected
- If there is failure of treatment

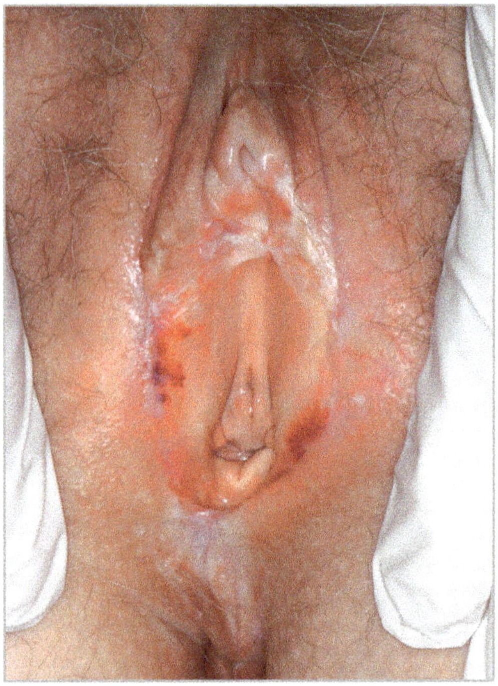

Figure 19.7 Ecchymoses indicate active lichen sclerosus and are caused by capillary fragility.

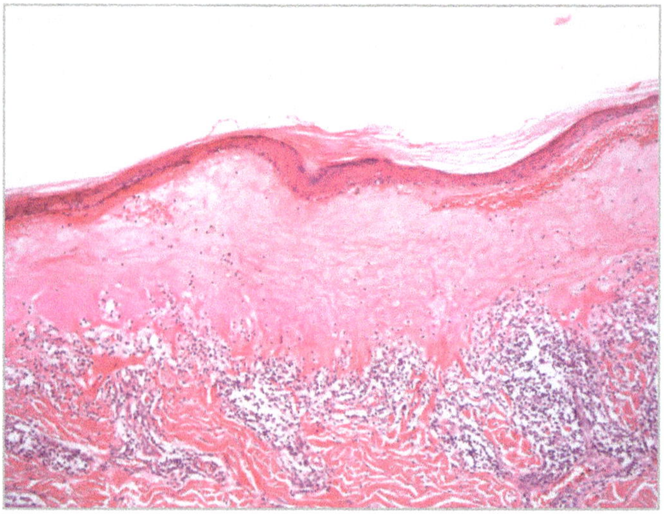

Figure 19.9 Histopathology of lichen sclerosus showing epidermal atrophy, hyaline band in the upper dermis and basal cell degeneration. By courtesy of Fraser Charlton, UK.

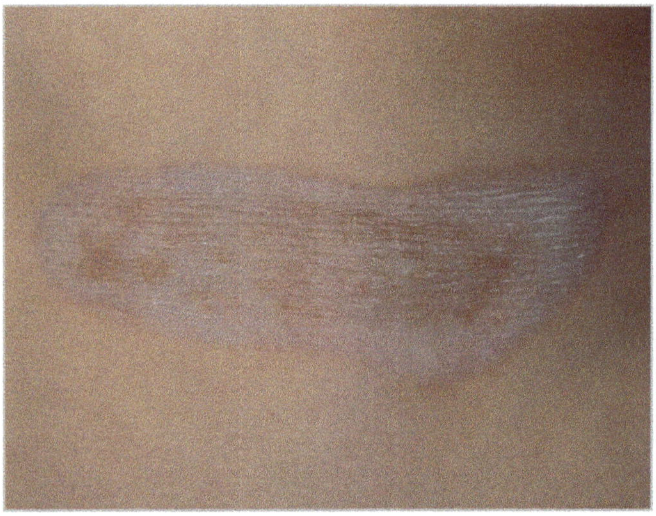

Figure 19.8 Extragenital lichen sclerosus with typical cigarette-paper appearance.

HISTOPATHOLOGY

Key points

- Clinical and pathological correlation is essential
- The biopsy has to be taken from a typical lesion
- In typical cases a biopsy may not be needed, but many clinicians prefer to take a biopsy at presentation
- A biopsy should be performed if the clinical diagnosis is uncertain, dysplasia is suspected, or there is failure of first-line treatment

LS s is characterized by changes in both the epidermis and dermis (**Figure 19.9**) (Calonje et al. 2011).

Key histopathologic features of LS

- Hyperkeratosis
- Atrophic epidermis
- Basal hydropic degeneration +/– pigmentary incontinence
- Edema and homogenization of collagen in upper dermis with loss of elastic tissue
- Band-like lymphohistiocytic infiltrate underneath hyaline band +/– dilated blood and lymphatic vessels
- Follicular plugging in hair bearing skin

In early LS some features like the hyalinization/homogenization of the upper dermis may be lacking and a firm diagnosis cannot be made. Also, mucosal/erosive vulvar lichen planus may show similar clinical and histological features, making a distinction between the two diseases impossible in some cases (see Chapter 20).

DIFFERENTIAL DIAGNOSES

The main differential diagnoses are lichen planus and vitiligo (**Table 19.1**). Vitiligo results in pallor but does not show the textural changes of LS and there is no structural change; it is typically asymptomatic. Vitiligo and LS may occur together. Bullous disorders, e.g. mucous membrane pemphigoid may be considered but vaginal, oral, or ocular lesions would help to clinically establish that diagnosis (see Chapter 26). Lichen planus and Graft versus Host Disease may be confused or coexist (see Chapters 20 and 18). In children sexual abuse may have to be considered and the two may coexist, possibly due to Köbnerization after trauma (Warrington & de san Lazaro 1996). In early inflammatory LS skin may be red and appear eczematous before the typical pallor develops.

Table 19.1 Main differential diagnoses of lichen sclerosus

Differential diagnosis	Clinical key features	Diagnostic test
Lichen planus	Erosions at the entrance to the vagina, lacy reticulation, evidence of lichen planus elsewhere, e.g. mouth, scalp, and vagina	Biopsy
Vitiligo	Well-demarcated depigmentation, no change of skin texture, no symptoms	Wood lamp helpful Biopsy
Eczema	Erythema +/− scale around the anogenital site with itch	Clinical history Biopsy

PRINCIPLES OF MANAGEMENT

Establish diagnosis

- Inform the patient about the diagnosis and implications

Educate patient

- Emollients and soap substitutes can be helpful
- Lubricants (preferably greasy) may aid penetration in sexual intercourse
- Advise that the disease may continue indefinitely
- Warn about the risk (about 4%) of developing SCC and lumps or ulcers lasting > 2 weeks should be referred urgently

Implement treatment

- Potent or very potent topical corticosteroids are the mainstay of treatment
- Other topicals, surgery, or systemic treatment may need to be considered

TREATMENT

Topical treatments (Table 19.2)

Moisturizers and soap substitutes often help any discomfort, and lubricants may make sexual intercourse more comfortable. Once remission has been established emollients can be useful for maintenance treatment. Silk knickers have been reported to be better than cotton.

Topical corticosteroids are effective (Wallace 1971). Very potent topical corticosteroids, e.g. clobetasol propionate 0.05% (Dalziel et al.1991, Kirtschig et al. 2015), have been shown to be effective and safe for long-term use. Cooper et al. did a retrospective study of 253 women and 74 girls and found that symptoms were relieved in most and signs were reversed in 20% (Cooper et al. 2004). A prospective trial of 54 patients (Virgili et al. 2014) randomized to mometasone furoate or clobetasol propionate for 12 weeks found that both were similarly efficacious and well tolerated. The frequency of application both initially and for maintenance after improvement varies between guidelines, but a reasonable regime would be to use potent to very potent topical steroids daily for 3 months followed by maintenance treatment with once or twice weekly application to prevent relapses, scar formation and cancer development (Kirtschig et al. 2015, Lee et al. 2015a). Application at night is often more practical as the ointment or cream is not wiped off after urination.

The calcineurin inhibitors tacrolimus and pimecrolimus have been used topically in small trials (Hengge et al. 2006). They often produce initial stinging, but theoretical concerns about the risk of malignancy do not seem to have been justified in practice. Pimecrolimus and tacrolimus (Funaro et al. 2014) are, however, significantly less effective than clobetasol propionate.

Topical tretinoin 0.025% cream, with an alternate-day regimen for 24 weeks may represent a useful alternative to corticosteroids in the treatment of active vulvar LS, acting particularly on hyperkeratosis and pallor (Borghi et al. 2015).

There is good evidence that topical sex hormones (testosterone and progesterone) are of minimal benefit if at all, certainly compared with topical corticosteroids; topical testosterone has androgenic side effects and is not recommended for use.

Injections

A study of 88 patients who had responded poorly to topical steroids (Baggish & Ventolini 2006) found that monthly subdermal steroid injections in addition to topical treatment led to improvement in 62 of them. A response to injections of adipose-derived stem cells and platelet-rich plasma is described by one investigator; however, this requires confirmation (Casabona et al. 2010).

Phototherapy

Topical PUVA and narrow-band UVB have been tried in small series. Phototherapy may be of some value, but a randomized clinical trial of 30 patients treated with either UV-A1 phototherapy or clobetasol propionate found that although UV-A1 produced a significant clinical improvement, it was inferior to clobetasol propionate with respect to relief of itch, improvement in quality of life, and practicability (Terras et al. 2014).

Extracorporeal photochemotherapy and photodynamic therapy have also been reported in small studies to be of benefit.

Systemic treatments

The oral retinoids etretinate and acitretin have been shown to be of benefit in small studies including a double-blind placebo-controlled trial of acitretin (Bousema et al. 1994).

Small studies and case reports have been published suggesting beneficial response to pulsed methylprednisolone with methotrexate, cyclosporine, methotrexate and hydroxyurea.

Surgical intervention

Vulvectomy was performed in the past, but the disease often recurred and it is now considered poor practice for the treatment of LS. Surgery to divide labial adhesions or Fenton procedure for introital stenosis may be helpful in selected cases (see also Chapter 40) (Gurumurthy et al. 2012).

Carbon dioxide laser vaporization has been used with some success in highly selected patients (Lee et al. 2015b).

Psychological

Studies show that having LS results in an impaired health-related quality of life. The majority of women of all ages with LS report that LS has a detrimental effect on sexual function, with problems including dyspareunia, apareunia, and difficulty achieving orgasm. The symptoms may relate to continuing inflammatory disease as well as to anatomic changes and scarring from long-standing active disease (Dalziel 1995). Many affected women feel embarrassed; some have persistent itch

Table 19.2 Outline of treatment for vulvar lichen sclerosus (see also Kirtschig et al. EDF guideline 2014)

Treatment modality		Main adverse effects	Evidence level/grade of recommendation
Topical steroids	Clobetasol propionate 0.05% ointment	Candidosis, skin atrophy	RCT 1–2/A (first line)
	Mometasone furoate 0.1% ointment	Candidosis, skin atrophy	RCT 1–2/A (first line)
Injections	Triamcinolone	Skin atrophy	1+/B
	Stem cells and platelet rich plasma	Local irritation	3–4/D (needs confirmation, not currently recommended)
Calcineurin inhibitors	Tacrolimus 0.1% ointment	Burning	2+/C (second line)
	Pimecrolimus 1% cream	Transient burning	1+/B (second line)
Phototherapy	UVA 1 / PUVA	Burning	1+/B (recommended in extragenital but not genital lichen sclerosus)
Systemic	Acitretin	Dryness, effect on lipids	1+/B
	Cyclosporine	Hypertension, nephrotoxicity	3/D
	Methotrexate 10–15 mg/week	Bone marrow suppression, hepatotoxicity	3/D
	Hydroxycarbamide (hydroxyurea) 1 g daily	Bone marrow suppression	3/D
Topical vitamin D analogs	Calcipotriol 0.005%	Irritation	3/D (extragenital)
Surgery	Vulvar adhesiolysis Z-plasty/perineotomy	Reoccurrence of adhesions	3D
The level of evidence varies between 1 and 4 and grade of recommendation between A and D, '1' (very good studies) and 'A' indicating best grades, and 4 and D worst.			

and pain despite successful control of the inflammation, and many are concerned about how the disorder may progress. This affects daily private life and work. Psychological support or psychosexual counseling may be helpful to deal with the emotional consequences of the disease (Lansdorp et al. 2013).

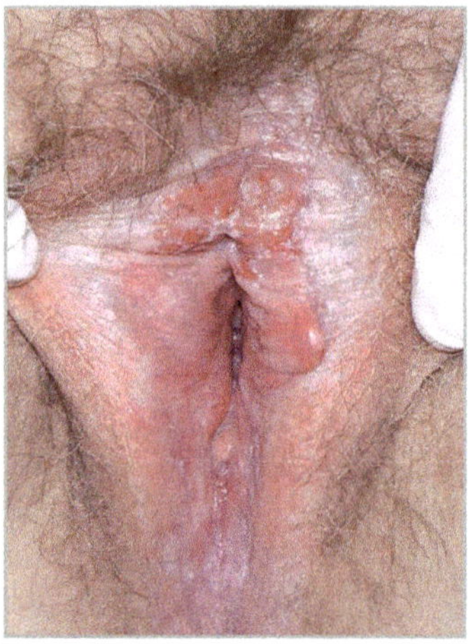

Figure 19.10 Squamous cell carcinoma (SCC) in lichen sclerosus: a nodule is seen anteriorly, which is a common site for an SCC in lichen sclerosus.

ASSOCIATION WITH MALIGNANCY

SCC has been described in association with male and female genital disease (Wallace & Whimster 1951) but not with extragenital LS. The incidence of SCC in LS is about 4%, i.e. 12 out of 290 patients with an average follow-up of 12.5 years (Meyrick Thomas et al. 1996, Wallace 1971). The risk of developing anogenital cancer may be higher in familial LS (Sherman et al. 2010) than in cases without a family history. SCC presents as an erythematous nodule or ulcer, which is painful and often rapidly growing (**Figure 19.10**). Recently, Lee and colleagues have demonstrated that good compliance with treatment of LS is associated with a reduced risk of SCC compared to poor compliance (Lee et al. 2015a).

COURSE AND PROGNOSIS

The LS of the vulva usually persists indefinitely but may in some cases become asymptomatic or resolve spontaneously; however, early treatment of LS, even if asymptomatic, is recommended in adults and children. Treatment improves symptoms in 80–90% of patients, although treatment will usually not lead to complete remission in women (Cooper et al. 2004). In 244 out of 255 patients symptoms improved and 168 became symptom free. Fifty-eight out of the 253 responders had a return to normal skin texture and color (22% of girls, 23% of women). Further long-term prospective studies need to confirm whether initial and maintenance treatment prevents scarring or the development of SCC.

Follow-up may not be essential for all patients in secondary care, but all patients should be advised to present to their doctor urgently with symptoms or signs that could indicate the development of an SCC.

REFERENCES

Baggish MS, Ventolini G. Lichen sclerosus: subdermal steroid injection therapy. A large, long-term follow-up study. J Gynecol Surg 2006; 22:137–141.

Baldo M, Ali I, Wojnarowska F. The contribution of drugs to lichen sclerosus. Clin Exp Dermatol 2014; 39:234.

Baldo M, Bailey A, Bhogal B, Groves RW, et al. T cells reactive with the NC16A domain of BP180 are present in vulval lichen sclerosus and lichen planus. J Eur Acad Dermatol Venereol 2010; 24:186–190.

Borghi A, Corazza M, Minghetti S, Virgili A. Topical tretinoin in the treatment of vulvar lichen sclerosus: an advisable option? Eur J Dermatol 2015 Aug 3. [Epub ahead of print]

Bousema MT, Rompannen U, Geiger J-M, et al. Acitretin in the treatment of severe lichen sclerosus et atrophicus of the vulva: a double-blind placebo-controlled study. J Am Acad Dermatol 1994; 30:225–231.

Calonje JE, Brenn T, Lazar AJ, McKee PH (eds). McKee's pathology of the skin, 4th edn. Philadelphia, PA: Saunders, 2011.

Casabona F, Priano V, Vallerino V, Cogliandro A, Lavagnino G. New surgical approach to lichen sclerosus of the vulva: the role of adipose-derived mesenchymal cells and platelet-rich plasma in tissue regeneration Plast Reconstr Surg 2010; 126:210–211.

Cooper SM, Ali I, Baldo M, Wojnarowska F. The association of lichen sclerosus and erosive lichen planus of the vulva with autoimmune disease: a case-control study. Arch Dermatol 2008; 144:1432–1435.

Cooper SM, Gao X-H, Powell JJ, Wojnarowska F. Does treatment of vulvar lichen sclerosus influence its prognosis? Arch Dermatol 2004; 140:702–706.

Dalziel KL. Effect of lichen sclerosus on sexual function and parturition, J Reprod Med 1995;40:351–354.

Dalziel KL, Millard PR, Wojnarowska F. The treatment of vulval lichen sclerosus with a very potent topical steroid (clobetasol propionate 0.05%) cream. Br J Dermatol 1991; 124:461–464.

Funaro D, Lovett A, Leroux N, Powell J. A double-blind, randomized prospective study evaluating topical clobetasol propionate 0.05% versus topical tacrolimus 0.1% in patients with vulvar lichen sclerosus [published online ahead of print April 13, 2014]. J Am Acad Dermatol.

Gambichler T, Sktygan M, Czempiel V, et al. Differential expression of connective tissue growth factor and extracellular matrix proteins in lichen sclerosus. J Eur Acad Dermatol Venereol 2012; 25:207–212.

Gambichler T, Terras S, Kreuter A, Skrygan M. Altered global methylation and hydroxymethylation status in vulvar lichen sclerosus: further support for epigenetic mechanisms. Br J Dermatol 2014; 170:687–693.

Gao XH, Barnardo MC, Winsey S, et al. The association between HLA DR, DQ antigens, and vulval lichen sclerosus in the UK: HLA DRB112 and its associated DRB112/DQB10301/04/09/010 haplotype confers susceptibility to vulval lichen sclerosus, and HLA DRB10301/04 and its associated DRB10301/04/DQB10201/02/03 haplotype protects from vulval lichen sclerosus. J Invest Dermatol 2005; 125:895–899.

Goldstein AT, Marinoff SC, Christopher K, Srodon M. Prevalence of vulvar lichen sclerosus in a general gynecology practice. J Reprod Med 2005; 50:477–480.

Goolamali SK, Barnes EW, Irvine WJ, Shuster S. Organ-specific antibodies in patients with lichen sclerosus. BMJ 1974; 4:78–79.

Gurumurthy M, Morah N, Gioffre G, Cruickshank ME. The surgical management of complications of vulval lichen sclerosus. Eur J Obstet Gynecol Reprod Biol 2012; 162:79–82.

Günthert AR, Faber M, Knappe G, Hellriegel S, Emons G. Early onset vulvar lichen sclerosus in premenopausal women and oral contraceptives. Eur J Obstet Gynecol Reprod Biol 2008; 137:56–60.

Hengge UR, Krause W ,Hofmann H, et al. Multicentre, phase 11 trial on the safety and efficacy of topical tacrolimus ointment for the treatment of lichen sclerosus. Br J Dermatol 2006; 155:1021–1028.

Higgins CA, Cruickshank ME. A population-based case-control study of aetiological factors associated with vulval lichen sclerosus. J Obstet Gynaecol 2012; 32:271–275.

Hofer MD, Meeks JJ, Mehdiratta N, et al. Lichen sclerosus in men is associated with elevated body mass index, diabetes mellitus, coronary artery disease and smoking. World J Urol 2014; 32:105–108.

Kirtschig G, Becker K, Günthert A, et al. Evidence-based (S3) Guideline on (anogenital) Lichen sclerosus. J Eur Acad Dermatol Venereol 2015; 29:e1–e43.

Kirtschig G, Kuik DJ. A Dutch cohort study confirms familial occurrence of anogenital lichen sclerosus. J Women's Health Care 2014; 3:209–211.

Lansdorp CA, van den Hondel KE, Korfage IJ, van Gestel MJ, van der Meijden WI. Quality of life in Dutch women with lichen sclerosus. Br J Dermatol 2013; 168:787–793.

Lee A, Bradford J, Fischer G. Long-term management of adult vulvar lichen cclerosus. A prospective cohort study of 507 women. JAMA Dermatol 2015a;151: 1061–1067.

Lee A, Lim A, Fischer G. Fractional carbon dioxide laser in recalcitrant vulval lichen sclerosus. Australas J Dermatol. 2015b Mar 5 [Epub ahead of print].

Leibovitz A, Kaplun VV, Saposhnicov N, Habot B. Vulvovaginal examinations in elderly nursing home women residents. Arch Gerontol Geriatr 2000; 31:1–4.

Marren P, Yell J, Charnock FM, et al. The association of lichen sclerosus and antigens of the HLA system. Br J Dermatol 1995; 131:197–203.

Meyrick Thomas RH, Ridley CM, McGibbon DH, Black MM. Anogenital lichen sclerosus in women. J Roy Soc Med 1996; 89:694–698.

Oyama N, Chan I, Neill SM, et al. Autoantibodies to extracellular matrix protein 1 in lichen sclerosus. Lancet 2003; 362:118–123.

Sherman V, McPherson T, Baldo M, et al. The high rate of familial lichen sclerosus suggests a genetic contribution: an observational cohort study. J Eur Acad Dermatol Venereol 2010; 24:1031–1034.

Tan S-H, Derrick E, McKee PH, et al. Altered p53 expression and epidermal cell proliferation is seen in vulval lichen sclerosus. J Cutaneous Pathol 1994; 21:316–323.

Terlou A, Santegoets LA, van der Meijden WI, et al. An autoimmune phenotype in vulvar lichen sclerosus and lichen planus: a Th1 response and high levels of micro-RNA-155. J Invest Dermatol 2012; 132:658–666.

Terras S, Gambichler T, Moritz RK, Stucker M, Kreuter A. UV-A1 phototherapy vs clobetasol propionate, 0.05%, in the treatment of vulvar lichen sclerosus: a randomised clinical trial [published online ahead of print Apr 2, 2014. JAMA Dermatol.

Virgili A, Borghi A, Toni G, Minghetti S, Corazza M. First randomized trial on clobetasol propionate and mometasone furoate in the treatment of vulvar lichen sclerosus: results of efficacy and tolerability [published online ahead of print Feb 21, 2014]. Br J Dermatol.

Wallace HJ . Lichen sclerosus and atrophicus. Trans St Johns Hosp Dermatol Society 1971; 57:9–30.

Wallace HJ, Whimster IW. Vulval atrophy and leukoplakia. Br J Dermatol 1951; 63:241–257.

Warrington SA, de san Lazaro C. Lichen sclerosus et atrophicus and sexual abuse. Arch Dis Child 1996; 75:512–516.

Chapter 20 Lichen planus

Gudula Kirtschig, Susan M Cooper

Synonyms

Lichen ruber planus

Key features

- Inflammatory disease of the skin, hair, nails and mucous membranes
- Clinical variants affect the skin and mucous membranes to different degrees
- Single or multiple sites may be affected; usually symmetrical distribution
- If present, oral and nail changes give diagnostic clues
- If mucous membranes are affected, scarring often occurs
- Mainly seen in middle aged adults, but the disease exists in children
- Mucosal LP usually takes a chronic course; spontaneous remission is possible

INTRODUCTION

Lichen planus is a mucocutaneous inflammatory disease of unknown origin. Approximately 50% of women with cutaneous lichen planus have vulvar involvement (Lewis 1996). When a diagnosis of vulvar lichen planus is considered it is very important to look for involvement at other sites with a full examination including skin, hair, nails and mucous membranes (McPherson 2010). If possible, the clinical diagnosis should be confirmed histologically.

EPIDEMIOLOGY

Lichen planus affects between 0.22 and 1% of the adult population. It is slightly more common in females than males. The prevalence for oral LP is estimated between 0.5 and 4%. The incidence and prevalence of mucosal vulvar lichen planus are not known. Classical cutaneous papulosquamous LP may occur at any age including childhood but most frequently occurs around 40-60 years of age. Mucosal vulvar lichen planus presents in peri- and postmenopausal women with a mean age of onset between 50 and 60 years (Helgesen 2010, Kirtschig 2005); mucosal LP is very rare in children (Pandhi 2014). There are no known racial differences in the prevalence for vulvar LP; although classical LP in children is commonly reported from India.

PATHOGENESIS

Lichen planus is thought to be a T-cell mediated mucocutaneous disorder. The exact pathogenesis is not known; however, it is proposed that there is damage to epidermal cells that express altered self or foreign antigens.

Immunology

T cells/autoimmune

There is an autoimmune phenotype in vulvar lichen planus, characterized by increased levels of Th1-specific cytokines, a dense T-cell infiltrate, and enhanced BIC/miR-155 expression, a microRNA involved in regulation of the immune response (Terlou 2012). Patients are often diagnosed with autoimmune conditions and have significantly higher frequencies of serum autoantibodies (ANA, anti-thyroid, anti-BP 180 antibodies) compared to controls (Cooper 2008, Cooper 2005).

Disease associations

Subsequently, autoimmune diseases like thyroid disease, vitiligo, alopecia areata, autoimmune bowel disease, rheumatoid arthritis, primary biliary cirrhosis, and systemic lupus erythematosus are more common in vulvar LP patients (Cooper 2008, Santegoets 2010). **Table 20.1** summarizes clinical tests to consider in diseases more commonly associated with LP.

Genetics

Familial

There are reports of familial cutaneous LP but no familial vulvar cases have been reported in the literature.

HLA

An association between the class II HLA DQB10201 allele and the vulvovaginal-gingival syndrome is reported once (Setterfield 2006).

Environmental factors/triggers

Mechanical factors

Trauma is a well-known trigger in cutaneous LP (Köbner phenomenon) but the role of mechanical triggers in genital LP is not investigated.

Infectious triggers

Hepatitis C virus (HCV) infection is associated with oral LP in some parts of the world such as the USA, the Mediterranean, South Asia,

Table 20.1 Clinical tests on clinical indication in diseases more commonly associated with LP

Associated disease	Recommended investigations
Thyroid disease	History, examination, TSH/FT4, autoantibodies
Autoimmune gastritis/pernicious anaemia	History, examination, full blood count, serum vitamin B12, autoantibodies
Hepatitis C	History, examination, liver function test, antibodies

and Africa; however, there is only limited evidence for an association for isolated cutaneous LP. There is a single study demonstrating no association in vulvar LP, however, this study was done in a part of the UK with a very low prevalence of HCV (Cooper 2004). HCV infection should be considered and HCV screening performed if there are risk factors or clinical hints. Vulvar LP after hepatitis B vaccination is not reported, in contrast to cutaneous LP. The role of an (oncogenic) mucosal human papillomavirus (HPV) in the aetiology and the possible premalignant character of erosive vulvar LP was discounted (Kirtschig 2005).

Drugs

Although there are many drugs reported to cause lichenoid drug eruptions there are no definite triggers for vulvar LP. A study in mucosal (oral and vulvar) lichen planus in women found angiotensin-converting enzyme inhibitors protective for the development of LP; in contrast beta-blockers and non-steroidal anti-inflammatory drugs were associated with LP (Clayton 2010).

Contact allergens

Oral lichen planus is described to be triggered by dental metallic restoration material (e.g. amalgam, copper, cobalt, and gold). Equivalent triggers are not described in cutaneous or vulvar LP.

Psychological factors

In patients with genital and erosive oral LP daily life may be severely affected. Depression, anxiety and stress may be more common in erosive LP. An interdisciplinary approach and counsellors/psychologists are sometimes needed (Lundquvist 2006).

CLINICAL PRESENTATION

Sites involved and key features

- **Vulva:** See box: Clinical features of LP variants affecting the anogenital site
- **Vagina:** Erosions, desquamative vaginitis; scarring may lead to stenosis
- **Urethra:** Erosions and stenosis leading to painful and impaired urination
- **Anus:** Painful defecation, scarring may lead to stenosis of the anus
- **Oral cavity:** Including buccal mucosa, tongue, gingiva and lips (rarely on the palate): The asymptomatic reticulate variant (Wickham striae) may be a diagnostic hint. Desquamative gingivitis may be seen in the vulvovaginal-gingival syndrome
- **Conjunctiva including lacrimal duct:** Conjunctivitis (sandpaper feeling), possibly scarring with pterygium formation
- **Aural/auditory canal (meatus externus):** Erosions and crusts, possibly narrowing
- **Nasal mucosa:** Erosions and crusts
- **Larynx and oesophagus:** Erosions and scarring (web formation) leading to dysphagia
- **Scalp:** Inflamed hair follicles, scarring alopecia
- **Nails:** Nail matrix damage leading to longitudinal ridges and fissures; possibly scarring (pterygium)

The oral cavity is possibly the site most commonly affected by LP. Reticulate (Wickham striae), erosive/ulcerative, plaque, and bullous forms are differentiated. Reticulate oral LP often affecting the buccal mucosa (**Figure 20.1**) is usually not symptomatic and does not require treatment. However, if present it may be a key feature for the diagnosis. Desquamative gingivitis (**Figure 20.2**) is a painful variant, possibly leading to early loss of teeth (**Figure 20.3**). It is associated with vulvar and vaginal disease in the vulvovaginal-gingival syndrome (Pelisse 1982).

Nail LP is found in about 10% of patients and may occur in isolation or in connection with skin or mucous membrane disease. There are longitudinal ridges or pterygium formation (**Figure 20.4**) this may be a diagnostic hint if present.

Lichen planus affecting the anogenital site

There are four main types of lichen planus affecting the anogenital site:

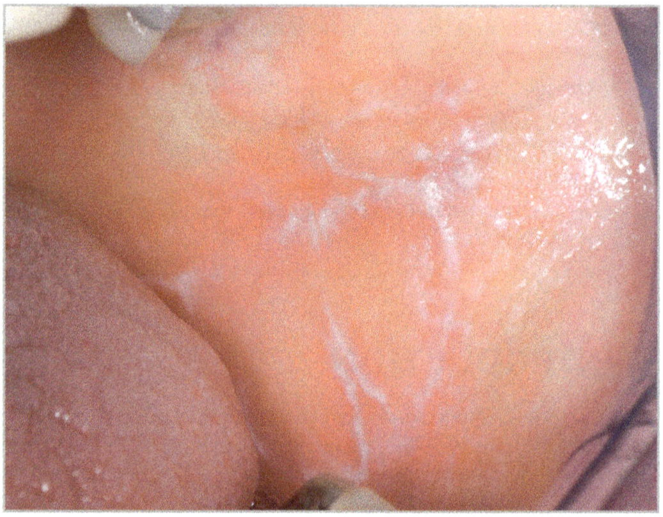

Figure 20.1 Typical Wickham striae in buccal lichen planus.

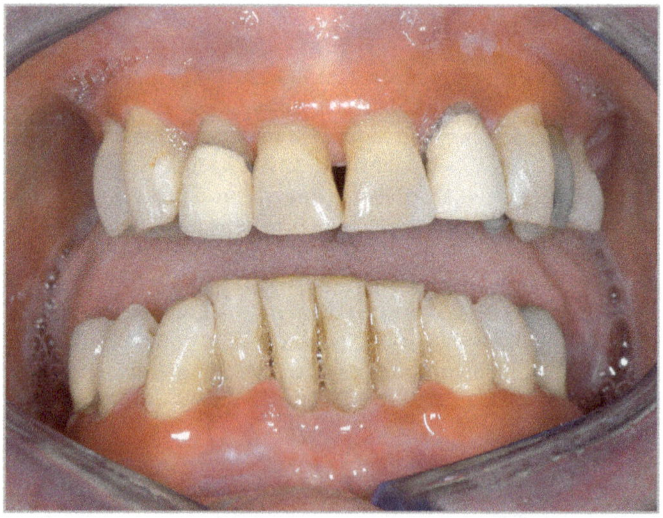

Figure 20.2 Desquamative gingivitis.

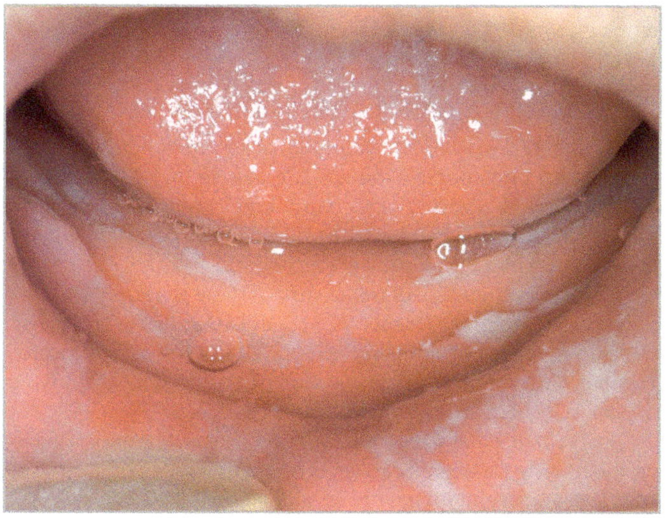

Figure 20.3 Erosive lesions in oral lichen planus with loss of teeth.

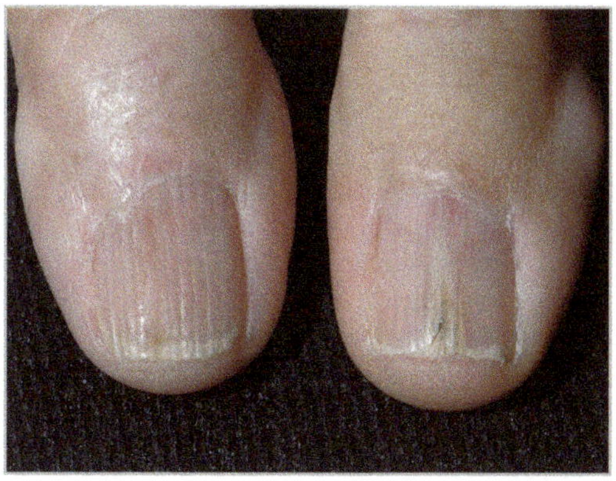

Figure 20.4 Longitudinal ridges or pterygium formation in lichen planus of the nails.

Clinical features of LP variants affecting the anogenital site

- **Classical** ('cutaneous' LP)
  Violaceous, flat-topped, itchy papules with whitish surface (Wickham striae) affecting the genitalia (labia majora and outer aspect labia minora)
- **Hypertrophic** ('verrucous' LP)
  Thick, very itchy, hyperkeratotic plaques with whitish surface (Wickham striae); occur over labia majora most frequently but can occur anywhere on the vulva
- **Lichen planopilaris** (LP of the hair-bearing site)
  Fine hyperkeratotic papules and erythema around the hair follicle, affecting the hair bearing aspects of the labia majora and the mons pubis, often leading to scarring alopecia
- **Atrophic/Erosive/Ulcerative** ('mucosal' LP)
  Glazed erythema, erosions or ulcers; commonly surrounded by a very fine white border usually painful, less itchy; at inner aspects of labia minora and vagina. Frequently results in scarring

Classical papulosquamous lichen planus

This is the most frequent form of lichen planus; but because it is usually self-limiting it is only rarely seen in specialist vulvar clinics. Patients with papulosquamous LP (**Figure 20.5**) usually complain of pruritus. Violaceous, polygonal, flat-topped papules may coalesce into plaques affecting labia majora, outer aspects of labia minora and the perianal area. Papules display white reticulations, the Wickham striae (Lewis 1998). It very often occurs in conjunction with episodes of cutaneous lichen planus at other sites, as well as reticulate oral LP. Although itch may be severe the disease is usually self-limiting and resolves after a few weeks or months. Rarely repeated episodes may be observed. No long term follow-up is required for this condition as there is no increased risk of malignant transformation with this type of lichen planus.

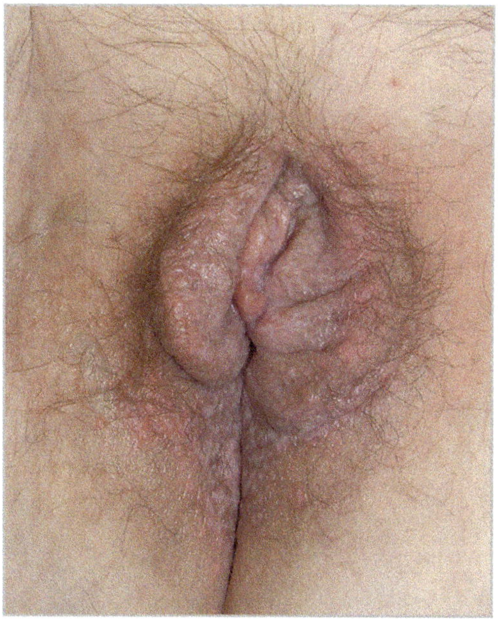

Figure 20.5 Classical papulosquamous lichen planus.

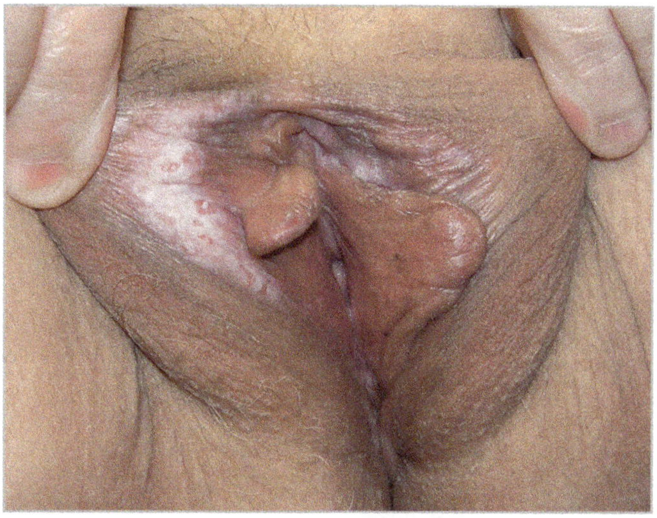

Figure 20.6 Hypertrophic lichen planus of the right labium.

Hypertrophic lichen planus

This variant is also called LP verrucosus. Small papular lesions coalesce to form thick white plaques over the vulva, similar to hypertrophic lesions seen on the shins although the lesions in the vulvar site are rarely violaceous (**Figure 20.6**). Hypertrophic LP is often intensely itchy and sore and the lesions may become more prominent with scratching (Köbner phenomenon). This type of lichen planus has a tendency to recur. It must be distinguished from vulvar intraepithelial neoplasia or malignancy and biopsy is essential (Lewis 1998).

Lichen planopilaris

In lichen planopilaris hair follicles are affected, it is also called follicular LP. It is usually seen on the scalp (**Figure 20.7**) but hair-bearing sites of the vulva including the mons pubis (**Figure 20.8**) and the outer surfaces of the labia majorae, buttocks and other body sites may be affected. Multiple keratotic plugs at the follicle opening and perifollicular violaceous erythema are observed. Itch and soreness are the main symptoms but often patients will be aware of a roughness of the skin and a prickly feeling when sitting. There is often scarring with permanent loss of hair. Some patients may get repeated attacks. It may occur in association with other types of lichen planus (Grunald 1998).

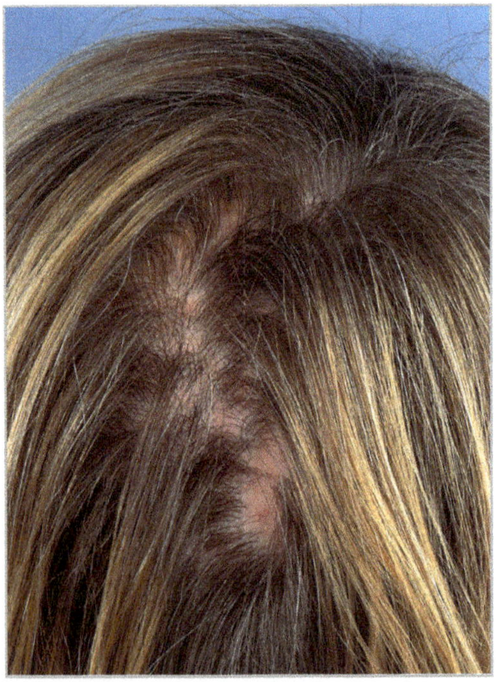

Figure 20.7 Scarring alopecia of the scalp in lichen planus.

'Erosive' mucosal lichen planus

Most women present with symptoms of severe pain, dysuria and soreness on intercourse although intercourse may be impossible due to pain and scarring of the vulva and vagina; pruritus is less frequently reported. Erosions are not seen in all patients with mucosal LP, they may develop but are secondary. Thus the term erosive, as this form is often called, is inaccurate. There is usually a sharply demarcated erythema (**Figure 20.9**) or erosion (**Figure 20.10**) over the inner aspects of the labia minora and vestibule or introitus vaginae. The erythema or erosions are often edged by a lacy white border, Wickham striae.

The erythema may have a glistening appearance, termed a glazed erythema (**Figure 20.9**). Scarring is frequently seen in mucosal LP with loss and agglutination of the labia minora possibly leading to midline fusion with loss of the clitoral hood and narrowing of the vaginal introitus in vulvar involvement (**Figure 20.10 and 20.11**). A severe complication is complete fusion of the labia minora.

There may be perianal involvement showing erythema with a whitish reticulate surface, erosions, or scarring possibly leading to anal stenosis (**Figure 20.12**) (Cooper 2006).

The vagina is affected in up to 70% of the reported cases of vulvar LP. Patients often report of vaginal discharge which may be bloody or mucopurulent or bleeding at intercourse; this is very distressing and may cause a great deal of discomfort to the patient. The prevalence of vaginal lichen planus may have been underestimated as the vagina is not always examined due to pain (Helgesen 2010). Sometimes examination and biopsies of the vagina must be done under general anesthesia. Typical features in vaginal LP include erythema, erosions and ulceration of the vaginal mucosa possibly bleeding on touching or a desquamative vaginitis (**Figure 20.13**).

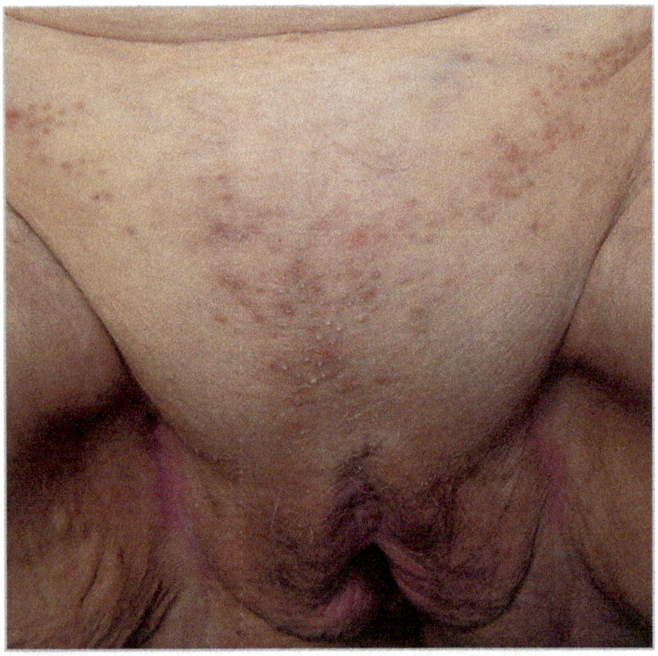

Figure 20.8 Scarring alopecia of the mons pubis in lichen planus.

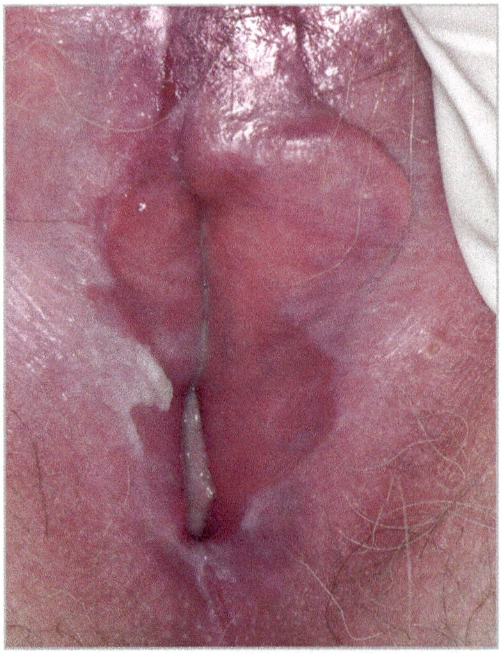

Figure 20.9 Sharply demarcated erythema with white hyperkeratotic border.

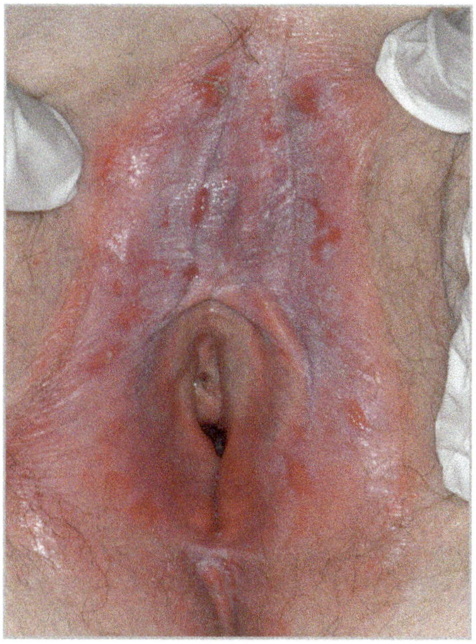

Figure 20.10 Erosive lichen planus of the vulva before treatment.

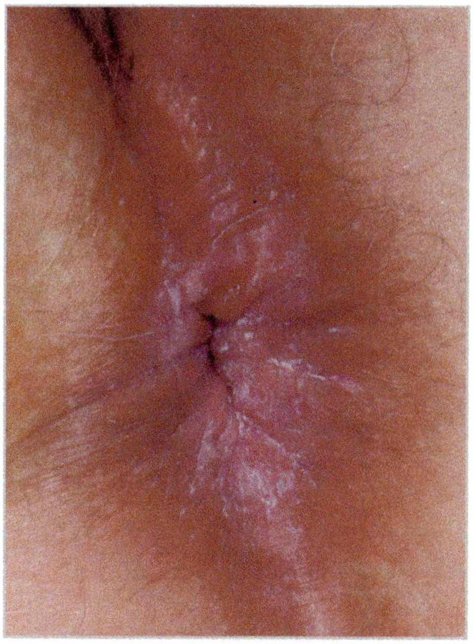

Figure 20.12 Perianal involvement showing pallor.

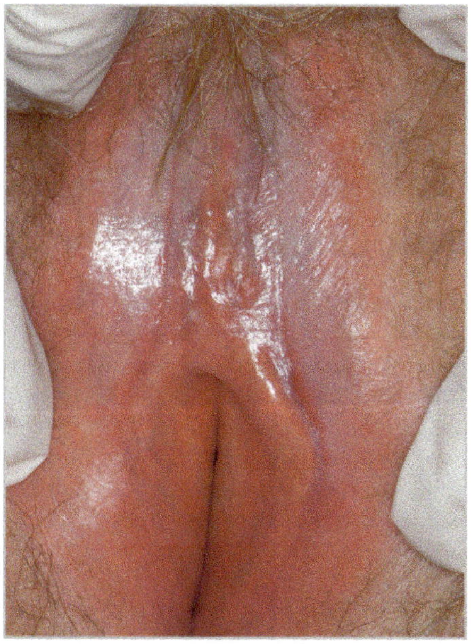

Figure 20.11 Erosive lichen planus in the same patient as Figure 20.10 three months after treatment with prednisolone and cyclosporine.

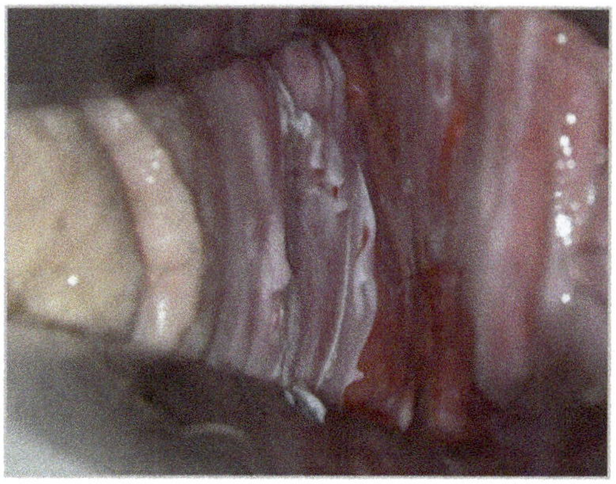

Figure 20.13 Desquamative vaginitis in vaginal lichen planus.

The whole vagina may not be involved but more usually there is a patchy erythema with areas of normal mucosa. Scarring may occur with adhesions and shortening of the vagina with almost total obliteration of the vaginal cavity in severe cases. Annular rings of narrowing may be observed.

If the vulva, vagina and gingiva are affected by erythematous or erosive LP it is called the **vulvovaginal-gingival syndrome**. Pelisse et al. first described in 1982 that LP often occurs simultaneously at those three mucosal sites (Pelisse 1982). It tends to be more chronic and severe than other forms of LP.

'Erosive' mucosal LP can be a difficult diagnosis to make and correlation between the clinical features and histopathology is necessary. A diagnostic data set has been agreed for diagnosis. A diagnosis of vulvar LP involving the mucosal site requires 3 out of the 9 following criteria (Simpson 2013):

Diagnostic criteria for mucous membrane/erosive vulvar lichen planus

1. Presence of well demarcated erosions or glazed erythema at the introitus
2. Presence of a hyperkeratotic white border to erythematous areas/erosions (Wickham striae)
3. Symptoms of pain/burning
4. Scarring/loss of normal architecture
5. Presence of vaginal inflammation
6. Involvement of other mucosal sites
7. Presence of a well-defined inflammatory band in the superficial connective tissue involving the dermo-epidermal junction
8. Presence of an inflammatory band that consists predominantly of lymphocytes
9. Signs of basal layer degeneration e.g. Civatte bodies, abnormal keratinocytes or basal apoptosis

HISTOPATHOLOGY

Key points

- Clinical and pathological correlation is essential
- The biopsy has to be taken from a longstanding, typical lesion
- In erythematous/erosive disease biopsy the edge (white rim) of a lesion not the centre
- In erosive disease don't expect the biopsy to be fully diagnostic

Despite its different clinical manifestations, the histopathology of LP is fairly uniform (**Figure 20.14** and **20.15**).

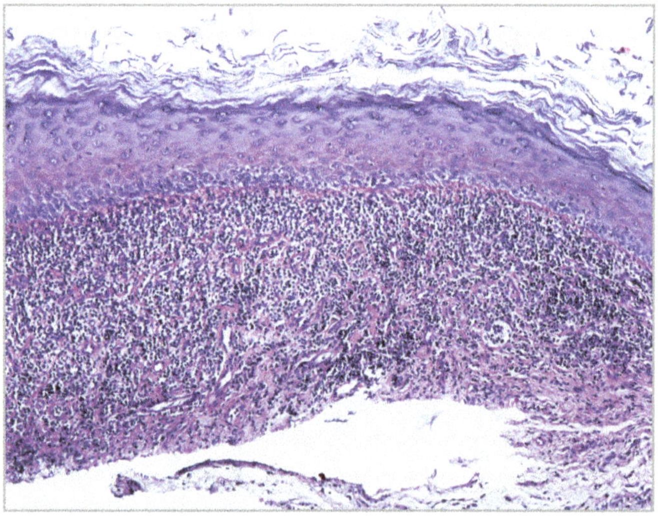

Figure 20.14 Histology of vulvar lichen planus showing hyperkeratosis, an atrophic epidermis with loss of rete ridges, hypergranulosis, basal cell vacuolization and a dense band-like infiltrate of lymphocytes hugging the basal layer.

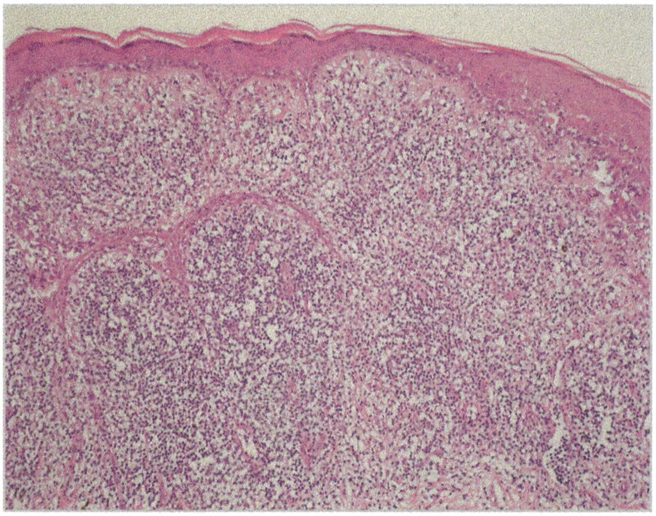

Figure 20.15 Histology of highly active vulvar lichen planus showing hyperkeratosis, hypergranulosis, pointed rete ridges, a dense lichenoid lymphocytic infiltrate along the basement membrane producing a vacuolar interphase dermatitis (courtesy of Sigrid Regauer, Graz, Austria).

Key histopathological features of lichen planus

- Hyperkeratosis (may be lacking in atrophic/erosive LP)
- Irregular acanthosis (pointed rete ridges/'sawtooth' appearance; may be lacking in atrophic/erosive LP)
- Wedge-shaped hypergranulosis
- Liquefactive/vacuolar degeneration of the basal layer
- Band-like infiltrate of lymphocytes hugging the basal layer
- Scattered Civatte/Colloid bodies (apoptotic or dyskeratotic keratinocytes)

In lichen planopilaris the inflammatory infiltrate extends around the hair follicles involving the infundibulum and the isthmus of the follicle. Lost follicles are replaced by linear tracts of fibrosis.

However, in **mucosal erythemous/erosive LP** histology may not be straight forward. The characteristic band-like inflammatory infiltrate is usually present, but it does not always have features such as pointed rete ridges, wedge-shaped hypergranulosis and cytoid bodies as observed in non-vulvar sites (Niamh 2009) (**Figure 20.14**). Plasma cells may be observed, a common feature of mucosa; if they are numerous other differential diagnoses must be considered. Histopathology should be considered as one component of the diagnosis and clinical-pathological correlation is essential. Furthermore, early lichen sclerosus and lichen planus may be indistinguishable histologically. Hyalanisation is characteristic of lichen sclerosus, however, may occasionally be seen in LP.

DIFFERENTIAL DIAGNOSES

The main differential diagnosis is vulvar lichen sclerosus (LS) (**Table 20.2**) which shares some clinical and histopathological features with lichen planus and early LS and LP can be hard to differentiate. There may be some pallor of the vulvar skin in LP but the ivory atrophic changes typical of lichen sclerosus are not observed. Ecchymoses seen commonly in lichen sclerosus are rarely observed in lichen planus.

The two conditions can coexist, e.g. simultaneous occurrence of oral LP and genital LS. Some patients with lichen sclerosus can develop erosive lichen planus after many years of disease.

PRINCIPLES OF MANAGEMENT

- Confirm diagnosis
- Check for potential triggers
- Inform the patient about the chronic course of the condition in mucosal more than in cutaneous disease
- Soothing emollients and soap substitutes are advised, particularly in erosive disease
- Any fluid (urine, water etc.) on eroded areas is painful: prior to bathing/swimming/urination, protection of the site with a petroleum jelly or very greasy emollient can be helpful
- In general, therapeutic ointments appear to be better tolerated and are less likely to cause allergy
- Tight clothing and other sources of mechanical irritation should be avoided

Table 20.2 Differential diagnosis of vulvar lichen planus

Differential diagnosis	Diagnostic test
Lichen sclerosus	Biopsy
Graft versus Host Disease (GvHD)	History (histology similar to LP)
(Autoimmune) bullous disease	Biopsy, DIF, IIF
Lupus erythematosus	Other sites?, biopsy, DIF, ANA
Inverse psoriasis	Other sites?, history, biopsy
Plasma cell vulvitis/Zoon disease	Histology similar to LP; but increased numbers of plasma cells
Behçet disease	History, clinical (other sites?)
Granulomatous vulvitis, e.g. Crohn disease	History, bowel disease?, biopsy
Erythema multiforme/TEN	History, clinical picture, biopsy
Fixed/lichenoid-drug eruption	History, biopsy, allergy test
Eczema (irritant, allergic, seborrheic)	History, biopsy, allergy test
Lichen simplex	Clinical picture: unilateral, biopsy
Squamous hyperplasia	Biopsy
Vulvar intraepithelial neoplasia	Biopsy
Squamous cell carcinoma	Biopsy
Paget disease	Biopsy
Infections	Swab (bacterial, viral, fungal)
Trauma	History
ANA, anti-nuclear antibodies; DIF, direct immunofluorescence; IIF, indirect immunofluorescence.	

TREATMENT

- **Classical and hypertrophic** LP are usually well treated with a potent or very potent topical steroid ointment daily for about 8 weeks and then as required next to an emollient. In troublesome hyperkeratotic plaques intra-lesional steroid injections with triamcinolone may be helpful; a topical steroid under occlusion, helpful at other sites, is unpractical at the vulva. An oral retinoid, e.g. acitretin 10-30mg/d, may help to thin plaques but must be used with caution in erosive disease because an adverse effect of acitretin is skin fragility which may worsen erosions. Retinoids have a high teratogenic potential, they should be avoided or only used with effective contraception in fertile women.
- **Vulvar lichen planopilaris** may be part of more widespread LP affecting the scalp and other body areas. Topical potent steroids may help reduce inflammation and may reduce scarring alopecia.
- **Erosive mucosal LP** is the most challenging form of LP to treat; but there is no reliable treatment advice possible as good studies are lacking (Cheng 2012 , Davari P et al. 2014, Simpson R et al. 2016). **Table 20.3** outlines the treatment of mucosal lichen planus.

Topical treatments

Treatment regimens with very potent topical steroids were adopted from treatment for lichen sclerosus. However, there is no overwhelming evidence for the efficacy of a single treatment, including topical steroids which are the widely accepted first-line therapy for mucosal erosive LP. Topical calcineurin inhibitors seem as effective as topical

Table 20.3 Treatment of mucosal lichen planus: there are only two randomized controlled trials (RCT) for vulvar LP (Rajar 2008, Helgesen 2015)

	Treatment modality	Main adverse effects	Evidence level/grade of recommendation
Topical steroids	Clobetasol propionate 0.05% ointment	Candidosis, skin atrophy	RCT oral: 1+ Case series vulvar: 3/D
	Triamcinolone acetonide 0.1% paste (e.g.)	Candidosis, skin atrophy	
	Topical steroids in oral LP	Candidiasis	RCT oral: 1+
Topical calcineurin inhibitors	Cyclosporine 1.5% gel	Oral application: skin rashes, parotid swelling, dyspepsia	RCT oral: 1- Case series vulvar: 3/D
	Tacrolimus 0.1% ointment	Burning	
	Pimecrolimus 1% cream	Transient burning	
Other topical preparations	Mesalazine gel 5%		RCT oral: 1-
	Aloe vera gel	Mild stinging	RCT oral/vulvar: 1+/B
Systemic treatment	Prednisolone 15mg/d	Typical steroid adverse effects	RCT oral
	Levamisol 150mg/d plus oral steroids	Mild gastrointestinal effects	3/D
	Hydroxychloroquine	Gastrointestinal effects, ophthalmopathy	3/D
	Mycophenolate mofetil	Bone marrow suppression	3/D
	Methotrexate 7.5 mg/wk, plus topical steroids/tacrolimus after vaginal adhesiolysis	Bone marrow suppression, hepatotoxicity	Case series vulvar: 3/D
	Cyclosporine 2–3 mg/kg/d	Hypertension, nephrotoxicity	3/D
Surgery	Vulvar/vaginal adhesiolysis in conjunction with anti-inflammatory treatment	Re-occurrence of adhesions	Case reports: 3/D
Photodynamic therapy (PDT)	Hexyl-5-aminolevulinate PDT	Soreness, vaginal bleeding	RCT vulval: 1+/B
Ongoing trials	Amevive (Alefacept) vs placebo		
	Topical sirolimus and petrolatum in orabase (Rapamune) 1 mg/ml bid 3 months vs topical betamethasone 0.05% in orabase and phosal (Diprolene) bid		
	Quercetin (flavonoid anti-inflammatory and antioxidant action) vs placebo		
Consult local guidelines for adverse reactions. Evidence levels and grade of recommendations are given according to GRADE (http://www.gradeworkinggroup.org/)			

steroids; topical aloe vera gel is more likely to reduce pain compared to placebo in oral LP. Several adverse effects of topical treatments are reported, but none are serious.

The following regimens are practiced:

- Super potent **topical steroid** such as clobetasol propionate 0.05% ointment, weaker steroids may be as effective, applied once or twice daily for 3 months initially. Maintenance treatment may consist of twice weekly topical steroid ointment, stepping up to daily treatment for a few days at a time if symptoms return.
- **Topical tacrolimus** 0.1% ointment (alternatively 0.03% or pimecrolimus 1%) twice daily for 4–12 weeks is useful in some patients. However, topical tacrolimus stings and may therefore not be tolerated.
- A **combination** of topical clobetasol propionate 0.05% ointment simultaneously applied with tacrolimus 0.1% ointment (a combination preparation is available in some countries) once or twice daily for at least 4 weeks is better tolerated; if this regimen is more effective than single preparations needs to be proven. Once the symptoms improve the application will be tapered to once daily application for a few weeks aiming for twice weekly maintenance treatment with either tacrolimus or steroid ointment.

The carcinogenic potential of topical tacrolimus is a matter of debate. This is a theoretical risk but the clinical evidence is not supportive of an increased risk of malignancies in vulvar LP after treatment with topical calcineurin inhibitors. However, there are several reports of the occurrence of herpes simplex infections after topical tacrolimus treatment. A careful history has to be taken and treatment interrupted if clinical signs of a viral infection arise.

Systemic treatments

Vulvar erosions may be so painful that topical application of ointments is not possible. In these cases a short course of oral prednisolone over three weeks can be helpful to reduce inflammation allowing topical treatment to be commenced. Some clinicians will use a slow release injection of steroid instead. Several systemic treatments including azathioprine, dapsone, griseofulvin, chloroquine, fumarate, anti-inflammatory acting tetracyclines (minocycline, doxycycline), low dose methotrexate, mycophenolate mofetil, azathioprin and alitretinoin are all tried empirically in the vulvovaginal-gingival syndrome (Bradford 2013). Biological agents, namely basiliximab, a monoclonal antibody against interleukin-2 receptor (CD25) and rituximab, which depletes CD20+B cells, are reported to be effective in erosive LP (Rebora 2002, Heelan 2015). Vulvovaginal photodynamic therapy was was more effective after 24 weeks than topical steroids in a randomized trial of 40 women (Helgesen 2015).

- **Oral steroids** are used, for example prednisolone 40 mg/day, tapered off over a few weeks; courses can be repeated as necessary for severe flares.
- **Oral cyclosporine** 2-3 mg/kg/day may be considered for severe flares; side effects usually prohibit long term use.
- **Oral methotrexate,** typically 10–15 mg per week for severe disease may be tried.

Vaginal lichen planus

Early detection and treatment of vaginal LP is recommended to try reducing the risk of vaginal scarring which can progress quickly. There are no licensed treatments for vaginal LP and the choice of treatment depends on what is available and whether a pharmacist will compound treatments. Treatment options include steroid foam such as hydrocortisone acetate foam or prednisolone foam, as used for rectal disease in inflammatory bowel disease, vaginal steroid tablets and pessaries.

One possible regime is to use steroid foam inserted into the vagina on alternate nights just as retiring to bed. Another option is to coat a vaginal tampon generously with clobetasol propionate 0.05% or tacrolimus 0.1% ointment nightly for 4 weeks.

Maintenance treatment with vaginal steroid or tacrolimus for example weekly or fortnightly application may be necessary. However, consideration must be given to bone protection as significant absorption of vaginal steroid may occur. Once ulcers and erosions are healed it is important to use vaginal dilators or have intercourse regularly to reduce the risk of vaginal narrowing.

Surgical intervention

This is sometimes necessary to treat adhesions, however, they may reoccur (Fairchield 2015). If a surgical intervention is decided for it should be performed in a phase with little inflammation. After the procedure anti-inflammatory treatment, e.g. topical steroids, topical tacrolimus possibly combined with or methotrexate, should follow a few days after the operation to prevent immediate re-adhesion. If there is any suspicion of infection it is necessary to use intra-vaginal clindamycin or other appropriate anti-infective treatment.

COURSE AND PROGNOSIS

Classical LP tends to be self-limiting although it can reoccur (**Table 20.4**); hypertrophic LP is more treatment resistant. Lichen planopilaris often leads to scarring alopecia, early treatment may prevent this, however, it may relapse. Erosive disease, usually at mucosal sites, tends to be more treatment resistant and persistent although some relief in symptoms can be expected in the majority of patients any scaring will persist. Malignant transformation is seldom but described (Simpson 2012, Regauer 2014).

Table 20.4 Complications of mucosal vulvar lichen planus and its treatment

Complication	Frequency of occurrence
Scarring with architectural distortion	+++
Dys-/apareunia	++
Dysaesthetic pain	++
Dysuria/urinary retention	+
Psychosexual	++
Infection	+
Allergic contact dermatitis	+
Malignancy	+/-

REFERENCES

Bradford J, Fischer G. Management of vulvovaginal lichen planus: a new approach. J Low Genit Tract Dis 2013;17:28–32.

Cheng S, Kirtschig G, Cooper S, et al. Interventions for erosive lichen planus affecting mucosal sites. Cochrane Database Syst Rev 2012;2:CD008092

Clayton R, Chaudhry S, Ali I, Cooper S, Hodgson T, Wojnarowska F. Mucosal (oral and vulval) lichen planus in women: are angiotensin-converting enzyme inhibitors protective, and beta-blockers and non-steroidal anti-inflammatory drugs associated with the condition? Clin Exp Dermatol 2010;35:384–387.

Cooper SM, Kirtschig G, Jeffery KJ, Wojnarowska F. No association between hepatitis B or C viruses and vulval lichen planus in a UK population. BJOG 2004;111:271–273.

Cooper SM, Dean D, Allen J, Kirtschig G, Wojnarowska F. Erosive lichen planus of the vulva: weak circulating basement membrane zone antibodies are present. Clin Exp Dermato 2005;30:551–556.

Cooper SM, Wojnarowska F. Influence of treatment of erosive lichen planus of the vulva on its prognosis. Arch Dermatol 2006;142:289–294.

Cooper SM, Ali I, Baldo M, Wojnarowska F. The association of lichen sclerosus and erosive lichen planus of the vulva with autoimmune disease: a case control study. Arch Dermatol 2008;144:1432–1435.

Davari P, Hsiao HH, Fazel N. Mucosal lichen planus: an evidence-based treatment update. Am J Clin Dermatol 2014;15:181–195.

Fairchield PS, Haefner HK. Surgical management of vulvovaginal agglutination due to lichen planus. Am J Obstet Gynecol 2015 [Epub ahead of print].

Grunald MH, Zvulunov A, Halevy S. Lichen planopilaris of the vulva. Br J Dermatol 1998;136:477–478.

Heelan K, McAleer MA, Roche L, et al. Intractable erosive lichen planus treated successfully with rituximab. Br J Dermatol 2015; 172:538–540.

Helgesen AL, Gjersvik P, Jebsen P, Kirschner R, Tanbo T. Vaginal involvement in genital erosive lichen planus. Acta Obstet Gynecol Scand. 2010;89:966–970.

Helgesen AL, Warloe T, Pripp AH, et al. Vulvovaginal photodynamic therapy vs. topical corticosteroids in genital erosive lichen planus: a randomized controlled trial. Br J Dermatol 2015 [Epub ahead of print]

Kirtschig G, Brink AA, Scheper RJ, Jaspars EH. No oncogenic mucosal human papillomaviruses in erosive vulval lichen planus. Br J Dermatol 2005;152:1367–1368.

Kirtschig G, Wakelin SH, Wojnarowska F. Mucosal vulval lichen planus: outcome, clinical and laboratory features. J Europ Acad Dermatol Venereol 2005;19:301–307.

Lewis FM, Shah M, Harrington CI. Vulval involvment in lichen planus: a study of 37 women. Br J Dermatol 1996;135:89–91.

Lewis F. Vulval lichen planus. Br J Dermatol 1998;138:569–575.

Lundqvist EN, Wahlin YB, Bergdahl M, Bergdahl J. Psychological health in patients with genital and oral erosive lichen planus. J Eur Acad Dermatol Venereol 2006;20:661–666.

McPherson T, Cooper S. Vulval lichen sclerosus and Lichen planus. Dermatol Ther 2010;23:523–532.

Niamh L, Naveen S, Hazel B Diagnosis of vulval inflammatory dermatoses: A pathological study with clinical correlation. Int J Gynecol Pathol 2009;28:554–558.

Pandhi D, Singal A, Bhattacharya SN. Lichen planus in childhood: a series of 316 patients. Pediatr Dermatol 2014; 31:59–67.

Pelisse M, Leibowitch M, Sedel D, Hewitt J. [A new vulvovaginogingival syndrome. Plurimucous erosive lichen planus]. [Article in French] Ann Dermatol Venereol 1982;109:797–798.

Rajar UD, Majeed R, Parveen N, Sheikh I, Sushel C. Efficacy of aloe vera gel in the treatment of vulval lichen planus. J Coll Physicians Surg Pak. 2008;18:612-614.

Rebora A, Parodi A, Murialdo G. Basiliximab is effective for erosive lichen planus. Arch Dermatol 2002;138:1100–1101.

Regauer S, Reich O, Eberz B. Vulvar cancers in women with vulvar lichen planus: a clinicopathological study. J Am Acad Dermatol 2014; 71:698–707.

Santegoets LA, Helmerhorst TJ, van der Meijden WI. A retrospective study of 95 women with a clinical diagnosis of genital lichen planus. J Low Genit Tract Dis 2010;14:323–328.

Setterfield JF, Neill S, Shirlaw PJ, et al. The vulvovaginal gingival syndrome: a severe subgroup of lichen planus with characteristic clinical features and a novel association with the class II HLA DQB10201 allele. J Am Acad Dermatol 2006;55:98–113.

Simpson RC, Murphy R. Is vulval erosive lichen planus a premaligant condition? Arch Dermatol 2012;148:1314–1316.

Simpson RC, Thomas KS, Leighton P, Murphy R. Diagnostic criteria for erosive lichen planus affecting the vulva: an international electronic-Delphi consensus exercise. Br J Dermatol 2013;169:337–343.

Simpson RC, Murphy R, Bratton DJ, et al. Systemic therapy for vulval erosive lichen planus (the 'hELP' trial): study protocol for a randomised controlled trial. Trials 2016; 17:2.

Terlou A, Santegoets LA, van der Meijden WI, et al. An autoimmune phenotype in vulvar lichen sclerosus and lichen planus: a Th1 response and high levels of microRNA-155. J Invest Dermatol 2012;132:658–666.

Chapter 21 Plasma cell vulvitis

Anne Lise Ording Helgesen

Synonyms

Zoon vulvitis, vulvitis circumscripta plasmacellularis

Key features

- A rare benign inflammatory condition
- Clinical findings: erythematous well-demarcated shiny red/brown patches over the inner aspects of the labia minora
- Symptoms: burning, dyspareunia, pain
- Diagnosis: take a biopsy to confirm the clinical diagnosis and exclude malignancy
- Treatment: potent topical steroids
- Prognosis: usually improvement after treatment, relapses possible

INTRODUCTION

Plasma cell balanitis was first described by J. J. Zoon in 1952 on the glans penis, and the female equivalent condition, plasma cell vulvitis, was described by Garnier in 1954 (Kyriakou et al. 2014). Only about 50 cases have been reported worldwide.

EPIDEMIOLOGY

Plasma cell vulvitis is a rare benign inflammatory condition, mostly seen in adult women in the age group between 20 and 70 years, but most commonly in the postmenopausal woman.

PATHOGENESIS

The etiology is unknown. A number of suggested factors such as irritation from poor hygiene, sweating, trauma, and long-standing friction may play a role in the pathogenesis. Also viral, autoimmune, and hormonal factors may be involved.

CLINICAL FEATURES

The clinical findings include erythematous well-circumscribed shiny non-scaly patches over the inner aspects of the vulva, most often in the vestibule and periurethral epithelium; the vagina may also be involved (**Figure 21.1**).

The lesions are sometimes erosive and have a shiny, deep red, or brownish-colored surface due to hemosiderin deposits. Some lesions are asymptomatic but usually give symptoms of tenderness, burning, pain, dyspareunia, and sometimes pruritus (Virgili et al. 2008).

INVESTIGATIONS

A biopsy should always be taken to confirm the diagnosis and especially to exclude malignancies.

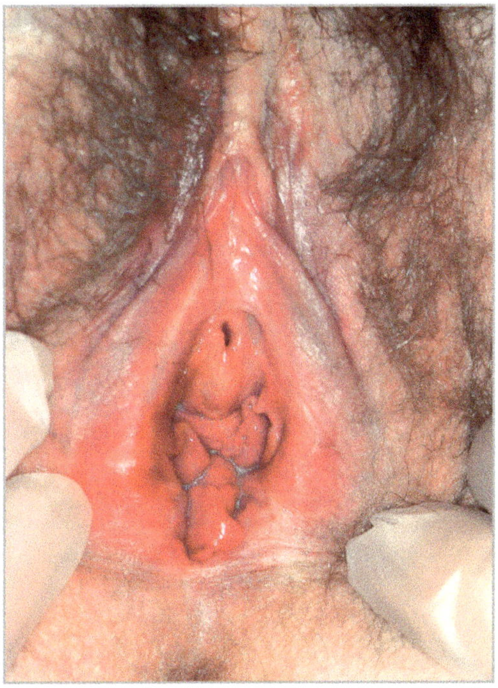

Figure 21.1 Typical clinical appearance of red/brown shiny patches at the inner aspects of the labia minora and entrance to the vagina.

HISTOPATHOLOGY

An attenuated epidermis and a dense band-like infiltrate in the upper and mid-dermis with mostly plasma cells (>50% is diagnostic) are typical. The epidermis may be ulcerated. Additional features include vascular proliferation, hemosiderin deposition, and erythrocyte extravasations (**Figure 21.2**).

DIFFERENTIAL DIAGNOSIS

Many of the clinical findings in plasma cell vulvitis are indistinguishable from those found in erosive/mucosal lichen planus, and some authors suggest it is the same disease (Virgili et al. 2008).

High-grade squamous intraepithelial lesions of the vulva, differentiated vulvar intraepithelial neoplasia or squamous cell carcinoma, bullous mucous membrane disorders, melanoma, fixed drug eruption, herpes simplex, syphilis, and lichen sclerosus are other differential diagnoses to be considered. Women in the postmenopause may develop purpuric changes indistinguishable from plasma cell vulvitis, but these changes usually respond to local estrogen.

MANAGEMENT AND TREATMENT

Effective treatment is often difficult. As only case reports exist, no evidence-based treatment advice can be given. Various treatment modalities have been used, and the traditional first-line treatment

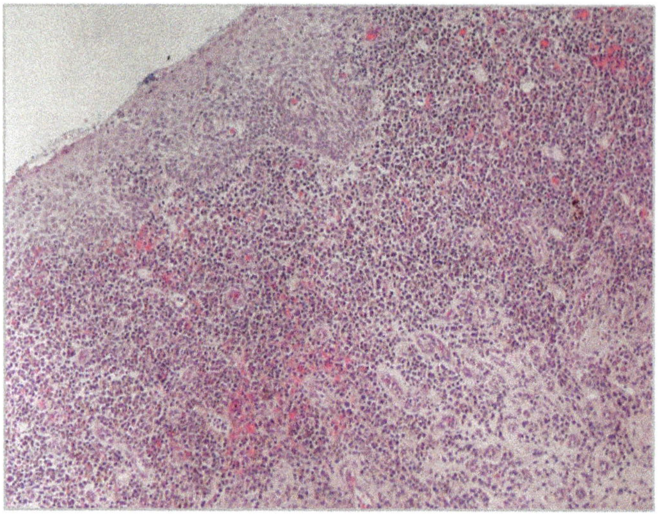

Figure 21.2 Dense band-like infiltrate of predominantly plasma cells within the superficial dermis. An increased number of blood vessels are also seen within the dermis as well as extravasated erythrocytes.

is high potent topical corticosteroid ointment or cream applied daily, sometimes for several months. Topical calcineurin inhibitors (pimecrolimus and tacrolimus), imiquimod, and estrogen (in postmenopausal women) have been used successfully, but skin irritation may be a limiting factor. Intralesional injections of steroids, retinoid therapy, interferon, surgical excision, electrocoagulation, and cryotherapy are also reported (Kyriakou et al. 2014).

COURSE AND PROGNOSIS

The lesions tend to heal slowly, often leaving a brownish rusty appearance in the involved area. Recurrence is common. Plasma cell vulvitis is regarded as a benign condition, with no malignant transformation.

REFERENCES

Kyriakou A, Patsatsi A, Patsialas C, Sotiriadis D.Therapeutic efficacy of topical calcineurin inhibitors in plasma cell balanitis: case series and review of the literature. Dermatology 2014; 228:18–23.

Virgili A, Mantovani L, Lauriola MM, Marzola A, Corazza M. Tacrolimus 0.1% ointment: is it really effective in plasma cell vulvitis? Report of four cases. Dermatology 2008; 216:243–246.

Chapter 22 Vulvar psoriasis

Michael Sticherling

Synonyms

Psoriasis vulgaris of inverse type, psoriasis of the folds, flexural psoriasis

Key features

- Psoriasis is a chronic inflammatory disease of cornifying skin, including the scalp, skin folds, and nails
- Mucous membrane involvement is still debated but may be underestimated or misinterpreted
- Genital manifestations are mostly non-characteristic, although a distinctly sharp delineation may be indicative
- The characteristic scaling is mostly missing at skin folds and mucous membranes, but involvement of other skin sites may be indicative of psoriasis
- Genital complaints should be sought by the physician as patients might not mention these due to embarrassment and possibly misinterpretation of symptoms

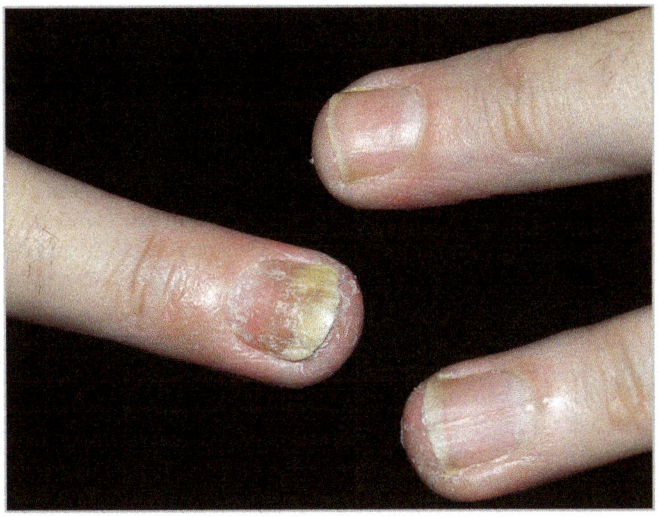

Figure 22.1 Psoriasis of the nails showing 'oil spots' and pitting of nails.

INTRODUCTION

Psoriasis is one of the most common chronic inflammatory skin diseases, which mostly affects the cornifying tissue of the body including the scalp and skin folds (Nestle et al. 2009). The disease may affect quality of life (Heller et al. 2012) and is often accompanied by comorbidities (Farley & Menter 2011). Severe itch is experienced by 60–70% of patients with psoriasis. Involvement of mucous membranes is still debated; however 'geographic' tongue and opalescent plaques of the mucous membranes are regarded as psoriatic manifestations at non-cornifying sites. The study of genital involvement has been neglected, and no good epidemiological or therapeutic data are available.

Physicians may overlook genital involvement as patients are often reluctant to report genital symptoms. Physicians may misdiagnose psoriasis in the genital site because the appearance may look different from psoriasis at other body sites. Inspection of the sites characteristically involved in psoriasis such as the elbows, knees, scalp, retroauricular, and lumbar regions as well as the umbilicus and gluteal crease is necessary if genital psoriasis is suspected (Farber & Nall 1992, Meeuwis et al. 2010, 2011a,b, 2012). There may be characteristic nail changes including nail plate grooves, oil patches, and nail dystrophy (**Figure 22.1**).

EPIDEMIOLOGY

The overall prevalence of psoriasis is estimated to be 2.5% in the Caucasian population but is rarer in Africans and Asians, with two peaks of onset around the third and around the fifth or sixth decade of life. Still, 20% of psoriatics will have their first signs before the age of 18. One-third of patients will have a single disease episode, but two thirds will have chronic disease. Clinical manifestations may vary over time and involve different body sites, though an increasing severity with increasing duration of disease episodes is not usual. Psoriatic arthritis, involving the joints (arthritis in the narrower sense, including distal finger joints, large joints, and/or axial spine), tendons (tendinitis), and their insertions (enthesitis) as well as fingers and toes (dactylitis), occurs after, on average, 10 years of skin involvement in about two-thirds of cases. Severe scalp and nail as well as skin fold involvement (psoriasis inversa) may indicate incipient psoriasis arthritis, although the overall disease severity of skin psoriasis is not related to the incidence of psoriatic arthritis. In fact, arthritis may appear without any prior skin involvement or may occur simultaneously, which is characteristic in juvenile psoriasis.

Vulvar involvement is estimated between 8% and 45% of psoriatic patients, the highest incidence was reported in a recent retrospective survey of members of the Dutch Psoriasis Society (Meeuwis et al. 2010). Three to five percent of patients may present with genital signs only; simultaneous involvement of other skin folds is found in two-thirds of patients with genital psoriasis. Accordingly, it is hypothesized that flexural and genital psoriasis present related, yet possibly separate 'entities.' Genital involvement can appear at any age (Kapila et al. 2012, van Eyk et al. 2009), although the cited Dutch study reported a mean age at first manifestation of 36 years and an interval between onset of psoriasis and onset of genital involvement of 8 years.

COMORBIDITIES

Another important issue is comorbidities with their incidence increased two to fivefold compared to the general population. Psoriasis is currently regarded as a systemic multiorgan inflammatory condition, not limited to the skin (Farley & Menter 2011).

Psoriasis

Psorisis is a condition associated with:

- Metabolic disorders, e.g. diabetes mellitus, hyperlipidemia, and hyperuricemia
- Cardiovascular disease, e.g. arterial hypertension and atherosclerosis
- Depression

PATHOGENESIS

Current evidence demonstrates that both the innate and specific immune systems are involved in pathogenesis. Psoriasis is regarded as a chronic inflammatory skin condition with involvement of sessile skin cells (keratinocytes) as well as migratory cells, prominently T lymphocytes and neutrophilic granulocytes. Some characteristics are shared with autoimmune disease; however, the one or possibly more pathogenetically relevant autoantigens remain to be found.

Various mediators including cytokines, namely, interleukin 2 (IL-2) and tumor necrosis factor alpha (TNF-α) as well as lipid mediators are involved. Currently, IL-23, TH17 cells and their secreted IL-17 is regarded as central to psoriasis pathogenesis underlined by dramatic clinical improvement upon use of specific therapeutic monoclonal antibodies (Nestle et al. 2009, Mease 2015).

Genetics

A genetic background is evident by frequent familial cases. If one parent is affected a child has a 30% chance of being affected, which rises to 60–70% if both parents have psoriasis. Recent genome wide association studies have broadened our genetic knowledge. Apart from human leukocyte antigens, especially Cw6, other genes coding for various inflammatory and immunological mediators of both the innate and adaptive immune system have been shown to play a role; however, no single one gene has been shown to be characteristic and specific for psoriasis. So far, there are no special clues with regard to the genetic background of genital psoriasis.

Environmental factors/triggers

In genetically predisposed individuals various environmental factors are suspected to trigger psoriasis, but only few have proven to be relevant triggers.

- Drugs
  - Beta-blockers, gold salts, antimalarials, and lithium
- Infections
  - Streptococcal as well as viral infections
- Psychological stress

If a drug is suspected to trigger psoriasis it should be replaced. Infections may cause seasonal peaks or exacerbation of psoriasis. Both inflammatory cytokines such as interferons induced during viral infections and streptococcal antigens have been experimentally shown to induce inflammation characteristic of psoriasis. For psychological stress no specific stressor is suspected to cause relapses or chronicity of psoriasis; it may be alleviated by individually adapted behavioral therapy. The question of whether psychological distress is a trigger or a consequence of psoriasis is still a matter of debate.

The well-known Köbner phenomenon, triggered by physical or chemical trauma, local irritation, or infections will result in psoriasis plaques at the exposed site within days to a few weeks. The Köbner phenomenon resulting from occlusion, humidity, or rubbing of underwear as well as local infections with bacteria or fungi may be a major cause of genital psoriasis in predisposed individuals. These factors should be avoided or reduced, and patients should be made aware of these. In addition, obesity may aggravate this phenomenon through increased occlusion and rubbing of skin folds though no relation of flexural psoriasis and increased body mass index was found.

CLINICAL PRESENTATION

General psoriasis manifestations

The term psoriasis comprises a group of clinically different signs and can be crudely separated into psoriasis vulgaris, with the often used, almost synonymous term plaque psoriasis, and pustular psoriasis. Eighty percent of psoriasis patients are plaque type, 20% show pustular features. Psoriatic scaling is white to silvery and firmly attached

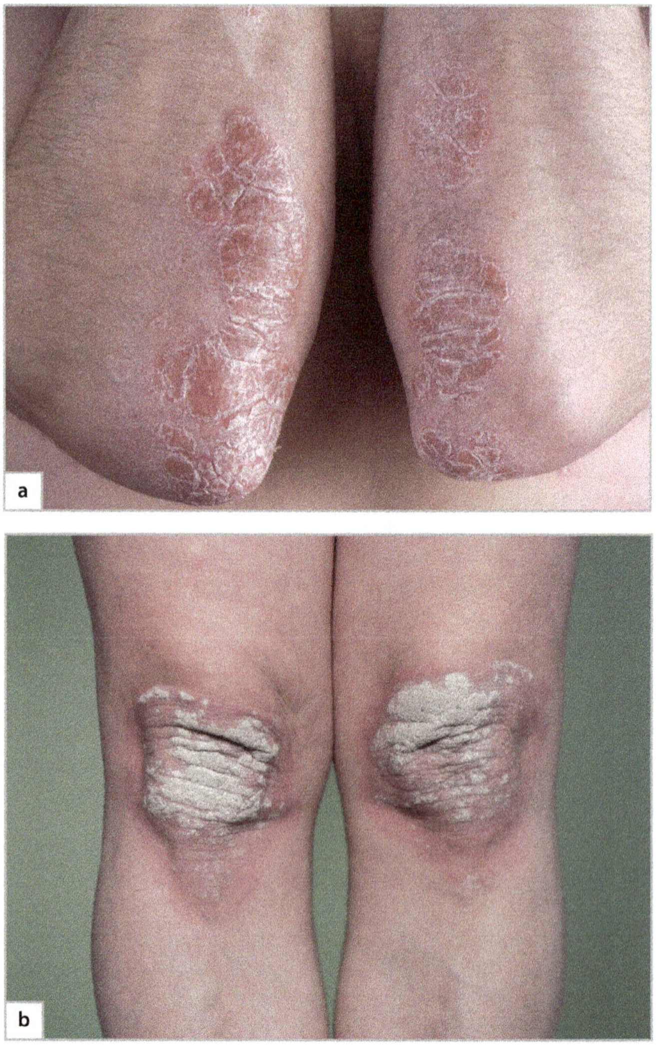

Figure 22.2 Typical scaly, erythematous lesions of (a) elbows and (b) knees in psoriasis.

(**Figure 22.2**) in contrast to eczematous scaling, which is finer and more loosely attached. Characteristic plaques are sharply demarcated and bright red in color. Guttate psoriasis (a form of psoriasis vulgaris) with multiple round to oval plaques of around 1 cm in diameter over trunk and limbs in exanthematous distribution is typically seen in childhood and adolescence following streptococcal infections of the upper airways.

Pustular psoriasis may involve only palms and soles (pustulosis palmoplantaris) or present with widespread and disseminated sterile pustules up to the maximal manifestation of von Zumbusch type pustular psoriasis seen in 2% of psoriasis cases.

In a subset of patients psoriasis is found at sites other than in the typical predilection sites, e.g. the face, palms and soles, axilla, groins as well as the perineal and genital area, this is referred to as inverse psoriasis (**Figures 22.3** and **22.4**). This group can further be subdivided into skin fold psoriasis or genital psoriasis whichever site is affected more prominently. However, all clinical forms of psoriasis may variably and individually be present next to each other or as single signs (Sticherling 2009).

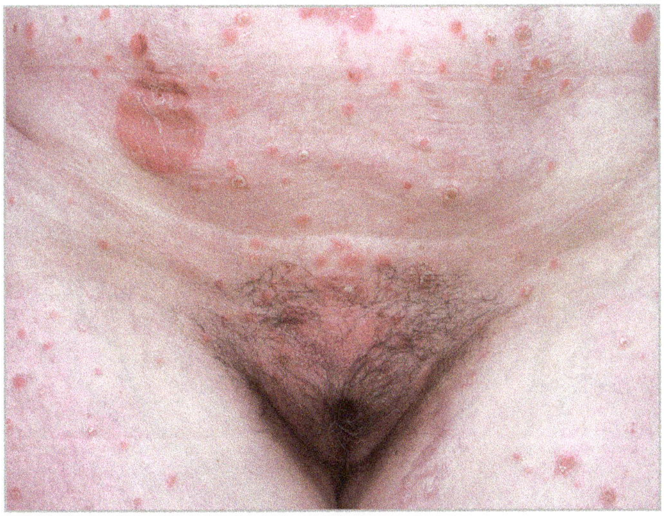

Figure 22.3 Genital psoriasis – plaques at the lower abdomen as well as genitally.

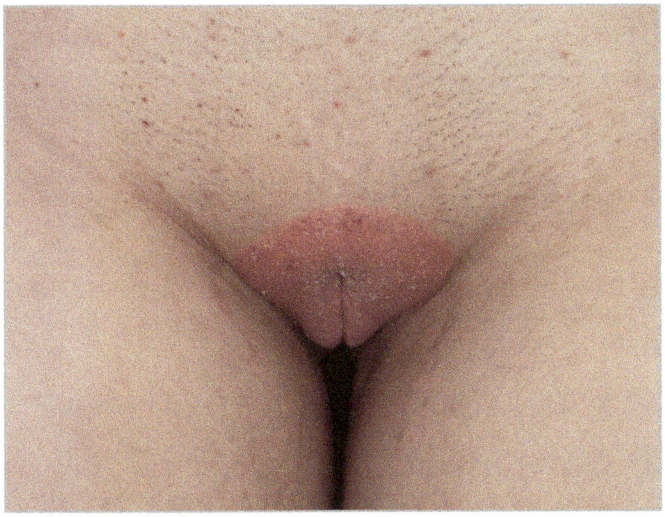

Figure 22.4 Genital psoriasis – sharply demarcated erythematous plaques.

Clinical signs typically seen in psoriasis

• Scalp	Well-demarcated redness and silvery scales, transgressing the hairline of scalp and forehead
• Nails	Pitting and 'oil spots' (subungual discoloration)
• Fissuring	Of folds, e.g. anal fold, interlabial sulci (**Figure 22.5**), back of ears
• Elbows and knees	Scaly plaques
• Auspitz phenomenon	Punctate bleeding upon scraping of a scale (see below)

Genital manifestations

Both plaque type and pustular psoriasis may occur in this site. The main symptoms are pruritus or pain and the effect on quality of life may be severe (Zamirska et al. 2008). Vulvar psoriasis is often symmetrical. It can vary from silvery scaling patches adjacent to the outer parts of the labia majora to moist grayish plaques or glossy red plaques without scaling in the skin folds. It may be non-specific in appearance; however, a sharply demarcated erythema is characteristic and should raise suspicion (**Figure 22.4**). In hairy areas erythematous, scaly papules and plaques are found but plaques on the labia are usually thin and moist, often without obvious scaling. The non-stratifying mucous membranes will show opalescent plaques or macules. A useful clinical sign is the Auspitz phenomenon that shows tiny punctate bleeding upon scraping of scaly psoriasis lesions. It is positive in many cases of genital psoriasis and should therefore be routinely examined for.

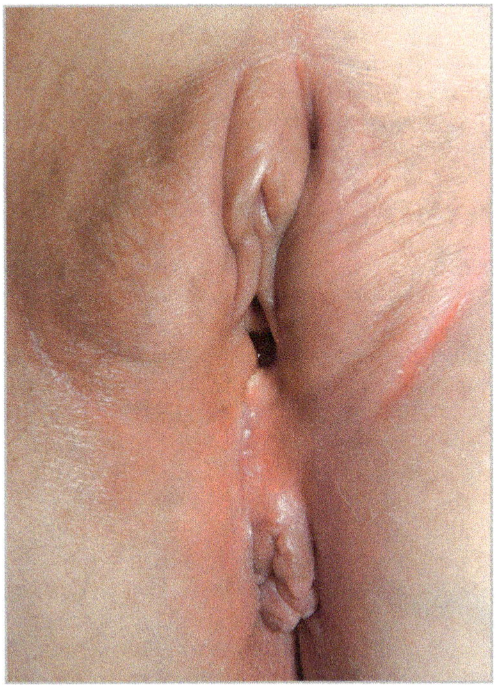

Figure 22.5 Psoriasis causing fissuring of folds. By courtesy of Dr Jennifer Yell, Manchester, United Kingdom.

Key features of genital psoriasis

Hairy sites (outer surface labia majora) • Sharply demarcated redness • Scaly papules and plaques • Whitish scales
Inner aspects of labia majora and labia minora • Thin, sharply demarcated redness • Moist surface • Fissuring of folds, e.g. sulcus interlabialis
Natal cleft and groins • Sharply demarcated erythema, fissures
Non-stratifying mucous membranes • Opalescent plaques or macules

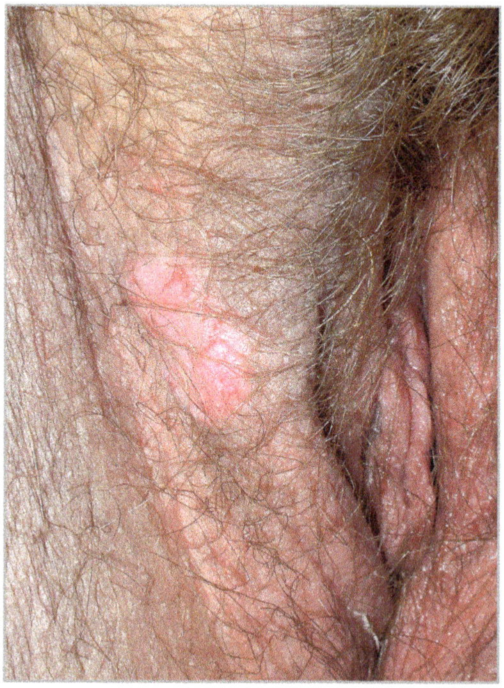

Figure 22.6 Vulvar eczema with partly oozing and scaly lesions.

INVESTIGATIONS

Biopsies are usually not needed but may be necessary to differentiate psoriasis, e.g. from eczema, lichen planus, and lichen sclerosus (LS), and Paget disease (Palamaras et al. 2006). Furthermore, microbiological examinations (skin swabs or examination of scales if present) should exclude bacterial, viral, or fungal infections.

HISTOPATHOLOGY

Histopathology of psoriasis is characteristic and distinguishes it from lichen planus and LS but may sometimes resemble eczema in psoriasiform dermatitis. Typically, the epidermis is thickened (acanthosis) with elongated lean papillae and shows disrupted keratinization with cell nuclei up to the stratum corneum (parakeratosis). Epidermal infiltration with lymphocytes and prominently neutrophilic granulocytes with the subcorneal accumulation as Munro abscesses is discriminative. In the dermis, papillae are elongated with capillary dilation and perivascular and periadnexal lymphohistiocytic infiltrates.

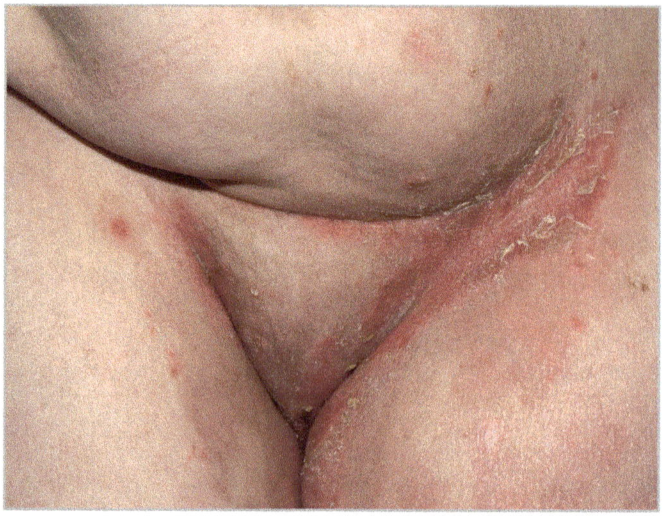

Figure 22.7 Seborrheic eczema of the vulva and groin.

DIFFERENTIAL DIAGNOSIS

A number of inflammatory conditions including acute and chronic atopic eczema (**Figure 22.6**), seborrheic eczema (**Figure 22.7**), contact dermatitis, infections (including syphilis and scabies), high-grade squamous intraepithelial lesions of the vulva, differentiated vulvar intraepithelial neoplasia, and Paget disease must be differentiated in the vulva (**Table 22.1**) (Andreassi & Bilenchi 2014).

Although itch may be present in both psoriasis and eczema, it is usually more severe in eczema (atopic, irritant, and allergic). A history and general inspection of the skin, possibly a skin biopsy or patch test, will help to differentiate.

Infections with yeasts or dermatophytes can be excluded by examining swabs or scales in culture or under the microscope. In *Candida* infections, satellites and follicular pustules around the immediate area of erythema are typically seen, but response to treatment with topical corticosteroids is unsatisfactory. Especially in cases of pustular genital psoriasis, herpes simplex infection should be excluded, though herpes simplex infection is usually more acute, painful, and transient.

Differential diagnoses may, however, be hampered by superinfection of psoriasis, which is common at this site.

Long-standing chronic inflammatory plaques resistant to anti-inflammatory treatment should be biopsied to exclude squamous cell carcinoma. Extramammary Paget disease is usually refractory or only partially responsive to topical corticosteroids.

MANAGEMENT AND TREATMENT

General care

- Treatment should start with education about good vulvar care including avoidance of soaps and inappropriate products. Atraumatic cleansing using fragrance-free liquid soaps or soap substitutes such as oils or emollients and careful drying is advised

Table 22.1 Criteria for the differential diagnoses and key features

Disease	Itch	Erythema	Scaling	Demarcation	Diagnostic clues
Psoriasis	Moderate	Bright to dull	Absent Silvery, attached	Sharp	Extragenital sites: scalp, nails, elbows/knees
Seborrheic dermatitis	Moderate	Yellowish	Yellowish, greasy	Not as sharp	Eye brows, nasolabial folds, scalp, V-area trunk
Allergic contact eczema	Severe	Bright	Absent, fine, loosely attached	Diffuse	History of allergies?
Irritant contact eczema	Severe	Variable	Absent or very fine	Not as sharp	Washing habits, other irritants?
Candida infection	Severe	Intense	Not usually	Diffuse to sharp, satellites	Islands of white pustules with glazed appearance
Lichen planus	Severe	Violaceous papules or glazed erythema	None	Variable, rather sharp	Extragenital sites, oral, and nail changes
Lichen sclerosus	Severe	Red, may resemble eczema	None	Not as sharp	Possibly scarring, itch
Neoplasia	Mild	Mild to severe	Possible but not typical	Sharp	Recent development
Paget disease	Possible	Mild to severe	Variable	Rather sharp	Asymmetrical

- Local irritating factors like tight clothing should be avoided; loosely fitting non-occlusive underwear (preferably cotton or silk) and its daily change are recommended (Beecker 2013, Goldnau et al. 2010)
- Emollients moisturize, soften, and protect the skin. They may reduce redness, itch, and pain and belong to the basic daily genital psoriasis therapy
- Suspected concurrent bacterial or fungal infections of the genital area should be treated with topical antibiotics or antimycotics; this may minimize a possible Köbner effect

Specific treatment

- Topical corticosteroids of low and medium strength are first-line therapy. The vulva is thought to be relatively steroid resistant, whereas inguinal folds, perineum, and perianal regions are steroid sensitive. At these sites, excessive use of topical corticosteroids of higher strength should be avoided because of possible skin atrophy. Hydrocortisone is mostly ineffective and moderately potent steroids are often required, e.g. methylprednisolone aceponate and mometasone, alternatively betamethasone are recommended. Superpotent steroid such as clobetasol propionate 0.05% ointment is only necessary in severe or recalcitrant cases. Topical corticosteroids should be started at higher strength and applied daily for, e.g. 2–4 weeks to be weaned down stepwise as soon as the lesions heal. Proactive therapy may be continued with applications twice weekly at the originally affected sites even in disease-free periods
- Topical calcineurin inhibitors including tacrolimus ointment and pimecrolimus cream may be useful treatments in the genital site; however, they may sting initially if the skin is open, and patients should be warned about this potential side effect. They are usually used twice daily for 4 weeks to be reduced to once daily thereafter followed by proactive therapy (see above)
- Vitamin D derivatives may be used cautiously; calcipotriol is usually too irritant in the genital folds. Calcitriol is better tolerated. Initial treatment is applied twice daily if possible; maintenance treatment may be used once a day; it may be combined with topical corticosteroids as part of the weekly treatment (e.g. 4 days calcitriol, 3 days glucocorticosteroids per week)
- Topical tar applications should be cautiously used as they may lead to local irritation and folliculitis
- UV light (UVB or cream or bath PUVA) is technically difficult to apply at the vulva and apart from acute UV burn may result in chronic photodamage and cancerogenesis after extended use
- Photodynamic therapy and laser therapy have been described anecdotally
- In severe and recalcitrant cases, mainly in generalized disease, systemic therapy may be necessary. Fumarates (only licensed in Germany), methotrexate (15–20 mg once weekly), or short-term cyclosporine (2.5–5 mg/kg body weight) are available (American Academy of Dermatology Work Group 2011). For disseminated hyperkeratotic lesions acitretin can be used; skin and mucous membrane dryness and irritation may, however, limit its use. There are reports of effective treatment for inverse psoriasis with dapsone (Guglielmetti et al. 2012). Biologics, including TNF-α blockers or anti-IL-12/23 antibodies, may be used when the conventional systemic therapy failed, is not tolerated, or contraindicated. Ample pretreatment tests as well as therapy-accompanying blood tests should be performed regularly.

COURSE AND PROGNOSIS

Psoriasis is usually chronic and relapsing, especially at the genital site. If not scratched extensively, scarring or atrophy is not expected. Malignant transformation has not been described, but recurrent superinfection is possible.

REFERENCES

American Academy of Dermatology Work Group, Menter A, Korman NJ, et al. Guidelines of care for the management of psoriasis and psoriatic arthritis: section 6. Guidelines of care for the treatment of psoriasis and psoriatic arthritis: case-based presentations and evidence-based conclusions. J Am Acad Dermatol 2011; 65:137–174.

Andreassi L, Bilenchi R. Non-infectious inflammatory genital lesions. Clin Dermatol 2014; 32:307–314.

Beecker J. Therapeutic principles in vulvovaginal dermatology. Dermatol Clin 2013; 28:639–648.

Farber EM, Nall L. Genital psoriasis. Cutis 1992; 50:263–266.

Farley E, Menter A. Psoriasis: comorbidities and associations. G Ital Dermatol Venereol 2011; 146:9–15.

Goldnau C, Köninger A, Kimmig R. [The female external genitalia : pathologic findings and first steps in treatment]. Urologe A 2010; 49:1496–1502.

Guglielmetti A, Conlledo R, Bedoya J, Ianiszewski F, Correa J. Inverse psoriasis involving genital skin folds: successful therapy with dapsone. Dermatol Ther (Heidelb) 2012; 2:15.

Heller MM, Wong JW, Nguyen TV, et al. Quality-of-life instruments: evaluation of the impact of psoriasis on patients. Dermatol Clin 2012; 30:281–291.

Kapila S, Bradford J, Fischer G. Vulvar psoriasis in adults and children: a clinical audit of 194 cases and review of the literature. J Low Genit Tract Dis 2012; 16:364–371.

Mease PJ. Inhibition of interleukin-17, interleukin-23 and the TH17 cell pathway in the treatment of psoriatic arthritis and psoriasis. Curr Opin Rheumatol 2015; 27:127–133.

Meeuwis KAP, de Hullu JA, de Jager MEA, et al. Genital psoriasis: a questionnaire-based survey on a concealed skin disease in the Netherlands. J Eur Acad Dermatol Venereol 2010; 24:1425–1430.

Meeuwis KA, de Hullu JA, Massuger LF, van de Kerkhof PC, van Rossum MM. Genital psoriasis: a systematic literature review on this hidden skin disease. Acta Derm Venereol 2011a; 91:5–11.

Meeuwis KA, de Hullu JA, van de Nieuwenhof HP, et al. Quality of life and sexual health in patients with genital psoriasis. Br J Dermatol 2011b; 164:1247–1255.

Meeuwis KA, van de Kerkhof PC, Massuger LF, de Hullu JA, van Rossum MM. Patients' experience of psoriasis in the genital area. Dermatology 2012; 224:271–276.

Nestle FO, Kaplan DH, Barker J. Psoriasis. N Engl J Med 2009; 361:496–509.

Palamaras I, Hamill M, Sethi G, Wilkinson D, Lamba H. The usefulness of a diagnostic biopsy clinic in a genitourinary medicine setting: recent experience and a review of the literature. J Eur Acad Dermatol Venereol 2006; 20:905–10.

Sticherling M. [Involvement of mucous membranes in papulosquamous diseases]. Hautarzt 2009; 60:891–897.

van Eyk N, Allen L, Giesbrecht E, et al. Pediatric vulvovaginal disorders: a diagnostic approach and review of the literature. J Obstet Gynaecol Can 2009; 31:850–862.

Zamirska A, Reich A, Berny-Moreno J, Salomon J, Szepietowski JC. Vulvar pruritus and burning sensation in women with psoriasis. Acta Derm Venereol 2008; 88:132–135.

Chapter 23 Hidradenitis suppurativa

Ditte M Saunte, Gregor B E Jemec

Synonyms

Acne inversa, Verneuil disease

Key features

- History of recurrent painful inflammatory lesions restricted to axillae, inframammary and perigenital areas
- Often premenstrual flares
- Signs of inflammation and scarring
- Pathogens rarely found
- Treatment includes antibiotics and immunosuppressants for disease control and surgery

INTRODUCTION

Hidradenitis suppurativa (HS) is a chronic, inflammatory, recurrent, debilitating skin disease that usually presents after puberty.

EPIDEMIOLOGY

A range of prevalence estimates exist with the figures varying significantly with the sources and methods used. Retrospective studies based on registered diagnoses from insurance companies, predominantly in the United States, show very low prevalence rates among the patients treated (<0.1%), but a rising incidence over time. In contrast, cross-sectional studies using either validated questionnaires for self-reported diagnosis or physician examination show much higher prevalence rates. Questionnaire-based studies in France and Denmark indicate an overall prevalence of 1–2.2% in general population samples. A prospective study involving physician-examined patients in Spain indicated a prevalence rate of 1%, and a Danish study of young adults attending a sexually transmitted disease (STD)-clinic found a point prevalence rate of 4%.

The majority of cases found in cross-sectional studies are mild, but data from patients seen in secondary care indicate a low level of recognition of the disease by primary physicians, and a substantial diagnostic delay in the majority of patients. These factors should be considered in the assessment of the prevalence rates reported using different approaches (Sung & Kimball 2013, Vinding et al. 2014).

PATHOGENESIS

The pathogenesis of HS is incompletely understood. It appears to be a follicular disease. Primary involvement of the apocrine glands, as previously suggested, is rare.

ETIOLOGY

The etiology is unknown, but an abnormal inflammatory reaction is suspected to propagate the lesions. It belongs to a group of autoinflammatory diseases that also includes pyoderma gangrenosum and acne. HS is not a simple infectious process, as pathogens are rarely found even in inflamed lesions.

Genetics may play a role as approximately one-third of patients report familial occurrence of the disease. Studies have suggested that the gamma-secretase complex may be involved in these cases. Deficient Notch signaling has been suggested as a communal mechanism (Melnik & Plewig 2013).

Analysis of the cytokine profiler of HS lesions has suggested that elevated levels of interleukin (IL)-1, tumor necrosis factor alpha (TNF-α), and IL-10 can be found. The IL-23/Th-17 pathway has also been implicated, as have mechanisms involving the innate immune response and antimicrobial peptides (van der Zee et al. 2012).

Histologically, subclinical changes have been described in non-involved skin, where sebaceous glands appear to have weaker periodic acid–Schiff staining, be smaller, or even absent. The folliculitis appears to involve an early lymphocytic infiltrate, followed by infundibular hyperkeratinization and a massive neutrophilic infiltrate destroying the architecture of the hair follicles and adjacent sebaceous glands and leading to the formation of intradermal or subcutaneous epithelialized sinus tracts and abundant granulation tissue.

CLINICAL PRESENTATION

Painful, deep-seated, inflamed lesions in the apocrine gland-bearing areas of the body most commonly affect the axillary, inguinal, and anogenital regions (Kelly et al. 2014).

It is associated with a short history of increased pain and suppuration, often preceded by stinging, and followed by increased suppuration. On examination, increased inflammation and/or suppuration is seen. Pustules can also present in and around superinfected lesions. Often, *Staphylococcus aureus* is cultured, although this is not the primary cause of HS, and antimicrobial treatment following sensitivity testing may help.

Diagnostic criteria

The following three criteria must be fulfilled:

1. Typical lesions: either deep-seated painful nodules (blind boils) in early primary lesions or abscesses, draining sinuses, bridged scars and 'tombstone' open comedones in secondary lesions (Figures 23.1–23.4)
2. Typical topography: axillae, groin, genitals, perineal and perianal region, buttocks, infra- and intermammary folds
3. Chronicity and recurrences

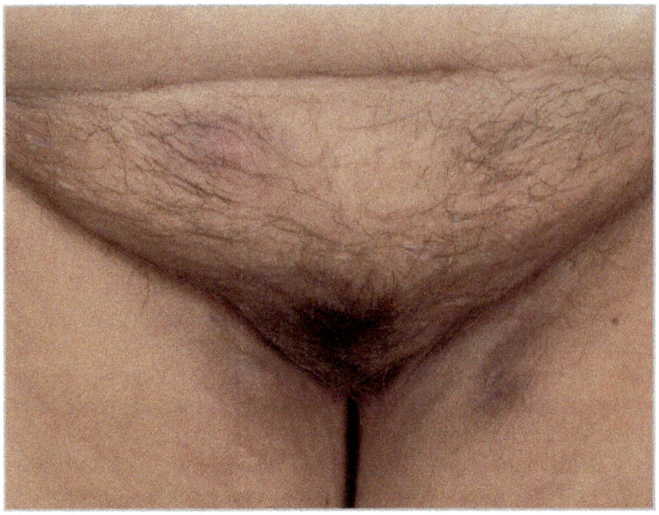

Figure 23.1 Hurley stage I: early hidradenitis suppurativa lesions are identified as crops of painful inflammatory lesions that appear restricted to perigenital areas, axillae, or inframammary folds. The inflammation subsides but leaves non-inflamed nodules and postinflammatory hyperpigmentation.

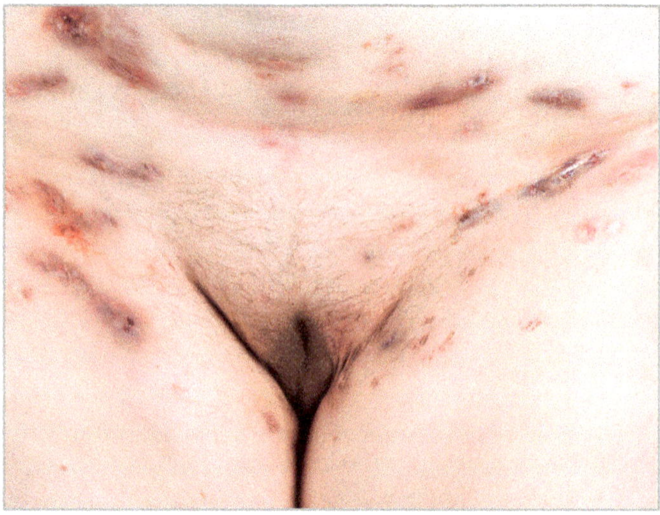

Figure 23.3 Hurley stage II: moderate disease. Inflamed lesions with scarring separated by normal looking skin.

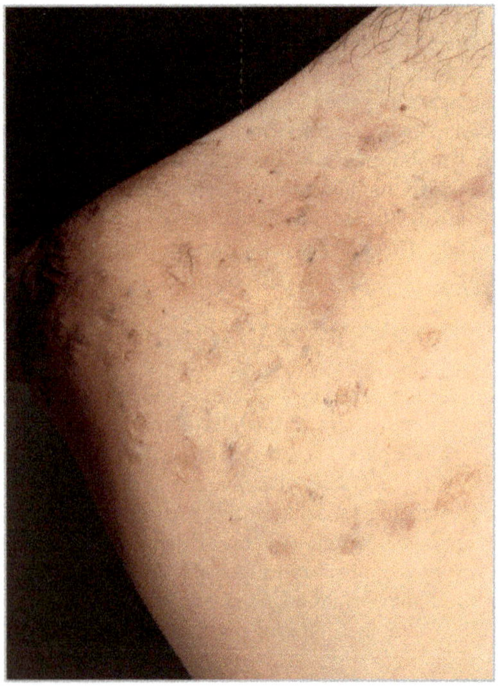

Figure 23.2 Burnt-out lesions leave scars and comedones.

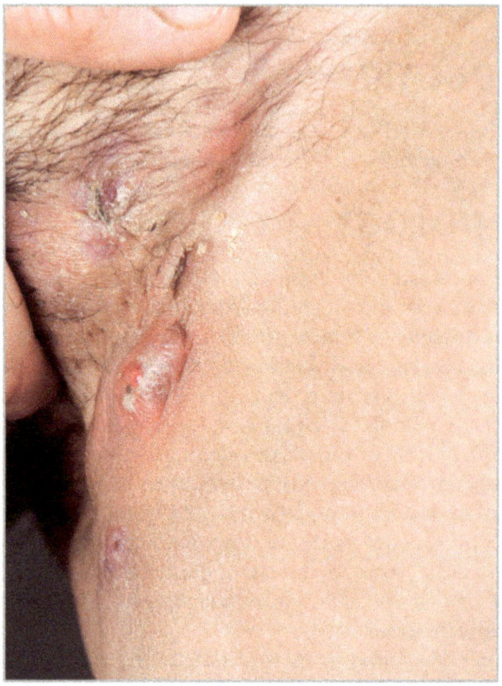

Figure 23.4 Hurley stage III: severe disease. Coalesced inflamed lesions and scarring, often with chronic drainage.

Disease severity assessment

Two different staging assessment tools are most often used:

- The 'Hurley stage' categorizes the disease severity into three stages
  - I, mild; II, moderate; III, severe (see Figures 23.1, 23.3 and 23.4)
- The 'Sartorius score' is an assessment tool used to assess treatment efficacy in an additive score (0 to infinity), it evaluates:
  - Hurley stage
  - The number of affected anatomical regions and presence of nodules, sinus tracts/fistula
  - The distance between them

Comorbidities

The coexistence of HS and other medical conditions or disease processes is well known.

Inflammatory bowel disease

In patients with inflammatory bowel disease (IBD) coexistence with HS has been reported in up to 26% of patients with Crohn disease and 18% of patients diagnosed with ulcerative colitis. Most patients with HS and associated IBD do not smoke, whereas patients with isolated HS often do. The buttocks are more frequently affected in patients with IBD (van der Zee et al. 2014).

Pyoderma gangrenosum

Pyoderma gangrenosum is also associated with HS. PASH (pyoderma gangrenosum, acne, and suppurativa hidradenitis) has recently been described as a new disease after bowel bypass surgery for obesity (Scheinfeld 2013).

Metabolic syndrome

Metabolic syndrome is a multifaceted disorder associated with chronic inflammatory diseases. It encompasses issues with dyslipidemia, obesity, hyperglycemia, and hypertension with increased risk for development of cardiovascular disease. The prevalence of metabolic syndrome is significantly higher in HS patients as compared with a control group (Gold et al. 2014).

Diseases of follicular occlusion

Diseases of follicular occlusion in the skin are often associated with HS. The triad/tetrad of acne conglobata, dissecting cellulitis (of the scalp), pinodal cysts, and HS is well reported. The component of the triad/tetrad might occur simultaneously or at different times. Acne vulgaris does not seem to be more common in HS patients (Scheinfeld 2013).

Cancer

Squamous cell carcinomas arising in chronic lesions (Marjolin ulcers) especially on the buttocks are associated with HS (Jemec 2012).

Psychiatric disorders

The psychiatric disorders, depression and anxiety, are significantly more frequent in HS patients as compared with controls, whereas psychoses, schizophrenia, and bipolar disorder are not (Shavit et al. 2014).

Complications of disease

Complications of long-standing untreated HS includes scarring, contractures leading to functional impairment, anemia, hypoalbuminemia, amyloidosis, lymphatic obstruction, fistula formation, reflex sympathetic dystrophy, and toxic shock syndrome (Ellis 2012).

Risk factors

Tobacco smoking is linked to the development of HS and clinical disease severity (Jemec 2012). The majority of patients are smokers (current or exsmokers) and a higher remission rate is found in non-smoking HS patients (Kromann et al. 2014a).

Obesity is also considered a risk factor and has been linked to the likelihood of developing HS. Weight reduction may improve HS symptoms. The proposed underlying mechanism include warm and humid milieu in the skin folds of obese patients as well as a shear forces from clothes and skin-to-skin contact (Jemec 2012, Kromann et al. 2014a, Kromann et al. 2014b).

DIAGNOSIS

The diagnosis is made clinically, and no pathognomonic test is currently available. It may, however, be helpful to swab lesions for bacteria, as superinfection may occur. Superinfections cause acute flares.

HISTOPATHOLOGY

Histopathological investigations of single lesions may be necessary to rule out malignancy in long-standing disease. Histology is not diagnostic in itself, but HS causes several, non-specific changes that may support the diagnosis. In milder cases, interfollicular psoriasiform epithelial hyperplasia associated with folliculitis containing a mixed infiltrate of lymphocytes and neutrophils are seen (von Laffert et al. 2011). In early lesions the infiltrate is predominantly lymphocytic. In Hurley stage II and III disease scarring and the formation of sinus tracts predominate the histology and appears associated with a chronic mixed inflammatory infiltrate (Jemec & Hansen 1996). Granulomatous foreign-body reactions are often seen, making the differential diagnosis from cutaneous Crohn disease a task for the specialist histopathologist with extensive experience of both diseases.

Ultrasound imaging may be useful in assessing the extent of lesions, particularly when closely associated with delicate structures.

DIFFERENTIAL DIAGNOSES

The differential diagnoses of HS most often considered are: abscesses, furuncles, carbuncles, lymphogranuloma venereum, cat scratch disease, infected epidermal cyst, Crohn disease, ulcerative colitis, tuberculosis, actinomycosis, pilonidal sinus, lymphadenitis, and granuloma inguinale.

MANAGEMENT

The management of HS is complex and depends on the severity of the disease. **Table 23.1** details treatment options for for HS.

Adjuvant therapy

- Weight loss
- Professional wound care
- Pain management
- Routine use of disinfectants is not recommended

Adjuvant treatment is strongly recommended. Epidemiology and observational studies of disease severity support the recommendation of weight loss. Disease prevalence and severity are both associated with increased body mass index. There is no evidence to suggest that routine use of disinfectants such chlorhexidine improves the outcome.

Patients benefit from contact with a wound-care nurse to assist and instruct in the use of dressings for management of symptoms such as leaking.

Pain management is not known to influence the course of the disease, but it is of great benefit to patients and may in combination with suitable bandaging reduce the impact of the disease. The need for pain management should be individually assessed for each patient.

Medical treatment

The disease is multifocal in nature and precursor lesions exist. Medical treatment is therefore warranted, even though surgery is often also needed for individual advanced lesions in a multimodal therapeutic approach. Clinical presentation is deceptively similar to simple infections, and most patients report having been treated with antibiotics usually to no avail. Nevertheless, the two medical approaches that have been used in the treatment of HS are antibiotics and immunosuppressant therapy.

Antibiotics

There is a paucity of clinical trials in HS, but an early randomized-controlled trial (RCT) suggests that the topical use of clindamycin 10 mg/mL is beneficial (Clemmensen 1983). This may be particularly suitable for early lesions or mild cases. Another RCT found no difference in effect, comparing topical clindamycin bd with systemic

Table 23.1 Treatment for hidradenitis suppurativa

	Treatment modality	Recommended clinical circumstance	Side effect/disadvantage	Evidence level/ grade of recommendation
Topical antibiotics				
	Clindamycin 10 mg/mL	Early lesions or mild cases	Local irritation, allergy	I/B
Systemic antibiotics				
	Tetracycline 500 mg bid	Mild cases	GI upset, *Candida* infection, photoallergy and teratogenicity	I/B
	Clindamycin 300 mg bid and rifampin 300 mg bid	Moderate-to-severe cases	Colitis, GI upset, *Candida* infection, allergy and promotion of drug resistance in other bacteria	II/A
Combined treatment	Moxifloxacin, rifampin, and metronidazole	Moderate-to-severe cases	Colitis, GI upset, *Candida* infection, allergy and promotion of drug resistance in other bacteria	IV/B
Immunosuppressives/immunomodulating				
	Glucocorticosteroids	Acute flare	Intralesional: atrophy systemic: superinfection, weight gain, hypertension, diabetes, etc.	V/D
	TNF-α inhibitors	Moderate-to-severe cases	Flare of latent infections, e.g. TB, psoriasiform drug eruptions	I/A
Surgery				
	Deroofing	Sinus tracts	Only suitable for larger sinus tracts	II/A
	Excision	Single recalcitrant lesions	Recurrence in non-excised areas	II/A
	Laser treatment	Single recalcitrant lesions	Recurrence in non-excised areas. Long duration of secondary intention healing	II/A

GI, gastrointestinal

tetracycline 500 mg bd (Jemec & Wendelboe 1998). Open case-series indicate that treatment combinations with systemic Clindamycin 300 mg bd combined with rifampin 300 mg bd given for 10 weeks is effective, but the results have not been confirmed in an RCT (Bettoli et al. 2014). Intensive antibiotic treatment combining moxifloxacin, rifampin, and metronidazole have also been described as successful (Join-Lambert et al. 2011).

Immunosuppressives/ immunomodulating

In view of the paucity of bacteria found in HS lesions it is speculated that non-antimicrobial, immunomodulatory effects of these antibiotics may explain their efficacy. Accordingly, an alternative approach using immunosuppressive/immunomodulatory drugs has been pursued.

Glucocorticosteroids

Severe flares of lesions often benefit from systemic prednisolone (up to 0.5 mg/kg/day), although this treatment is not well supported by trials.

TNF-α inhibitors

More recently, RCTs have shown that the use of the TNF-α inhibitors adalimumab and infliximab are also beneficial. Infliximab at a dose of 5 mg/kg in a routine setting of treatments week 0, 2, 6, and thereafter every 8th week was shown to be effective in achieving secondary outcomes in an investigator initiated study (Grant et al. 2010). Two studies have investigated the effect of adalimumab, indicating that weekly dosing at 40 mg produces significant amelioration of disease (Kimball et al. 2012, Miller et al. 2011).

Miscellaneous

A wide range of other drugs have reportedly been used successfully in the treatment of HS in small case series, which await more substantial evidence before a firm recommendation can be made. These include topical resorcinol (15%), and systemic drugs such as acitretin, anakinra, dapsone, and metformin (Jemec 2012).

Superinfections occur and should be treated according to the resistance pattern of the offending organism.

Surgical treatment

Surgical management of recalcitrant lesions often results in local clearing. It includes deroofing, incision and drainage, excision with and without reconstruction, and laser treatment (Ellis 2012).

Incision

Incision is only suitable for soft, clearly fluctuating abscesses; it is not generally recommended. If acute painful lumps, which do not fluctuate, are incised, there is no relief and recurrence rate will be 100%. Acute painful lumps should be treated with either systemic antibiotics or intralesional glucocorticoids (e.g. triamcinolone 4–6 mg).

Deroofing

Deroofing and marsurpialization is a simple and minimally invasive procedure, where the 'roof' of an HS nodule or sinus tract is removed.

Methods used to this procedure are probe and electrosurgical cutting/blunt scissors and CO_2 laser. Usually, the wounds are left open for secondary-intension healing (Ellis 2012).

Excision

Excision is performed as either limited local excision or radical wide excision. Surgery can offer a curative intervention for scarred lesions. The results of a radical wide excision of all involved skin and tissue is the only curative treatment; however, it is challenging in the perianal areas, as preservation of the sphincter is important. Preoperative imaging (magnetic resonance imaging or ultrasound) or intraoperative color marking of sinus tracts can be used to define the operative area. Primary closure, secondary-intension to healing, immediate or delayed split-skin grafting, and fasciocutaneous and musculocutaneous flaps are all methods used to reconstruction. Recurrence rate vary between the reconstruction methods and surgical location (Ellis 2012).

Laser treatment

The CO_2 laser has been used to excision and evaporation of the affected area. When using the excision technique, the laser works as a scalpel with a good vascular control and the possibility to send the excised tissue to a pathologist. When using the evaporation technique, the CO_2-laser evaporates the HS lesions layer by layer until all visualized inflamed tissue and sinus tracts are removed hereby minimizing the loss of healthy tissue. These wounds are often left for secondary-intension healing (Ellis 2012).

Other treatment options

Nd:YAG laser (1,064-nm neodymium-doped yttrium aluminum garnet), Smoothbeam (1,450-nm diode laser), non-ablative radiofrequency device, radiation treatment, cryotherapy, photodynamic therapy, botulinum toxin treatment have all been used to treat HS patients; however, more research and validation in larger studies are required (Ellis 2012).

PROGNOSIS

Long-term follow-up of patients in routine treatment (median follow-up 22 years, range 12–32 years) suggests that approximately one-third go into remission, one-third continue unchanged or worse, and one-third report some degree of amelioration (unspecified), which may, however, reflect increased acceptance of disease symptoms (Kromann et al. 2014a).

REFERENCES

Bettoli V, Zauli S, Borghi A, et al. Oral clindamycin and rifampicin in the treatment of hidradenitis suppurativa-acne inversa: a prospective study on 23 patients. J Eur Acad Dermatol Venereol 2014; 28:125–126.

Clemmensen OJ. Topical treatment of hidradenitis suppurativa with clindamycin. Int J Dermatol 1983; 22:325–328.

Ellis LZ. Hidradenitis suppurativa: surgical and other management techniques. Dermatol Surg 2012; 38:517–536. Review.

Gold DA, Reeder VJ, Mahan MG, Hamzavi IH. The prevalence of metabolic syndrome in patients with hidradenitis suppurativa. J Am Acad Dermatol 2014; 70: 699–703.

Grant A, Gonzalez T, Montgomery MO, Cardenas V, Kerdel FA. Infliximab therapy for patients with moderate to severe hidradenitis suppurativa: a randomized, double-blind, placebo-controlled crossover trial. J Am Acad Dermatol 2010; 62:205–217.

Jemec GB. Clinical practice. Hidradenitis suppurativa. N Engl J Med 2012; 366:158–164. Review.

Jemec GB, Hansen U. Histology of hidradenitis suppurativa. J Am Acad Dermatol 1996; 34:994–999.

Jemec GB, Wendelboe P. Topical clindamycin versus systemic tetracycline in the treatment of hidradenitis suppurativa. J Am Acad Dermatol 1998; 39:971–974.

Join-Lambert O, Coignard H, Jais JP, et al. Efficacy of rifampin-moxifloxacin-metronidazole combination therapy in hidradenitis suppurativa. Dermatology 2011; 222:49–58.

Kelly G, Sweeney CM, Tobin AM, Kirby B. Hidradenitis suppurativa: the role of immune dysregulation. Int J Dermatol 2014; 53:1186–1196.

Kimball AB, Kerdel F, Adams D, et al. Adalimumab for the treatment of moderate to severe hidradenitis suppurativa: a parallel randomized trial. Ann Intern Med 2012; 157:846–855.

Kromann CB, Deckers IE, Esmann S, Boer J, Prens EP, Jemec GB. Risk-factors, clinical course and long-term prognosis in hidradenitis suppurativa: a cross-sectional study. Br J Dermatol 2014a; 171:819–824.

Kromann C, Ibler KS, Kristiansen V, Jemec GBE. The influence of body weight on the prevalence and severity of hidradenitis suppurativa. Acta Derm Venerol 2014b; 94: 553–557.

Melnik BC, Plewig G. Impaired Notch-MKP-1 signalling in hidradenitis suppurativa: an approach to pathogenesis by evidence from translational biology. Exp Dermatol 2013; 22:172–177.

Miller I, Lynggaard CD, Lophaven S, et al. A double-blind placebo-controlled randomized trial of adalimumab in the treatment of hidradenitis suppurativa. Br J Dermatol 2011; 165:391–398.

Scheinfeld N. Diseases associated with hidradenitis suppurativa: part 2 of a series on hidradenitis. Dermatol Online J 2013; 19: 18558

Shavit E, Dreiher J, Freud T, et al. Psychiatric comorbidities in 3207 patients with hidradenitis suppurativa [published online ahead of print June 9, 2014]. J Eur Acad Dermatol Venereol 2015; 29:371–376.

Sung S, Kimball AB. Counterpoint: analysis of patient claims data to determine the prevalence of hidradenitis suppurativa in the United States. J Am Acad Dermatol 2013; 69:818–819.

van der Zee HH, Laman JD, Boer J, Prens EP. Hidradenitis suppurativa: viewpoint on clinical phenotyping, pathogenesis and novel treatments. Exp Dermatol 2012; 21:735–739.

van der Zee HH, de Winter K, van der Woude CJ, Prens EP. The prevalence of hidradenitis suppurativa in 1093 patients with inflammatory bowel disease. Br J Dermatol 2014;171:673–675.

Vinding GR, Miller IM, Zarchi K, et al. The prevalence of inverse recurrent suppuration: a population-based study of possible hidradenitis suppurativa. Br J Dermatol 2014; 170:884–889.

von Laffert M, Stadie V, Wohlrab J, Marsch WC. Hidradenitis suppurativa/acne inversa: bilocated epithelial hyperplasia with very different sequelae. Br J Dermatol 2011; 164:367–371.

Chapter 24 Granulomatous conditions of the vulva

Michael A Hambardzumyan, Ad A van Bodegraven, Tom J Stoof

Key features

- A cluster of inflammatory diseases with specific histological features (granulomas) of various etiologies, involving skin, mucous membranes of the vulva, and gastrointestinal tract
- Single or multiple sites may be affected
- Primarily seen in, but not confined to, young adults, as it may also occur in children or older adults
- Diagnosis is made when there are characteristic histological features (granulomas) and typical clinical, serological, and microbiological findings

INTRODUCTION

Granulomatous inflammatory diseases may affect many organs, the skin being one of them. The etiology of granulomatous conditions is variable, involving infectious and non-infectious causes. Four common granulomatous conditions potentially affecting the vulva are as follows:

- Crohn disease (CD)
- Sarcoidosis
- Melkersson–Rosenthal syndrome (MRS)
- Idiopathic granulomatous vulvitis (GV)

CROHN DISEASE – CUTANEOUS MANIFESTATIONS OF THE VULVA

Synonyms

Metastatic Crohn disease of the vulva, vulvar Crohn disease

Introduction

Inflammatory bowel disease (IBD) is an idiopathic group of chronic, relapsing inflammatory diseases of the gastrointestinal tract, comprising chiefly CD and ulcerative colitis (UC). CD may affect any part of the digestive system from mouth to the anus. CD with cutaneous involvement was first described by Parks et al. in 1965 (Parks et al. 1965).

Subsequently, it was named metastatic CD (metastatic as in away from the gastrointestinal tract). When characteristic non-caseating granulomatous inflammatory lesions occur non-contiguously to the gastrointestinal tract, these may be referred to as metastatic CD.

Apart from this entity, continuous lesions with the gastrointestinal tract confined to the anal area are known and described in literature as perianal CD. This perianal involvement occurs in about 30% of CD cases, being a clinical feature distinguishing CD from other IBDs in which perianal involvement is rare (Berkowitz & Lebwohl 2000, Burgdorf 1981, Corbett et al. 2010, Parks et al. 1965).

The most common granulomatous condition affecting the vulva is due to CD. Vulvar lesions have been described in patients with luminal (intestinal) CD but may precede gastrointestinal disease. Clinical signs of vulvar granulomatous inflammation are non-specific, including swelling of the labia, ulcers, fissures, and mucosal tags. In addition, involvement of the mouth may be observed in CD, sometimes difficult to distinguish from Behçet disease. CD occurs mostly in young and middle-aged individuals (20–40 years), with slightly more affected women than men (Palamaras et al. 2008).

Key features

- Affected sites: intestine (with a predilection for the ileum, colon, or anus), vulvar skin, oral mucosa
- Clinical features: swelling, ulcers, fissures of vulvar skin/mouth, an array of abdominal complaints including pain, diarrhea, and loss of weight
- Affected age group: 20–40 years, but affects all ages
- Sex distribution: more common in females than in males
- Course of intestinal disease: chronic, relapsing
- Course of extraintestinal disease: not necessarily in line with activity of intestinal disease

Epidemiology

The prevalence of CD in Europe is about 100–250 in 100,000 with a possible decreasing north-south gradient but overall rising. The incidence of IBD is worldwide steadily rising as well, although primarily confined to Westernized countries, thus rapidly increasing in countries such as China. The disease usually develops between the second and fourth decade of life, but it also occurs in children and seniors, with an incidence of pediatric CD ranging from 0.2 to 8.5 per 100,000. There is a rise in incidence, which is also seen in children similar to the trend seen in adults; this is in contrast to UC, where a more stable pattern of incidence is manifested, at least in the conventional Westernized countries, such as in the USA, Canada, and western Europe (Sathiyasekaran & Shivbalan 2006). Among extraintestinal manifestations of IBD, occurring in 30–40% of patients, cutaneous lesions are commonly observed (in 5–10% of patients). Both oral and vulvar (granulomatous) lesions may precede CD.

Pathogenesis

Despite extensive study, the exact cause of CD has yet to be elucidated. A combination of environmental, immunological, and genetic factors is thought to induce a dysregulation (essentially an overactivation) of the gastrointestinal (mucosal) immune system.

Microorganisms such as *Mycobacterium avium* subspecies paratuberculosis, the measles virus, Helicobacter pylori, and adherent-invasive strains of Escherichia coli have been considered to be of etiopathogenic importance but are found not to be causative factors (Molodecky & Kaplan 2010). Currently, dysbiosis of the intestinal microbiome is focus of investigational interest (Jostins et al. 2012). Several other risk factors have been described, e.g. a deleterious course of CD is directly associated with smoking while that of UC is not; they are summarized in **Table 24.1**.

More than 150 genetic risk factors have been identified, most of which appear to be involved in bacterial recognition and immunological handling, most notably, several polymorphisms of the NOD-2 gene (Jostins et al. 2012).

Immunological changes of the intestinal mucosa, involving several sets of the immune cells and its cytokine network have been well characterized (Neurath 2014).

Clinical manifestations and features of vulvar Crohn disease

Crohn disease may, among others, affect the oral cavity, lips, skin, including vulva and anus, eyes, and joints (arthropathy/arthritis). The vulva seems more commonly affected than other cutaneous sites, but it is almost never routinely examined in patients, in particular not when seen by a gastroenterologist. Involvement of the lower extremities and soles is seen in 38%, the trunk and abdomen in 24%, the upper extremities and palms in 15%, face and lips in 11%, and intertriginous areas in 8% of patients. Therefore, any patient with IBD should be carefully examined for cutaneous manifestations (Barret et al. 2014, Georgiou et al. 2006).

Patients with cutaneous manifestations of CD may be subdivided into three groups according to the sites involved:

1. Perianal cutaneous lesions (erythema, abscesses, fissures, fistulas, subcutaneous nodules, pseudocondylomata, and ulceration) occur in 25–36% patients. These manifestations develop commonly following presentation of intestinal lesions but may precede intestinal disease. This group also includes patients with (ulcerative) lesions of the oral cavity
2. Metastatic (specific) cutaneous lesions, including vulvar lesions - metastatic cutaneous CD is characterized by non-caseating, granulomatous, cutaneous lesions lacking continuity with diseased areas of the gastrointestinal tract. Metastatic cutaneous CD usually presents after manifestation of gastrointestinal tract symptoms (Berkowitz & Lebwohl 2000, Burgdorf 1981), but it may also precede intestinal disease. It may involve lips, upper and lower limbs, and buttocks. Metastatic CD is not frequently described in literature.
3. Non-specific cutaneous lesions - histologically, these lesions are characterized by non-sarcoidal inflammatory changes.

Furthermore, cutaneous CD can be subdivided into a genital and an extragenital group (**Table 24.2**). If children are affected by cutaneous manifestations of CD, the genital form is more likely to occur, that is two third, as contrasted to adults, in which half suffers from purely genital manifestations.

Table 24.1 Environmental risk factors for Crohn disease (Molodecky & Kaplan 2010)

- Smoking
- Perinatal infections
- Use of antibiotics (in childhood)
- Appendectomy
- Gastrointestinal infections
- Human environment ('too' hygienic)
- Diet

Vulvar involvement may be discerned by swelling of one or both labia, 'knife cut' ulceration (both or one side), papules, and vulvar distortion. Patients may complain of local burning, and an array of abdominal complaints including pain, diarrhea, and loss of weight.

Diagnostic criteria

A clinically suspected diagnosis should be confirmed by histopathological examination of a cutaneous lesion. Ileocolonoscopy and sometimes gastroscopy and small bowel imaging, preferably with magnetic resonance imaging. Whenever possible, sampling of biopsy specimens of the (ileo) colon or other affected intestinal segments is indicated in addition.

Recognition of cutaneous manifestations, including those of the vulva, fitting in with a diagnosis CD can therefore provide guidance to a proper diagnosis. Of note, at the time of primary manifestation of CD, the general health of a patient is usually considered to be good. Clinical manifestations like genital induration and swelling, especially

Table 24.2 Characteristics of clinical cutaneous manifestations in genital and extragenital cutaneous Crohn disease

Signs regularly seen in genital lesions

- Vulvar swelling or edema/lymphedema/lymphangiectasia (unilateral or bilateral) (**Figures 24.1** and **24.2**)
- Fissures and tags
- Ulceration (knife cut) (**Figure 24.3**)
- Vulvar distortion
- Vulvovaginal burning sensation/discomfort
- Dyspareunia
- Dysuria
- A feeling of 'heaviness' in the pubic area

Signs commonly seen in extragenital manifestations

- Papules or nodules
- Plaques with or without ulceration
- Abscesses/sinuses
- Hidradenitis suppurativa
- Lobular panniculitis and scars

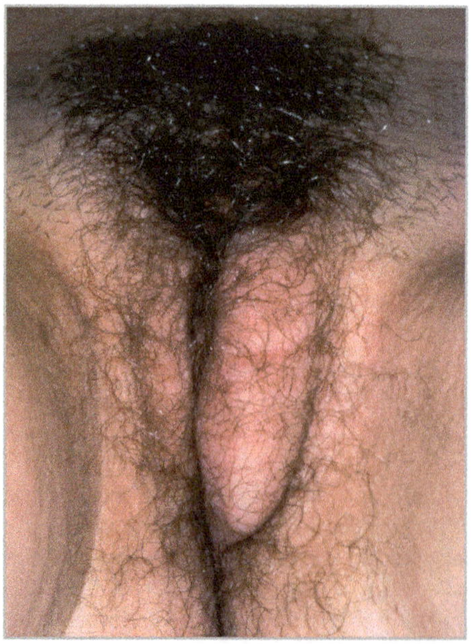

Figure 24.1 Firm swelling of the left labium majus in a patient with Crohn disease.
Copied with kind permission by Wiley, ©European Academy of Dermatology and Venereology 2003: van de Scheur MR, van der Waal RI, van der Waal I, Stoof TJ, van Deventer SJ. Anogenital granulomatosis: the counterpart of orofacial granulomatosis. J Eur Acad Dermatol Venereol 2003; 17:184–189.

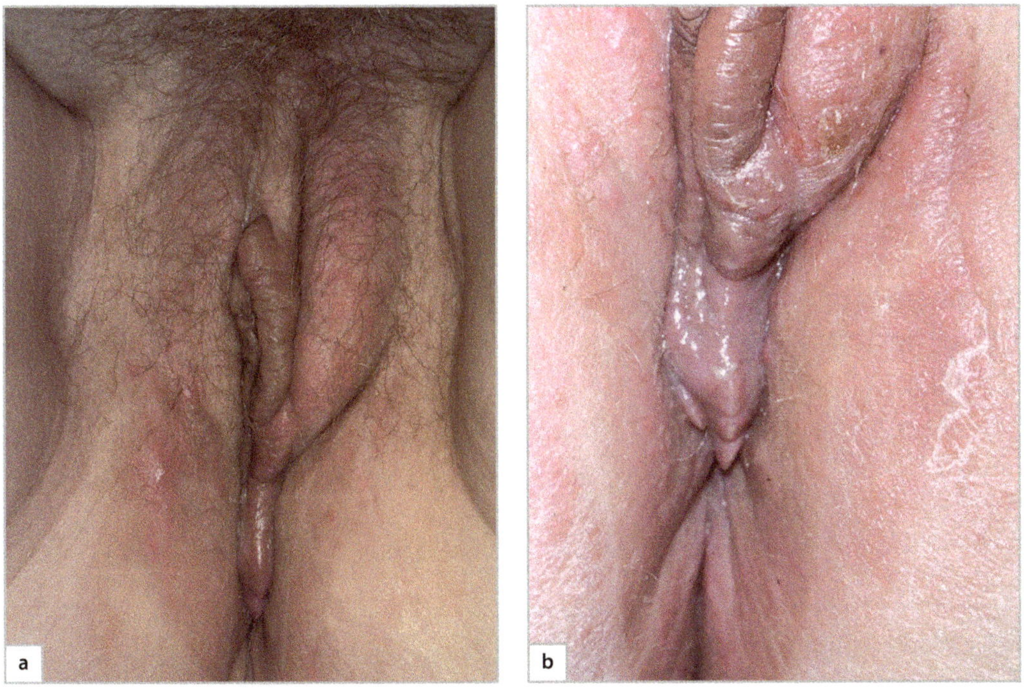

Figure 24.2 Firm swelling of (a) the vulva and (b) the anoperineal region in a patient with Crohn disease.

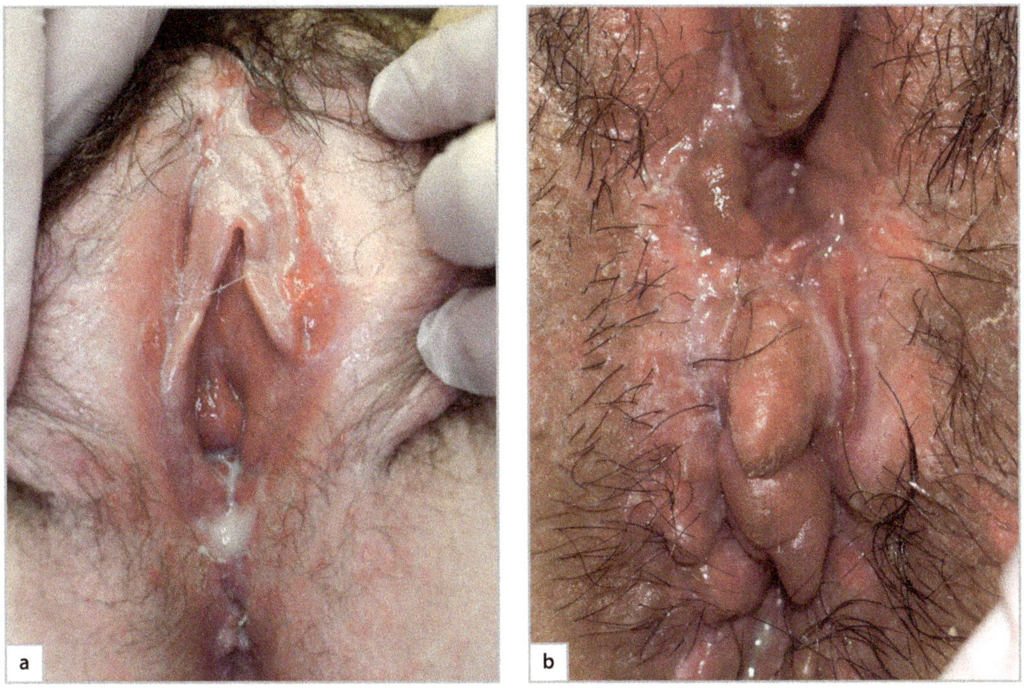

Figure 24.3 Typical 'knife-cut' ulcer in cutaneous Crohn disease. By courtesy of Professor Emmanuel Delaporte, Lille, France (a) and Dr Pablo Lázaro Ochaita, Spain (b).

in a young patient, should therefore in any case be extensively investigated, including analysis of the gastrointestinal tract, to demonstrate or exclude a presentation of metastatic CD.

Early diagnosis (and treatment) of CD may prevent retardation of growth in the (very) young patients, one of the main concerns of (untreated) CD in children, and prevent disabling lesions or loss of gastrointestinal function in more adult patients.

Therefore, any child or adult with labial swelling, hemorrhage, diarrhea or with a provisional diagnosis for pyoderma gangrenosum, Behçet disease or lymphedema is a possible candidate for CD, necessitating proper diagnostic work-up.

Fecal calprotectin is being used as a biomarker of intestinal inflammation; it is not a specific diagnostic test for CD. It is comparable to blood tests such as C-reactive protein measurement or the erythrocyte sedimentation rate, but this test is confined to stools, reflecting 'a state of inflammation' of any part of the intestine.

Histopathology

Histopathological examination of a biopsy of vulvar lesional skin typically shows infiltration of histiocytes, monocytes, and lymphocytes, often perivascular, and additionally scattered multinucleated giant cells forming 'non-caseating granulomas,' consistent with findings of CD (**Figure 24.4**).

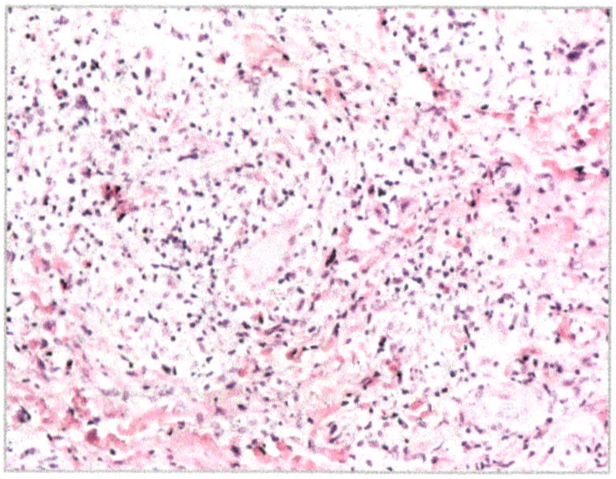

Figure 24.4 Histologic pattern of active Crohn disease showing focal granulomatous inflammation.

Differential diagnosis

There is a range of differential diagnoses of skin manifestations associated with CD. A detailed list of differential diagnoses is shown in **Table 24.3.**

Management and treatment options for vulvar Crohn disease

Key points

- First treat luminal CD to induce remission
- Follow a sequential (step-up) approach
- Maintenance therapy will keep it under control
- Site-specific topical therapy may support local problems

Because granulomatous conditions like CD and sarcoidosis are systemic diseases topical treatment alone is not usually successful (Barret et al. 2014, Mayberry 2013, Escher et al. 2002, Thiriar 1988). Therefore, the extent of the disease has to be carefully evaluated and the treatment approach decided accordingly. Furthermore, the disease may start with disease at one site such as the vulva (or penis as demonstrated in **Figure 24.5**, corresponding histology in **Figure 24.6**, and perianal fissuring **Figure 24.7** years later the patient developed intestinal CD) but will then affect other sites in its course. It depends on the experience of the treating physician as to when systemic treatment for a 'local' problem will be introduced. Systemic treatment is usually accompanied by more side effects; however, for many patients this may be the only option to treat a 'local' problem. The second consensus on CD provides detailed information on its diagnosis and management (Dignass et al. 2012b).

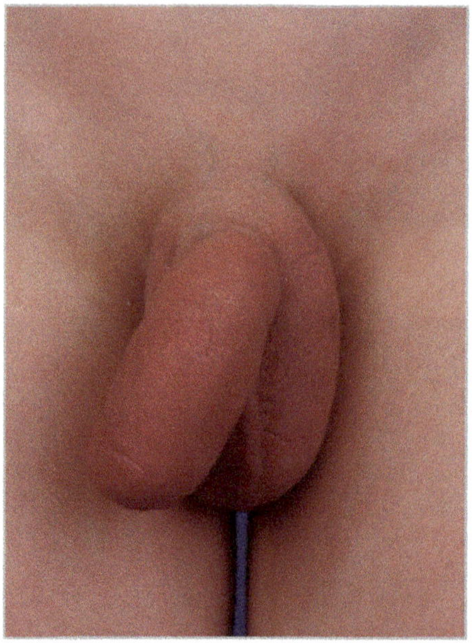

Figure 24.5 A 10-year-old boy with swelling of penis and scrotum as the only manifestation of metastatic Crohn disease. After several years he developed full blown and severe intestinal Crohn disease, particularly affecting his colon, which finally had to be removed surgically.

Table 24.3 Clinical important differential diagnosis of most common granulomatous and non-granulomatous conditions

Granulomatous		Non-granulomatous	
Disease	**Clinical/histological features**	**Disease**	**Clinical signs**
Tuberculosis	Inflammatory, caseous necrosis	Pyoderma gangrenosum	Ulceration with possibly undermined purple border
Sarcoidosis	Non-caseating granuloma	Behçet disease	Multiple ulcerations, arthralgia, pathergy
Melkersson–Rosenthal syndrome	Non-caseating granuloma	Infectious vulvovaginitis (venereal and non-venereal, deep bacterial/fungal)	Ulceration, nodules, swelling, vaginal discharge
Idiopathic granulomatous vulvitis	Non-caseating granuloma	Bartholinitis/Bartholin cyst	Painful swelling labia majora
Foreign body granuloma	Foreign body granuloma	Condylomata acuminata	Exophytic painless lesions
Lymphogranuloma venereum	A small, non-indurated ulcer or papule, inguinal lymph nodes	Hidradenitis suppurativa	Nodular abscess, multiple lesions
Syphilis	Solitary painless ulceration	Rosacea	Pustules, erythema
Langerhans cell histiocytosis CD1a positive with eosinophilia	Shortness of breath, joint pain and arthritis, red bumps on the skin, enlarged liver and dry eyes (asymptomatic in various cases)	Vulvar edema/lymphedema	Patient history postradiotherapy, neoplastic lymphatic vessel obstruction
Allergic granulomatous reactions	Itchy, more generalized skin eruption; patch test	Lymphangioma	Swelling
		Traumatic hemorrhage	Aching pain, feeling of local heaviness

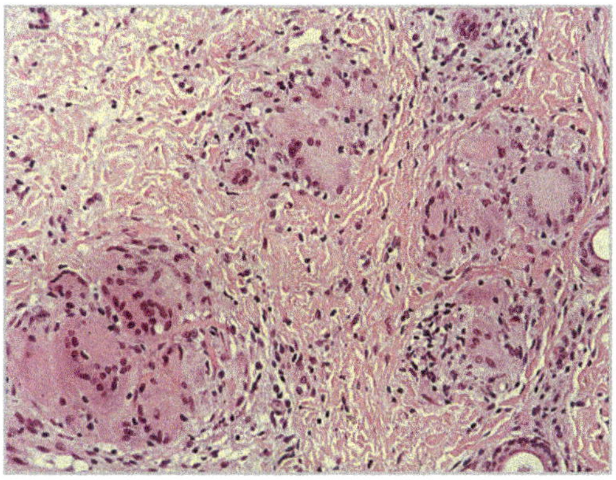

Figure 24.6 Histopathology of penile skin biopsy showing granulomatous inflammation.

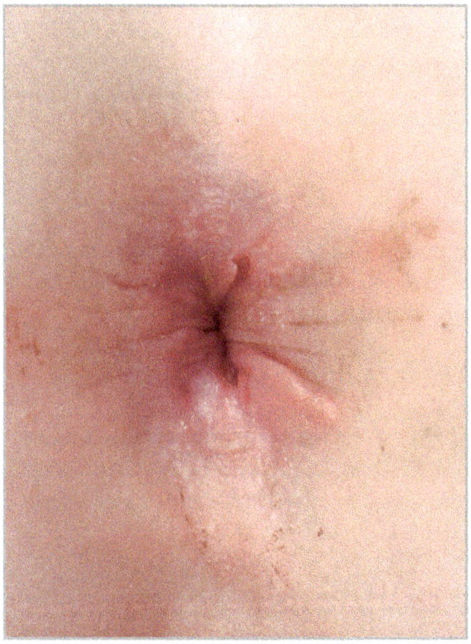

Figure 24.7 Swelling and fissuring of the (peri) anal region.

Corticosteroids

Since corticosteroids are the cornerstone of the treatment of CD, the use of corticosteroids is widely reported (Mayberry 2013).

- Topical treatment with clobetasol propionate 0.05% ointment can be tried alone (once daily at 4 consecutive days) or in combination with a calcineurin inhibitor (tacrolimus 0.1% ointment): clobetasol 0.05% once daily for 4 days and tacrolimus 0.1% twice daily for 3 days. However, most cases do probably not respond to topical treatment, have also luminal CD, and will therefore need systemic treatment.
- Systemic treatment with prednisolone 60 mg/day alone, tapered off over time, or in combination with azathioprine (1–2 mg/kg/day).
- Intralesional treatment with corticosteroid steroid injections, e.g. in granulomatous cheilitis (GC), is tried but the results are generally poor (Duan et al. 2014).

Systemic corticosteroids may be combined with other immunosuppressives or anti-inflammatory drugs to reduce steroid-specific adverse effects if used long term or if steroids alone are not sufficiently effective.

Other systemic treatments

Anti-inflammatory/immunosuppressive/immunomodulatory

1. Azathioprine alone (1–2 mg/kg/day, depending on the tolerability)
2. Metronidazole (10–20 mg/kg/day)
3. Sulfalazine (3–6 g/day in divided doses)
4. Tetracycline (100–200 mg/day)

Biologics

As in luminal CD, anti-tumor necrosis factor (TNF)-α treatment is increasingly used in vulvar CD, especially in refractory cases.

1. Infliximab (5 mg/kg infusions at weeks 0, 4, and 12, followed by maintenance treatment with an infusion every 6–8 weeks)
2. Adalimumab (40 mg subcutaneous every other week)

New developments include vedolizumab, an α4β7 blocker (=lymphocyte homing molecule), etrolizumab (binds the β7 subunit of the integrins α4β7 and αEβ7), ustekinumab (anti IL-12 and IL-23), tofacitinib (janus kinase inhibitor), and antisense therapy with oral SMAD7 antisense oligonucleotides, mongersen, targeting ileal, and colonic SMAD7, an inhibitor of transforming growth factor β1 (TGF-β1) signaling. SMAD7 is a potential target for suppression of CD-associated inflammation, which is characterized by reduced activity of the immunosuppressive cytokine TGF-β1 due to high levels of SMAD7 (Monteleone et al. 2015). However, it is not known if any is effective in vulvar CD.

Nutrition

There have been no sufficiently statistically powered placebo-controlled trials of nutritional therapy for active CD in adults. Based on limited data, elemental or polymeric diets appear less effective than corticosteroids. Unlike in the management of pediatric/adolescent CD, enteral therapy is regarded as only appropriate for adjunctive treatment to support nutrition and not for primary therapy. However, it is important not to underestimate the role of nutrition as supportive care in patients with CD, even if there is limited evidence to support its use as a primary therapy to induce remission (Gassull & Cabre 2001). Total parenteral nutrition may sometimes be an appropriate adjunctive therapy in complex, fistulating disease.

Surgery

The surgical management of CD has changed considerably during the last decade as a result of developments in medical therapy. Although most patients will still, eventually, have surgery, the care of CD is now primarily in the hands of medical gastroenterologists.

Local superinfection is not usually a problem, swabs and appropriate treatment need to be performed if clinically indicated. Vulvar lymphedema in CD is not associated with a high risk of infection; prophylactic low-dose antibiotics are not indicated.

Course and prognosis

The CD is a chronic (lifelong) inflammatory disease with episodes of flares and remission. CD is well known for its diagnostic delay, even in the stage with presence of cutaneous manifestations, which easily can be erroneously diagnosed as a primarily gynecological disorder (Assche van et al. 2010, Dignass et al. 2012a).

There is an increased risk of colorectal adenocarcinoma in areas of chronic inflammation due to CD and also for adenocarcinoma of the small bowel, although the latter is seldom diagnosed (Jess et al. 2013). Many patients live with a considerable burden of symptoms despite medical treatment in the absence of a curative therapy.

Concluding remarks

The CD of the vulva, vagina and to the perianal region is a well-known extraintestinal manifestation complicating intestinal CD and it is simply recognized by vigilant dermatologists, gynecologists, gastroenterologists, and proctologists, in particular when fistulizing on clinical presentation.

Metastatic vulvar CD on the other hand is a rare condition and a diagnostic challenge, because the symptoms and the clinical lesions are non-specific.

A multidisciplinary approach is required, involving gastroenterologists, dermatologists, gynecologists, pathologists, and proctologists/intestinal surgeons.

Treatment currently relies on systemic steroids (often combined with other immunosuppressive drugs and metronidazole), oral metronidazole, anti-TNF-α or, in refractory cases, surgery.

SARCOIDOSIS

Synonyms

Morbus Besnier-Boeck-Schaumann

Key features

- Schaumann bodies on histology
- Non-necrotizing granulomas

Introduction

Sarcoidosis, a rare inflammatory condition, results from an abnormal immune response to an unspecified or unidentified inflammatory trigger. It may affect multiple organs, predominantly lungs, lymph nodes, liver, and skin. Formation of abnormal nodules, called granulomas, which may readily destruction affected organ, is caused by sarcoidosis.

Epidemiology

The disease can affect people of any ethnic background and age, but mostly those aged under 40 and more common in women, rarely in children. Sarcoidosis is common in the Afro-American population of the USA.

Clinical features

The symptoms of sarcoidosis vary according to the affected organ, age, and gender of the patient. The disease can wax and wane unpredictably, as can its symptoms. Cutaneous manifestations may be found in up to an estimated 35% cases. Vulvar involvement with infiltrated plaques, although a rare condition, has been described (Tatnall et al.1985, Vera et al. 2013). The typical skin manifestation is a red patch with a yellowish brown tint. General signs may be headache, tiredness, painful joints, enlarged lymph glands, enlarged liver, meningitis, arrhythmias, and heart failure and depression. There are many cases without symptoms, in which sarcoidosis is 'accidently' diagnosed following chest X-ray examination for other reasons. In rare cases, the disease may affect heart and brain, including severe symptoms due to heart failure and brain damage. The frequency of organ manifestations varies, in 75–90% a liver biopsy will be positive but only 5% of brain biopsies show typical features of sarcoidosis.

Pathogenesis

Sarcoidosis is an inflammatory disease of unknown cause. It has been suggested that sarcoidosis results from an exaggerated immune response to an unknown infection (virus or specific bacteria, but this is unlikely due to the therapeutic response to immunosuppressive treatment), some other unidentified inflammatory trigger, such as chemicals, or a dysbalanced immune system.

In the majority of people diagnosed with sarcoidosis, this condition resolves spontaneously; this contrasts patients who are refractory to extensive anti-inflammatory treatment, and subsequently get chronic disease with organ damage.

Histopathology

Histopathological examination (usually of a lung biopsy harvested via bronchoscopy or mediatinoscopy or a skin biopsy if the skin is involved) may reveal non-caseating granulomas.

Diagnosis

The diagnosis of sarcoidosis can be made following (bronchoscopically guided) needle or punch biopsy, X-ray, or computed tomography scan, dependent on the localization of the disease and organs affected. The family history of patients is usually positive.

Differential diagnosis

Microbial or fungal infections, particularly tuberculosis, lymphoma, CD, and lung cancer are common differential diagnoses.

Treatment

Prednisolone or other corticosteroid medication, sometimes combined with immunosuppressive drugs, may be prescribed. Use of extensive immune suppression, including anti-TNF-α therapy and antimetabolites, is reserved for refractory cases. Many patients with sarcoidosis require no treatment as the condition is spontaneously remitting and relapsing. Vulvar disease may respond to topical steroids (Vera et al. 2013).

In general, patients are additionally being advised to change lifestyle, to obtain healthy diet habits, a regular sleep pattern, and to refrain from smoking, more as a general rule that due to its etiological or therapeutic properties.

Prognosis

Many patients with sarcoidosis do not need any medication. Specifically, mild disease may disappear after an episode lasting from months to years. Mortality rate is low and confined to cerebral and severely aggressive clinical forms.

MELKERSSON–ROSENTHAL SYNDROME

Synonyms

Miescher-Melkersson-Rosenthal syndrome, granulomatous cheilitis, orofacial granulomatosis

Key features

- Orofacial swelling (predominantly involving the lips)
- GC on histology
- Furrowed tongue
- Recurrent facial nerve palsy or paralysis

Introduction

Melkersson-Rosenthal syndrome is a rare neurological triad of disorders recognized in 1931. Facial edema and paralysis was described by E. Melkersson in 1928 and fissure of the tongue by C. Rosenthal. It is characterized by the triad of orofacial swelling (predominantly involving the lips), recurrent facial palsy or paralysis, and a furrowed tongue. Nevertheless, the diagnosis is difficult as the triad itself is a rare condition. The most frequent presentation is orofacial swelling (GC of Miescher) a monosymptomatic variant.

Recent studies have suggested an association between orofacial granulomatosis (GC) and CD (van de Scheur et al. 2003).

Vulvar MRS presents with indurated painless swelling of the labia majora (Kambil et al. 2013).

Epidemiology

Reliable epidemiological data are lacking. It may occur in childhood likewise in early adolescence.

Clinical features

The most common feature of MRS syndrome is orofacial swelling, which includes the face and lips (soft and nodular); in most cases abrupt swelling of the upper lip occurs. The lip is reddish-brown and may become hard and fissured after several recurrences. The disease waxes and wanes and will finally lead to sometimes painful, enlarged, firm lips. The periods of swelling may last for days initially; the periods of swelling will increase and finally hardly remit. MRS of the vulva has rarely been described and shows indurated papules or plaques at the vulva and groins (Kambil et al. 2013, Knopf et al. 1992).

Pathogenesis

Pathogenesis is unknown. There may be a genetic predisposition.

Histopathology

Histopathology of biopsy specimens from the lip reveals Langerhans giant cells, non-caseating granulomas with mononuclear inflammatory cell infiltration and lymphedema.

These granulomas are not invariably present, and their absence does not exclude the diagnosis of MRS (Rogers 1996).

Diagnostic criteria

Diagnosis is based on clinical symptoms and confirmed histopathologically. MRS may be diagnosed when only one or two components of the MRS triad are found (mono or bisymptomatic).

Differential diagnosis

Differential diagnoses are similar to that of sarcoidosis, comprising microbial or fungal infections, lymphoma, Behçet disease, and CD.

Treatment

Treatment is symptomatic and may include corticosteroids (topical, intralesional, or systemic in refractory cases), immunosuppressives and non-steroidal anti-inflammatory medications to reduce swelling. Also, (plastic) surgery may finally be indicated.

Prognosis

The MRS may become a chronic disorder, accompanied by increasing pain and discomfort in each recurrence period.

IDIOPATHIC GRANULOMATOUS VULVITIS

Introduction

Granulomatous vulvitis and GC are uncommon, localized inflammatory disorders, which may occur in adults and children. Only a few cases have been reported in the literature (Guerrieri et al. 1995, Rowan & Jones 2004).

Etiology

The etiology is unknown.

Pathogenesis

Pathogenesis is obviously 'idiopathic,' as to whether it is an entity is debated, some cases may develop into CD.

Clinical features

Clinical features of GV and GC include pain, swelling, distortion, and induration of the oral mucosa or vulva. In the reported cases gastrointestinal symptoms were absent, unlike to what is usually seen in Crohn or Behçet disease. However, cutaneous manifestations may precede luminal inflammation.

Histopathology

In both disorders (GV and GC) non-caseating granulomas may be observed on histopathology. Typical features consist of epithelioid cell granulomas with Langerhans giant cell and mononuclear cells, an inflammatory infiltrate may be seen in early stage. GV may have histological similarities with MRS and CD (Handa et al. 2003).

Diagnosis

The diagnosis is made histopathologically in addition to the clinical features.

Differential diagnosis

Crohn disease, Behçet disease, MRS, sarcoidosis, bartholinitis or abscess in Bartholin gland cyst, mycobacterial infection, lupus vulgaris, metastatic, and foreign body granuloma form part of the differential diagnosis of GV. In case of GC, local variations of this list are applicable.

Treatment

Although treatment of GV is generally disappointing, medical therapy with metronidazole, corticosteroids, sulfasalazine, danazol, and mesalazine has been proposed.

REFERENCES

Assche van G, Dignass A, Panes J, et al. for the European Crohn's and Colitis Organisation (ECCO). The second European evidence-based Consensus on the diagnosis and management of Crohn's disease: Definitions and diagnosis. J Crohn Colitis 2010; 4:7–27.

Barret M, de Parades V, Battistella M, et al. Crohn's disease of the vulva. J Crohn Colitis 2014; 8:563–570.

Berkowitz EZ, Lebwohl M. Cutaneous manifestations of inflammatory bowel disease. J Eur Acad Dermatol Venereol 2000; 14:349–350.

Burgdorf W. Cutaneous manifestations of Crohn's disease. J Am Acad Dermatol 1981; 5:689–695.

Corbett SN, Walsh CM, Spitzer RF, et al. Vulvar inflammation as the only manifestation of Crohn's disease in an 8-year-old girl. Pediatrics 2010; 125:e1518–e1522.

Dignass A, Eliakim R, Magro F, et al. Second European evidence-based consensus on the diagnosis and management of ulcerative colitis part 1: definitions and diagnosis. J Crohn Colitis 2012a;6:965–990.

Dignass A, Lindsay JO, Sturm A, et al. Second European evidence-based consensus on the diagnosis and management of ulcerative colitis part 2: current management. J Crohn Colitis. 2012b; 6:991–1030.

Duan D, Stevenson ML, Malter LB, et al. Cutaneous Crohn's disease of the vulva. BMJ Case Reports 2014.doi.1136/bcr-2014-204507.

Escher JC, Stoof TJ, van Deventer SJ, van Furth AM. Successful treatment of metastatic Crohn's disease with infliximab. J Pediatr Gastroenterol Nutr 2002; 34:420–423.

Gassull MA, Cabre E. Nutrition in inflammatory bowel disease. Curr Opin Nutr Metab Care 2001; 4:561–569.

Georgiou S, Pasmatzi E, Monastirli A, Tsambaos D. Cutaneous manifestations of inflammatory bowel disease. Hospital Chronicles 2006; 1:158–168.

Guerrieri C, Ohlsson E, Ryden G, Westermark P. Vulvitis granulomatosa: a cryptogenic chronic inflammatory hypertrophy of vulvar labia related to cheilitis granulomatosa and Crohn's disease. Int J Gynecol Pathol 1995; 14:352–359.

Handa S, Saraswat A, Radotra BD, Kumar B. Chronic macrocheilia: a clinico-pathological study of 28 patients. Clin Exp Dermatol 2003; 28:245–250.

Jess T, Horváth-Puhó E, Fallingborg J, Rasmussen HH, Jacobsen BA. Cancer risk in inflammatory bowel disease according to patient phenotype and treatment: a Danish population-based cohort study. Am J Gastroenterol 2013; 108:1869–1876.

Jostins L, Ripke S, Weersma RK, et al. Host-microbe interactions have shaped the genetic architecture of inflammatory bowel disease. Nature 2012; 491:119–124.

Kambil SM, Bhat RM, Dandakeri S, Bisen N. Granulomatous cheilitis with granulomatous vulvitis: a rare association. Indian J Dermatol Venereol Leprol 2013; 79:799–801.

Knopf B, Schaarschmidt H, Wollina U. Monosymptomatisches melkersson-Rosentha-Syndrom mit nachfolgender Vulvitis und perivulvitis granulomatosa. Hautarzt 1992; 43:711–713.

Mayberry JF, Lobo A, Ford AC, Thomas A. NICE clinical guideline (CG152): the management of Crohn's disease in adults, children and young people. Aliment Pharmacol Ther 2013; 37:195–203.

Molodecky NA, Kaplan GG. Environmental risk factors for inflammatory bowel disease. Gastroenterol Hepatol (N Y) 2010; 6:339–346.

Monteleone G, Neurath MF, Ardizzone S, et al. Mongersen, an oral SMAD7 antisense oligonucleotide, and Crohn's disease. N Engl J Med 2015; 372:1104–1113.

Neurath MF. Cytokines in inflammatory bowel disease. Nat Rev Immunol 2014; 14:329–342.

Palamaras I, El-Jabbour J, Pietropaolo N, et al. Metastatic Crohn's disease: a review. J Eur Acad Dermatol Venereol 2008; 22:1033–1043.

Parks AG, Morson BC, Pegum JS. Crohn's disease with cutaneous involvement. Proc R Soc Med 1965; 58:241–242.

Rogers RS 3rd. Melkersson-Rosenthal syndrome and orofacial granulomatosis. Dermatol Clin 1996; 14:371–379.

Rowan DM, Jones RW. Idiopathic granulomatous vulvitis. Australas J Dermatol 2004; 45:181–183.

Sathiyasekaran M, Shivbalan S. Crohn's disease. Indian J Pediatr 2006; 73:723–729.

Tatnall FM, Barnes HM, Sarkany I. Sarcoidosis of the vulva. Clin Exp Dermatol 1985; 10:384–385.

Thiriar S, Deroux E, Dourov N, et al. Granulomatous vulvitis, granulomatous cheilitis: a single diagnosis? Dermatology 1998; 196:455–458.

Van de Scheur MR, van der Waal RIF, Völker-Dieben HJ, et al. Orofacial granulomatosis in a patient with Crohn's disease. J Am Acad Dermatol 2003; 49:952–954.

Vera C, Funaro D, Bouffard D. Vulvar sarcoidosis: a case report and review of the literature. J Cutan Med Surg 2013; 17:287–290.

Chapter 25

Scleroderma, systemic lupus erythematosus, and Sjögren syndrome

Christiane Pfeiffer

INTRODUCTION

Scleroderma, systemic lupus erythematosus (SLE), and Sjögren syndrome are connective tissue diseases affecting women predominantly. They are characterized by inflammation and autoimmune features, specific skin signs, and systemic involvement. Although each disease has distinct features (**Table 25.1**), there can be overlap between scleroderma, SLE, and Sjögren syndrome in any combination. There is also an overlap of scleroderma with polymyositis in up to a fifth of patients. Another subgroup of patients is affected by 'mixed connective tissue disease' (MCTD), a distinct disease entity. Vulva and perineum involvement affecting sexual function may be found in scleroderma, SLE, and Sjögren either from disease-specific manifestations or from an increased risk of infection and neoplasia.

Morphea is a distinct entity without systemic involvement; however, it may exhibit histopathological features similar to scleroderma, namely, dermal fibrosis and atrophy of skin appendages in affected areas and will therefore also be covered in this chapter.

Table 25.1 Key features of the connective tissue diseases

	SSc	SLE	Sjögren	MCTD
Age at disease onset	40–50 years	20–40 years	40–50 years	30–50 years
Female:male	8:1	9:1	9:1	4:1
Antinuclear autoantibodies	+++	+++	+++	++
Hallmark extractable nuclear antigens recognized	Topoisomerase (SCL-70) Centromere (CENP-B)	Double-stranded DNA Ro (SS-A), La (SS-B)	Ro (SS-A), La (SS-B)	U1-RNP U3-snRNP
Other (auto)antibodies		Anti-phospholipid antibodies, CCP, RF, cryoglobulins	Cryoglobulins, RF, monoclonal gammopathy	
Chronic B cell-stimulation with hypergammaglobulinemia	–	+++	++++	+
Complement-activation	+	+++	+	+
Typical organ involvement	Raynaud, skin fibrosis, calcinosis, telangiectasia, puffy handy, esophagus, lung, kidney, pulmonary hypertension	Arthritis, serositis (pleura, pericardium), kidney, central nervous system, mucocutaneous disease, ultraviolet-sensitivity	Exocrine (salivary) glands, Sicca-syndrome (eye, nose, mouth, vagina), parotis swelling, interstitial lung disease, arthralgia, peripheral neuropathies	Raynaud, puffy hands, arthritis, esophagus, UV-sensitivity, mucocutaneous disease, kidney, pulmonary hypertension
Basic therapy strategy	Symptomatic therapy, immunosuppressants: not in all patients, not continuously	Continuous therapy with GCS or GCS-sparing agents	Symptomatic therapy, if lung involvement: immunosuppressants	Often continuous therapy with hydroxychloroquine (and low dose GCS)
Commonly employed immunosuppressant agents	Cyclophosphamide, methotrexate, azathioprine,	GCS, azathioprine, cyclophosphamide, mycophenolate mofetil, hydroxychloroquine, biologics (rituximab, belimumab)	Hydroxychloroquine, cyclosporine A, azathioprine, mycophenolate mofetil, methotrexate, rituximab	GCS, hydroxychloroquine, methotrexate, azathioprine
Age at disease onset	40–60 years	20–40 years	40–50 years	30–50 years
Cancer risk	Increased lung, liver, lymphoma	Increased lymphoma (especially non-Hodgkin lymphoma); lung; vulvar carcinoma	Increased lymphoma (especially MALT)	?

GCS, glucocorticosteroids; MCTD, mixed connective tissue disease; SLE, systemic lupus erythematosus; SSc, systemic sclerosis

Key features

- Scleroderma, SLE, and Sjögren syndrome are autoimmune multisystem diseases affecting women predominantly
- Vulvar disease is secondary to autoimmune processes affecting mucus production and epithelial integrity; in SLE ulceration may occur
- Dyspareunia is more frequent in patients with connective tissue diseases and should be sought and treated
- Treatment is symptomatic in the majority of patients; causal treatment is on the horizon for Sjögren syndrome

SCLERODERMA

Synonyms

Systemic sclerosis (SSc), limited cutaneous systemic sclerosis (lSSc), diffuse cutaneous systemic sclerosis (dSSc)

Key features

- Scleroderma is a systemic disease characterized by autoimmune, fibrotic, and vascular processes, typically with a loss of capillaries in the superficial capillary plexus of the dermis, clinically visible over the nail folds and gingiva
- Limited cutaneous scleroderma takes a slowly progressive course dominated by Raynaud phenomenon, esophageal dysmotility, telangiectasia, arthritis, sicca symptoms (e.g. dry mouth, dry eyes, dry vagina), and in late stages pulmonary arterial hypertension
- Diffuse cutaneous scleroderma is often highly aggressive with lung fibrosis and pulmonary hypertension arising early, up to 15% of patients develop renal arterial hypertension
- Vulvar sicca symptoms and dyspareunia are frequent in both types
- Perineal fibrosis may impair sexual function and complicate delivery

Introduction

Scleroderma is a rare connective tissue disease of unknown etiology, with strong female preponderance. At onset, most patients show an inflammatory phase with dermal swelling and Raynaud phenomenon followed by a tight induration and fibrosis. Two major clinical subtypes can be differentiated according to skin involvement:

- Limited cutaneous scleroderma with induration of distal extremities and facial involvement often shows a slower progression of disease and exhibits a specific pattern of systemic involvement
- Diffuse cutaneous scleroderma is characterized by induration of the skin on trunk, face, and extremities. Diffuse cutaneous scleroderma often progresses within the first 2 years of disease involving lung, heart, and/or kidney and warrants more aggressive, immunosuppressive treatment. Life expectancy has greatly improved during the past decades due to successful management of scleroderma renal crisis with angiotensin-converting-enzyme inhibitors and improvement in the management of pulmonary arterial hypertension

Epidemiology

Prevalence of scleroderma is estimated at 3–24/100,000.with 60% having lSSc, 30% dSSc, and 10% MCTD and overlap diseases. There is a decreased life expectancy in dSSc, mostly due to lung involvement.

Pathogenesis

In scleroderma, autoimmunity leading to fibrosis and endothelial dysfunction results in vasculopathy in the presence of strong angiogenic signals. Secondary Raynaud disease occurs in all organs, even on genital surfaces if exposed, e.g. in the setting of examination. Capillaries and small arteries may occlude (Doss et al. 2002) and give rise to ulcers. Salivary glands are occluded by fibrosis and secondary sicca syndrome with dry eye-dry mouth-dry vagina ensues.

Immunosuppression may tip the scale toward angiogenesis but cannot restore the glandular function.

Clinical presentation and differential diagnosis

As patients are very cold intolerant, care should be taken to perform the examination in a warm setting (ideally with an infrared lamp) and with prewarmed instruments, preferably of small size. Typically, most patients with vulvar complaints related to scleroderma have established cutaneous scleroderma.

Key complaints of vulvar scleroderma

- Dryness
- Dyspareunia

Most patients have no vulvar clinical signs, but some may exhibit visible perineal fibrosis with vaginal stenosis. Calcinosis may appear on thighs and vulva, with ulceration in 23% (Bhadauria et al. 1995). Sixty percent of patients complain of sexual dysfunction (Levis et al. 2012), which is strongly correlated with fingertip ulceration, a hallmark of progressive vaso-occlusive disease (Rosato et al. 2014) (**Figure 25.1**).

Differential diagnoses include drug-induced perineal fibrosis after tamoxifen treatment, stiff-man disease, porphyria, scleredema adultorum, lichen myxedematosus, eosinophilic fasciitis, nephrogenic fibrosing dermopathy, vinyl chloride disease, Graft versus Host Disease, and pansclerotic morphea.

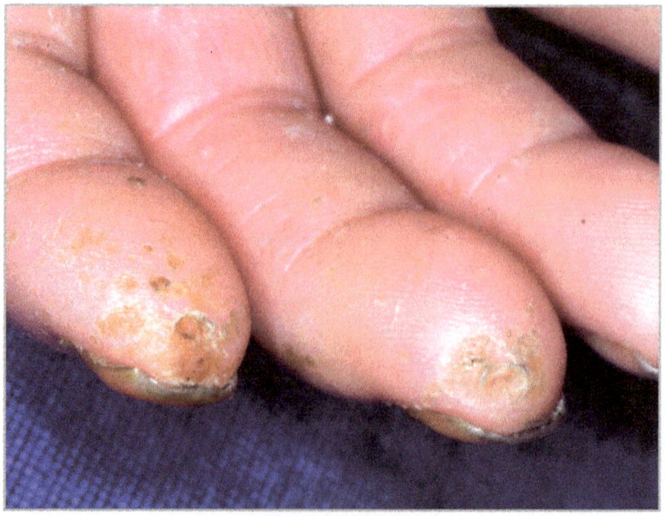

Figure 25.1 Digital fingertip ulcers in a patient with diffuse scleroderma and contractures of the fingers.

Morphea

Morphea, i.e. localised scleroderma, is a skin disease characterized by inflammation, fibrosis, and loss of skin appendages, and may be histologically difficult to differentiate from scleroderma. Its prevalence is about tenfold higher than scleroderma, and women are predominantly affected. There is no systemic involvement , and in one subtype alone (linear scleroderma), antinuclear autoantibodies (ANA) may be detected.

The most common type is the plaque-form, with single or multiple, indurated, plaques, which have an inflammatory purple rim (lilac ring) in active disease. Morphea has a strong association with lichen sclerosus (LS) (Farrell et al. 2000). About one fifth of individuals with morphea will also have cutaneous LS sometimes arising within plaques of morphea (**Figure 25.2**).

Key features

- Morphea is a common skin disease whose skin features may mimic scleroderma
- It frequently coexists with LS
- All patients with morphea should be examined for LS and vice versa

Histopathology of scleroderma and morphea

Histology is not useful for establishing the diagnosis in systemic scleroderma, which is based on the clinical criteria outlined in **Table 25.2**. Histology may help to diagnose morphea. A deep incisional biopsy of an established lesion is necessary to find the characteristic features, which involve the dermis and subcutaneous fatty tissue underneath a normal epidermis and papillary dermis. Intensely eosinophilic and thickened collagen bundles are oriented in parallel to the surface in the reticular dermis. Hair follicles and sebaceous glands may be atrophic or absent. The subcutaneous fat is replaced by collagen fibers. Thus, eccrine glands appear situated abnormally high within the dermis, whereas eccrine ducts appear compressed in the densely sclerotic dermis. A biopsy taken from an active lilac ring may reveal a dense inflammatory lymphohistiocytic infiltrate with interspersed plasma cells, accentuated in the dermis close to the subcutaneous fat and perivascularly.

There are no histopathological features that distinguish an established morphea lesion from systemic sclerosis. In scleroderma, the

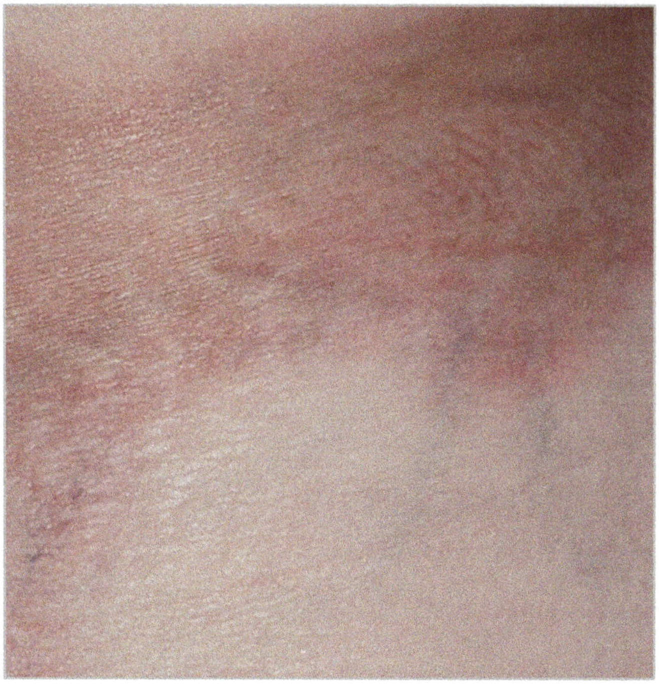

Figure 25.2 Simultaneous occurrence of morphea and lichen sclerosus in a patient with generalized morphea. (Note whitish opalescent small confetti-like plaques on livid brownish morphea plaque).

Table 25.2 Classification criteria for systemic sclerosis (Van den Hoogen et al. 2013)

Item	Subitem(s)	Weight/score
Skin thickening of the fingers of both hands extending proximal to the metacarpophalangeal joints (sufficient criterion)	-	9
Skin thickening of the fingers (only count the higher score)	Puffy fingers	2
	Sclerodactyly of the fingers (distal to the metacarpophalangeal joints but proximal to the proximal interphalangeal joints)	4
Fingertip lesions (only count the higher score)	Digital tip ulcers	2
	Fingertip pitting scars	3
Telangiectasia	-	2
Abnormal nailfold capillaries	-	2
Pulmonary arterial hypertension and/or interstitial lung disease (maximum score is 2)	Pulmonary arterial hypertension	2
	Interstitial lung disease	2
Raynaud phenomenon	-	3
SSc-related autoantibodies (maximum score is 3)	Anti-centromere (CENP-B) Anti-topoisomerase I (SLC-70) Anti-RNA-polymerase III	3

The total score is determined by adding the maximum weight (score) in each category. Patients with a total score of ≥ 9 are classified as having definite SSc.
SSc, systemic sclerosis

dermis is thickened containing swollen eosinophilic collagen bundles organized in parallel, entrapping fat cells, and accompanied by loss of skin appendages. Rarely, affected vessels may be present in the specimen, either with endothelial cell swelling, intimal thickening, and medial hypertrophy or occluded with fibrin.

Diagnosis

Scleroderma is a clinical diagnosis. The diagnostic criteria established in 1980 did not apply to many patients with lSSc. Therefore, a revision process has been undertaken, giving rise to new classification criteria that, though not yet validated for diagnostic purposes, are already applied when diagnosing the disease (**Table 25.2**).

Management of vulvar complaints

Therapy in scleroderma is guided by systemic involvement. Vulvar dryness can be alleviated by lubricants. It is observed clinically that patients undergoing vasoactive therapy for Raynaud symptoms or pulmonary hypertension with prostanoid infusions (e.g. epoprostenol) or oral phosphodiesterase-5-inhibition (e.g. sildenafil or tadalafil) experience improvement of vulvovaginal dryness and softening of perineal stiffness.

Rarely, perineal fibrosis progresses to stenosis of the vaginal opening and/or the anus, which may warrant surgery.

SYSTEMIC LUPUS ERYTHEMATOSUS

Key features

- SLE is an immune-complex disease with B-cell stimulation, high titers of autoantibodies (ANA, dsDNA, Ro, La, Sm, CCP, anti-phospholipids), complement activation, T-cell deviation
- Mucosal lesions include immune complex deposits and appear as poikilodermic CDLE-like plaques or ulcers
- Increased susceptibility to viruses, especially human papilloma virus (HPV)
- The HPV-related disease may take an aggressive course with widespread condylomata acuminata, giant and/or destructive condylomata, or atypical disease such as intraepithelial neoplasia (Bowenoid papulosis)
- Increased risk of vulvar squamous intraepithelial neoplasia (mostly HPV positive) and vulvar cancer, which may occur in young women
- Management of HPV-induced lesions in SLE should include careful monitoring for malignant transformation

Introduction

The SLE typically occurs in young women. Chronic B-cell stimulation results in production of (auto)antibodies, high titers of circulating immune complexes and complement activation on basement membranes of skin, mucosa, and serosa causes chronic inflammation. Immune defense is reduced against viruses, specifically against HPV. Chronic immune stimulation confers an increased risk to develop neoplasms, especially lymphoma.

Epidemiology

Ninety percent of all patients with SLE are women with an estimated prevalence of 12.5/100,000 European women. Due to modern immunosuppressive therapy, life expectancy has improved but there is an increased susceptibility to cancer, chiefly lymphoma (non-Hodgkin lymphoma and leukemia), but also lung cancers in smokers, and vulvar cancer (SIR 3.27-3.78) in younger women, in whom the risk is increased up to 24-fold. In a Californian study this risk was increased even further in women with Hispanic or Asian ethnicity (Parikh-Patel et al. 2008, Bernatsky et al. 2013). Mucocutaneous involvement is a diagnostic feature, even though it is not often observed clinically.

Pathogenesis

T-, B- and NK-cell function is impaired. There is a greatly increased susceptibility to HPV (Santana et al. 2011). HPV manifestations include common warts, epidermodysplasia verruciformis-like disease and high risk HPV 16 and 18 lesions. The exact reason for the inability to clear HPV is unknown. Normal immune response to HPV depends on B-cell-dependent formation of specific antibodies as well as CD8 function. In SLE, B-cells are hyperstimulated and produce a plethora of autoantibodies, while CD8-response is low. Hypothetical predisposing factors include NK- or T-cell dysfunction as well as effects of the immunosuppressant therapies applied in SLE patients. Abud-Mendoza et al. observed a significant decrease in B-cell and NK-cell numbers in SLE patients with HPV lesions, markedly in patients treated with mycophenolate mofetil (Abud-Mendoza et al. 2013). Other studies demonstrated more HPV lesions in patients having undergone cyclophosphamide or azathioprine treatments.

Clinical presentation

Chronic cutaneous lesions

The SLE-specific skin lesions include chronic cutaneous lupus erythematosus lesions, psoriasiform, and annular lesions, as well as oral ulcers.

Similar to lesions of cutaneous discoid lupus, chronic cutaneous mucosal lesions are characterized by poikilodermic plaques with whitish epidermal atrophy and scarring with telangiectasia. They arise on the mucosal surface of the mouth and genitals (**Figure 25.3**). In the labia majora hypo-and hyperpigmentation may be observed.

Similar to mouth ulcers affecting the palate, genital ulcers usually present as a single, highly painful, often recalcitrant lesion resolving with a small scar (Jolly & Patel 2006).

HPV-associated lesions

- Condylomata acuminata
- Intraepithelial neoplasia
- Vulvar carcinoma

Vulvar HPV lesions usually present as condylomata acuminata and are often HPV6/11 positive; however they are often widespread and recalcitrant to therapy. Giant condylomata and destructive condylomata may occur, especially during disease flares. Intraepithelial neoplasia (Bowenoid papulosis) may present as discrete velvet-like, sharply

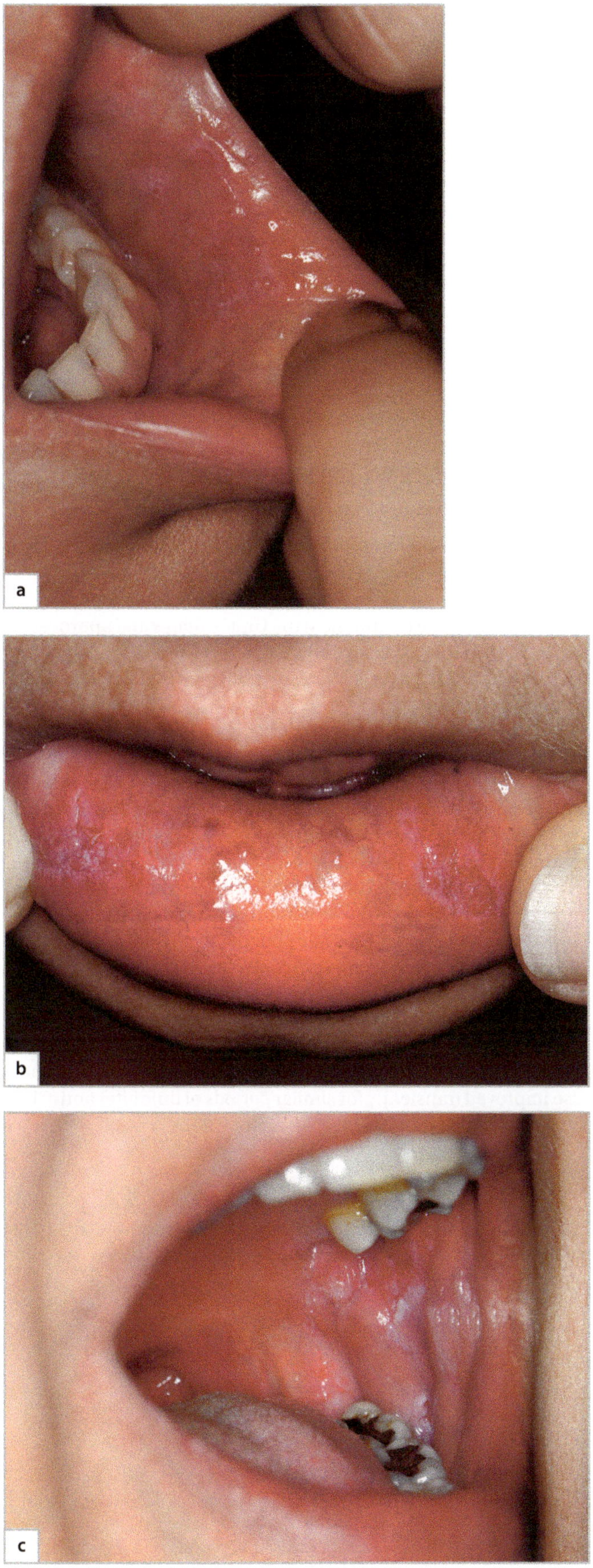

Figure 25.3 (a–c) Oral discoid lupus erythematosus lesions in a patient with systemic lupus erythematosus.

but irregularly demarcated brownish papules or patches involving the vulvar and/or perianal region. Any superficially ulcerated lesion as well as any raised papules should be biopsied to rule out vulvar intraepithelial neoplasia or vulvar carcinoma. The risk of HPV-related vulvar carcinoma is greatly increased in SLE (about 3.5-fold) and may occur in young patients.

Other viral disease

The SLE patients may suffer from recurrent genital herpes, which is difficult to treat especially in patients on mycophenolate mofetil, which in itself induces higher susceptibility to herpes infections. Widespread mollusca contagiosa and giant mollusca may occur.

Diagnosis

The diagnoses are based on their typical clinical picture and should be confirmed histologically. The histopathological features are the same as in non-SLE patients (see text books of dermatology or histopathology of the skin).

The SLE should be diagnosed according to the 1997 ACR update of the 1982 ARA classification (Hochberg 1997).

Management

Prevention

The quadrivalent HPV vaccine provides protection against HPV lesions caused by HPV 6 / 11 and HPV 16 / 18 infections (see Chapter 30). Once a woman is infected by a particular HPV virus the vaccination is of no further value.

Therapeutic options

Because of the high risk for vulvar intraepithelial neoplasia and vulvar carcinoma, HPV-induced lesions should be treated. Often destructive therapy with CO_2-laser or cryotherapy is warranted. However, therapy of HPV-related lesions may be difficult (Chapter 30); therefore, immunomodulatory treatment, such as imiquimod or sinecatechins, should be considered in conjunction with the destructive therapies. Use of emollients such as almond oil-based ointments is recommended, this seems to prevent further spread of lesions. Combined therapy of oral zinc sulfate with conventional treatments of vulvar warts appears to reduce the relapse rate (Akhavan et al. 2014) and systemic treatment with zinc compounds has been applied in patients with epidermodysplasia verruciformis (such as zinc sulfate up to 10 mg/kg body weight). Zinc levels are low in many SLE patients; oral zinc supplements aim to raise levels to the upper normal range.

In giant molluscum contagiosum cidofovir can be applied topically. Nephrotoxicity, even after topical application, limits its use.

SJÖGREN SYNDROME

Introduction

Sjögren syndrome is a systemic autoimmune disease with autoantibody formation, which affects eccrine glands, thereby causing the sicca syndrome; major organ involvement can occur.

Key features

- Sjögren is a B-cell stimulatory disease occurring in perimenopausal women affecting eccrine glands
- Characteristic features include: dry eye, dry mouth, dry vulva/vagina
- Dyspareunia
- Extraglandular disease can be present

Epidemiology

Sjögren syndrome is regarded as the second most frequent connective tissue disease (after rheumatoid arthritis), with an estimated prevalence of up to 4.8% and a female to male ratio of 9:1.

Pathogenesis

Sjögren syndrome is characterized by a destructive inflammation of eccrine glands associated with a production of Ro- and La-antibodies. Current knowledge infers interplay between genetic, especially HLA-driven, environmental, viral and hormonal factors (hormonal changes related to menopause) triggering polyclonal B-cell stimulation. Affected glands include lacrimal, salivary, and vulvar vestibular glands. Xerophthalmia with keratoconjunctivitis sicca, xerostomia with resultant increased periodontitis and caries risk, parotid swelling, and vulvar dryness are hallmarks of the disease. Extraglandular disease manifestations include interstitial lung disease, arthralgia, interstitial nephritis, and neurological disease. Sjögren syndrome may be primary, or arise as a secondary disease to underlying connective tissue diseases such as SLE or rheumatoid arthritis. About 15% of patients initially classified as primary Sjögren will develop SLE over time. In SSc Sicca-syndrome can be observed either as an overlap, with the presence of Ro/La-antibodies or as a consequence of gland destruction by fibrosis without lymphocytic infiltrates.

Clinical presentation

About 60% of patients complain of vaginal dryness, often described as itchiness and a sandpaper-like feeling. There are no characteristic signs apart from possible atrophy. Dryness may be more pronounced during sexual foreplay, as the vestibular glands provide secretion during arousal, thus, dyspareunia is a common complaint.

Diagnosis

The diagnosis is based on the symptoms of vaginal dryness in conjunction with the criteria for Sjögren syndrome.

Diagnostic features (at least two are necessary for diagnosis)(Shiboski et al. 2012)

- Keratoconjunctivitis sicca with a score > 3 (in an individual not taking glaucoma eye drops, nor having undergone eye surgery within the past 5 years)
- Histopathology in minor salivary gland biopsy: focal lymphocytic sialadenitis with a focus score ≥ 1 (a focus: ≥50 lymphocytes per 4 mm^2 glandular tissue adjacent to normal acini)
- Positive anti-SSA/Ro- and/or anti-SSB/La-antibodies or (positive rheumatoid factor and ANA ≥ 320)

Differential diagnosis

Sicca symptoms may also be present after irradiation treatment, in patients with hepatitis C infection, AIDS, sarcoidosis, amyloidosis, Graft versus Host Disease, or IgG4-related disease.

Principles of management

Therapeutic options

The mainstay of therapy is symptomatic. Keratoconjunctivitis is treated with frequent application of artificial tear drops, containing hydoxymethyl cellulose, hydrocolloid, or carbomer or topical cyclosporine A (first-line treatment in the United States and approved by the Food and Drug Administration, not by the European Medicines Agency) to prevent complications such as corneal ulceration, opacification, or perforation.

No evaluation of vaginal lubricant has been performed in a systematic way. Clinical evidence supports application of paraffin/ Vaseline-based emollients. Patients have reported lessening of symptoms by regular use of perineal massage oils, such as lavender or roman coriander oil (*Nigella sativa*). Dyspareunia can be alleviated by using lubricants and lubricated condoms.

Systemic secretagogue therapy (a substance that causes another substance to be secreted) with pilocarpine (and cevimeline in the United States) is being used for patients with keratoconjunctival ulcers, but effectiveness in vaginal disease has not even been reported anecdotally. Anti-B cell therapy (anti-CD20) with biologics, however, has been tested in larger case series and been demonstrated to induce remission of xerophthalmia for a mean of 24 weeks after the first cycle. We have observed patients in whom vaginal dryness also improved transiently for similar periods of time after anti-CD20 treatment.

Course of disease

Without treatment the course is chronic progressive. Anti-CD20 therapy shows some promise.

REFERENCES

Abud-Mendoza C, Cuevas-Orta E, Santillan-Guerrero EN, et al. Decreased blood levels of B lymphocytes and NK cells in patients with systemic lupus erythematosus (SLE) infected with papillomavirus (HPV). Arch Dermatol Res 2013; 305:117–123.

Akhavan S, Mohammadi SR, Modarres Gillani M, et al. Efficacy of combination therapy of oral zinc sulfate with imiquimod, podophyllin or cryotherapy in the treatment of vulvar warts. J Obstet Gynaecol Res 2014; 40:2110–2113.

Bernatsky S, Ramsey-Goldman R, Labreque J, et al. Cancer risk in systemic lupus: an updated international multicenter cohort study. J Autoimm 2013; 42:130–135.

Bhadauria S, Moser DK, Clements PJ, et al. Genital tract abnormalities and female sexual function impairment in systemic sclerosis. Am J Obstetr Gynecol 1995; 172:580–587.

Doss BJ, Qureshi F, Mayes MD, Jacques SM. Vascular and connective tissue histopathologic alterations of the female lower genital tract in scleroderma. J Rheumatol 2002; 29:1384–1387.

Farrell AM, Marren PM, Wojnarowska F. Genital lichen sclerosus associated with morphoea or systemic sclerosis: clinical and HLA-characteristics. Br J Dermatol 2000; 143:598–603.

Hochberg MC. Updating the American College of Rheumatology revised criteria for the classification of systemic lupus erythematosus [letter]. Arthritis Rheum 1997; 40:1725.

Jolly M, Patel P. Looking beyond the ordinary: genital lupus. Arthritis Rheum 2006;55:821-822.

Levis B, Hudson M, Knafo R, et al. Rates and correlates of sexual activity and impairment among women with systemic sclerosis. Arthritis Care Res 2012; 64:340–350

Parikh-Patel A, White RH, Allen M, Cress R. Cancer risk in a cohort of patients with systemic lupus erythematosus (SLE) in California. Cancer Causes Control 2008; 19:887–894.

Rosato E, Rossi C, Molinaro I, et al. Sexual distress, sexual dysfunction and relationship quality in women with systemic sclerosis: correlation with clinical variables. Int J Immunopathol Pharmacol 2014; 27:279 -285.

Santana IU, Gomes AD, Lyrio LD, Rios Grassi MF, Santiago MB. Systemic lupus erythematosus, human papillomavirus infection, cervical pre-malignant and malignant lesions: a systematic review. Clin Rheumatol 2011; 30:665–672.

Shiboski SC, Shiboski CH, Criswell LA, et al. ACR classification criteria for Sjögren's syndrome: a data-driven, expert consensus approach in the Sjögren's international collaborative clinical alliance cohort. Arthritis Care Res 2012; 64:475–487.

Van den Hoogen F, Khanna D, Fransen J, et al. 2013 classification criteria for systemic sclerosis: an ACR/EULAR collaborative initiative. Ann Rheum Dis 2013; 72:1747–1755.

Chapter 26 Autoimmune bullous diseases

Kathy Taghipour, Gudula Kirtschig

INTRODUCTION

Key features

- Autoimmune bullous diseases should be considered in the presence of blistering and erosions
- They are a heterogeneous group divided into subepidermal and intraepidermal blistering diseases
- Mucosal involvement is more prominent in some diseases, whereas cutaneous involvement is more prominent in others
- Diseases may be divided into scarring and non-scarring
- Autoantibodies are either primarily of the immunoglobulin G (IgG) or IgA class
- Immunofluorescence tests confirm the diagnosis

Autoimmune bullous diseases are a heterogeneous group of diseases characterized by blisters, leading to erosions and crusts of the skin and mucous membranes. The blistering is caused by autoantibodies that bind various antigens of the epithelium or the basement membrane zone (BMZ) of epithelia. The autoantibodies are tissue bound and may circulate in patient's serum. In addition to antibody interaction, complement activation and possibly T-cell activity play a role in the pathogenesis.

Depending on the location of the antigen in the skin, the antigen-antibody interaction leads to a cleft either subepithelially (pemphigoid group) or intraepithelially (pemphigus group) of skin or mucosa (**Figure 26.1**). Thus, autoimmune bullous diseases are usually classified into subepidermal and intraepidermal blistering disease groups.

Although rare, autoimmune bullous diseases are important differential diagnoses (DD) to consider in cases of erosions and scarring in the genital area. **Tables 26.1** to **26.6** summarize the clinical and immunopathological characteristics of autoimmune bullous diseases. All bullous diseases may present in the genitals; however, the genital site is more commonly affected in certain conditions, as shown in the box below.

- Bullous pemphigoid (BP) in children
- Linear IgA disease (LAD) in children
- Mucous membrane pemphigoid (MMP)
- Epidermolysis bullosa acquisita (EBA)
- Pemphigus vulgaris (PV)
- Paraneoplastic pemphigus (PNP)

DIAGNOSIS OF AUTOIMMUNE BULLOUS DISEASES

Diagnosis is based on a combination of clinical features and immunological characteristics of each disease. Investigations are usually performed by specialist laboratories as testing is complex. It is best to request expert opinion and to liaise with your laboratory before requesting these tests as there are special considerations.

Direct immunofluorescence

A skin biopsy (usually a 4 mm punch biopsy) of uninvolved perilesional skin, usually 1–2 cm away from a lesion, is tested for autoantibody binding in the tissue; see **Figure 26.2** for the principle of the test. This biopsy is normally frozen in liquid nitrogen immediately after taking or transported to the laboratory in a special transport medium or normal (0.9% NaCl) saline.

Indirect immunofluorescence

This serum test is recommended if an autoimmune blistering disease is strongly suspected but may not yield positive results in diseases with undetectable levels of circulating antibodies. In the subepidermal group, indirect immunofluorescence (IIF) is performed on 1 M NaCl split skin that leads to a separation of the skin through the lamina lucida lifting certain antigens to the top of the artificial blister (epidermal side) and others to the bottom (dermal side) (**Figure 26.1**). This helps to distinguish, e.g. BP from EBA and certain variants of MMP; this method is also thought to be more sensitive compared to the non-split tissue test.

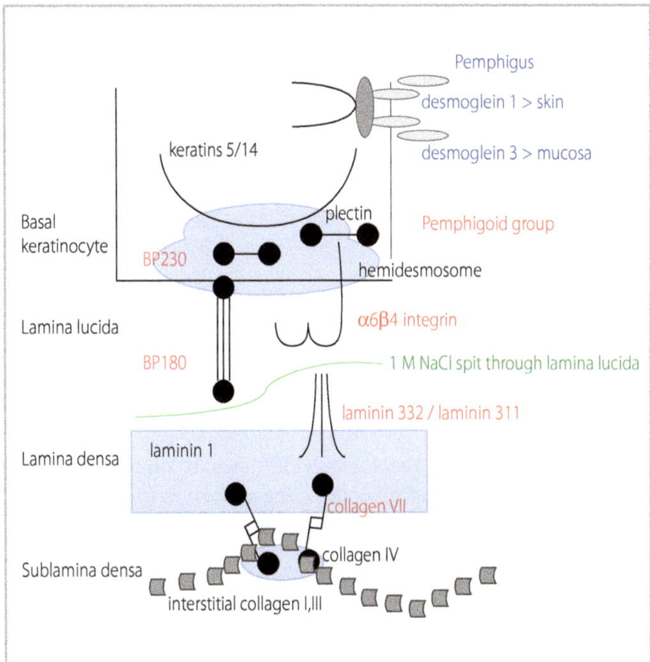

Figure 26.1 Autoantigens in autoimmune bullous diseases.

Table 26.1 Clinical characteristics of subepithelial autoimmune bullous diseases

Autoimmune bullous disease	Age group	Clinical distribution	Scarring	Primary treatment option
BP	Elderly, rarely children	Limbs, trunk, flexures, rarely vulva in children; minor oral lesions	No	Topical or systemic steroids; tetracyclines
MMP	Middle age and elderly; rarely children	Oral, esophagus, ocular, genital, and airway mucosae with or without skin involvement	Yes	Systemic steroids; dapsone, cyclophosphamide
LAD/CBDC	All ages	Trunk and limbs (face and genitals in children) with frequent mucosal involvement	No; if scarring occurs the disease should be classified as MMP or possibly EBA	Dapsone, systemic steroids, sulfonamides, erythromycin in children (spontaneous remission expected)
EBA	All ages	Inflamed generalized or mechanobullous +/– mucosal involvement	Yes	Systemic steroids, immunosuppressants dapsone, colchicine and intravenous immunoglobulins. Children are mainly treated with steroids and dapsone, spontaneous remission can be expected
DH	Young adults, rarely children and elderly	Extensor areas, e.g. elbows, knees, buttocks	No	Gluten free diet, dapsone, sulfonamides

BP, bullous pemphigoid; MMP, mucous membrane pemphigoid; LAD, linear IgA disease; CBDC, chronic bullous disease of childhood; EBA, epidermolysis bullosa acquisita; DH, dermatitis herpetiformis

Table 26.2 Immunopathological characteristics of subepithelial autoimmune bullous diseases

Autoimmune bullous disease	IF antibody deposition on salt-split skin	Target antigens	Antibody isotype
BP	Linear along BMZ, epidermal	BP180, BP230, rarely P200	IgG, less commonly IgA, IgM, IgE
MMP	Linear along BMZ, may be epidermal or dermal	BP180 (collagen XVII), BP230, laminin 332 (laminin 5/epiligrin), α6ß4 integrin, collagen VII	IgG, IgA
LAD/CBDC	Linear along BMZ, epidermal	BP180, LAD285, BP230	IgA
EBA	Linear along BMZ, dermal	Collagen VII	IgG, (IgA?)
DH	(granular IgA at BMZ on DIF only)	Possibly epidermal tissue transglutaminase	IgA

BMZ, basement membrane zone; BP, bullous pemphigoid; CBDC, chronic bullous disease of childhood; DH, dermatitis herpetiformis; DIF, direct immunofluorescence; EBA, epidermolysis bullosa acquisita; IgG, immunoglobulin G; LAD, linear IgA disease; MMP, mucous membrane pemphigoid

Table 26.3 Classification and management in subepidermal bullous disease based on clinicopathological signs

Good response to treatment	Refractory disease
• Localized disease • Non-scarring disease • Predominant IgA, usually responsive to dapsone	• Generalized disease • Predominantly mucosal disease • Scarring disease

Table 26.4 Key clinical and immunopathological features in the differential diagnosis (DD) of subepidermal diseases

Clinical features	Main DD	Alternative DD
Predominant mucosal involvement	MMP	LAD if sole IgA? EBA if antibodies to collagen VII
Scarring of mucosae	MMP	LAD if sole IgA? EBA if antibodies to collagen VII
Predominant skin lesions, no scarring	BP	LAD if sole IgA
Predominant skin lesions with scarring	EBA	LAD if sole IgA?

BP, bullous pemphigoid; MMP, mucous membrane pemphigoid; LAD, linear IgA disease; EBA, epidermolysis bullosa acquisita; IgA, immunoglobulin A

ELISA

Enzyme linked immunosorbent assay (ELISA) using recombinant epitopes of antigens has the advantage of detecting antibodies to specific target antigens/epitopes but may be negative in the case of unknown epitopes.

Histopathology

Investigation of lesional skin (intact blister if possible or edge of erosion) gives diagnostic clues, but the diagnosis of an autoimmune bullous disease cannot be made by histopathology only. Features such as the level of the split and the nature of the inflammatory infiltrate distinguish certain diseases.

Table 26.5 Immunopathological characteristics of intraepithelial autoimmune bullous diseases.

Autoimmune bullous disease	IF antibody deposition pattern	Target antigens
Pemphigus vulgaris/vegetans (PV)	Epidermal/intercellular	Desmoglein 3 (130 kD) Desmoglein 1 (110 kD)
Pemphigus foliaceus (PF)	Epidermal/intercellular: in the upper layer of epidermis below stratum corneum	Desmoglein 1
Paraneoplastic pemphigus (PNP)	Epidermal/intercellular and subepidermal	Plakins: desmoplakin I (250 kD), BPag1 (230 kD), desmoplakin II (210 kD), envoplakin (210 kD), periplakin (190 kD), plectin (500 kD) and a 170-kD protein

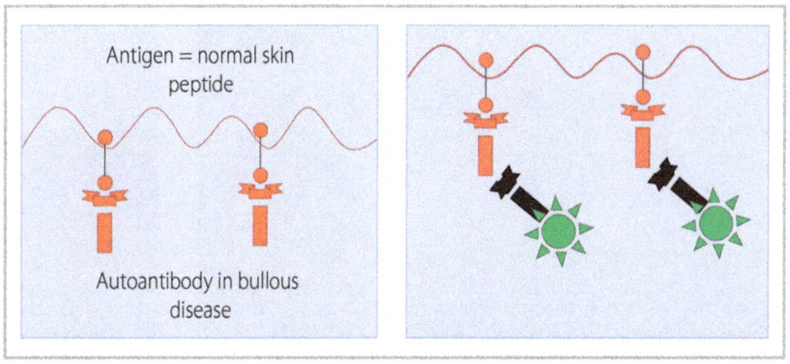

Figure 26.2 Direct Immunofluorescence: patient's skin containing the autoantigen bound by specific autoantibodies. Visualization with FITC labelled anti-immunoglobulin antibody (one step procedure).

Table 26.6 Clinical characteristics of intraepithelial autoimmune bullous diseases

Autoimmune bullous disease	Age group	Clinical distribution
Pemphigus vulgaris (PV)	Middle age but with a peak at 70 years	Face, scalp, and trunk are common; often generalized; mucosae always affected
Pemphigus vegetans	As PV	Flexural including inguinal and oral mucosa
Pemphigus foliaceus (PF)	As PV, children and young adults in endemic form	Scalp, chest, back, or generalized; no mucosal involvement
Paraneoplastic pemphigus (PNP)	All ages	Upper body, palmoplantar, genital, generalized with severe mucosal involvement

SUBEPIDERMAL AUTOIMMUNE BULLOUS DISEASES

These encompass mainly the pemphigoid group with two major entities: BP that predominantly affects the skin and MMP that affects the mucous membranes but may also involve the skin. The autoantigens and antibody class (IgG/IgA) partly overlap. The clinical features are therefore an important criterion when making the diagnosis. LAD and EBA are subepidermal bullous diseases that partly overlap with BP and MMP; as to whether they are separate entities is still debated and needs to be further defined (Chan et al. 2002). A distinct entity of the subepidermal bullous disease group is dermatitis herpetiformis (DH). DH is associated with gluten sensitivity disease of the bowel, Coeliac disease, and tissue-bound autoantibodies of IgA class targeting tissue transglutaminase of the skin (**Tables 26.1** and **26.2**).

There are overlapping clinical and immunopathological features in autoimmune subepidermal bullous diseases. **Table 26.3** summarizes the classification and management of subepidermal diseases based on clinico-pathological features and **Table 26.4** shows the key clinical and immunopathological features in the differential diagnosis of subepidermal diseases.

Bullous pemphigoid

Epidemiology

BP affects mainly the elderly with an average age of 80 years. It is the most common bullous disease in Western Europe with reported incidences of 6.6-43 per million persons per year. The incidence seems to be rising, and this has been attributed to an aging population. A female predilection is suggested.

Pathogenesis

Blister formation is caused by antigen–antibody binding and complement activation along the dermo-epidermal junction (**Figure 26.3**). The main BP antigens are BPag1 (BP230) and BPag2 (BP180/collagen XVII) that are structural components of the hemidesmosomes of the basal keratinocytes providing adherence to the underlying dermis.

Recently, it has been shown that BP is associated with neurological diseases such as cerebrovascular disease, dementia, Parkinson disease, epilepsy, and multiple sclerosis (Langan et al. 2011, Taghipour et al. 2010). The diseases pre-date BP and are considered to be risk factors. An association between BP and some drugs in particular neuroleptic drugs, spironolactone, and furosemide has been described, although it is not yet clear if these drugs can trigger BP (Lloyd-Lavery et al. 2013).

Clinical presentation

BP often starts with itch followed by an urticated and/or eczematous-looking rash and tense blisters on erythematous or normal-looking skin. The blisters may develop months after the initial symptoms. BP frequently affects the skin of limbs and trunk (with an affinity to flexural sites) (**Figure 26.4a** and **b**) but the oral mucosa may also be affected. Other mucosal sites (e.g. eyes and esophagus) are not involved in BP. The vulva may be affected (**Figure 26.5**) and is indeed the main affected site in childhood. Blisters and erosions heal without scarring.

Histopathology

A biopsy of a fresh blister stained with hematoxylin and eosin (H&E) usually shows subepidermal cleavage with a dermal inflammatory infiltrate consisting of eosinophils and neutrophils.

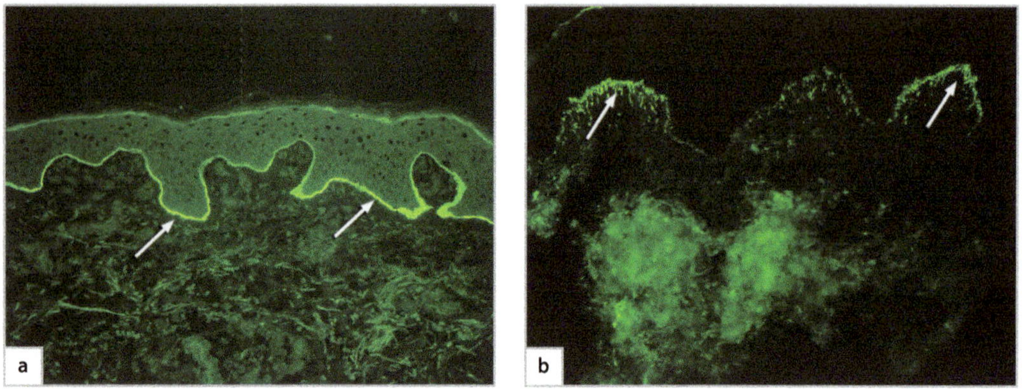

Figure 26.3 Immunofluorescence showing linear IgG deposition at the basement membrane zone, typically seen in the pemphigoid group (a) and granular IgA clustered at dermal papillae in dermatitis herpetiformis (b).

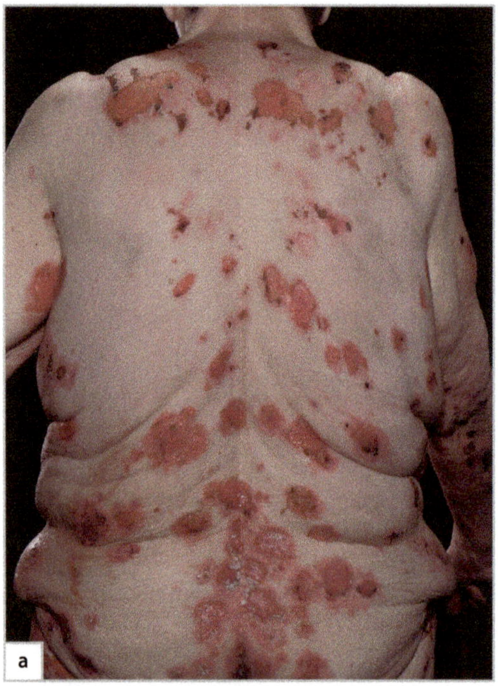

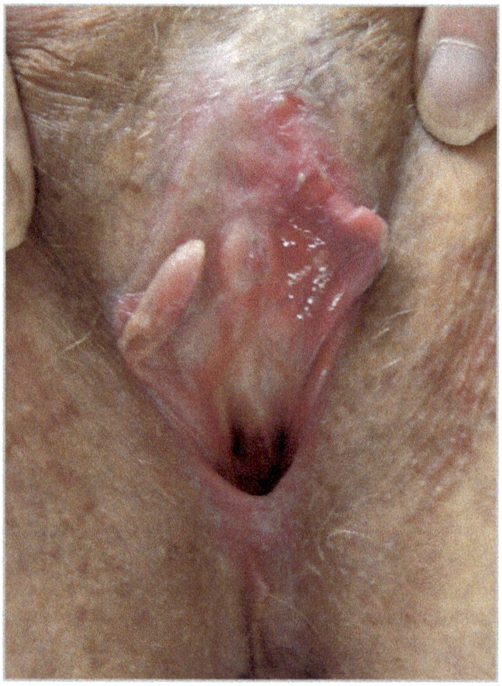

Figure 26.5 Localized pemphigoid of the vulva in a young woman showing erosions.

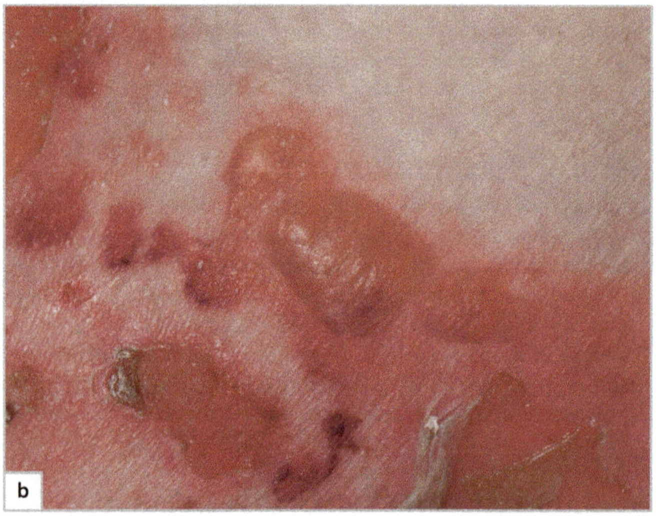

Figure 26.4 Generalized bullous pemphigoid (a) and close-up of tense blisters and erosions (b).

Diagnosis

Typical clinical features and laboratory findings confirm the diagnosis of BP. The gold diagnostic standard is direct immunofluorescence (DIF) showing linear deposition of IgG (less commonly IgA, IgE, and IgM) and/or C3 along the BMZ (**Figure 26.3a**). IIF on 1 M salt-split skin usually shows binding of antibodies to the epidermal aspect of split skin (**Figure 26.6**). ELISA (using recombinant epitopes) identifies specific antibodies to e.g. BPag1 and BPag2 and quantifies the antibody titer that may give clues with regard to disease activity.

Treatment

Blisters in occluded areas such as the vulva will usually burst leaving painful erosions that may be difficult to take care of. The principle of general care for blisters and erosions in the vulvar area is the same for all blistering and erosive disease.

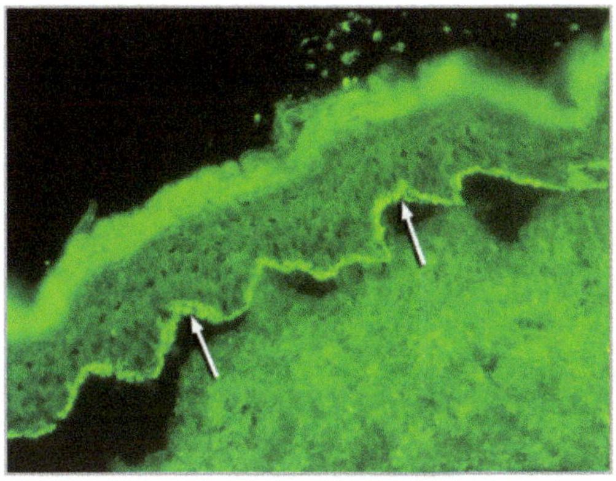

Figure 26.6 Indirect immunofluorescence of salt-split skin showing epidermal binding of immunoglobulin G.

General care of vulvar blisters and erosions

- Tight clothing and other mechanical irritation should be avoided
- The roof of blisters should be kept intact if possible as this provides protection
- Soothing emollients and soap substitutes improve the symptoms
- Any fluid (urine, water, etc.) on eroded areas is painful; prior to bathing, swimming or urination protection of the site with a petroleum jelly or a very greasy emollient can be helpful
- In general, therapeutic ointments seem better tolerated than creams and are less likely to cause allergy
- Antiseptic washing fluids, e.g. containing chlorhexidine, may prevent secondary infection

Specific treatment options can be divided into anti-inflammatory drugs, immunosuppressive/immunomodulating drugs, and procedures that remove circulating autoantibodies and inflammatory mediators (Venning et al. 2012; Kirtschig et al. 2008). For mild and localized disease, daily application of super potent topical steroids such as 0.05% clobetasol propionate ointment is usually effective. Systemic steroids are the mainstay for the treatment of BP in more extensive disease. Prednisolone 0.5 mg/kg body weight is typically used until the blisters stop evolving, then the dose can be tapered. Long-term applications and high doses of glucocorticosteroids are associated with significant toxicity in the elderly population. Anti-inflammatory antibiotics, e.g. tetracycline/doxycycline, are an alternative treatment; they are generally less toxic and effective for the treatment of BP. Topical tacrolimus 0.1% has been used to treat localized BP and vulvar BP (Lebeau et al. 2004). It is associated with a stinging sensation that may subside with continuous use. Although topical tacrolimus may not be as effective as super potent topical steroids; it causes less skin atrophy. Other treatment modalities to treat refractory and generalized BP include immunosuppressive agents; specific regimens are detailed in treatment guidelines (Venning et al. 2012).

Course and prognosis

BP is usually a self-limiting disease and resolves in most patients after months to a few years. During the active stage, generalized BP is associated with considerable morbidity and a mortality twice that of the general elderly population, in particular in the first year of disease when treated with high doses of systemic steroids. Treatment should therefore aim to control the symptoms with minimum adverse effects.

Childhood pemphigoid

BP is rare in children but localized vulvar involvement is well recognized. In particular, the IgA-mediated variant (chronic bullous disease of childhood/LAD) is more common in children. The immunopathological characteristics of childhood pemphigoid are the same as in adult disease. The main differential diagnoses include other acquired (MMP/pemphigus) or hereditary bullous diseases, including the various forms of epidermolysis bullosa (Chapter 27). The prognosis of childhood BP is favorable. It responds well to treatment with oral corticosteroids (1–2 mg/kg body weight/day) or very potent topical corticosteroids. Oral erythromycin with or without nicotinamide and dapsone (in IgA predominant disease) may be an alternative in some children, in particular to avoid long-term systemic steroids if the disease course is protracted (Venning et al. 2012).

Mucous membrane pemphigoid

Synonyms

Cicatricial pemphigoid; antiepiligrin cicatricial pemphigoid; anti-laminin 5 pemphigoid; benign MMP; oral pemphigoid; ocular (cicatricial) pemphigoid

Introduction

MMP is a rare, chronic subepidermal bullous disease that predominantly affects the mucous membranes but may also involve the skin (Chan et al. 2002). Blisters leading to erosions and ulcerations may be present in oral, nasopharyngeal, laryngeal, esophageal, ocular, and genital mucosae where they may lead to scarring. Life-threatening respiratory tract stenosis and blindness may follow scarring that is an important feature of MMP. Involvement of the vulva may be associated with changes that mimic other inflammatory conditions such as lichen planus (LP) and lichen sclerosus (LS).

Epidemiology

There are few reports of incidence; 1–2 cases per million population per year have been estimated in Western Europe. MMP is more common in middle-aged to older individuals, with women more frequently affected.

Pathogenesis

Autoantibodies of IgG and/or IgA type are directed against a number of antigens of the BMZ of epithelia (**Table 26.2**) and are shown to cause blistering in mice. The main antigens are BP180 (BPag2) and laminin 332 and less frequently BP230 (BPag1), collagen VII, and $\alpha6\beta4$ integrin.

Clinical features

MMP usually affects the oral and ocular mucosa and less frequently the skin. Oral involvement consists of frank blisters and erosions or a desquamative gingivitis (**Figure 26.7**), very similar to mucosal LP (Chapter 19). Esophageal involvement is possible and may lead to painful swallowing. Vulvar MMP presents with soreness, erosions, inflammation, and possibly scarring that may rarely lead to architectural changes. Intact blisters may occasionally be seen in the genitals; however, they often burst at this site and patients may rarely only present with erosions that may lead to a delay in diagnosis. It is important that the skin and other mucosal sites are examined for further erosions, blistering, or scarring. Urinary and sexual dysfunctions are important sequelae.

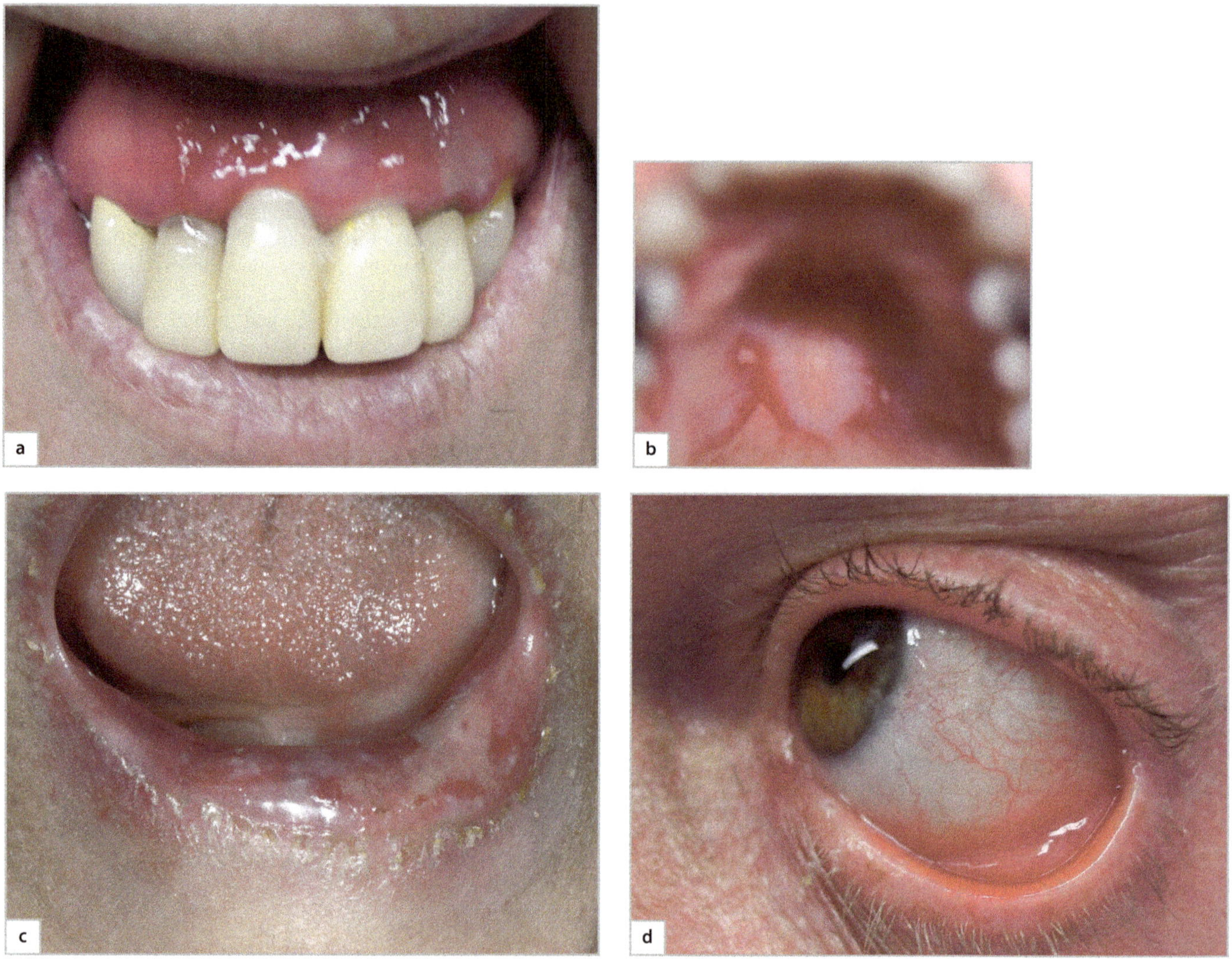

Figure 26.7 Mucosal lesions in mucous membrane pemphigoid showing gingivitis (a), erosions at the palate (b) and lips (c), and conjunctival injections (d).

Diagnosis

The diagnosis is made using defined clinical and immunopathological features (Chan et al. 2002). Histological and immunopathological examination shows a similar picture to that of BP, i.e. a subepidermal blister with a linear deposition of IgG and/or IgA along the dermo-epidermal junction. Circulating BMZ antibodies may be absent or detected in low titers by IIF or ELISA. Clinically, mucosal lesions in MMP and LP may be indistinguishable; the DIF test is diagnostic.

Treatment

Treatment is aimed at relieving symptoms and prevention of scarring, although scarring may develop despite treatment. MMP is more difficult to control than BP. Mild disease may be treated with super potent topical steroids, dapsone (50–200 mg/day), oral tetracycline (2 g/day), or doxycycline (200 mg/day) with or without nicotinamide (1000–2500 mg/day). Moderate and severe cases require systemic steroids possibly combined with cyclophosphamide in ocular or esophageal disease (Chan et al. 2002; Kirtschig et al. 2003, 2008). Other treatments of refractory disease include intravenous immunoglobulin and rituximab, a monoclonal anti-CD20 antibody that targets pathological B cells. These treatments may stabilize the disease but do not reverse scarring.

Linear IgA disease

Synonym

Chronic bullous disease of childhood in children

LAD is characterized by autoantibodies of the IgA type targeting various antigens of the BMZ (**Table 26.2**). However, it is not determined whether LAD is a separate entity as there is considerable overlap with BP, MMP, and EBA (Chan et al. 2002). LAD may affect both adults and children. Urticated, annular, and polycyclic plaques may be surrounded by blisters ('string of pearls') (**Figure 26.8**). Mucosal involvement is common and in children anogenital sites are often affected. The disease usually responds well to treatment with dapsone (similar to other diseases with an IgA response), sulfonamides and erythromycin (in children); thus it is important to investigate all autoimmune bullous diseases for the presence of both IgG and IgA as this may influence the treatment choice. Occasionally, LAD may take a refractory course despite treatment (Wojnarowska et al. 1988).

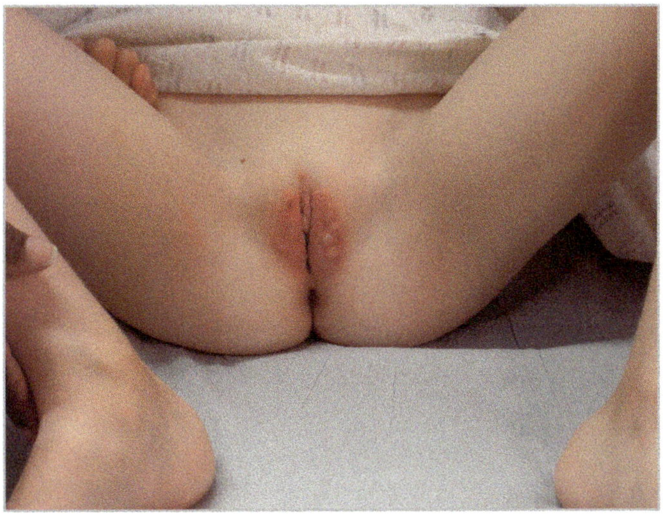

Figure 26.8 Linear IgA disease of childhood showing an erythema with blisters towards the edge. By courtesy of Dr Vanessa Venning, Oxford, UK.

Epidermolysis bullosa acquisita

Synonyms

Acquired epidermolysis bullosa, dermolytic pemphigoid

EBA is a very rare autoimmune blistering disease that is defined by autoantibodies (IgG and rarely IgA) to collagen type VII of the epithelia (Caux 2011). However, there is considerable overlap with MMP and LAD and a clear disease definition is awaited. Two main clinical subtypes are described: a mechanobullous type that tends to localize to areas of trauma (feet/knees etc.) resembling the hereditary dystrophic form of epidermolysis bullosa and an inflammatory (BP-like) type that is clinically indistinguishable from other subepidermal diseases like BP. Mucosal involvement including the genital tract is common (Iranzo et al. 2014). The clinical course is often protracted and immunosuppressants, systemic steroids, and dapsone are commonly used as treatment agents (Caux et al. 2011, Kirtschig et al. 2003).

Dermatitis herpetiformis

Synonyms

Dermatitis herpetiformis Duhring, Duhring disease, Morbus Duhring, Duhring-Brocq disease

DH is an autoimmune subepidermal bullous disease that is associated with intolerance to gluten, IgA autoantibodies to tissue transglutaminase of the epithelial BMZ (**Figure 26.3b**), and Coeliac disease (gluten sensitive bowel disease). It does not usually affect the vulva. However, key features are unbearable itch and an eczema-like rash with small vesicles typically distributed over elbows, knees, buttocks, and possibly the scalp. It may be a rare DD in women presenting with vulvar pruritus or an eczema-like clinical picture (Caproni et al. 2009, Clarindo et al. 2014). Coeliac disease is also described to be associated with LS (Jacobs et al. 2014).

INTRAEPIDERMAL AUTOIMMUNE BULLOUS DISEASES

Pemphigus

The pemphigus group is characterized by flaccid blisters or erosions of the skin and mucous membranes. The most common type of pemphigus is PV with frequent mucosal involvement; a subtype known as pemphigus vegetans is particularly seen at the vulva. Pemphigus foliaceus (PF) only affects the skin, and may be sporadic or endemic (Fogo selvagem). Paraneoplastic pemphigus (PNP) is a distinct disease that can affect multiple organs other than the skin, as outlined below.

Main subtypes of pemphigus

- Pemphigus vulgaris (PV)
- Pemphigus vegetans (clinical variant of PV often affecting the genitals)
- Pemphigus foliaceus (PF)
- Paraneoplastic pemphigus (PNP)

Epidemiology

Pemphigus is more common in the Middle East, India, North Africa, and the Mediterranean region compared with Northern Europe (Marazza et al. 2009). The UK incidence is estimated at 7 per million population per year (Langan et al. 2008). It is generally a disease of the middle-aged individuals, but peaks of incidence in the seventh decade have been reported (Langan et al. 2008). Both sexes are affected.

Pathology

Intraepithelial separation of keratinocytes is mediated by autoantibodies against two main desmosomal cadherins that provide cell adhesion. Desmoglein 3 is mainly present in the mucosa and lower layers of the skin, whereas desmoglein 1 is expressed more frequently in the upper layers of the skin that is an explanation for the development of blisters at different sites. IgG antibodies are directly pathogenic, leading to separation of cells (acantholysis) that is clinically manifested as flaccid blisters and/or erosions.

Clinical features

PV usually affects the mucosa and the skin (**Figure 26.9**). It may present with erosions in the oral mucosa and intact flaccid or burst blisters leading to cutaneous erosions. Vulvovaginal and cervical involvement have been described (Akhyani et al. 2008, Batta et al. 1999, Fairbanks Barbosa et al. 2012, Marren et al. 1993) (**Figure 26.10**). In general, patients with genital mucosal involvement have a tendency to have widespread and recurrent disease with multiple sites involvement (Malik & Ahmed et al. 2005). Pemphigus vegetans (**Figure 26.11**) is a clinical variant characterized by hyperkeratotic and vegetating lesions that are found predominantly in the flexural areas such as the groins with frequent mucosal involvement. PF does not affect the mucosal surfaces. Pemphigus lesions heal without scarring.

Histopathology

Skin biopsy shows suprabasal clefting with acantholysis and mixed inflammatory cell infiltrate. The basal cell layer that remains attached to the BMZ forms a single row of cells in a pattern known as 'tombstoning'.

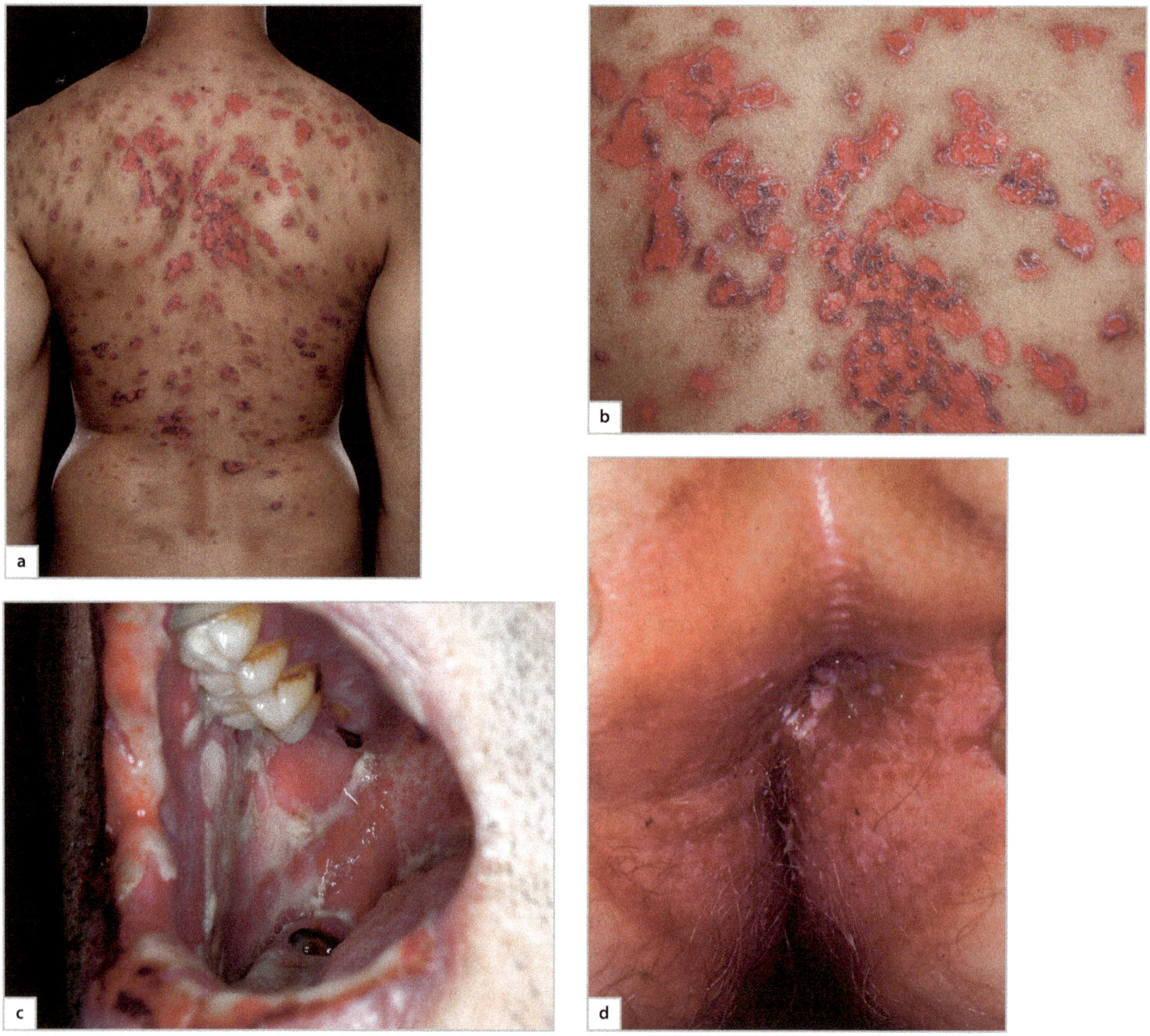

Figure 26.9 Generalized pemphigus vulgaris (a), in close-up (b), oral lesions (c), and anal lesions (d).

Immunopathology

DIF of perilesional skin and IIF (using monkey/rabbit esophagus (rich in desmoglein 3) and normal human skin (rich in desmoglein1) show intercellular deposition of IgG on the keratinocyte surfaces (**Figure 26.12**).

ELISA is used to detect and quantify specific antibodies in sera. Disease activity has been related to circulating antibody titers.

Diagnosis

Clues in the diagnosis of pemphigus

- Typical clinical picture with flaccid blisters and erosions of skin and/or mucosa
- Acantholysis on histology
- Intercellular IgG +/– other immunoglobulins on DIF/IIF
- ELISA shows antibodies to Desmoglein 1 (PF) or 3 (PV)

Treatment

General aspects of vulvar care in blistering diseases are discussed in subepidermal disease. Therapeutic agents used in the treatment of pemphigus are detailed in **Table 26.7**. Potent topical steroids are useful especially in localized and limited disease; however, systemic steroids are the mainstay of treatment, and in the initial stages of the disease high doses (prednisone equivalent 1 mg/kg/day) are often necessary. Other agents (see below) may be necessary in combination with or instead of systemic steroids.

A consensus report has recommended disease definition and treatment end points and outcome measures (Murrell et al. 2008). The aim is to control the disease with the lowest dose of systemic steroids and/or immunosuppressants. Pemphigus autoantibody titer in serum is useful in monitoring the disease activity and adjusting the treatment dosage. Concomitant bone and gastric protection is important in patients who are treated with systemic steroids.

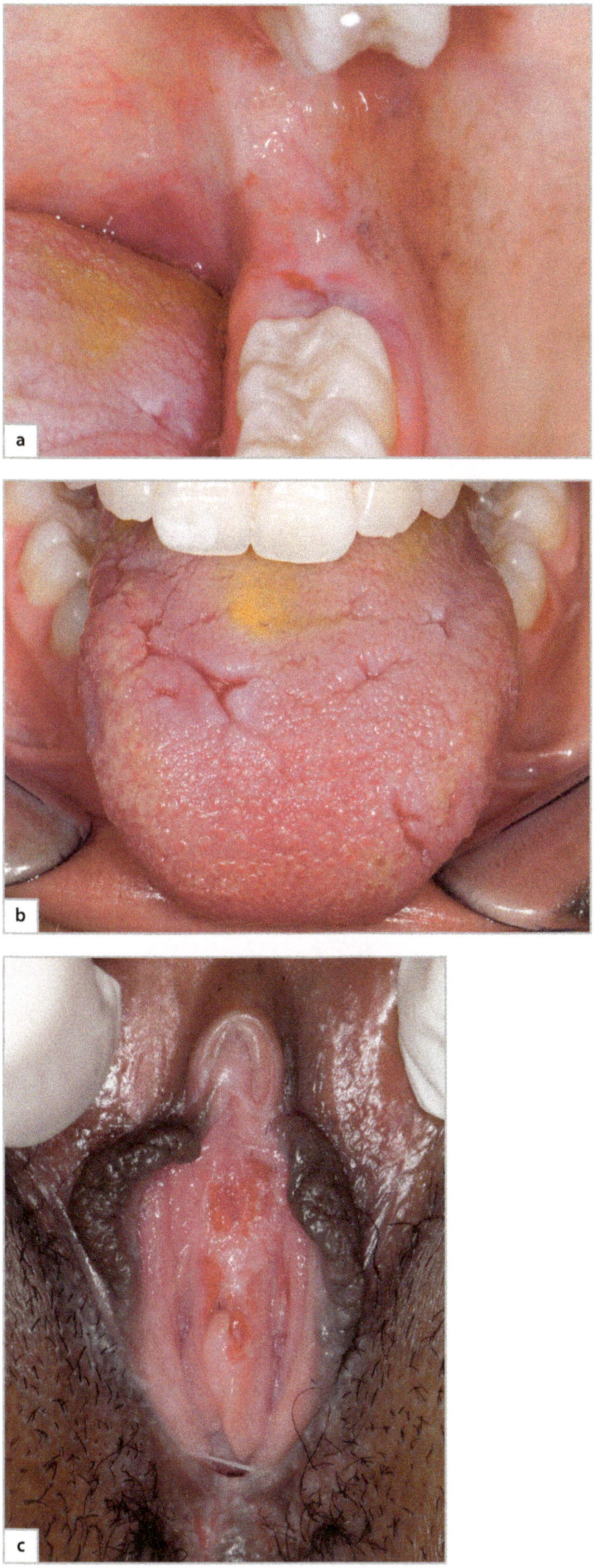

Figure 26.10 Autoimmune pemphigus showing erosions and fissures of the oral mucosa (a, b), and vulva (c) in one patient.

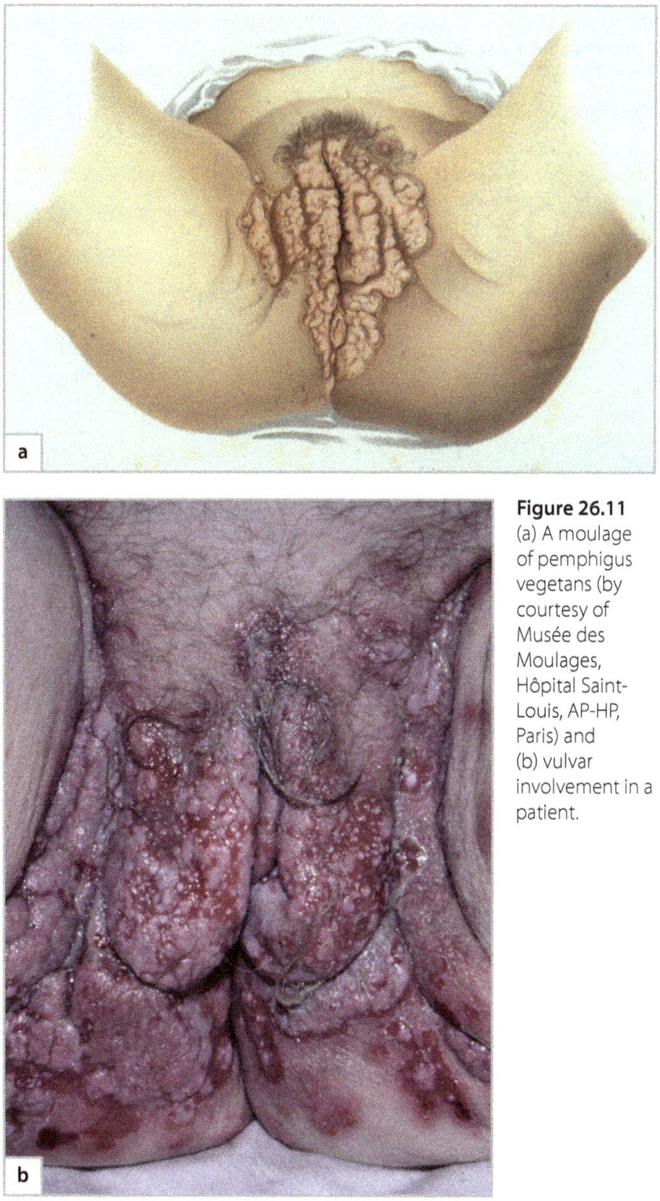

Figure 26.11 (a) A moulage of pemphigus vegetans (by courtesy of Musée des Moulages, Hôpital Saint-Louis, AP-HP, Paris) and (b) vulvar involvement in a patient.

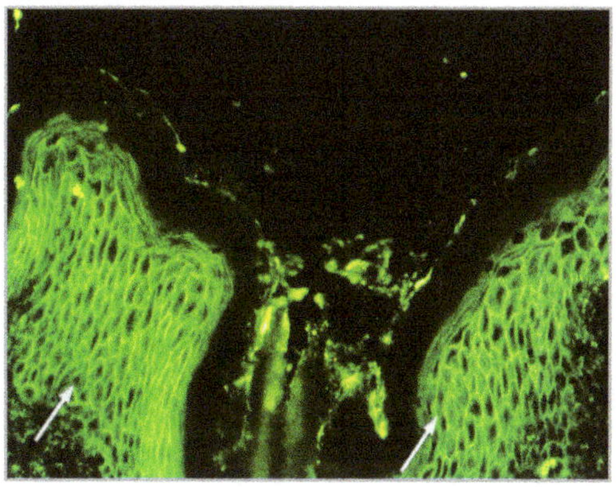

Figure 26.12 Direct immunofluorescence showing intercellular depositions of IgG, diagnostic for autoimmune pemphigus.

Table 26.7 Treatment in pemphigus (Sperber et al. 2008)

Treatment	Application
Potent topical steroids	To single lesions, possibly in addition to systemic treatment
Systemic steroids	Mainstay of treatment; initial dose prednisone ≤1 mg/kg/day to achieve disease control
Steroid sparing agents/ immunosuppressants	Used in combination with or instead of systemic steroids
Azathioprine	1–3 mg/kg/day
Mycophenolate mofetil	2–3 g/day
Dapsone	50–200 mg/day
Cyclophosphamide	50–200 mg/day: 2000 mg/kg infusion divided in daily doses for up to 5 days, usually repeated monthly
Methotrexate	10–25 mg/week
Tetracycline	2 g/day, effectiveness from prospective trials requested
Intravenous immunoglobulin	In refractory disease; various dosing regimens are reported
Rituximab (anti-CD20 antibody that depletes pathogenic B-cells)	In refractory disease; various dosing regimens, e.g. 375 mg/week for 4 weeks
Plasmapheresis/ immunoadsorption (aims to remove circulating pathogenic antibodies)	In refractory disease combined with systemic steroids or immunosuppressants

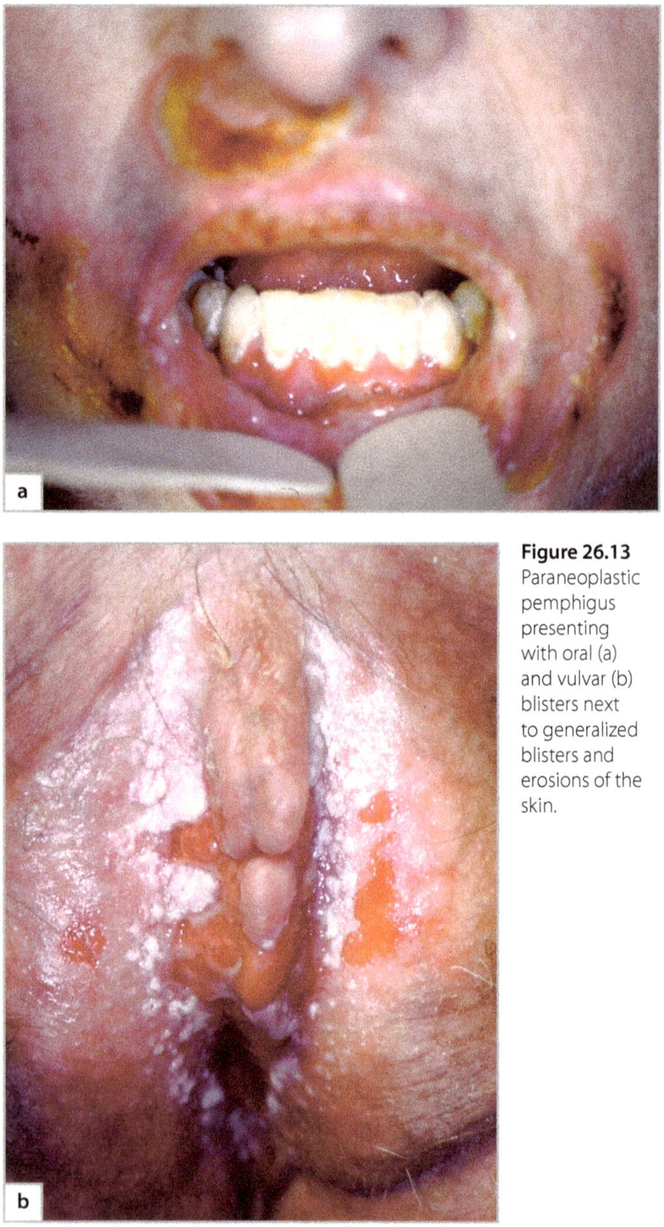

Figure 26.13 Paraneoplastic pemphigus presenting with oral (a) and vulvar (b) blisters next to generalized blisters and erosions of the skin.

Paraneoplastic pemphigus

Clinical features

PNP is a paraneoplastic syndrome that causes severe mucosal and cutaneous eruptions. It is associated with an underlying neoplasm that is most commonly hematological, such as non-Hodgkin lymphoma, Castleman disease, and chronic lymphocytic leukemia. PNP typically presents with painful, severe oral erosions that may be accompanied by a generalized cutaneous eruption. The clinical picture is variable, consisting of lesions that may resemble pemphigus (**Figure 26.13**), pemphigoid, erythema multiforme, Graft versus Host Disease (GvHD), as well as LP.

Histopathology

The histological findings not only show considerable variability with features of pemphigus but also basal cell necrosis indistinguishable from that seen in toxic epidermal necrolysis (**Figure 26.14**).

Immunopathology

PNP is characterized by the presence of autoantibodies against various antigens. Antibody-binding can be visualized by DIF of patient's perilesional skin or by IIF using rodent bladder epithelium as substrate (**Figure 26.15**).

Treatment and prognosis

The prognosis of PNP is poor and the disease is often fatal. Immunosuppressive agents are often required to decrease blistering, and treating the underlying malignancy may control autoantibody production.

DIFFERENTIAL DIAGNOSES OF AUTOIMMUNE BULLOUS DISEASES

There is significant overlap between autoimmune bullous diseases and a number of other diseases that may have similar clinical pictures when affecting the genitals (**Table 26.8**). Vulvar LP and LS are important to be considered because BP antibodies are occasionally found in the serum of patients with LS and LP; histopathology and DIF studies will distinguish these diseases (Chapters 19 and 20). Genetic bullous diseases such as epidermolysis bullosa and Hailey-Hailey disease must be differentiated (Chapter 27), and infections can be identified microbiologically taking a swab. GvHD

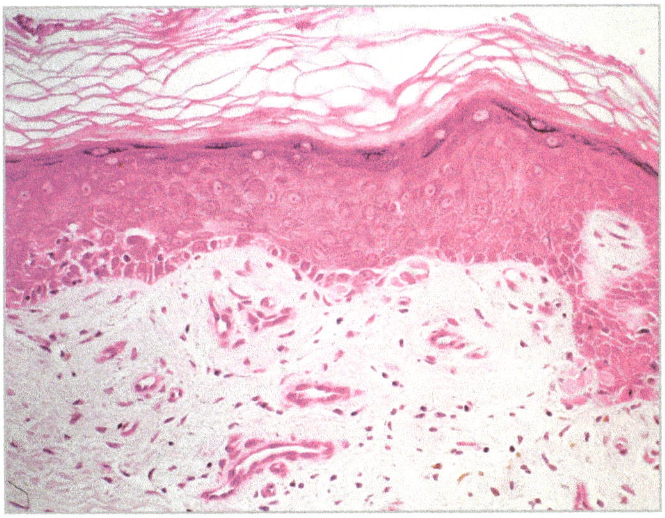

Figure 26.14 Histopathology of paraneoplastic pemphigus showing slight vacuolization of the basal keratinocytes, edematous, and slightly fibrotic dermis with lymphocytic infiltrate. No obvious acantholysis, but only reduced cohesion of keratinocytes, apoptosis and Civatte bodies. By courtesy of Dr Hannelore Mittag, Marburg, Germany.

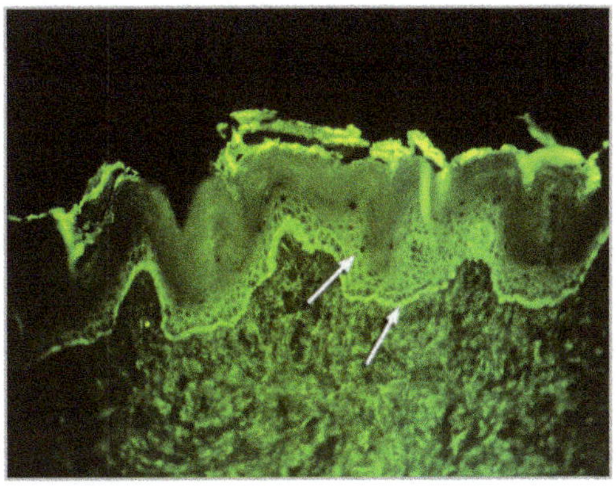

Figure 26.15 Direct immunofluorescence of paraneoplastic pemphigus with IgG depositions at the basement membrane zone and intercellularly.

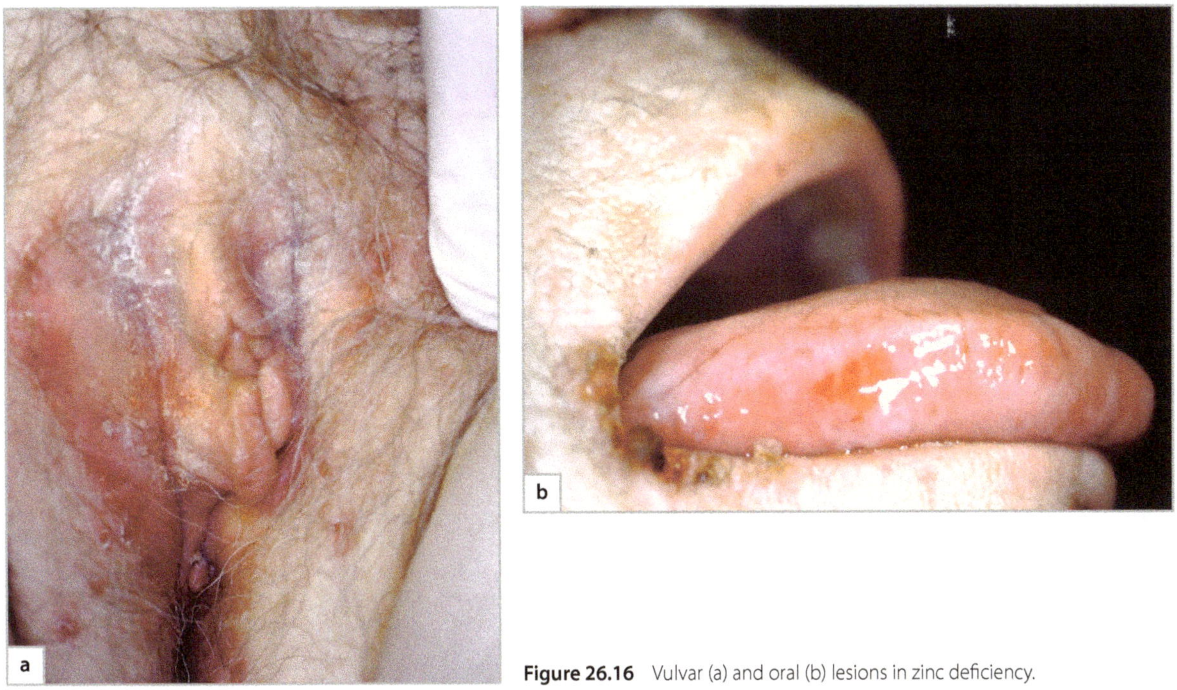

Figure 26.16 Vulvar (a) and oral (b) lesions in zinc deficiency.

may develop in patients with bone marrow or solid organ transplants and may mimic LP, LS, or a bullous disease. Erosive vulvar intraepithelial neoplasia can be differentiated histologically. A thorough history and examination of the skin and mucous membranes followed by histopathological and immunofluorescence studies, if indicated, will lead to a diagnosis in patients with vulvar blisters or erosions.

Table 26.8 Differential diagnoses of erosive and bullous diseases affecting the vulva

Disease group	Examples of diseases
Inflammatory diseases	Lichen planus, lichen sclerosus, atopic eczema, contact dermatitis, Behçet disease, Aphthous ulcers, Pyoderma gangrenosum, Graft versus Host Disease, Crohn disease
Genetic diseases	Epidermolysis bullosa group, Hailey-Hailey disease
Infections	*Staphylococcus aureus*, staphylococcal scalded skin syndrome, *Candida* infection, herpes simplex/varicella infection
Malignant/premalignant diseases	Vulvar intraepithelial neoplasia, squamous cell carcinoma, Paget disease
Drugs	Fixed drug eruption, Stevens-Johnson syndrome, toxic epidermal necrolysis
Physical causes	Excoriations, burns, sexual abuse
Deficiency disorders	Zinc deficiency (**Figure 26.16**)

REFERENCES

Akhyani M, Chams-Davatchi C, Naraghi Z, et al. Cervicovaginal involvement in pemphigus vulgaris: a clinical study of 77 cases. Br J Dermatol 2008; 158:478–482.

Batta K, Munday PE, Tatnall FM. Pemphigus vulgaris localized to the vagina presenting as chronic vaginal discharge. Br J Dermatol 1999; 140:945–947.

Caproni M, Antiga E, Melani L, et al; Italian Group for Cutaneous Immunopathology. Guidelines for the diagnosis and treatment of dermatitis herpetiformis. J Eur Acad Dermatol Venereol 2009; 23:633–638.

Caux F. Diagnosis and clinical features of epidermolysis bullosa acquisita. Dermatol Clin 2011; 29:485–491.

Chan LS, Ahmed AR, Anhalt GJ, et al. The first international consensus on mucous membrane pemphigoid: definition, diagnostic criteria, pathogenic factors, medical treatment, and prognostic indicators. Arch Dermatol 2002; 138:370–379.

Clarindo MV, Possebon AT, Soligo EM, et al. Dermatitis herpetiformis: pathophysiology, clinical presentation, diagnosis and treatment. An Bras Dermatol 2014; 89:865–877.

Fairbanks Barbosa ND, de Aguiar LM, Maruta CW, et al. Vulvo-cervico-vaginal manifestations and evaluation of Papanicolaou smears in pemphigus vulgaris and pemphigus foliaceus. J Am Acad Dermatol 2012; 67:409–416.

Iranzo P, Herrero-Gonzalez JE, Mascaro-Galy JM, et al. Epidermolysis bullosa acquisita: a retrospective analysis of 12 patients evaluated in four tertiary hospitals in Spain. Br J Dermatol 2014; 171:1022–1030.

Jacobs L, Gilliam A, Khavari N, et al. Association between lichen sclerosus and celiac disease: a report of three pediatric cases. Pediatr Dermatol 2014; 31:e128–e131.

Kirtschig G, Murrell D, Wojnarowska F, et al. Interventions for mucous membrane pemphigoid and epidermolysis bullosa acquisita. Cochrane Database Syst Rev 2003 (1):CD004056.

Kirtschig G, Khumalo NP, Venning V, et al. Acquired subepidermal bullous diseases. In: Williams H, Bigby M, Diepgen T, et al. (eds). Evidence based dermatology, 2nd edn. BMJI Books, Blackwell Publishing Group Ltd, USA, UK, Australia 2008:573–580.

Langan SM, Groves RW, West J. The relationship between neurological disease and bullous pemphigoid: a population-based case-control study. J Invest Dermatol 2011; 131:631-636.

Langan SM, Smeeth L, Hubbard R, et al. Bullous pemphigoid and pemphigus vulgaris--incidence and mortality in the UK: population based cohort study. BMJ 2008; 337:a180.

Lebeau S, Mainetti C, Masouye I, et al. Localized childhood vulval pemphigoid treated with tacrolimus ointment. Dermatology 2004; 208:273–275.

Lloyd-Lavery A, Chi CC, Wojnarowska F, et al. The associations between bullous pemphigoid and drug use: a UK case-control study. JAMA Dermatol 2013; 149:58–62.

Marazza G, Pham HC, Schärer L, et al. Autoimmune bullous disease Swiss study group. Incidence of bullous pemphigoid and pemphigus in Switzerland: a 2-year prospective study. Br J Dermatol 2009; 161:861–868.

Malik M, Ahmed AR. Involvement of the female genital tract in pemphigus vulgaris. Obstet Gynecol 2005; 106:1005–1012.

Marren P, Wojnarowska F, Venning V, et al. Vulvar involvement in autoimmune bullous diseases. J Reprod Med 1993; 38:101–107.

Murrell DF, Dick S, Ahmed AR, et al. Consensus statement on definitions of disease, end points, and therapeutic response for pemphigus. J Am Acad Dermatol 2008; 58:1043–1046.

Sperber BR, Martin LK, Murrell DF, et al. Pemphigus. In: Williams H, Bigby M, Diepgen T, et al (eds), Evidence based dermatology, 2nd edn. BMJI Books, Blackwell Publishing Group Ltd USA, UK, Australia 2008:581–594.

Taghipour K, Chi CC, Vincent A, et al. The association of bullous pemphigoid with cerebrovascular disease and dementia: a case-control study. Arch Dermatol 2010; 146:1251–1254.

Venning VA, Taghipour K, Mohd Mustapa MF, et al. British Association of Dermatologists' guidelines for the management of bullous pemphigoid 2012. Br J Dermatol 2012; 167:1200–1214.

Wojnarowska F, Marsden RA, Bhogal B, et al. Chronic bullous disease of childhood, childhood cicatricial pemphigoid, and linear IgA disease of adults. A comparative study demonstrating clinical and immunopathologic overlap. J Am Acad Dermatol 1988; 19:792–805.

Chapter 27 Inherited bullous diseases

Kathy Taghipour, Gudula Kirtschig

Mutations in the genes that encode for some structural and functional proteins of the epithelium can lead to separation of keratinocytes from each other or the basement membrane zone, and cause erosions, blisters, and fragility of the skin and mucosa. This is associated with pain, discomfort, and restriction of daily activities. The main inherited bullous diseases that can affect the vulva are Darier disease (DD), Hailey–Hailey disease (HH), and the epidermolysis bullosa (EB) group.

DARIER DISEASE

Synonyms

Keratosis follicularis, dyskeratosis follicularis, Darier–White disease

Key features

- Autosomal dominant
- Mutation in ATP2A2 leads to abnormal intercellular calcium signaling
- Acantholysis and characteristic 'corps ronds' and 'grains' are seen on histology
- Keratotic papules in a seborrheic distribution, palmar pits, and characteristic nail changes are the key clinical features

Introduction

DD is a rare autosomal dominant skin disease with an estimated worldwide prevalence of 1: 30,000 to 1: 100,000. It is caused by abnormal function of Ca^{2+} ATPase and a subsequent defect in calcium signaling between the cells that results in separation and death of keratinocytes (acantholysis and dyskeratosis).

Etiology

Mutation in the gene ATP2A2 leads to dysfunction of the sarco/endoplasmic reticulum Ca^{2+} ATPase isoform 2 pump and subsequently impaired calcium transport to the endoplasmic reticulum (Sakuntabhai et al. 1999). Reduced calcium stores in the endoplasmic reticulum results in separation of keratinocytes from each other (acantholysis), abnormal keratinization, and cell death (apoptosis) (Savignac et al. 2011).

Clinical presentation

The disease usually presents in the first decade, but symptoms may not be noticed until the second decade (Burge and Wilkinson 1992). Keratotic papules and crusts appear typically on the chest, upper back, groin, and the face, and there may be erosions in the vulvar area (**Figure 27.1**). Typical nail changes include longitudinal ridges and onycholysis (**Figure 27.2**). Keratotic papules in DD may coalesce forming large, crusting, vegetating plaques that are malodorous and prone to infection especially in intertriginous areas. Mild itch may occur but the main complaint is usually malodor that may lead to distress, embarrassment, and social isolation. Factors that worsen disease include heat, friction, and ultraviolet radiation. Flares are therefore not only common in summer but also in the premenstrual period. Vaginal involvement has been rarely reported and may be a cause of abnormal cervical cytology (Adam 1996).

Summary of the clinical features in Darier disease

Skin

- Keratotic, skin-colored or yellow-brown papules on face, scalp, trunk, and skinfolds
- Inguinal, anogenital, and vulvar areas may be eroded and macerated
- Small scattered papules on dorsa of hands and feet
- Pits or fine keratotic papules on palms and soles

Nails

- Brittle with longitudinal red or white lines
- Typical V-shaped notch on distal nail plate

Mucosa

- Asymptomatic white papules on the palate
- Vaginal involvement is rare

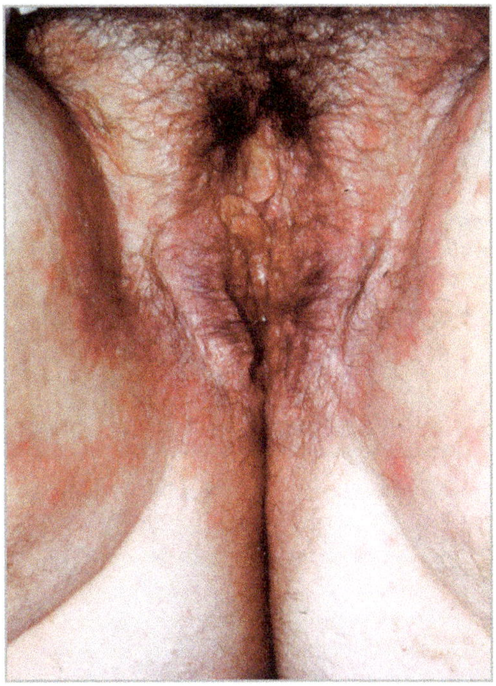

Figure 27.1 Darier disease showing erythema and erosions of the groins. By courtesy of Dr Jennifer Yell, Manchester, UK.

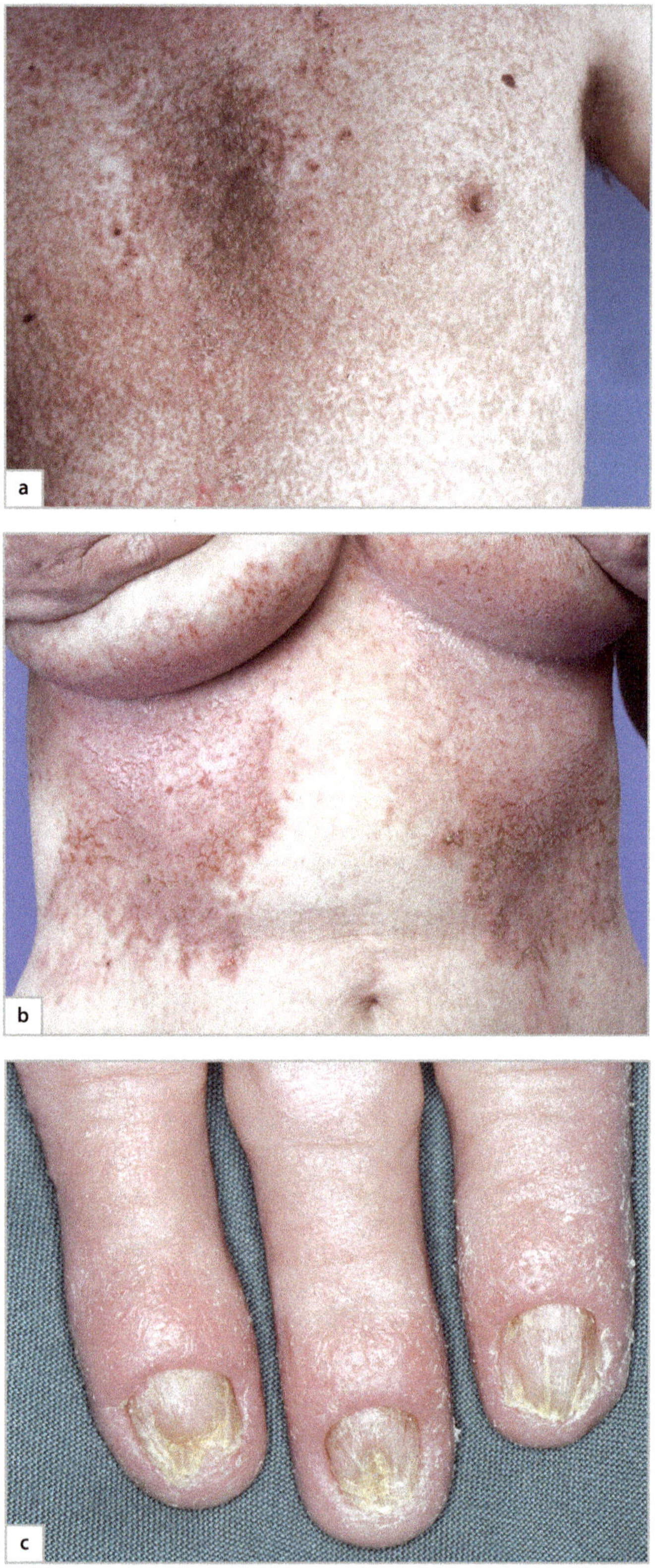

Figure 27.2 Typical papular rash (a and b) and nail dystrophy with pterygium formation (c) in Darier disease. By courtesy of Professor Theo Starink, the Netherlands.

Histopathology

The two main characteristic findings are acantholysis (separation of keratinocytes) and dyskeratosis (abnormal keratinization). Dyskeratotic cells appear as 'corps ronds' that are acantholytic keratinocytes with dark nuclei and a clear perinuclear halo with a bright surrounding ring, and 'grains,' which are small cells located in the upper layer of epidermis with elongated and grain-shaped nuclei (**Figure 27.3**). There is often an epidermal and superficial dermal inflammatory process comprising lymphocytes.

Differential diagnosis

There is clinical and histological overlap with HH, but the presence of characteristic clinical signs such as nail changes, palmar pits, and papules in the mouth helps to differentiate DD. Dyskeratosis with corps ronds and grains are more typical of DD, although acantholysis is present in both. Other differential diagnoses of DD and HH are summarized in **Table 27.1**.

Table 27.1 Differential diagnosis of vulvar Darier and Hailey-Hailey diseases

Differential diagnosis	Diagnostic features
Inflammatory dermatoses • Eczema • Seborrheic dermatitis • Flexural psoriasis • Lichen simplex chronicus	• Characteristic signs such as distal nail notches and palmar pits seen in DD are absent • No acantholysis in histology as seen in DD and HH
Autoimmune bullous diseases • Autoimmune pemphigus	• Immunofluorescence shows intercellular IgG/IgA/C3 deposition in pemphigus but not in DD or HH
Infections • Intertrigo • Impetigo • Herpes simplex NB: infections may be superimposed	• No family history • No acantholysis in histology • Resolves with treatment
Other acantholytic disorders • Papular acantholytic dyskeratosis in the genitocrural region	• Consists of focal skin colored or whitish papules but no erosions or crusts in intertriginous or seborrheic areas • Histology is similar to HH and DD • There is no family history • However, it is debated if this is a minimal variant of HH

DD, Darier disease; HH, Hailey-Hailey disease; IgG, immunoglobulin G

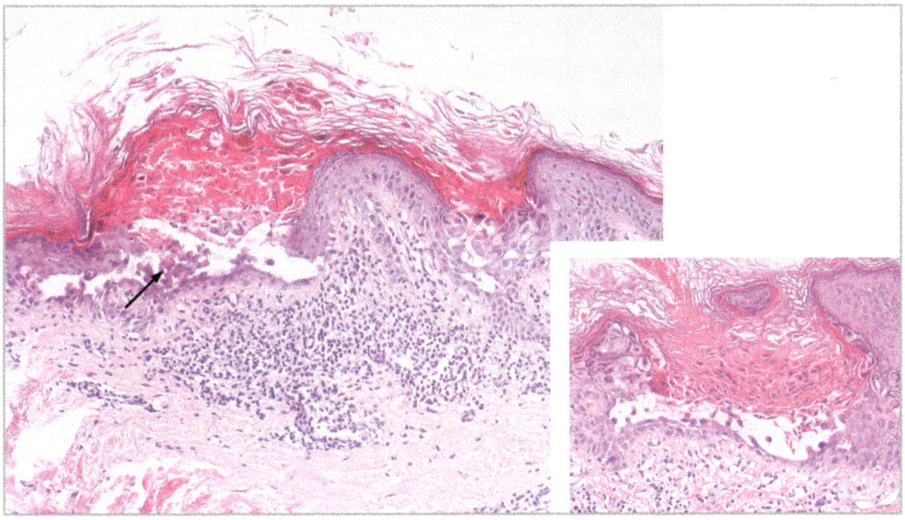

Figure 27.3 Histopathology in Darier disease showing epidermal acantholysis with vesicle formation and corps ronds (arrow). By courtesy of Professor Theo Starink, the Netherlands.

Treatment

General measures for the treatment of DD and HH

- Wearing loose and lightweight underwear reduces friction and sweating
- Antiseptic washes help to prevent malodor and colonization of bacteria
- Use of regular emollients may be soothing
- Secondary infection can be treated with topical antibiotic or antifungal agents, which may be combined with topical steroids
- Oral antibiotics and/or antivirals may be necessary to treat infection
- Consider patch testing as development of allergic contact dermatitis is frequent

Apart from the general treatment measures in the vulvar area, topical retinoids are effective, but their use in genital skin is limited by irritant effects. Severe disease requires systemic treatment with retinoids (acitretin and isotretinoin). Cyclosporine may be considered for patients who are unable to take oral retinoids. It is important for the sun-exposed skin to be protected with sunscreen.

Surgery

For focal, persistent areas surgical excision followed by split-skin grafting, dermabrasion and treatment with CO_2 or erbium:Yag lasers may be beneficial (Beier & Kaufmann 1999, McElroy et al. 1990, Zachariae 1979) and the effect may last several years.

Specific treatment recommendations

Topical disinfectants/antibiotics to diminish bacteria causing malodor:

- Mupirocin, fusidic acid, or silver sulfadiazine containing creams and Povidone iodine or chlorhexidine containing wash fluids
- Metronidazole 2% cream has an additional anti-inflammatory effect

Topical calcineurin inhibitors and topical corticosteroids:

- Topical tacrolimus and pimecrolimus cream or topical steroids may diminish the inflammation

Topical retinoids:

- Vitamin A derivatives, e.g. 0.025–0.05% tretinoin or isotretinoin cream may diminish hyperkeratosis after several months. To avoid irritation, they may be combined with topical steroids

Antimicrobials may be combined with steroids to minimize inflammation:

- Mild to moderately potent topical steroid creams

Crusts may be removed with:

- Salicylic acid 2-6% in vaseline or urea 5–20% cream or ointment

Oral retinoids:

- Oral retinoids are effective, but are teratogenic (contraception in fertile women) and accompanied by side effects
- Acitretin 0.25–0.75 mg/kg/day, starting at 10–25 mg/day and increasing to 0.3–0.6 mg/kg/day (max. 1.5 mg/kg/day) after 2–4 weeks. Once improvement is seen, reduce to the smallest effective dose
- Isotretinoin 0.5–1 mg/kg/day is possibly also effective but not suitable for long-term use

Other options:

- 5-fluorouracil cream has been tried in combination with oral retinoids
- Cyclosporine (initial dose 5 mg/kg body weight) can be tried in severe disease if retinoids cannot be used
- Ultraviolet (UV) light B treatment is effective in some patients but may trigger the disease in others; UV light is difficult to deliver in vulvar disease; photodynamic therapy has been used

HAILEY–HAILEY DISEASE

Synonyms

Familial benign chronic pemphigus

Key features

- Autosomal dominant
- Mutation of ATP2C1 gene interferes with intracellular calcium signaling
- Acantholysis in histology
- Flaccid blisters/erosions in intertriginous sites

Introduction

HH is a rare autosomal dominant, blistering dermatosis that affects the intertriginous skin. The age of onset and clinical manifestations can vary widely within families. The onset is usually in the third or fourth decade and childhood disease is uncommon. There is no recorded difference in prevalence among ethnic groups. Patients present with flaccid blisters that burst easily leaving macerated and crusted lesions. There is clinical and pathological overlap with DD.

Etiology

Mutations in the ATP2C1 gene that encodes the Golgi membrane Calcium ATPase (human secretory pathway Ca^{2+}/Mn^{2+} ATPase isoform 1, hSPCA1) are causative, leading to abnormal calcium signaling and loss of keratinocyte adhesion (acantholysis).

Clinical presentation

Flaccid vesicles, erosions, and erythematous plaques are apparent in flexural areas such as axillae, groins, neck, submammary, and perianal area (**Figures 27.4 and 27.5**). Lesions worsen with heat, friction, sweating, infection, and UV exposure. Isolated vulvar disease is rare, and patients with genital involvement usually present with other affected flexural areas (Wieselthier & Pincus 1993). The lesions tend to expand peripherally and heal in the center and may develop into hypertrophic and fissured vegetations. Vaginal, oral, and conjunctival involvement is rare. Longitudinal white bands may be present on the nails but brittle nails, as seen in DD, are not observed. The main symptoms are itch, pain, and malodor, which may impact on physical activity and quality of life (Harris et al. 1996).

Histopathology

The main histopathological feature is suprabasal acantholysis that is more widespread within the epidermis compared with DD. Clumps of partially acantholytic cells that float in the suprabasal space have an appearance similar to a 'dilapidated brick wall.' Epidermal hyperplasia and parakeratosis (persistence of nuclei in keratinocytes as they migrate to the uppermost layer of the epidermis, stratum corneum) may be seen in chronic lesions (**Figure 27.6**).

Differential diagnosis

The main histological differential diagnosis of HH is DD and acquired acantholytic dermatoses, e.g. autoimmune pemphigus (Chapter 26). However, at the initial presentation, macerated intertriginous areas resemble intertrigo. A family history will provide a first diagnostic clue. A swab and a biopsy should follow to diagnose HH. Immunofluorescence tests of patient's skin will exclude autoimmune pemphigus (see Chapter 6 and 26).

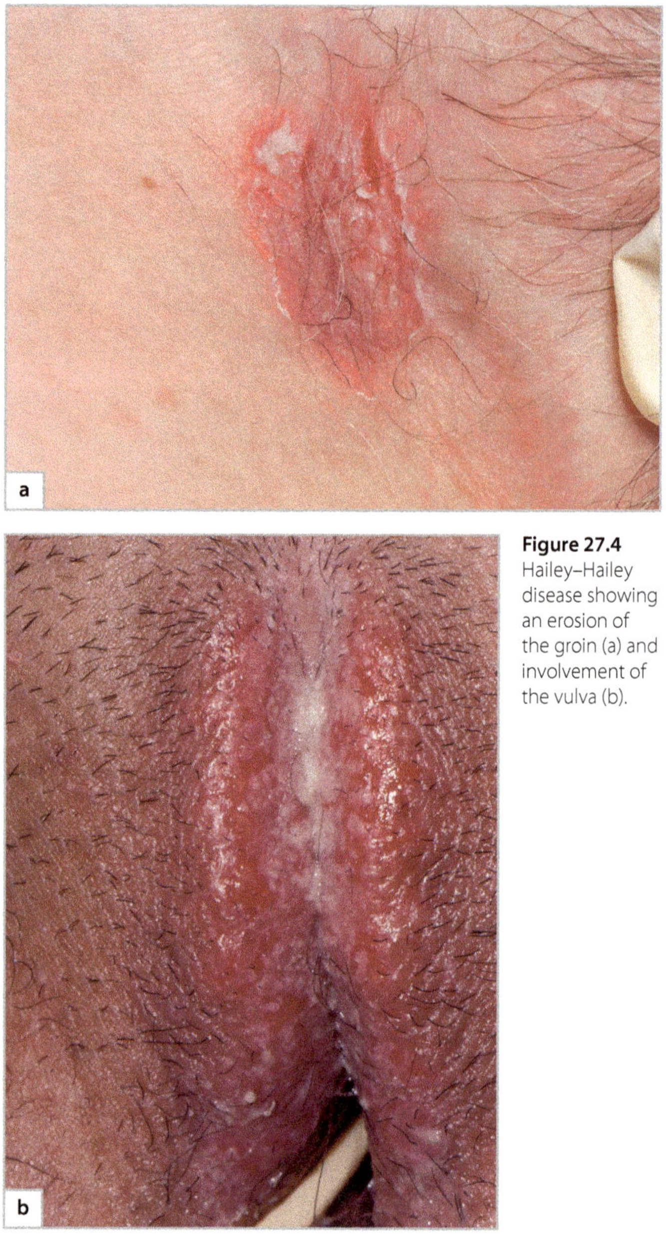

Figure 27.4 Hailey–Hailey disease showing an erosion of the groin (a) and involvement of the vulva (b).

Treatment

In addition to the general measures, combined topical steroids and antimicrobial agents are effective treatment modalities and if applied early may prevent a lesion from developing. To prevent skin atrophy and striae in flexural areas, application of potent topical steroids should be avoided or limited. Oral antibiotics such as tetracyclines and erythromycin are also beneficial. In persistent and painful disease, diagnosis and treatment of superadded herpes simplex infection should be considered. Similar to DD, surgical treatment with excision and skin grafting, dermabrasion and treatment with CO_2 and erbium:YAG lasers have been reported to be successful in recalcitrant HH (Beier & Kaufmann 1999, Christian & Moy 1999, Hamm et al. 1994, Menz et al. 1987).

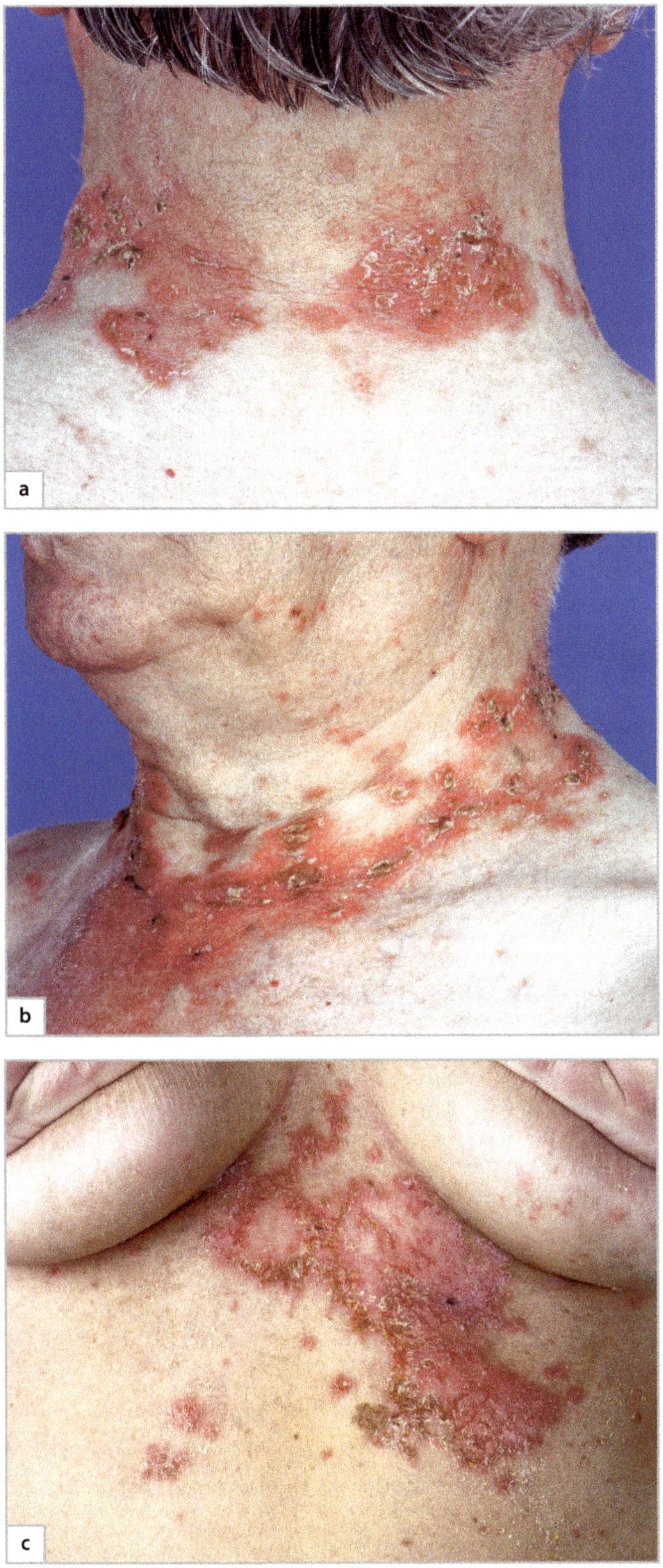

Figure 27.5 Erosions and crusts affecting various sites with friction in Hailey–Hailey disease. By courtesy of Professor Theo Starink, the Netherlands.

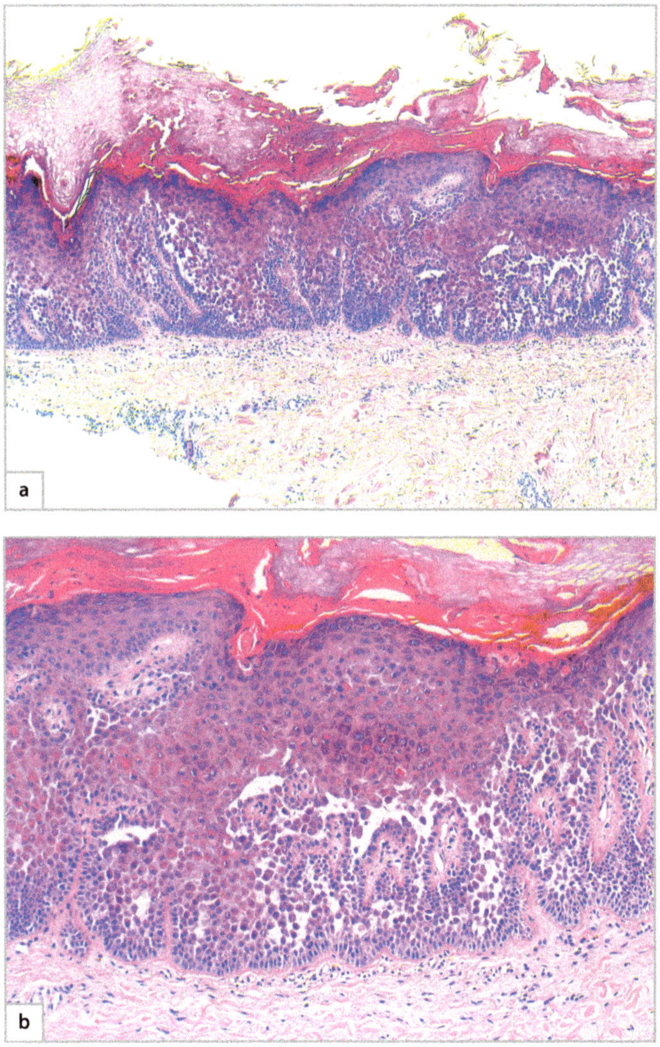

Figure 27.6 Histopathology in Hailey–Hailey disease showing acantholysis. By courtesy of Professor Theo Starink, the Netherlands.

Specific treatment recommendations

First choice
Topical treatment:
Topical antimicrobials, e.g. chlorhexidine, fusidic acid, tetracycline (topical 3% cream or ointment)
Topical corticosteroids, be aware of skin atrophy in flexural sites after long-term use
Systemic treatment:
A combination of topical corticosteroids and antimicrobials often leads to a good response. Hydrocortison acetate 1% or triamcinolone cream/ointment 0.1% may be combined with chlorhexidine digluconate 1%, tetracycline 3% or fusidic acid
Systemic antibiotics (erythromycin, broad spectrum penicillin, minocycline), antimycotics (terbinafine) or antivirals in herpes infection
Second choice
Topical treatment:
Topical tacrolimus or calcitriol, possibly alternating with topical steroids. Botulinum toxin A injection into axillary lesions may lead to reduced sweating and less troublesome disease
Systemic treatment:
Systemic corticosteroids in generalized disease, however, a rapid relapse may be experienced when stopping steroids. Dapsone, cyclosporine (maximum 5 mg/kg) and methotrexate (in one case report 15 mg/ week used successfully), oral retinoids, e.g. acitretin 30 mg dd have all been tried
Surgery:
Dermabrasion or CO_2 laser ablation of superficial skin layers; re-epithelialization occurs via (uninvolved?) appendages
Total excision of the affected skin followed by skin transplantation. Recurrences may be seen at the edges of the excised skin

Prognosis

HH is a benign but disabling chronic disease. There is often an exacerbation during summer months. The disease becomes usually less troublesome with age.

EPIDERMOLYSIS BULLOSA GROUP

Key features

- EB is inherited in an autosomal dominant or autosomal recessive manner
- A mechanobullous clinical picture is characterized by trauma-induced skin and mucosal fragility
- Genitourinary system may be involved in some subtypes of EB. Erosions and scarring will be painful and may compromise functionality
- EB is classified according to the ultrastructural level of blister formation into four main types:
  - EB simplex
  - Junctional EB
  - Dystrophic EB
  - Kindler syndrome
- Diagnosis is mainly made with immunofluorescence antigen mapping and transmission electron microscopy on a skin biopsy from a newly induced blister
- No specific treatment is available yet and most measures aim to prevent shearing of the skin and treat superadded infection and complications

Introduction

EB encompasses a group of inherited skin diseases that are characterized by skin fragility and blisters on skin and mucosal membranes that appear after minor trauma. Mutations occur in the genes that encode proteins involved in skin integrity, and this results in 'mechanobullous' disease in form of erosions and blisters after friction, pressure or trauma. There are four main forms of inherited EB according to the level of skin cleavage. There are a number of clinical subtypes and EB classification is continuously updated to include newly discovered gene mutations and phenotypes (Fine et al. 2014).

Etiology

Skin fragility in EB is caused by genetic mutations within a number of genes that encode structural proteins in the epithelium and dermo-epithelial junction zone. The location of these proteins determines the blister level and types of EB. Target polypeptides for different types of EB are summarized in **Table 27.2** and their location in the skin is illustrated in **Figure 27.7**.

Clinical presentation

In all forms of EB, patients suffer from fragility of the skin and presence of blisters, erosions, and crusts at the site of friction, pressure, or trauma (**Figure 27.8 a** and **b**). Atrophic scarring may be present, in particular in recessive dystrophic EB, and scarring of the vulva and vagina can cause strictures and reflux of urine into the eroded vagina (Holbrook 1988). The epithelia in other organs are often affected, and extracutaneous involvement in various types of EB is summarized in **Table 27.3**. During pregnancy, blisters may extend as the abdominal skin stretches. Vulvovaginal lesions complicate vaginal delivery, and caesarian section may be indicated in severe cases. However, normal vaginal delivery with episiotomy has been reported to be safe and without further complications such as vaginal stenosis, in women with recessive dystrophic EB without extensive genital blistering. Breastfeeding also seems to be possible when there is no areoral involvement (Hanafusa et al. 2012).

Histopathology

Depending on the type of EB, a split through either epithelial basal keratinocytes (EB simplex) or underneath the basal keratinocytes (junctional and dystrophic EB) is seen on histology. There is usually no inflammatory infiltrate; however, histopathology is not diagnostic in EB.

Diagnosis

Helpful clues in the diagnosis of epidermolysis bullosa

- Presentation at birth or in infancy
- Positive family history
- Mechanical skin fragility

When EB is suspected, a thorough clinical examination should be performed to include skin, nails, teeth, oral, and genital mucosa. In the majority of EB types, blisters can be induced by gentle rubbing of the skin.

Disease classification relies on the identification of the polypeptide defect (caused by a genetic mutation) within the skin, resulting

Table 27.2 Genetic transmission mode, cleavage levels, mutated polypeptides, and skin structures affected in main types of epidermolysis bullosa

Main EB type	Mode of inheritance	Level of blister formation	Mutated polypeptides	Target structure
EB simplex	Mainly AD, rarely AR	Within the basal keratinocytes or suprabasal (intraepithelial)	Keratin 5 and 14, plectin, desmoplakin, plakoglobin, plakophillin1, transglutaminase 5, exophilin 5 (AR), BPag1 (AR)	Keratin tonofilaments, hemidesmosome
Junctional EB	AR	Through the junction or middle part of BMZ (lamina lucida)	Laminin 332, collagen XVII, α6β4 integrin, α3 integrin subunit	Anchoring filaments, hemidesmosome
Dystrophic EB	AD and AR	Uppermost part of the dermis and lower BMZ (lamina densa)	Collagen VII	Anchoring fibrils
Kindler syndrome	AR	Mixed, within or beneath the BMZ	Kindlin-1	Anchorage of actin cytoskeleton to extracellular matrix

EB, epidermolysis bullosa; AD, autosomal dominant; AR, autosomal recessive; BMZ, basement membrane zone

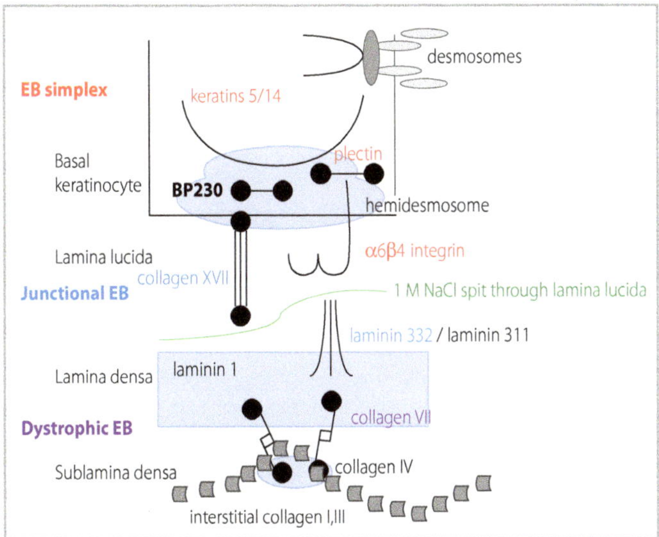

Figure 27.7 Schematic view of the basement membrane zone including basal keratinocyte showing structures and polypeptides involved in epidermolysis bullosa.

in a particular level of cleavage (**Table 27.2** and **Figure 27.7**). The two diagnostic methods that are most commonly used are immunofluorescence antigen mapping and transmission electron microscopy using a skin biopsy from a freshly induced blister after gentle rubbing. Once the diagnosis is made, mutational analysis provides more accurate information required for subclassification of the disease; this is important in genetic counseling especially in severe disease forms.

Differential diagnosis

There are few other blistering conditions that present at birth, and although reaching a diagnosis in infancy may be challenging, a clinical diagnosis of EB can usually be made based on clinical signs and family history.

Treatment

At present, there is no definitive treatment or cure for EB. Current treatments mainly aim to prevent blistering and treat the complications such as infection and extracutaneous disease.

Supporting treatment

Trauma to the skin needs to be avoided at any time. Tight clothes/shoes, the use of tourniquets and other instruments that apply direct pressure on the skin, adhesive tapes, intravenous cannula fixtures and electrocardiogram electrodes may all lead to shearing of the skin and must be avoided if possible.

Pain management, especially prior to dressing changes, is an important aspect of the treatment. The affected areas should be cleaned with saline or an antiseptic solution, and non-adhesive dressings (e.g. silicon-based, vaseline-impregnated, or hydrocolloid) should be applied. Loose-fitting underwear helps to reduce friction and topical antibiotics and antiseptic agents treat secondary bacterial infection.

Treatment of complications

Scarring and stenosis may require surgical intervention with reconstruction and dilatation when function is compromised, although repeated procedures may be necessary. Painful perianal erosions resulting in constipation can be helped by using topical anesthetic agents, laxatives, and a high fiber diet.

The significant risk of developing squamous cell carcinomas in recessive dystrophic EB necessitates careful examination and regular surveillance of these patients. Histologically, these tumors are usually well differentiated; however, wide surgical excision is advised as the risk of recurrence is high and the response to other treatments such as radiotherapy is poor.

There is no conclusive evidence for the use of systemic treatment in EB, although phenytoin, tetracycline, and retinoids have all been suggested.

Emerging treatments

Although an effective therapy for EB is not yet established, important work has been done to potentially make treatment a reality in the near future. Examples of recent advancements in this field include gene therapy, gene-corrected keratinocytes grafted on patients' skin, protein replacement therapy with recombinant proteins, injection of allogeneic fibroblasts in the dermis of affected skin, and bone marrow stem cell therapy (Hsu et al. 2014).

Prognosis

EB simplex usually causes only minor problems in daily life, whereas junctional and dystrophic forms may be mutilating diseases and may cause major morbidity. Multiple and recurrent cutaneous squamous cell carcinomas within the erosions and

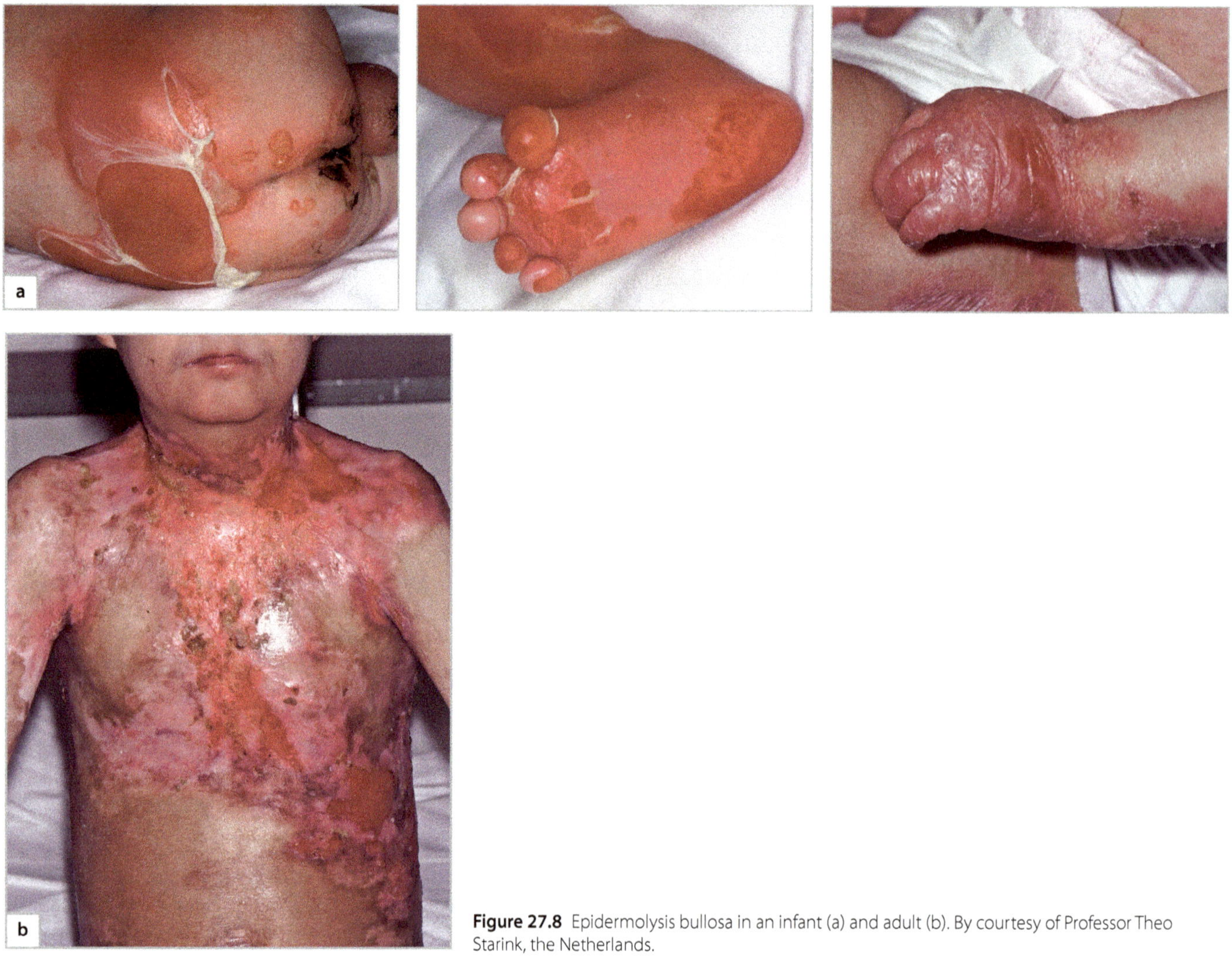

Figure 27.8 Epidermolysis bullosa in an infant (a) and adult (b). By courtesy of Professor Theo Starink, the Netherlands.

Table 27.3 Urogenital and other extracutaneous involvement in major types of EB

EB type	Involvement of urogenital system	Other extracutaneous involvement
EB simplex	Only in rare AR forms namely EB simplex with muscular dystrophy and acantholytic EB; the latter is usually lethal in neonatal period	• Oral cavity • GI tract • Respiratory tract • Cardiac system
Junctional EB	Usually in generalized form but not localized disease	• Oral cavity with extensive caries • GI tract (e.g. pyloric atresia) • Respiratory/renal tract
Dystrophic EB	Not present with AD subtype. Recessive dystrophic EB inversa affects the genital and intertriginous areas with blisters, milia and atrophic scarring.	• Oral cavity • Nails • Growth retardation • Anemia • Pseudosyndactyly (fusion of digital web spaces in generalized recessive dystrophic EB)
Kindler syndrome*	Urethral stricture	• Oral cavity • GI tract (colitis, esophageal stricture)

AD, autosomal dominant; AR, autosomal recessive; BMZ, basement membrane zone; EB, epidermolysis bullosa; GI, gastrointenstinal
*Kindler syndrome is associated with photosensitivity and poikiloderma (reticulate pigmentation, telangiectasia and skin atrophy)

chronic wounds complicate recessive dystrophic EB and are a common cause of death in adolescence. Careful clinical examination and regular surveillance are needed in this group of patients.

While beyond the scope of this book, perinatal diagnosis in EB is a possibility. There are specialized support groups for EB in many countries (e.g. DEBRA).

REFERENCES

Adam AE. Ectopic Darier's disease of the cervix: an extraordinary cause of an abnormal smear. Cytopathology 1996; 7:414–421.

Beier C, Kaufmann R. Efficacy of erbium:YAG laser ablation in Darier disease and Hailey-Hailey disease. Arch Dermatol 1999; 135:423–427.

Burge SM, Wilkinson JD. Darier-White disease: a review of the clinical features in 163 patients. J Am Acad Dermatol 1992; 27:40–50.

Christian MM, Moy RL. Treatment of Hailey-Hailey disease (or benign familial pemphigus) using short pulsed and short dwell time carbon dioxide lasers. Dermatol Surg 1999; 25:661–663.

Fine JD, Bruckner-Tuderman L, Eady RA, et al. Inherited epidermolysis bullosa: updated recommendations on diagnosis and classification. J Am Acad Dermatol 2014; 70:1103–1126.

Hamm H, Metze D, Brocker EB. Hailey-Hailey disease. Eradication by dermabrasion. Arch Dermatol 1994; 130:1143–1149.

Hanafusa T, Tamai K, Umegaki N, et al. The course of pregnancy and childbirth in three mothers with recessive dystrophic epidermolysis bullosa. Clin Exp Dermatol 2012; 37:10–14.

Harris A, Burge SM, Dykes PJ, et al. Handicap in Darier's disease and Hailey-Hailey disease. Br J Dermatol 1996; 135:959–963.

Holbrook KA. Extracutaneous epithelial involvement in inherited epidermolysis bullosa. Arch Dermatol 1988; 124:726–731.

Hsu CK, Wang SP, Lee JY, et al. Treatment of hereditary epidermolysis bullosa: updates and future prospects. Am J Clin Dermatol 2014; 15:1–6.

McElroy JA, Mehregan DA, Roenigk RK. Carbon dioxide laser vaporization of recalcitrant symptomatic plaques of Hailey-Hailey disease and Darier's disease. J Am Acad Dermatol 1990; 23:893–897.

Menz P, Jackson IT, Connolly S. Surgical control of Hailey-Hailey disease. Br J Plast Surg 1987; 40:557–561.

Sakuntabhai A, Ruiz-Perez V, Carter S, et al. Mutations in ATP2A2, encoding a Ca2+ pump, cause Darier disease. Nat Genet 1999; 21:271–277.

Savignac M, Edir A, Simon M, et al. Darier disease: a disease model of impaired calcium homeostasis in the skin. Biochim Biophys Acta 2011; 1813:1111–1117.

Wieselthier JS, Pincus SH. Hailey-Hailey disease of the vulva. Arch Dermatol 1993; 129:1344–1345.

Zachariae H. Dermabrasion in Darier's disease. Acta Derm Venereol 1979; 59:184–186.

Chapter 28 Vulvar ulcers

Jennifer Anne Yell, Aysha Javed

INTRODUCTION

There are many causes of vulvar ulceration. The most common are aphthosis (non-infectious) and herpes simplex virus infection.

Key features

- Ulcers may be infectious or non-infectious
  - Primary genital
  - Part of a more widespread skin disease
  - A manifestation of systemic disease
- The chronicity (acute, chronic, or recurrent) may be a clue to diagnosis

Ulcers should be distinguished from erosions. An erosion is a superficial defect of the skin with loss of the epithelium, whereas an ulcer is a deeper tissue defect exhibiting complete loss of the epithelium extending below the papillary dermis. Ulcers often heal with scarring of the skin, but scarring in the oral mucosa is very rare. Ulcers are often secondary; e.g. erosions can become ulcers due to trauma or secondary infection. The initial clinical finding may be a blister (herpes simplex) or pustule (neutrophilic dermatoses) which will be a pointer towards the correct diagnosis of an ulcer.

Ulcers may be due to sexually transmitted diseases (STD) (Chapters 30 and 31), other non-sexually transmitted infections, or non-infectious causes. Non-infectious ulcers are the most frequent cause of ulceration and may present in isolation at the genital site (e.g. aphthous ulcers) or may be part of a generalized dermatosis (e.g. pyoderma gangrenosum) or systemic disease (e.g. Behçet disease) (**Table 28.1**). This chapter concentrates on the most common genital ulcers not due to STD; other diseases presenting with ulcers are outlined in other chapters and will be referred to.

Separating the many causes of ulcers into categories of acute, chronic, and recurrent, with information about chronicity and speed of onset is a simple and effective tool, which forms the basis of this chapter (**Table 28.2**).

HISTORY

A good history (personal/family/sexual activity) and clinical examination including full cutaneous, mucosal, nail and hair assessments, the presence of prodromal symptoms, and systemic symptoms and underlying medical conditions will identify diagnostic clues.

INVESTIGATIONS

To identify an ulcer caused by an infection, a swab for bacterial and viral cultures or polymerase chain reaction (PCR), and blood tests, searching for antimicrobial antibodies should be performed early with the patient's consent (Chapters 30 and 31). A routine blood screen

Table 28.1 Infectious/non-infectious diseases causing genital ulcers

Infectious		Non-infectious	
Diseasew	**Features**	**Disease**	**Features**
Ecthyma	Deep skin infection with streptococcus pyogenes +/- *Staphylococcus aureus*	**Idiopathic** • Aphthous ulcers • Lipschütz ulcer	• Idiopathic acute or recurrent ulcer • Reactive ulcer, possibly a type of aphthous ulcer however, association with primary EBV and *Borrelia burgorferi* infection is reported
Other infections	Tuberculosis, typhoid, pneumonia, brucellosis etc. are not further discussed	**Neutrophilic dermatoses** • Behçet disease • Pyoderma gangrenosum • Sweet syndrome • Pyodermatitis/pyostomatitis vegetans	• Autoinflammatory disease • Trauma induced, painful • Raised temperature • IgE, eosinophils, neutrophils, malignancies
Sexually transmitted diseases	(see Chapters 30 and 31)	**Granulomatous conditions** Crohn disease	Knife-cut ulcers (Chapter 24)
		Vasculitis • Churg- Strauss • Wegener granulomatosis	• Allergic granulomatosis • Necrotizing vasculitis
		Neoplasms Skin tumors, i.e. SCC, BCC, Paget disease	Biopsy required
		Langerhans cell histiocytosis	Rare clonal cell proliferation
		Traumatic ulcers	Trauma/artefact
		Erythema multiforme / TEN	Drugs/infective cause
		Drugs	i.e. nicorandil, methotrexate

Table 28.2 Commonest causes of acute, recurrent, and chronic ulcers

Acute	Recurrent	Chronic
Infectious: • STDs • Ecthyma	• Herpes simplex infection	
Non-infectious: • Aphthous ulcers • Lipschütz ulcer • Dermatitis artefacta	• Aphthous ulcers • Behçet disease	• Pyoderma gangrenosum • Crohn disease • Dermatitis artefacta • Tumor

may detect anemia or deficiency disorders; a biopsy is indicated if blistering or systemic diseases are suspected.

Key investigations to consider

- Swab for *Candida*, bacterial, herpes simplex virus culture or PCR
- Serology for Epstein–Barr virus (EBV), *Mycoplasma pneumoniae*, syphilis, HIV screen
- Blood/serum for full blood count, ferritin, B12, folate and zinc
- Biopsy for hematoxylin and eosin +/– immunofluorescence to check for autoimmune blistering diseases, Crohn disease

Key factors in the history and examination

General medical

- Systemic symptoms, e.g. fever, headache, malaise
- Lymphadenopathy
- Systemic disease
- Immune status
- Extragenital skin problems

Exposure to microbes

- Travel and sexual exposure
- Previous or current sexually transmitted infection

Pattern of ulcer occurrence

- Speed of onset, acute or chronic, pattern of recurrence
- Number of lesions (single, multiple, other sites)

ACUTE ULCERS

Aphthous ulcers are the most common cause of acute ulcers; however, it is important to exclude STD, e.g. herpes simplex and syphilis; if suspected, tests need to be performed.

Causes of acute ulcers

- Aphthous ulceration (see recurrent ulcers)
- Lipschütz ulcers
- Sexually transmitted diseases, e.g. herpes simplex primary infection (Chapter 30) and syphilis (Chapter 31)
- Non-sexually transmitted infectious ulcers
- Trauma
- Erythema multiforme/Steven–Johnson syndrome/TEN (Chapter 18)

Lipschütz ulcer

Synonyms

Non-sexually acquired genital ulceration, complex aphthosis

Lipschütz ulcers are characterized by the rapid appearance of a large, deep, and painful solitary ulcer on the labia minora (Kinyó et al. 2014) and frequently occur in adolescent girls who are not sexually active but have been reported in women in their fourth decade. Some authors classify Lipschütz ulcers as a type of aphthous ulcer.

Pathogenesis

Although of unknown etiology, they are sometimes associated with an infection such as EBV, mycoplasma, streptococcus, salmonella, cytomegalovirus, typhoid, or paratyphoid (Farhi et al. 2009).

Clinical features

This ulcer normally presents with acute, rapidly-developing pain. There may be preceding fever and malaise. Lesions are usually solitary but may be multiple and are surrounded by a reddish areola, with a white/gray, firmly adherent membrane (slough) that separates in a few days (**Figure 28.1**). The lymphatic glands are usually enlarged. Occasionally, there may be involvement of the vagina or urethra.

Diagnosis

A biopsy is usually not indicated. The diagnosis is clinical and based on the exclusion of other causes for vulvar ulceration. However, a swab and serology to exclude infectious causes that may need treatment is recommended.

Treatment and prognosis

The ulcer is self-limiting and resolves spontaneously within 6 weeks; however, scarring often results. Treatment is aimed at pain relief. Symptomatic treatment includes analgesics, e.g. 5% lidocaine ointment or gel and topical glucocorticosteroids. In severe acute ulceration, pain can be so severe that patients may need to be admitted to hospital and catheterized. Urinating in a warm bath may be more comfortable. In cases of identified infection, treatment may be needed but often these ulcers are reactive.

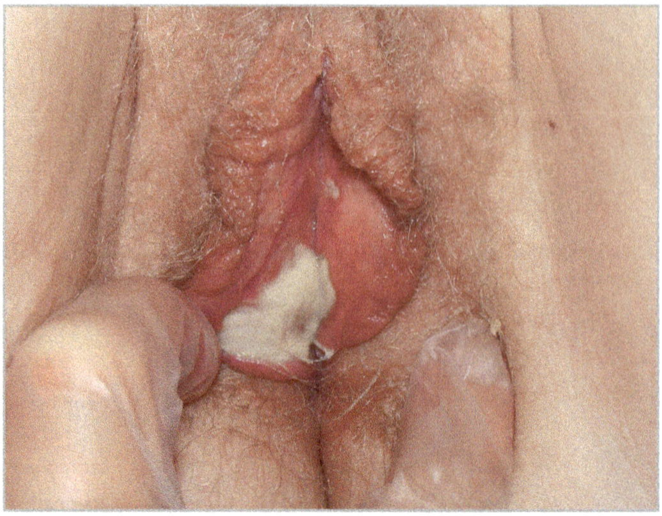

Figure 28.1 Large painful ulcer covered with a gray membrane typical of a Lipschütz ulcer. This 17-year-old had a fever and felt generally unwell for 2 weeks before presenting with this painful ulceration.

Infectious non-sexually transmitted ulcer

Ulceration rarely occurs in tuberculosis, streptococcus, brucellosis, typhoid and paratyphoid infections, and Lyme disease (Finch et al. 2014).

CHRONIC ULCERS

Chronic ulceration is defined as ulceration lasting >6 weeks. It may occur as part of a generalized dermatosis or systemic condition.

Causes of chronic ulcers

- Neutrophilic dermatoses, e.g. PG and Sweet syndrome
- Malignancy including Langerhans cell histiocytosis (LCH)
- Drugs
- Vasculitis
- Dermatitis artefacta

Neutrophilic dermatoses

The neutrophilic dermatoses are characterized by neutrophilic sterile cutaneous infiltrates and sometimes sterile pustules.

The location of the neutrophilic infiltrate results in distinct clinicopathologic entities:

- Subcorneal pustular dermatosis in the epidermis
- Sweet syndrome in the dermis
- PG in the deep dermis/subcutis
- Neutrophilic panniculitis in the subcutis

Although some of these conditions may occasionally show features of small vessel vasculitis, all dermatoses with primary leukocytoclastic vasculitis (polyarteritis nodosa, microscopic polyangiitis, hypersensitivity angiitis) are excluded. Systemic symptoms can be present and include fever, malaise, myalgia, and arthralgia. The disorders are frequently associated with underlying internal diseases such as inflammatory bowel disease, hematological malignancies, and rheumatoid arthritis. Extracutaneous involvement can occur and may involve the lungs, eyes, bones, muscles, heart, joints, bowels, kidneys, and lymph nodes (Vignon-Pennamen 2000).

Sweet syndrome

Synonyms

Acute febrile neutrophilic dermatosis

Sweet syndrome, the commonest form of the neutrophilic dermatoses, is a reactive process characterized by abrupt onset of tender, red-to-purple papules, and nodules often accompanied by systemic symptoms including fever, malaise, myalgia, and arthralgia (Sweet 1964). Sweet syndrome ranges from classic Sweet disease, which occurs in young women after a mild respiratory illness, to a more aggressive neutrophilic process, which may be associated with other inflammatory diseases or malignancy. In fact, the lesions may be the first evidence of an underlying disorder and should prompt further investigation. Disorders frequently associated with Sweet are inflammatory bowel disease, hematological malignancies, and rheumatoid arthritis.

Clinical features

It is characterized by cutaneous red-to-purple papules and nodules that coalesce to form plaques (Vignon-Pennamen & Wallach 1991). The plaques usually occur on the upper extremities, face, or neck and are typically accompanied by fever and peripheral neutrophilia.

Vulvar involvement (**Figure 28.2a–d**) is rare (Keefe et al. 1988). It is one to be distinguished from other diseases that commonly affect the eyes, mouth, and skin (**Table 28.3**).

Extracutaneous involvement can occur and may involve the lungs, eyes, bones, muscles, heart, joints, bowels, kidneys, and lymph nodes (Vignon-Pennamen 2000). Ocular involvement may occur in up to a third of patients with Sweet syndrome and may consist of iritis, episcleritis, conjunctivitis, and ulcerative keratitis. Behçet, PG, and Sweet all share the phenomenon of pathergy (new ulceration occurring after trauma or injury to the skin).

Diagnosis and differential diagnosis

Peripheral neutrophilia and an infiltrate of sterile neutrophils in the dermis are characteristic features. It needs to be distinguished from other diseases that commonly affect the eyes, mouth, and skin (**Table 28.3**).

Treatment and prognosis

In general, Sweet syndrome responds dramatically to oral corticosteroids and may improve or resolve with treatment of the underlying condition. Steroid-resistant cases have been treated with dapsone, colchicine, doxycycline, cyclosporine, retinoids, and methotrexate (von den Driesch 1994). Without treatment, the syndrome may persist for weeks or months and then improves without leaving scars. Recurrences are common.

Pyoderma gangrenosum

Pyoderma gangrenosum (PG), a neutrophilic dermatosis, is associated with systemic diseases in around 50% of cases.

Disorders associated with pyoderma gangrenosum

• Gastrointestinal	Crohn disease, ulcerative colitis
• Joint	Rheumatoid arthritis, psoriatic arthritis, spondyloarthropathy, symmetrical polyarthritis
• Hematologic	Myeloma (usually IgA), leukemia, monoclonal gammopathy
• Hepatic	Chronic active hepatitis, primary biliary cirrhosis
• Autoimmune	Systemic lupus erythematosus (SLE), Sjögren syndrome

Clinical features

The ulcers in PG typically begin as a pustule or nodule, which soon breaks down to form a rapidly enlarging ulcer, with a raised necrotic/purple 'overhanging' inflammatory border and a boggy, necrotic base. It typically affects the lower limbs and dorsum of the hands and is very painful. PG has an atypical variant that may involve the vulva (**Figure 28.3**), penis, and scrotum. It heals with scarring. Pathergy (an exaggerated skin injury occurring after minor trauma such as scratch or venepuncture) occurs in 30%.

Diagnosis

This rare genital presentation of PG should be considered in cases of refractory genital ulceration and diagnosis is based on exclusion of other pathology (Satoh & Yamamoto 2013). A biopsy for histology and tissue

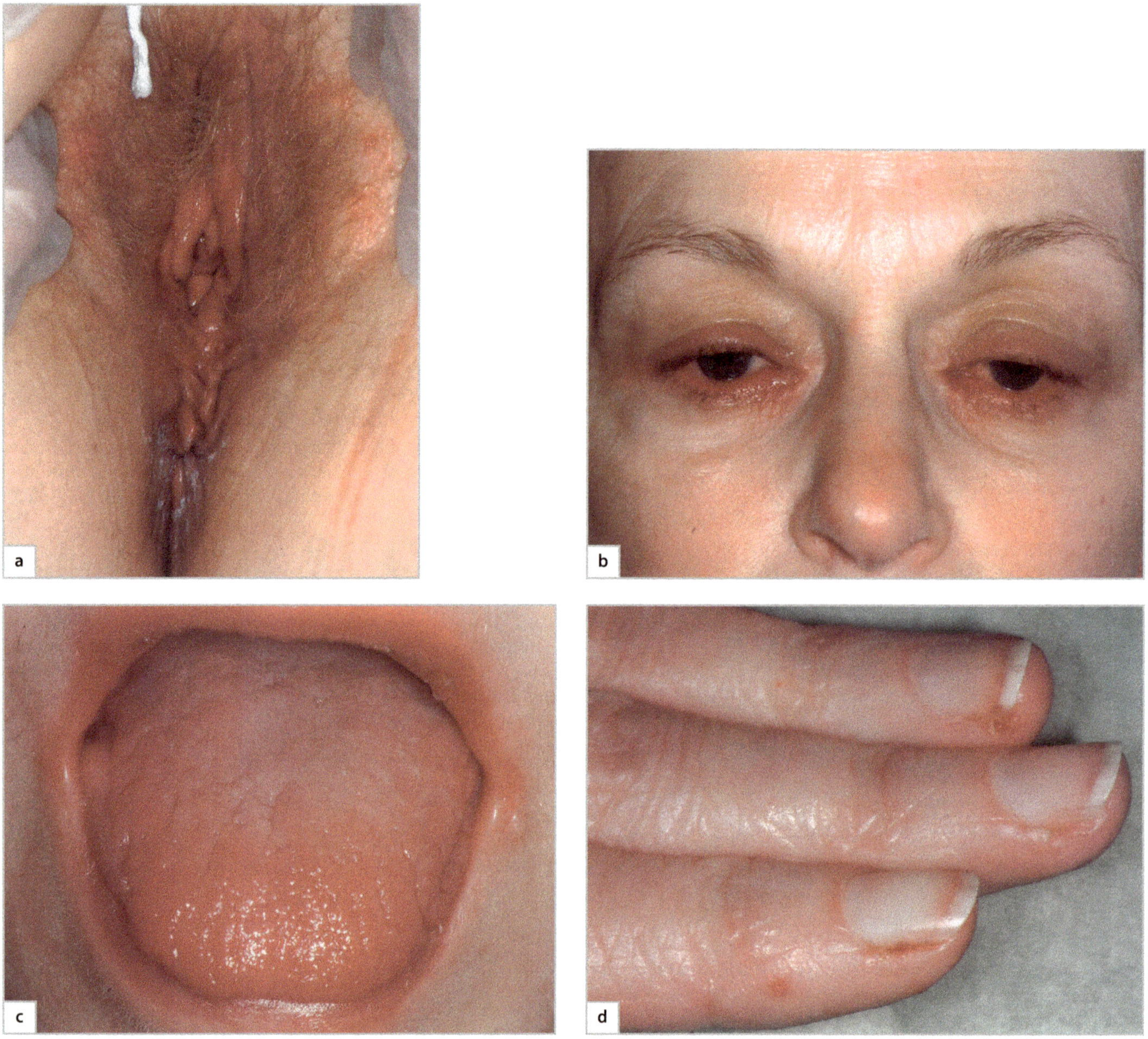

Figure 28.2 (a) Vulvar erythematous glazing and vulvar aphthous ulceration in a patient with Sweet syndrome. She was systemically unwell. (b) Eye involvement in same patient with blepharitis and conjunctivitis. (c) Desquamative stomatitis. (d) 8 weeks later, she developed erythema and scaling of the finger tips and nail folds.

culture is necessary for bacteria, fungi, atypical mycobacteria, and viruses. A workup is required to rule out associated underlying conditions.

Treatment

Treatment with high dosage systemic steroids and other immunosuppressants are usually indicated. Potent topical steroids, tacrolimus, and tetracycline antibiotics may also be helpful in less severe cases.

Solid malignant tumors

Malignancy must be excluded in any ulcer without an obvious cause. Ulcerated tumors occurring in the vulva include squamous cell carcinomas, basal cell carcinomas, and lymphomas.

Langerhans cell histiocytosis

LCH is thought to be clonal proliferation of Langerhans cells (CD1a positive with Birbeck granules) with an infiltrate deposited in the bone marrow, skin, and lymph nodes, often occurring in childhood. However, recent studies have called into question the Langerhans cell as the cell of origin. This condition may very rarely present in the vulva (Kurt et al. 2013). Nodulo-ulcerative lesions occur in the oral, perineal, vulvar, or retroauricular regions. In adults with LCH, the pulmonary system is the most frequently involved organ system; so, there may be associated systemic symptoms including chronic cough, dyspnea, and chest pain.

Table 28.3 Oculomucocutaneous syndromes with oral ulcerations

	Ocular manifestations	Cutaneous features	Treatment
Sweet syndrome	• Conjunctivitis/episcleritis • Uveitis or iritis • Limbal nodules • Glaucoma • Subconjunctival hemorrhage • Sudden visual loss	• Violaceous papules, plaques or nodules • Dorsal hand lesions • Lesion can be studded with pustules • Ulcers and bullae	Oral prednisolone
Behçet disease	• Anterior uveitis • Posterior uveitis • Cells in corpus vitreum • Retinal vasculitis	• Erythema nodosum • Pseudofolliculitis • Papulopustular lesions • Acneiform lesions	Immunosuppressant medication frequently needed
Reiter syndrome	• Conjunctivitis • Anterior uveitis	• Keratoderma blenorrhagica	

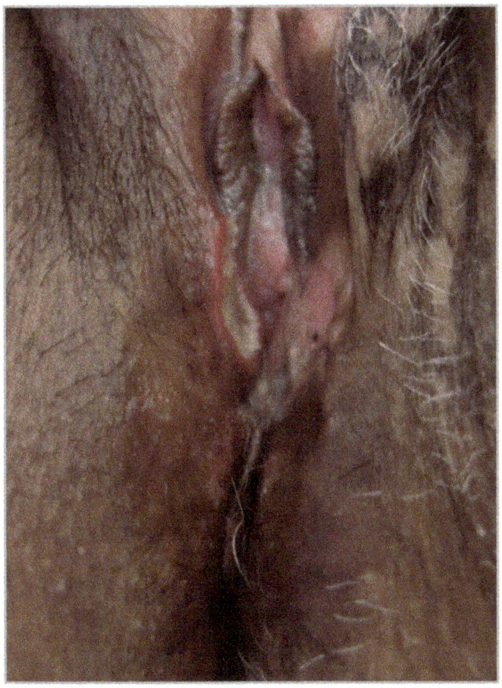

Figure 28.3 Cribriform ulcer of pyoderma gangrenosum that presented with significant pain. By courtesy of Dr Gudula Kirtschig, Tübingen, Germany.

Medications

A number of medications may induce ulceration including nicorandil and methotrexate possibly as a first sign of an adverse drug effect. Typically ulcerations will not heal until the drug is withdrawn.

Vasculitis

A number of rare vasculitic conditions including granulomatosis with polyangitis (Wegener granulomatosis) and Churg-Strauss syndrome may present in the vulva (Lewis 2002). Dermatological manifestations of granulomatosis with polyangitis include subcutaneous nodules, papules, vesicles, and ulcers.

Dermatitis artefacta

This is usually a diagnosis of exclusion as women rarely admit to harming themselves. A biopsy is usually needed to exclude other causes of ulceration.

RECURRENT ULCERS

Key causes of recurrent ulceration

- Herpes simplex infection
- Aphthous ulcers
- Behçet disease

Recurrent herpes simplex infection

This is a frequent cause of recurrent ulceration (see Chapter 30).

Recurrent idiopathic aphthosis

Recurrent aphthosis (RAS) describes a common condition affecting up to 50% of the population, confined to mucosal surfaces mainly affecting the mouth but sometimes affecting the vulvar area (**Figure 28.4a** and **b**).

Pathogenesis

The cause is unknown; however, there may be a genetic predisposition in 40%. Other contributory factors include localized trauma, menstrual cycle hormone changes, stress, and a foaming agent in toothpaste, sodium lauryl sulfate. Systemic diseases associated include Behçet disease (see later), iron deficiency, and some gastroenterological diseases including gluten sensitive enteropathy, inflammatory bowel disease, HIV infection, and SLE. Some medications, including non-steroidal anti-inflammatory agents, predispose.

Clinical features

Aphthous ulcers usually first occur in childhood or adolescence and tend to resolve or abate spontaneously with age. An underlying cause is particularly likely where RAS commences or worsens in adult life.

RAS is classified into three categories (**Table 28.4**):

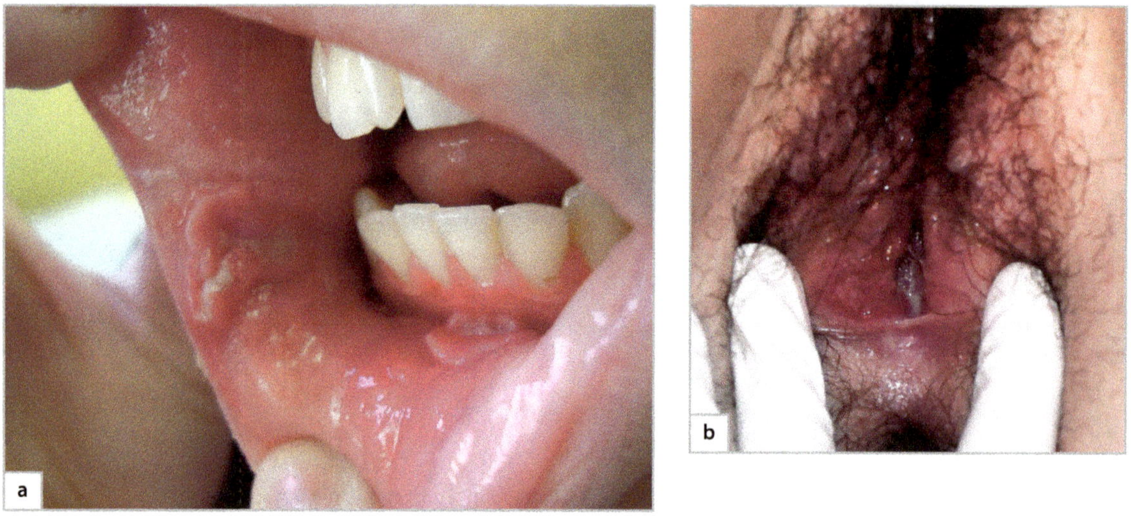

Figure 28.4 (a) Oral aphthous ulcer showing an ovoid ulcer reaching 1 cm in diameter, with surrounding edema. Concurrent vulvar ulcer in this patient was morphologically identical. (b) Typical major aphthous genital ulcer. By courtesy of Dr Gayle Fischer Associate Professor of Dermatology, Northern Clinical School, Sydney, Australia.

Table 28.4 Types of aphthous ulcers

	Minor recurrent aphthosis (RAS)	**Major RAS**	**Herpetiform RAS**	**Lipschütz ulcer**
Chronology	Recurrent every 1–4 months	Recurrent more frequently than other RAS	Almost continuous	Acute <6 weeks
Number of ulcers	Few	Multiple	Multiple	Single or sparse
Morphology	Small, round or ovoid ulcers, well circumscribed margin, red halo	Large lesions 1 cm or larger with scarring when healed	Typical of herpes simplex, without a viral etiology	Sparse lesions are surrounded by a reddish areola, with a dirty, firmly adherent membrane that separates in a few days
Associations	• Family history • Hematinic deficiency (iron, folic acid, B12) • Gastrointestinal disease (coeliac, Crohn) • Endocrine (premenstrual) • Immunodeficiency (HIV) • Other (trauma, foods, stress, cessation of smoking) • Cyclical neutropenia	As per minor RAS	As per minor RAS	Infection (typhoid, paratyphoid, infectious mononucleosis)
Systemic manifestations	Minimal symptoms	Painful	Extremely painful	May have fever Enlarged lymph nodes
Age	10–40 years	From childhood or adolescence	Older population Females > males	Adolescent girls >50%
Duration	Rapid healing without scarring in a few days	Slow healing over 10–40 days	Continuous	6 weeks before spontaneous regression

1. **Minor aphthous** (synonym: Mikulicz ulcers) (**Figure 28.5**)

These represent approximately 80% of all cases of aphthous ulceration usually during the age 10-40 with minor symptoms. They are small round or oval ulcers 2-4 mm in diameter and have a yellowish/gray pseudomembrane surrounded by an erythematous halo and edema. They occur in crops of 1-6 lesions at 1-4 monthly intervals, are self-limiting, healing within 7–10 days without scarring.

2. **Major aphthous** (synonym: Sutton ulcers, periadenitis mucosa necrotica recurrens)

These account for 10% of cases of RAS. They are more severe than minor RAS, have a longer duration, recur more frequently and are painful. Round/ovoid groups of 1-6 ulcers reaching 1 cm in diameter, or larger are associated with surrounding edema. Healing is slow over 10-40 days with scarring. There may be a prodromal illness with fever or malaise in some (Dixit et al. 2013).

3. **Herpetiform ulcers**

This subtype occurs in 1–10% of RAS and mainly in older females. They are characterized by multiple vesicles that rapidly progress to minute, small, deep, painful superficial ulcers, which then coalesce forming larger ulcerations with irregular/jagged edges. The name is misleading because there is no herpes simplex infection. Healing takes 10 days or longer and episodes are so frequent that ulceration may be continuous.

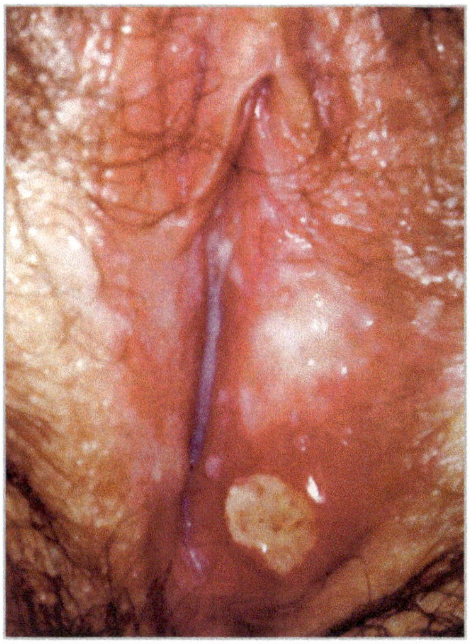

Figure 28.5 Simple aphthous ulcer with erythematous halo of the vulva.

Diagnosis

The diagnosis is clinical. Biopsy is indicated only where another form of ulceration is suspected. A check of full blood count, ferritin, B12, and folate is prudent.

Treatment

Treatment of minor RAS is usually straightforward (Belenguer-Guallar et al. 2014) and aims at symptom control (**Table 28.5**). Symptomatic treatment includes analgesics, e.g. 5% lidocaine ointment or benzdymine spray or topical glucocorticosteroids. A short course of oral glucocorticosteroids (e.g. prednisolone commencing at 30 mg for a 70 kg adult and dropping by 5 mg daily over 6 days) will settle most exquisitely painful aphthous ulcers.

The evidence for systemic treatment resides primarily in the oral medicine literature (Brocklehurst et al. 2012). Oral tetracyclines (e.g. Doxycycline 100 mg bd) are the best tolerated and therefore usually used first line (Preshaw et al. 2007, Dixit et al. 2013). Dapsone and Colchicine may be necessary in the case of failure of tetracyclines (Mimura et al. 2009). Colchicine is commenced at 500 µg 2x/day. Increasing the dose to 500 µg 3x/day may be limited by diarrhea. Thalidomide is very effective in refractory severe cases (Hello et al. 2010) but baseline and interval nerve conduction studies are necessary because of potential irreversible peripheral neuropathy. It is unusual to require other systemic immunosuppressives such as cyclosporine, azathioprine, or mycophenolate mofetil, in uncomplicated aphthosis.

Behçet disease

Behçet disease is a rare, complex, multisystem disorder characterized by a triad of recurrent oral aphthous ulceration, genital ulcers, and uveitis.

Pathogenesis

It is of unknown etiology but thought to be due to an abnormal immune reaction to infection. It is one of the oculomucocutaneous syndromes. It occurs most frequently in the Mediterranean, Far East, and Middle East. The presence of HLA-B51/B5 alleles increases the risk of developing the condition (Calamia et al. 2009).

Table 28.5 Treatment options for recurrent aphthous ulceration

Treatment modality	Preparation/strength
Topical	• Corticosteroids: hydrocortisone hemisuccinate pellets, triamcinolone acetonide paste 0.05-5%, fluocinolone acetonide 0.025–0.05%, clobetasol proprionate 0.025%, betamethasone sodium phosphate • Topical anesthetics: 2% lidocaine gel or spray • Topical tetracyclines: doxycycline 100 mg in 10 mL water, or as a fixed dose gel adhesive • Antiseptics, analgesics and anti-inflammatory agents: amlexanox 5%, diclofenac 3%, chlorhexidine 0.2% wash/gel • Hyaluronic acid gel 0.2%
Systemic	• Multivitamins and B_{12} orally • Corticosteroids: prednisolone 25 mg/day • Tetracyclines: doxycycline 100 mg od, minocycline 100 mg od, tetracycline 500 mg 3 times/day • Colchicine 500 µg 2–3 times/day • Pentoxifylline 400mg 3 times/day • Dapsone 50–100 mg/day • Zinc sulfate 150 mg/day • Clofazimine 100 mg/day • Immunomodulating: thalidomide 50–100 mg/day • Levamisole 150 mg 3 times/week
Laser	• Nd:YAG laser
Natural remedies/ homeopathy	• Myrtle • Quercetin • Licorice hydrogel • Damask rose

Clinical features

The morphology of genital ulcers in Behçet disease is not diagnostic (**Figure 28.6a** and **b**) as they show many features of recurrent aphthous ulceration. Other dermatological manifestations include pathergy, papulopustular eruptions, erythema nodosum-like lesions, Sweet-like lesions, PG, bullous necrotizing vasculitis, and thrombophlebitis (Calamia et al. 2009).

A history of general malaise, anorexia, lymphadenopathy, weakness, and headache may precede the onset by years. Tonsillitis, myalgia, joint pain, and recurrent sore throats are common. In addition to cutaneous and ocular features, systemic involvement may include cardiovascular, GI, progressive central nervous system, renal, pulmonary, vascular, and urologic. Potential life-threatening problems include blindness, thromboembolism, aneurysms, GI ulceration, and encephalitis.

Diagnosis

The diagnosis of Behçet is notoriously difficult as there are no universally accepted diagnostic criteria. The current internationally recognized criteria are based on the revised guidelines from the International Study Group for Behçet disease (**Table 28.6**). The diagnosis of Behçet disease requires the presence of recurrent oral aphthous ulceration at least 3 times in 12 months plus 2 of the following listed criteria.

Histopathology

The distinguishing histopathology of Behçet is a vasculitis, involving any size of vessel, including veins (unusual) as well as arteries. Early mucosal and cutaneous lesions show a leukocytoclastic vasculitis (endothelial swelling, extravasation of red blood

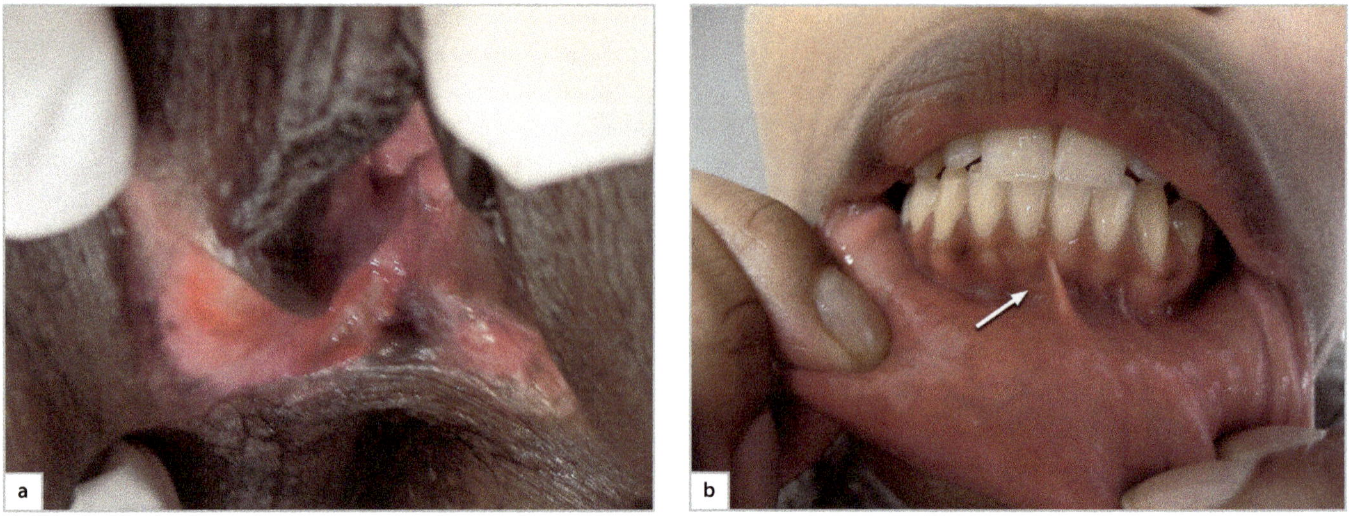

Figure 28.6 Behçet disease. This patient had recurrent large painful genital (a) and oral (b) ulcers and optic neuritis. By courtesy of Dr Gudula Kirtschig, Tübingen, Germany.

Table 28.6 International criteria for the classification of Behçet disease (1990). For diagnosis, one major and at least two minor criteria should be present

Site of involvement	Specific criteria
Genital (minor)	Recurrent genital ulceration, aphthous ulceration or scarring
Oral (required/major)	Recurrent oral ulceration, minor aphthous, major aphthous or herpetiform ulceration at least 3 times in one 12-month period
Ocular (minor)	Anterior uveitis, posterior uveitis, and cells in corpus vitreum upon slit-lamp examination or Retinal vasculitis observed by physician (ophthalmologist)
Dermatological (minor)	Erythema nodosum-like lesions, pseudofolliculitis, or papulopustular lesions or Acneiform nodules in post-adolescent patients not receiving corticosteroids
Positive pathergy test (minor)	An erythematous papule >2 mm at the prick site 48 hours after the application of a 20- to 22-gauge sterile needle

cells, fibrinoid necrosis) with a neutrophilic vascular reaction. Thrombophlebitis results from vessels being infiltrated by large numbers of lymphocytes.

Treatment

Treatment involves symptomatic treatment of ulceration similar to those used in RAS. Systemic treatments are usually required including colchicine or other immunosuppressants.

REFERENCES

Belenguer-Guallar I, Jiménez-Soriano Y, Claramunt-Lozano A. Treatment of recurrent aphthous stomatitis. A literature review. J Clin Exp Dent 2014; 1;6:e168–174.

Brocklehurst P, Tickle M, Glenny AM, et al. Systemic interventions for recurrent aphthous stomatitis (mouth ulcers). Cochrane Database Syst Rev 2012; 9:CD005411.

Calamia KT, Wilson FC, Icen M, et al. Epidemiology and clinical characteristics of Behçet's disease in the US: a population-based study. Arthritis Rheum 2009; 61:600-604.

Dixit S, Bradford J, Fischer G. Management of non-sexually acquired genital ulceration using oral ad topical corticosteroids followed by doxycycline prophylaxis. J Am Acad Dermatol 2013; 68:797-802.

Farhi D, Wendling J, Molinari E, et al. Non-sexually related acute genital ulcers in 13 pubertal girls: a clinical and microbiological study. Arch Dermatol 2009; 145:38.

Finch JJ, Wald J, Ferenczi K, et al. Disseminated lyme disease presenting with nonsexual acute genital ulcers. JAMA Dermatol. 2014; 150:1202–1204.

Hello M, Barbarot S, Bastuji-Garin S, et al. Use of thalidomide for severe recurrent aphthous stomatitis: a multicenter cohort analysis. Medicine (Baltimore) 2010; 89:176–182.

International Study Group for Behçet's Disease. Criteria for diagnosis of Behçet's disease. International Study Group for Behçet's Disease. Lancet 1990; 335:1078–1080.

Kurt S, Mehmet TC, Kopuz A, et al. Diagnosis of primary Langerhans cell histiocytosis of the vulva in a postmenopausal woman. Hindawi Publishing Corporation. Case Rep Obstet Gynecol 2013; 2013: 975196. Published online, 2013.

Lewis FM. Vulvar involvement in Wegener's granulomatosis. A case report. J Reprod Med 2002; 47:725-727.

Keefe M, Wakeel RA, Kerr RE. Sweet's syndrome, plantar pustulosis and vulval pustules. Clin Exp Derm 1988; 13:344–346.

Kinyó A, Nagy N, Oláh J, et al. Ulcus vulvae acutum Lipschütz in two young female patients. Eur J Dermatol 2014; 24:361–364.

Mimura MA, Hirota SK, Sugaya NN, et al. Systemic treatment in severe cases of recurrent aphthous stomatitis: an open trial. Clinics (Sao Paulo) 2009; 64:193–198.

Preshaw PM, Grainger P, Bradshaw MH, et al. Subantimicrobial dose doxycycline in the treatment of recurrent oral aphthous ulceration: a pilot study. J Oral Pathol Med 2007; 36:236–240.

Satoh M, Yamamoto T. Genital pyoderma gangrenosum: report of two cases and published work review of Japanese cases. J Dermatol 2013; 40:840-843.

Sweet RD. An acute febrile neutrophilic dermatosis. Br J Dermatol 1964; 76:349–356.

Vignon-Pennamen MD, Wallach D. Cutaneous manifestations of neutrophilic disease: a study of seven cases. Dermatologica 1991; 183:255–264.

Vignon-Pennamen MD. The extracutaneous involvement in the neutrophilic dermatoses. Clin Dermatol 2000; 18:339–347.

Von den Driesch P. Sweet's syndrome (acute febrile neutrophilic dermatosis). J Am Acad Dermatol 1994; 31:535-556.

Chapter 29 Primary bacterial and fungal vulvar and vulvovaginal infections

Mariola Pawlaczyk, Michał Pawlaczyk

Key features of vulvar bacterial and fungal infections

- Vulvar bacterial and fungal skin infections are usually superficial
- The vulva may be affected by infectious skin diseases specific to the location or occasionally by dermatoses with a predilection for other parts of the body
- Direct microscopic examination and Wood lamp examination are helpful diagnostic tools
- The diagnosis of vulvovaginal symptoms requires correlation of the medical history, clinical examination, and laboratory tests
- For healthy individuals, topical treatment is usually sufficient
- Pregnant women with asymptomatic candida vulvovaginitis and bacterial vaginosis (BV) should receive treatment
- Predisposing and precipitating factors need to be searched for

PRIMARY BACTERIAL AND FUNGAL VULVAR INFECTIONS

Introduction

The skin microbiota plays an important role in the skin immune function. Although resident flora can cause skin infection, these are generally linked with bacteria not normally present. The vulva and the surrounding skin may be affected by bacterial and fungal infections that are specific to this location, though other infectious dermatoses with a predilection for other body parts may occasionally be present.

Skin surface micro-organisms

Gram positive

- Aerobic bacteria, e.g. *Lactobacillus* species, *Diphtheroides (Corynebacterium* species), Staphylococci *(Staphylococcus epidermidis)*
- Anaerobic bacteria, e.g. *Diphteroides (Propionibacterium acnes)*

Gram negative

- *Escherichia coli*, *Pseudomonas* species, *Gardnerella vaginalis*

Commensal yeasts

- e.g. *Candida* species, *Malassezia* species

Impetigo

Impetigo is an acute superficial skin infection with a high prevalence in children and young adults, but it can develop at any age. It is caused by either *Staphylococcus aureus*, which is currently the most frequently isolated pathogen, or a group A β-hemolytic *Streptococcus* (GABHS) *(Streptococcus pyogenes)*. The disease is very contagious and spreads easily from person to person.

Bullous impetigo

Exfoliative toxins produced by *S. aureus* are responsible for acantholysis (loss of cell adhesion leading to blisters) within the most upper layers of the epidermis leading to bullous impetigo, the localized form of staphylococcal scaled skin syndrome (which causes generalized blistering). Lesions are preferentially located in the intertriginous and diaper area. During the early stages, small vesicles appear. They soon change into flaccid blisters 1–2 cm in diameter. Due to the thin roof of the blisters, they easily rupture, and lesions progress to superficial erosions with collarette of scale. The disease occurs most commonly in neonates and children aged 2–5 years.

Predisposing factors for impetigo

- Poor hygiene
- Warm weather/high humidity
- Malnutrition
- Skin injury
- Underlying pruritic dermatoses leading to scratching and skin injury, e.g. scabies
- Dermatoses with a disturbed immune system, e.g. patients with atopic eczema are prone to infections
- Immunosuppression

Clinical presentation

Non-bullous impetigo

Clinical features:

- Initially small erythematous macules, vesicles, and pustules
- Subsequently erosions covered with characteristic yellow 'honey-colored' crusts

Sites of predilection:

- Face and hands
- Satellite lesions caused by inoculation may be present in other body parts

Diagnosis

Impetigo is usually diagnosed clinically, but microbiological tests are helpful if the diagnosis is in doubt.

Treatment

Untreated non-bullous impetigo tends to resolve in 2–3 weeks. The deeper, ulcerated type (ecthyma) heals with scarring.

Topical antibiotics such as fusidic acid (twice daily for 10 days), mupirocin (the drug of choice in methicillin-resistant *Staphylococcus aureus* infections), or retapamulin offer a highly effective treatment.

Extensive or disseminated lesions should be treated with systemic antibiotics: erythromycin (the drug of choice), other macrolides (clarithromycin, roxithromycin, azithromycin), amoxicillin with clavulanic acid, and clindamycin, tetracyclines, and fluoroquinolones for methicillin resistant *S. aureus* (Pereira 2014).

Intertrigo

Intertrigo is an inflammatory condition of skinfolds, including the groin (**Figure 29.1**).

Predisposing factors:

- Obesity (occlusion)
- Hyperhidrosis
- Poor hygiene
- Urinary or fecal incontinence
- Vaginal discharge
- Diabetes mellitus
- Immunodeficiency
- Malnutrition

Age preference:

- Infants (occlusion due to diapers)
- Elderly (occlusion due to immobilization, reduced immunity)

Skin-on-skin friction leading to heat, maceration, moisture, and lack of air circulation in flexural sites are all contributing factors. Those circumstances may support secondary bacterial or fungal infections. *Staphylococcus aureus*, group A β-hemolytic streptococcus (GABHS), *Proteus mirabilis*, *Proteus vulgaris*, and *Pseudomonas aeruginosa* may aggravate the inflammation. Streptococcal intertrigo is common in children and is characterized by a 'weeping' appearance and offensive odor (Wolf et al. 2011). *Candida* intertrigo affects inguinal folds and vulvar skin, and may spread to the buttocks and medial thighs with characteristic satellite lesions (**Figure 29.2**). Patients may complain of burning, stinging, and itching.

Clinical presentation

Characteristics of lesions

- Erythema
- Erosions leading to oozing
- Fissures
- Crusts

Diagnosis and differential diagnosis

The diagnosis is usually based on clinical presentation but microbiological tests (swabs) may help to differentiate the cause of infection. Green fluorescence under Wood light is characteristic for *Pseudomonas* infection.

The most common disorders mimicking inguinal intertrigo are diaper dermatitis (skin irritation due to the nappy) in infants and small children, psoriasis, tinea inguinalis, erythrasma, seborrheic dermatitis, atopic dermatitis, contact dermatitis and Hailey-Hailey disease (Janigger et al. 2005).

Treatment

Patients should be advised to eliminate the triggering factors, minimize friction, and moisture with the use of absorptive powders and barrier creams (e.g. containing zinc oxide). Application of low potency glucocorticosteroids for a few days may help reduce inflammation. Secondary infection should be treated by washing with disinfectant

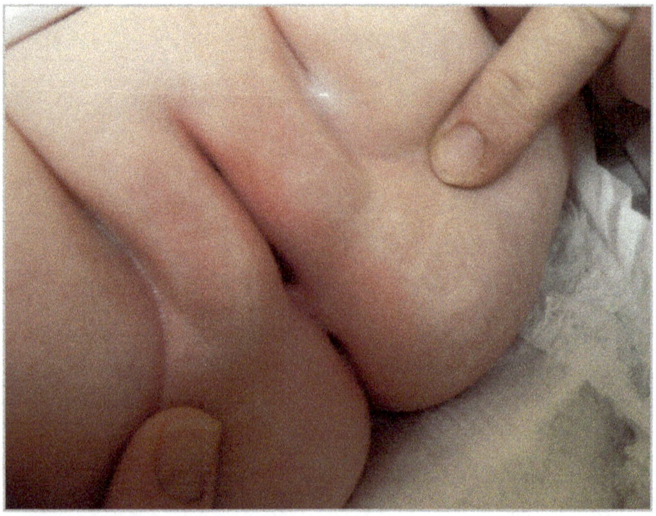

Figure 29.1 Intertrigo in the inguinal folds of a 16-month-old girl wearing diaper.

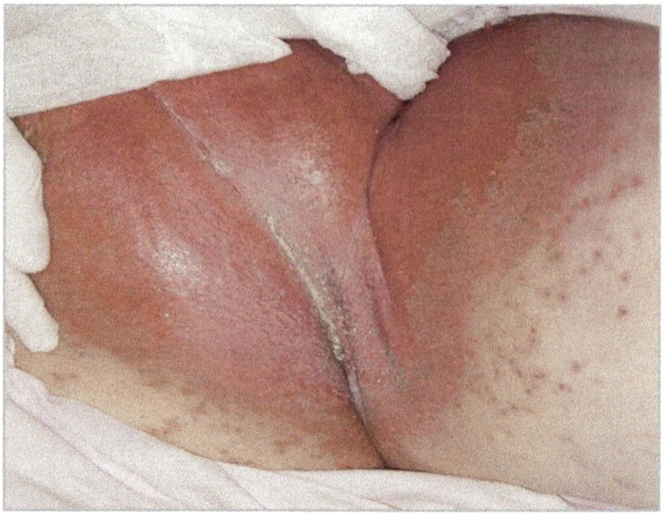

Figure 29.2 Candida intertrigo of the groin, characterized by collarette scales and satellite lesions in an obese diabetic woman. By courtesy of Prof. Z. Adamski, Poznan, Poland.

fluids (e.g. containing chlorhexidine) and the application of topical or oral antibiotics and antifungal medications.

Erythrasma

Erythrasma is a superficial bacterial infection caused by *Corynebacterium minutissimum* located in the intertriginous area such as the groin, axillae, and between the toes.

Clinical presentation

Key features

- Patches with well-defined border
- Initially pink or red
- Fade to uniform brown color

The brown coloration, along with a fine scale and wrinkled surface, distinguishes erythrasma from fungal infections. Lesions are confluent and usually asymptomatic, but sometimes mild pruritus may be reported. Although males and females are equally affected, the groin involvement is more often observed in men. A generalized disciform variant exists and is relevant to diabetes mellitus type 2. Erythrasma can occur in all ages or ethnicities, but is more common in warm, humid climates. Predisposing factors include old age, diabetes, obesity, excessive sweating, poor hygiene, and immune deficiency.

Diagnosis and differential diagnosis

Examination under Wood light with the characteristic coral-red fluorescence resulting from porphyrin production usually confirms erythrasma. Differential diagnosis includes tinea inguinalis, seborrheic dermatitis, inverse type psoriasis, and cutaneous candidosis.

Treatment

Topical treatment with clindamycin, erythromycin, miconazole, or Whitfield ointment is usually effective. Systemic therapy with erythromycin (4 times/day for 5 days) or a single dose of clarithromycin (1 g) is recommended in persistent or recurrent cases (Holdiness 2002).

Tinea cruris/inguinalis

Synonyms

Tinea inguinals (German-speaking countries; inguen=groin), Tinea cruris (a misnomer in Anglo-American countries as 'cruris' in Latin means 'of the lower leg')

Tinea cruris or tinea inguinalis is a dermatophyte infection of the inguinal region that mainly affects adult men. It is less common in women but can be transmitted through direct contact, including sexual contact, by autoinoculation from tinea pedis or onychomycosis, and indirectly from fomites, e.g. sponges. *Trichophyton rubrum* and *Trichophyton mentagrophytes varietas interdigitale* are the most common etiologic agents isolated in recent years, whereas *Epidermophyton floccosum* remains a rare occurrence. The infection is reported worldwide but is predominantly found in hot climates (Seebacher et al. 2008).

Clinical presentation

Key features

- Well-defined, slowly expanding erythematous plaques with central clearing, covered with scales accentuated on the margin
- Vesicles and pustules may be present in acute stages at the edge of the lesions
- Itching and burning

Tinea is usually restricted to skinfolds, but may spread to the thighs, buttock, labia majora, and mons if untreated or treated with glucocorticosteroids (tinea incognito). When progressing, the lesions change color and become hyperpigmented. Deep follicular invasion of dermatophytes may provoke follicular tinea with inflammation, papules, and pustules (**Figure 29.3**). More infiltrative lesions with nodules and papules within the erythematous plaque are known as the Majocchi granuloma. This form usually affects immunocompromised hosts; but women who shave their pubic hair, particularly pregnant women, may be at risk.

Diagnosis

The diagnosis is confirmed by microscopic examination of a potassium hydroxide (KOH) preparation of skin scrapings that shows hyphae. Mycological culture helps to distinguish the species present (Degreef 2008).

Treatment

Topical treatment with antifungal agents is usually effective and various medications may be used: ciclopirox, butenafine, azoles (clotrimazole, ketoconazole, miconazole, oxiconazole, sulconazole, luliconazole, sertaconazole), and allylamines (naftifine, terbinafine). The combination of antifungal agents and topical

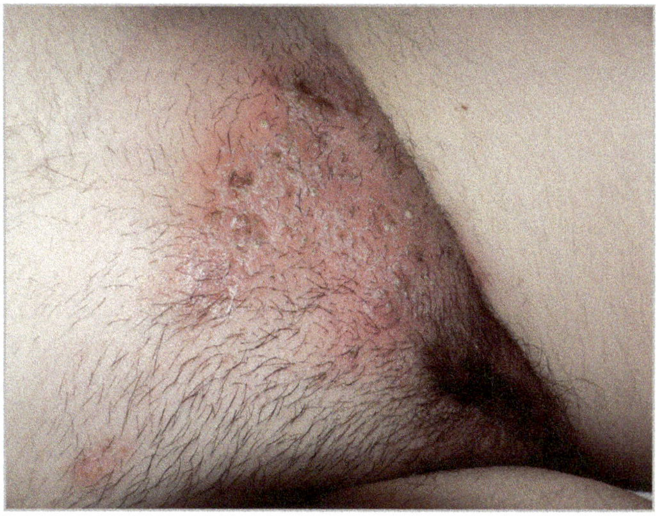

Figure 29.3 Follicular dermatophytosis located on the mons pubis and spreading to the labia majora in a pregnant woman.

corticosteroids for a few days helps to reduce inflammation. If lesions affect a large area, are recurrent, or are present in immunocompromised patients, systemic therapy should be administered (itraconazole 200 mg daily or terbinafine 250 mg daily for 2–4 weeks or fluconazole 150–300 mg once weekly for 2–4 weeks, orally) (Gupta & Cooper 2008).

Pityriasis versicolor

Pityriasis versicolor is a chronic superficial skin infection, restricted to stratum corneum, caused by *Malassezia sp.* yeasts. Those commensal microorganisms under some circumstances may change to mycelia phase and become invasive.

Predisposing factors

- Heat
- Humidity
- Occlusion
- Poor hygiene

Clinical presentation

Key features

- Light pink, brown
- Round or oval in shape, sharp margins
- Very fine scales
- Asymptomatic
- Patches become white after treatment—re-pigmentation after UV-exposure

Although the upper arms and trunk are the main sites of predilection, lesions may occasionally spread to the lower abdomen, vulva, and buttocks.

Diagnosis

The disease is easily recognized by clinical presentation (Pedrosa et al. 2014). Wood lamp examination reveals a yellow-orange color of active lesions and facilitates assessment of the infected area, providing that invasive *Malassezia* species fluoresce. Examination of skin scrapings with KOH by direct microscopy showing hyphae (characteristic 'spaghetti and meatballs' picture) confirms the diagnosis.

Treatment

Shampoos containing ketoconazole, zinc pyrithione, selenium sulfide 2.5%, ciclopirox olamine, as well as antifungal creams (ketoconazole, clotrimazole, miconazole, terbinafine) are recommended for topical therapy usually for 2 weeks, which is the first-line treatment. Systemic treatment should be considered if lesions are persistent or recurrent (fluconazole 300 mg weekly for 2–3 weeks or as a single dose of 400 mg). Due to possible side effects, itraconazole is the second choice and should be administered in a dose of 200 mg daily for 1 week or 100 mg daily for 2 weeks (Hald 2014).

PRIMARY VAGINAL INFECTIONS

Introduction

Vaginal infections are a common cause for women to seek medical advice. The three most prevalent vaginal infections are candidosis, trichomoniasis, and BV. Useful clinical manifestations and differences in laboratory tests for disease differentiation are presented in **Table 29.1.** Numerous vaginal infections occur due to bowel flora infection (*E. coli*, enterococci), GABHS, GBS, and other bacteria. Primary vaginal infections may lead to secondary vulvitis (especially candidal) that is important to be aware of otherwise treatment may be incomplete and/or ineffective.

Bacterial vaginosis

BV (often wrongly named non-specific vaginitis, bacterial vaginitis) is believed to be the main cause of vaginal discharge in women of the reproductive age.

Table 29.1 Differential diagnosis in most common vaginal infections

Feature	Bacterial vaginosis	Vaginal candidosis	Trichomoniasis
Discharge	Greyish-white, malodorous	Vary from cottage-cheese-like through watery to homogenously thick	Greenish yellow, frothy, malodorous
Symptoms	Malodor	Vaginal soreness, pruritus, burning, irritation, dyspareunia	Pruritus, pain, dyspareunia, malodor
Examination of vaginal walls	Normal	Erythema adherent off-white discharge	Erythema
Examination of vulva	Normal, sometimes erythema	Swelling, erythema, fissures and satellite lesions	Swelling, erythema
Vaginal pH	>4.7	4.0–4.5	5.0–6.0
Microscopic examination of saline preparation (0,9% NaCl)	Clue cells, lack of leucocytes and lactobacilli, numerous Gram negative, and curved rods	Normal bacterial flora, yeast cells, mycelia, low number or lack of lactobacilli, leucocytes	Motile trichomonades, leukocytes
Whiff test (with 10% KOH)	Positive fish-like odor	Negative	Sometimes positive
Microscopic examination of vaginal discharge with 10% KOH	Negative	Yeast, hyphae	Negative

Definition

- Disturbances in the vaginal ecosystem
- Reduction or abnormal function of *Lactobacillus* species
- Domination of anaerobic bacteria such as *G. vaginalis, Prevotella* species, *Prophyromonas* species, *Peptostreptococcus* species, *Mycoplasma hominis, Ureaplasma urealyticum, Bacteroides* species, *Mobiluncus* species, *Fusobacterium* species, *Atopobium vaginae*

The term 'vaginosis' signifies the absence of an inflammatory component. **Figure 29.4** illustrates the probable pathogenetic pathway of BV. Recent studies suggest that BV is a polymicrobial biofilm infection, with *G. vaginalis* playing a vital role in the formation of the biofilm. However, the pathogenesis of the disease remains to be fully elucidated (Verstraelen & Swidwinski 2013). Proper diagnosis and treatment are of great importance in this age group due to possible pregnancy-related complications such as miscarriages, preterm birth, and postpartum fever, development of pelvic inflammatory disease, plasma-cell endometritis, post-abortal infections, and infertility. Women with BV are also at a higher risk of sexually transmitted microorganisms, including HIV. Epidemiologic data are diverse, depending on the country, ethnicity, or population. The disease incidence is estimated to be between 7.5 and 60.8% depending on the population studied (Kenyon et al. 2013).

Predisposing factors

- Multiple partners
- Women who have sex with women
- Vaginal douching
- Younger age
- Smoking
- Black ethnicity

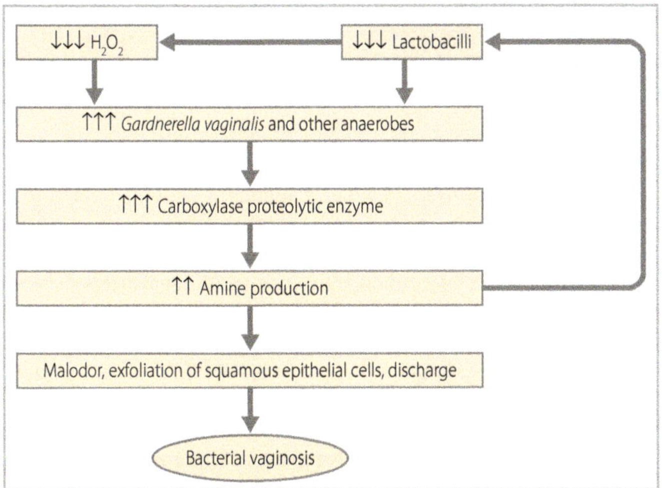

Figure 29.4 Correlations of biochemical phenomena in the pathogenesis of bacterial vaginosis.

Clinical presentation

Key features

- White, watery vaginal exudate
- 'Fishy' smell
- Absent inflammatory features (redness, edema): discharge may be present
- Asymptomatic in up to 75% of affected women

Diagnosis

Key features

- Amsel criteria
  - Characteristic thin, grayish-white vaginal discharge
  - Vaginal pH > 4.5
  - Positive whiff-amine test defined as the presence of a fishy odor when a drop of 10% KOH is added to a sample of vaginal discharge
  - >20% clue cells on microscopic examination: clue cells are vaginal epithelial cells studded with adherent coccobacilli that are best appreciated at the edge of the cell
- Nugent system: this is the gold standard (see below)

The diagnosis is based on the Amsel criteria if at least 3 out of 4 are met (**Table 29.1**). A more demanding method, the Nugent system, is based on microscopic examination of three selected morphotypes of bacteria identified as part of the BV flora: lactobacilli, *Gardnerella*, and curved bacteria (*Mobiluncus*) per high power field in Gram-stained vaginal smears. The count of each morphotype is assessed on a scale from 0 to 4, followed by calculation of the total score and classification of the bacterial flora on a 10-point scale, as normal (0–3), medium (4–6), and BV (7–10). The Nugent criteria are considered to be the gold standard in BV diagnosis. Commercial tests (Affirm VP III, OSOM BV Blue) may be used in centers without access to a microscope.

Treatment

Metronidazole or clindamycin are the drugs of choice, with similar effectiveness regardless of the route of administration. Metronidazole is administered orally (500 mg twice daily for 7 days) or as a 0.75% gel in vaginal therapy (5 g once daily for 5 days). Clindamycin is recommended as a 2% vaginal cream (5 g daily for 7 consecutive days), or orally (300 mg twice daily for 7 days), or as vaginal ovules (100 mg once daily for 3 days). The effectiveness of seconidazol (2 g orally in a single dose) has also been confirmed (Oduyebo et al. 2009). The recurrence rate reaches 30% and 80% at 3 and 9 months after completion of treatment. Maintenance therapy and probiotics have proven to be ineffective (Senok et al. 2009).

Candida infections

Introduction

Vulvar candidosis (VC) is frequently accompanied by vaginitis, thus the term 'vulvovaginal candidosis' (VVC) is often used. In premenopausal women, the involvement of the vulva is usually secondary to vaginal candidosis, while postmenopausal patients suffer from vulvar and/or intercrural candidosis. *C. albicans* is the most common pathogen of VVC, responsible for 85–95% of all infections but *C. glabrata*, C. krusei, *C. parapsilosis*, *C. tropicalis* may also be involved. Women with compromised immune system may get infected by other, rare types of fungi (Sobel 2007). Asymptomatic carriers of *Candida* species, which in most cases may be perceived as a typical commensal, account for 7.8–25.9% of the healthy population. Candidosis of the genital tract mostly results from endogenous infections. The vaginal flora plays a significant role in individual susceptibility (Hurley & Delouvois 1979, Marrazzo 2003, Xu & Sobel 2004).

Epidemiology

- Approximately 40% of all cases of vaginitis
- Epidemiologic data often ambiguous
- Approximately 50% of misdiagnosed cases due to lack of laboratory verification
- Half of the female population will have developed candidosis by the age of 25 years at least once
- Pre-puberty and postmenopausal infections are rare
- Incidence rapidly increases towards the end of the second decade of life and persists for the next 20 years
- Fungal colonization is extremely common in pregnancy

Promoting factors

- Pregnancy
- Antibiotic therapy
- Compromised general and local immunity
- Systemic diseases (especially uncontrolled diabetes)
- Poor diet/nutritional deficiency
- Inadequate hygiene
- High sexual activity
- Hormonal contraceptives

Clinical presentation

Key features

- Severe pruritus and burning
- Vulvar erythema and edema
- Satellite lesions including pustules may be seen
- White or creamy 'cottage-cheese-like' discharge
- Vaginal redness, itch, burning, and dyspareunia
- Dysuria appears in case of urinary tract involvement

Typical clinical manifestations are shown in **Figures 29.5** and **29.6.** Clinical examination reveals vaginal and cervical swelling and redness, disseminated white patches adjacent on the surface of the vaginal walls, erosions, profuse, thick, white or creamy 'cottage-cheese-like' discharge. Differentiation includes dermatophytoses and skin diseases (seborrheic dermatitis, lichen planus, contact, and atopic eczema, erythrasma) (Achkar & Fries 2010, Hurley & Delouvois 1979, Marrazzo 2003). Depending on symptom intensity, VVC may be classified into uncomplicated or complicated (Pappas et al. 2009). Mild VVC is characterized by sporadic inflammatory episodes in women with normal immune response, which are caused by *C. albicans*. Severe VVC is

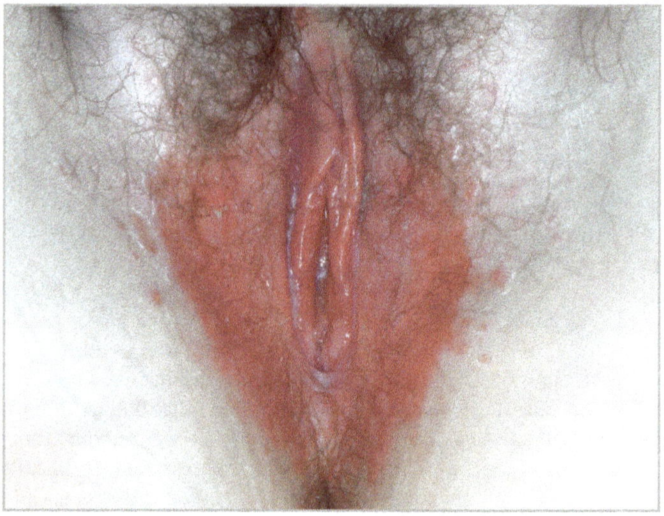

Figure 29.5 Vulvovaginal candidosis in an adolescent girl presenting with redness and edema of the modified mucous membranes and white vaginal secretion.

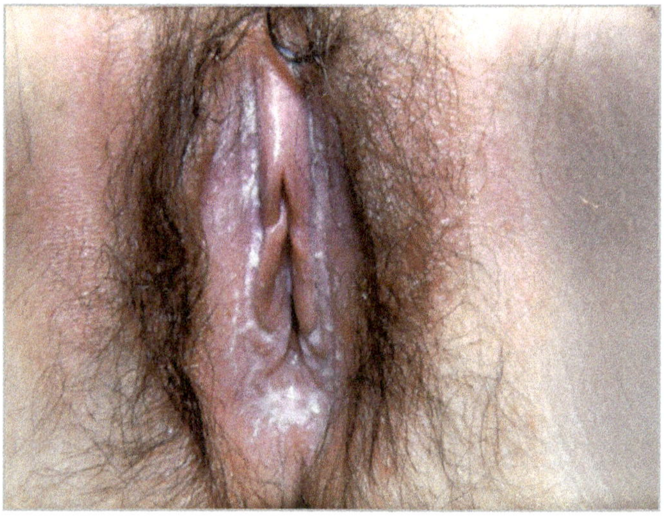

Figure 29.6 Vulvovaginal candidosis with characteristic vulvar edema and white discharge attached to the modified mucous membranes. By courtesy of Prof. Z. Adamski, Poznan, Poland.

associated with non-candida infections and consists in severe inflammatory manifestations in gravidas, diabetics or patients treated with immunosuppressants, and recurrent VVC (RVVC) among women with normal immune response, usually as a premenstrual exacerbation. *C. glabrata*, rarely *Saccharomyces cerevisiae*, or antifungal drugs resistant to *Candida* species are responsible for severe infections, observed in 10% of the affected individuals. RVVC is diagnosed in the event of at least 4 recurrences annually (Pappas et al. 2009). VVC is diagnosed on the basis of medical history, clinical symptoms, and laboratory results as presented in **Table 29.1.** Culture should be performed in symptomatic women with negative results of microscopic examination, RVVC and cases resistant to therapy. In asymptomatic patients, positive results may only confirm colonization and are not an indication to treatment (Sobel 2007). Asymptomatic *Candida* colonization in pregnancy should be treated in the last weeks of gestation (Mendling & Brusch 2012).

Treatment

The optimal drug to treat VVC should have a broad spectrum, no negative influence on vaginal flora, and good safety profile including in pregnancy. There is a wide range of medications available used either topically or systemically (**Table 29.2**). Current guidelines recommend monotherapy and intravaginal drug application. However, benefits of oral administration include high drug penetration into the vaginal mucosa, convenience, and short treatment duration. The medications used in the treatment of VVC are presented in **Table 29.2** (Mendling & Brusch 2012, Pappas et al. 2009, Sobel 2007). In severe infections where there is, e.g. immunosuppression, concomitant use of glucocorticosteroids or uncontrolled diabetes longer treatment (e.g. fluconazole 100 mg daily for 7 days) may be necessary. RVVC requires long-term suppressant antifungal treatment. A typical regime would be oral fluconazole weekly or either oral fluconazole or butoconazole nitrate ovula monthly on the 4th and 5th day of the menstrual cycle for 6-9 months, see Table 29.2 for details. In addition, an azole cream twice daily during the last week of the menstrual cycle may be applied. Nevertheless, recurrence is noted in 40–50% of patients after treatment cessation (Sobel 2007). Caution is advised in drug administration to children. Typically, mild VVC will subside after one-time or short-duration treatment, with no significant advantage of one particular medication over others (Pappas et al. 2009), except for topically applied azoles, which demonstrate higher efficacy as compared to nystatin. It is the recurrent infections, especially related to non-*Albicans* species, which present the real therapeutic challenge.

Treatment in pregnancy and lactation

Topical clotrimazole and miconazole are the drugs of first choice for the treatment of vulvovaginal candidosis in pregnancy; the other azole preparations are second choice treatments. Oral treatment is contraindicated in pregnancy and lactation. However, if unavoidable, and depending on pathogen spectrum, fluconazole or itraconazole (preferably after the first trimester) and fluconazole or amphotericin B (during lactation) are the drugs of choice.

Table 29.2 Therapeutic options for vulvovaginal candidosis

Topical treatment options	Systemic treatment options
Azoles or nystatin as • Intravaginal creams or ointments • Vaginal tablets • Vaginal suppositories • Creams for vulval use	Oral fluconazole Oral itraconazole
Specific regimens	
Mild disease	Vulvar cream usually twice daily for 7 (-14) days either topical butoconazole, clotrimazole, miconazole, econazole, tioconazole, tetraconazole, sertaconazole, terconazole, or nystatin Vaginal treatment, e.g. butoconazole ovula 100 mg for 3 days or clotrimazole, and econazole between 1 and 14 applications (depending on drug and formula) Oral fluconazole 150 mg single dose or itraconazole 200 mg for 3 days
Severe or complicated disease	7–14 days topical treatment plus Oral fluconazole 100 mg daily for 7 days
Recurrent disease	Maintenance treatment for 6-9 months with either: Oral fluconazole 150 mg weekly or monthly on the 4th and 5th day of the menstrual cycle or itraconazole 400 mg/day once a month or butoconazole nitrate 100 mg ovula monthly on the 4th and 5th day of the menstrual cycle
Candida glabrata	600 mg boric acid in a gelatin capsule for 14 days
Pregnancy	Topical clotrimazole or miconazole for 7–14 days If unavoidable, oral fluconazole or itraconazole
Lactation	Topical clotrimazole or miconazole for 7–14 days If unavoidable, oral fluconazole or amphotericin B

REFERENCES

Achkar JM, Fries BC. *Candida* infections of genitourinary tract. Clin Microbiol Rev 2010; 23:253–273.

Degreef H. Clinical forms of dermatophytosis (Ringworm infections). Mycopathologia 2008; 166:257–265.

Gupta AK, Cooper EA. Update of antifungal therapy of dermatophytosis. Mycopathologia 2008; 166:353–367.

Hald M, Arendrup MC, Svejgaard EL, et al. Evidence-based Danish Guidelines for the Treatment of *Malassezia*-related Skin Diseases. Acta Derm Venereol 2014 Acta Derm Venereol 2015; 95:12–19.

Holdiness MR. Management of cutaneous erythrasma. Drugs 2002; 62:1131–1141.

Hurley R, Delouvois J. *Candida* vaginitis. Postgrad Med J 1979; 55:645–647.

Janigger CK, Schwartz RA, Szepietowski J, et al. Intertrigo and common secondary skin infection. Am Fam Physician 2005; 72:833–838.

Kenyon C, Colebunders R, Crucitti T. The global epidemiology of bacterial vaginosis: a systematic review. Am J Obster Gynecol 2013; 209:505–523.

Marrazzo J. Candidiasis (vulvovaginal). Clin Evid 2003; 9:1980–1993.

Mendling W, Brusch J. Guideline vulvovaginal candidosis (2010) of the German Society for Gynecology and Obstetrics, the Working Group for Infections and Infect Immunology in Gynecology and Obstetrics, German Society of Dermatology, the Board of German Dermatologists and the German Speaking Mycological Society. Mycoses 2012; 55 (suppl.3):1–13.

Oduyebo OO, Anorlu RI, Ogunsola FT. The effects of antimicrobial therapy on bacterial vaginosis in non-pregnant women. Cochran Databaes Syst Rev 2009; 3:CD 006055.

Pappas PG, Kauffman CA, Andes D, et al. Clinical practice guidelines for the management of candidiasis: 2009 update by the Infectious Diseases Society of America. Clin Infect Dis 2009; 48:503–535.

Pedrosa AF, Lisboa C, Rodrigues AG. Malassezia infections: a medical conundrum. J Am Acad Dermatol 2014; 71:170–176.

Pereira LB. Impetigo-review. An Bras Dermatol 2014; 89:293–299.
Seebacher C, Bouchara JP, Mignon B. Updates on the epidemiology on dermatophyte infections. Mycopathologia 2008; 166:335–352.
Senok AC, Verstraelen H, Temerman M, et al. Probiotics for the treatment of bacterial vaginosis. Cochran Database Syst Rev 2009; 4:CD006289.
Sobel JD. Vulvovaginal candidosis. Lancet 2007; 369:1961–1971.
Verstraelen H, Świdwiński A. The biofilm in bacterial vaginosis: implications for epidemiology, diagnosis and treatment. Curr Opin Infect Dis 2013; 26:86–89.
Wolf R, Oumeish YJ, Parish LC. Intertriginous eruption. Clin Dermatol 2011; 29:173–179.
Xu J, Sobel JD. Candida vulvovaginitis in pregnancy. Curr Infect Dis Rep 2004; 6:445–449.

FURTHER READING

Christensen GJ, Brüggemann H. Bacterial skin commensals and their role as host guardians. Benef Microbes 2014; 5:201–215.
Fisher G. Chronic vulvovaginal candidiasis: what we know and what we have yet to learn? Austr J Dermatol 2012; 55:247–254.
Havlickova B, Czaika VA, Friedrich M. Epidemiological trends in skin mycoses worldwide. Mycoses 2008; 51:16–26.
Leppäluoto PA. Bacterial vaginosis: what is physiological in vaginal bacteriology? An update opinion. Acta Obstet Gynecol Scand 2011; 90:1302–1306.
Otero L, Palacio V, Vázquez F. Tinea cruris in female prostitutes. Mycopathologia 2002; 153:29–31.

Chapter 30 Viral diseases

Dominique Parent, Fanny Camus

INTRODUCTION

Viruses responsible for non-cancerous infections of the vulva include mollusciPoxvirus (MCV), human papillomavirus (HPV), herpes simplex virus (HSV), and varicella zoster virus (VZV). HPV and HSV infections are classical sexually transmitted diseases, and vulvar MCV is considered a sexually transmitted infection (STI) but VZV infections are not.

Key features

- Double-stranded DNA viruses
- Viruses able to infect the squamous stratified epithelia
- Transmission by direct contact
- Vertical transmission is possible
- Except for VZV infections, the anogenital localization is considered a STI
- Immunosuppression worsens the clinical manifestations and the prognosis

SEXUALLY TRANSMITTED INFECTIONS

Key features

- Risk factors: early age of first sexual intercourse, number of sexual partners, number of lifetime sexual partners of the male partner, unknown partner, previous history of STIs, HIV infection, unprotected sex
- HIV infection increases the risk of HPV or HSV acquisition. In HIV-infected patients, clinical infections due to MCV, HPV, and HSV worsen gradually as the patient's immunity decreases
- Management: both a physical examination and a screening for the other STI must be performed. For recurrences of genital herpes or anogenital warts (AGW), screening is not needed except if the patient has sex at risk. Condoms must be used but are not completely safe
- Educational and psychological aspects: women with chronic and sexually transmitted vulvar infections are frightened, anxious, depressed, and have little self-esteem. Education is mandatory and psychological support should be offered

MOLLUSCIPOXVIRUS INFECTIONS

Molluscum contagiosum

Key features

- Molluscum contagiosum (MC) is a cutaneous infection caused by the MCV, a Poxviridae virus
- In healthy adults, vulvar MC is considered a STI
- In immunocompromised adults, the transmission may be sexual or non-sexual
- Lesions are characteristic umbilicated papules
- MC infection is a self-limiting disease but the high risk of sexual transmission encourages treatment

Introduction

MC is a common lesion in the pediatric population. During the last 30 years, a rising incidence of MC has been observed in sexually active young adults and in immunocompromised individuals (mainly HIV-positive patients). In healthy females (except during pregnancy), lesions limited to the vulva, lower abdomen, upper thighs, and buttocks are usually considered to be STIs. In immunodeficient patients with a low CD4 T-lymphocytes count (children or adults), the MCs commonly involve other body regions (Chen et al. 2013).

Epidemiology/transmission

MCV1 is the most frequent viral subtype; MCV2 seems to be associated with HIV infection (Scholz et al. 1989).

MC is transmitted by direct skin contact or sometimes via fomites such as bath sponges, towels or tattooing procedures. Autoinoculation is common. Vertical transmission has been reported (Luke & Silverberg 2010).

Pathogenesis

Viral particles replicate in the cytoplasm of the basal layers. The viral inclusion bodies thrive in the stratum spinosum, gradually filling the infected cell that migrates through the granular and horny layers where they appear as large inclusion bodies. At the top of the lesion, the stratum corneum disintegrates, forming a central depression releasing numerous infective viruses (Chen et al. 2013). MCV has the capacity to remain undetected by the immune system for many years or indefinitely; therefore, a clinical manifestation may present many years after the acquisition of the virus. Specific antibodies are not always present and a reinfection is possible. Clinical resolution depends on the cutaneous cellular mediated response (Chen et al. 2013).

Risk factors

Mechanical factors

- Shaving, epilation, and scraping cause microscopic abrasions that facilitate MCV dissemination

Genetics

- Patients with atopic dermatitis are at higher risk of presenting MC
- Patients with DOCK8 deficiency, a genetic disorder, may have extensive MC (Chen et al. 2013)

Immunological factors

- Topical applications of immunosuppressive drugs, e.g. corticosteroids or calcineurin inhibitors
- Immunosuppressed individuals: after organ transplantation, HIV infection, etc.

Clinical presentation and differential diagnosis

The typical lesions are asymptomatic, firm, flesh-colored, umbilicated papules of 2–6 mm in diameter. Small lesions can be mistaken with chicken pox or plane warts. They are single to numerous, grouped, or scattered (**Figure 30.1**). Genital warts are the main differential diagnosis. Less frequently, MC is confused with scabies, lymphangiectasia, adnexal tumors, pyogenic granuloma, and basal cell carcinoma. In immunocompromised individuals, MCV acts as an opportunistic virus. The papules quickly disseminate and become larger, sometimes giant (**Figure 30.2**), recalcitrant and recurrent. In patients with AIDS, cutaneous cryptococcosis should be ruled out (Chen et al. 2013).

Histopathology

The histopathology is characteristic (**Figure 30.3**):

- Lobules resulting from endophytic hyperplasia
- Large intracytoplasmic inclusion bodies in stratum spinosum and granulosum
- Central invagination at the top of the lobule

Diagnosis

The diagnosis is made clinically. Atypical forms are identified by a histopathological examination.

Management of genital mollusca contagiosa

- Exclude an underlying immunosuppression
- In prepubertal girls, sexual transmission is unlikely
- Educate the patient and answer her questions
- In immunocompromised patients, inform that the disease is often recalcitrant

Course of disease

The incubation period lasts 2–7 weeks. The appearance of pustular lesions and inflammation are signs of spontaneous remission. In healthy individuals, the infection is self-limited. An individual papule remains generally for a maximum of 2 months and the cutaneous infection resolves spontaneously within 6 and 9 months, but sometimes lasts for 3 or 4 years. In immunocompromised individuals, eruptions have no tendency to heal spontaneously.

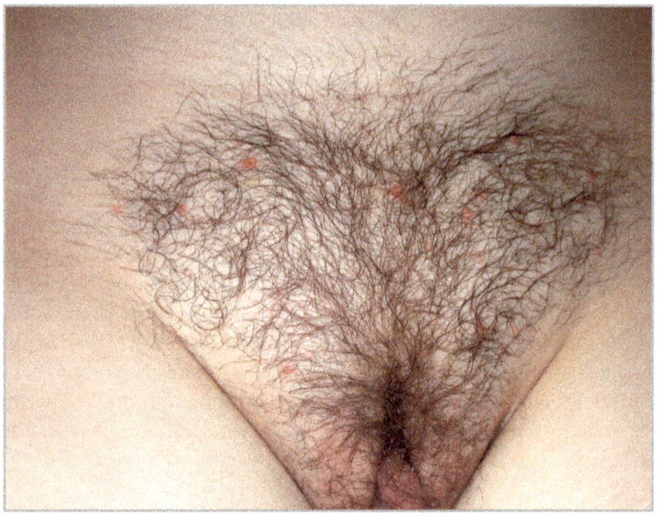

Figure 30.1 Numerous mollusca contagiosa scattered on the pubis.

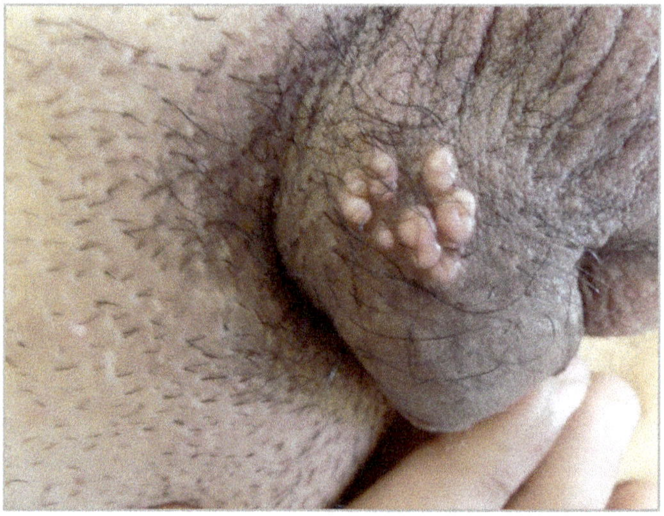

Figure 30.2 Giant genital mollusca contagiosa in a patient suffering from Crohn disease.

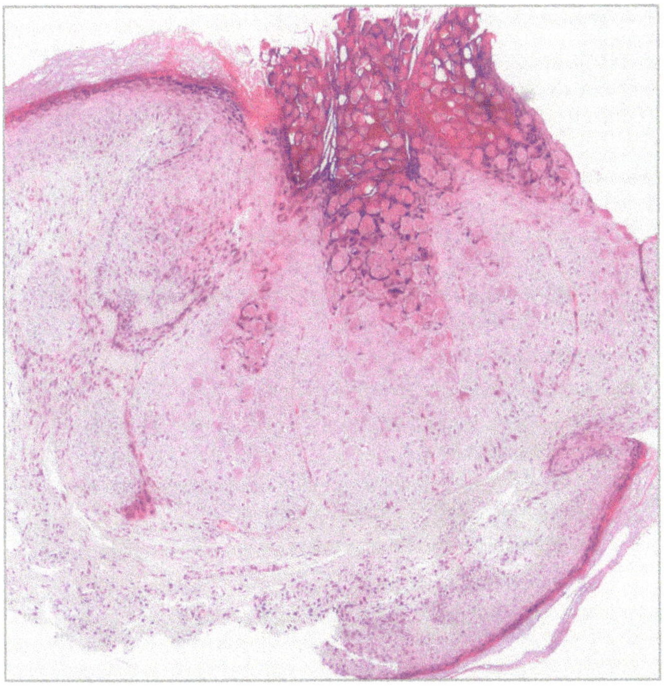

Figure 30.3 Histopathology of a molluscum contagiosum (× 4). Lobulated endophytic hyperplasia with central invagination is observed. The stratum spinosum and the granular layers show intracytoplasmic inclusion bodies. In this case, the basal membrane and dermis are not damaged. By Courtesy of Dr J André, MD, Hôpital St Pierre, Brussels, Belgium.

Therapeutic options

Table 30.1 outlines the treatment of MC (Chen et al. 2013, Tyring 2003). Studies on the management of genital MC are scarce. No evidence-based consensus has been obtained as for the best therapy for MC in immunocompetent patients (Chen et al. 2013, van der Wouden et al. 2009). In immunocompromised patients, the treatment is rarely efficient. In patients with AIDS, an effective antiretroviral therapy is required, but is often insufficient to eradicate the MC.

HUMAN PAPILLOMAVIRUS INFECTION

Anogenital warts

Synonym

Condylomata acuminata is a synonymous of the exophytic papillary variant of AGW.

Key features

- HPV infections are restricted to squamous stratified epithelia
- HPV 6 /11 are low-risk oncogenic viruses causing more than 95% of AGW (Lacey et al. 2013)
- HPV6 /11-associated lesions are STIs affecting the anogenital and oropharyngeal regions
- AGW in prepubertal girls are not always associated with a sexual abuse
- In immunocompromised patients, AGW are more severe and more recalcitrant to therapy
- Regardless of the treatment, the percentage of recurrence is significant (20–30% or more)

Introduction

It is estimated that 50–80% of sexually active women are infected by HPV at least once in their life. In females, the incidence peak is before 24 years old (Patel et al. 2013). Full screening for other STIs is required when a primary infection is diagnosed. All mucocutaneous regions likely to be infected by HPV should be examined. Cervical screening and colposcopy are mandatory. An associated vulvovaginal candidosis is commonly found and must be treated.

Table 30.1 Therapeutic options in the treatment of vulvar mollusca contagiosa

	Therapy	Posology	Location of therapy	Local side-effects
Physical modalities	Curettage	Topical anesthetic	Office	Pain, bleeding, scars (rare)
	Liquid nitrogen	10–20 seconds, weekly	Office	Pain, redness, blister
Chemical agents (applied with a cotton swab)	Potassium hydroxide aqueous solution 5–10%	Twice daily until inflammation/ulceration	Home	Irritation, erythema, depigmentation
	Trichloroacetic acid solution 80–90%	Two applications with 2 weeks' interval	Office	
Immune modulator	Imiquimod 5% cream*	Three to five times a week (maximum 16 weeks) Overnight (8 hours) Wash off in the morning	Home	Erythema, edema, ulceration (rare), burning, tenderness

*More data is needed before using imiquimod in pregnancy
None of the local therapy has been approved by the FDA
In extended or recurrent lesions, the combination of treatments can be helpful
Consider repeating the examination a few weeks after treatment

Epidemiology/transmission

HPV infection is the most frequent STI in the world. According to the type of population and the country studied, the HPV prevalence varies from 0.03% to 4%. Since the 2000s, both AGW annual incidence and HPV prevalence are on the rise (Patel et al. 2013).

In adults, sexual contamination rates between partners are evaluated close to 60-65% (Lacey et al. 2013). In children, AGW can be transmitted by sexual or non-sexual contact. Vertical transmission has been described either in utero (exceptional) or at delivery. The HPV subtypes that cause common warts have been identified in AGW of infants. Contamination by the infected hands of a caregiver has been demonstrated (Ornstein & Hatchette 2012).

Pathogenesis

HPV infects the human basal keratinocytes. HPV 6/11 never integrate into human DNA. In the latent period, HPV persists without any clinical manifestations for months or even for years. In episomal infection, HPV initiates cellular proliferation. It replicates and induces abnormal differentiation of keratinocytes with a characteristic cytopathogenic effect named koilocytosis. The viruses are shed from the upper layers of the lesions (Thornsberry & English 2012).

Seroconversion occurs in 60% of the infected women but the antibody levels are low and subsequent contamination by the same subtype is possible. HPV has several mechanisms to reduce both the effectiveness of innate immunity and the response of proinflammatory cytokines. The adaptive cell-mediated immune response plays a major role in AGW clearance (Frazer 2009).

Risk factors of the AGW are outlined in **Table 30.2.**

Behavior of AGW in pregnancy

- Vertical transmission during delivery is possible
- A caesarean section is not justified because it does not completely prevent the risk of contamination
- The AGW may be larger and more extensive
- Treatment is recommended because of the risk of AGW proliferation in mother and the risk of transmission to a partner
- In the last 2 months before delivery, therapies that induce large genital wounds should be avoided

Table 30.2 Risk factors and environmental factors for anogenital warts

Risk factors and environmental factors	Promoting
• Unprotected intercourse • More than one male partner • The number of lifetime sexual partners of the male partner • Unknown or anonymous partner • HIV infection	Contamination
• Micro-abrasions on the skin/mucous membranes • Shaving and epilation of the genital region	Transmission
• Pregnancy • Reduction of innate and cellular immunity • HIV infection • Grafted patients • Systemic immunosuppressive therapy • Topical anti-inflammatory therapy: corticosteroids, calcineurin inhibitors	Extension/growth (no treatment) of vulvar warts

Female pediatric population

Approximately one-third of children with AGW are likely to have been sexually abused. The associated risk of sexual abuse increases with age (Ornstein & Hatchette 2012).

Management of children with AGW

- Consider the age of the child and possible modes of transmission before investigating for sexual abuse
- Careful medical, familial, and social history together with a full physical examination
- Screening for other STI and for HPV typing
- Multidisciplinary care is recommended
- If abuse is suspected, hospitalize the girl and warn the child protection authority
- According to the clinical presentation, options for therapy are medical/surgical. Recurrences are frequent
- Medical, psychological, and social follow-up of the child and the family

Clinical presentation

AGW are symptomless; patients sometimes complain of itching, bleeding or pain. Lesions may vary in number (single, multiple, disseminated) and size from 0.1 to 1.0 cm. They may involve hair-bearing areas of skin as well as mucosa (vagina, cervix, and urethral meatus). In women, perianal warts can occur by self-inoculation in the absence of anal sex. Lesions predominate in sites traumatized by intercourse and in macerated areas (**Figure 30.4**). Condylomata acuminata are white grayish or pink-reddish depending on the degree of keratinization of the epithelium. Non-pigmented papules are lobulated with a smooth or slightly rough surface (**Figure 30.5**). Other clinical variants are sometimes more difficult to diagnose (**Figure 30.6**). Warts can proliferate in the form of cauliflower-like

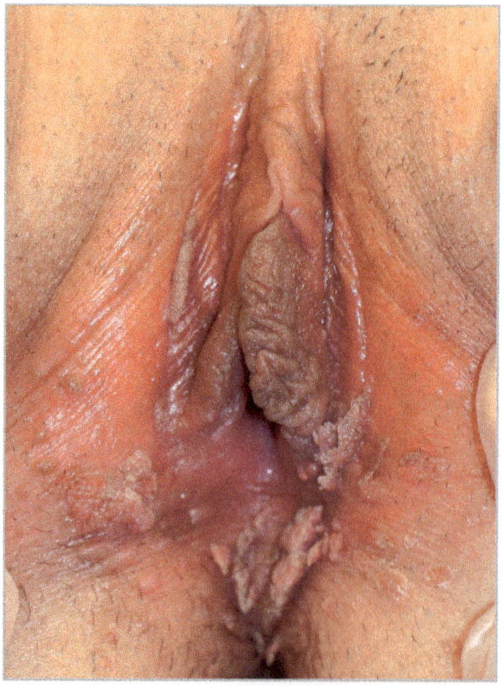

Figure 30.4 Exophytic papillary lesions (condylomata acuminata) predominating in sites traumatized by intercourse (fourchette, labia minora, introitus) and in macerated areas (interlabial or nymphohymeneal folds).

clusters that invade extended area (**Figure 30.7**). Large confluent lesions are more frequent in immunosuppressed patients. Vulvar warts and high-grade squamous intraepithelial lesions (HSIL) can coexist (**Figure 30.8**).

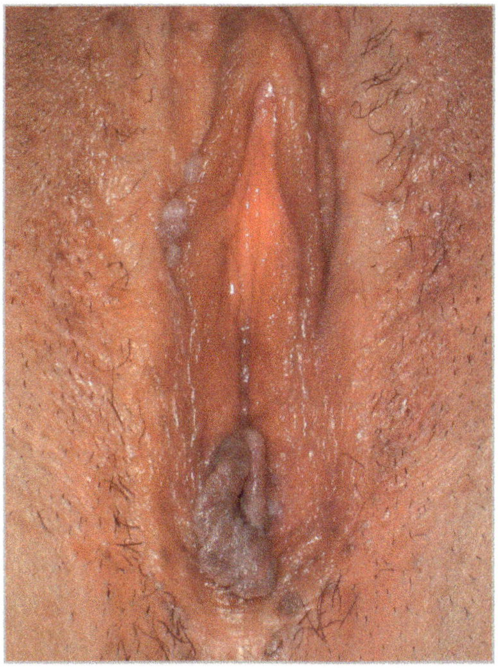

Figure 30.5 HPV6-associated non-pigmented papules and an inconspicuous vulvovaginal candidosis in the same patient.

Histopathology

Typical histopathology is illustrated in **Figures 30.9 a** and **b**.

Key features

- Hyperkeratosis +/ dyskeratosis
- Substantial acanthosis and papillomatosis
- Koilocytes in the upper epithelial layers (perinuclear vacuoles and condensed nuclei)

Diagnosis

The diagnosis of AGW is clinical. HPV serology and HPV cultivation are neither available nor useful. HPV subtyping is not appropriate except for children's AGW.

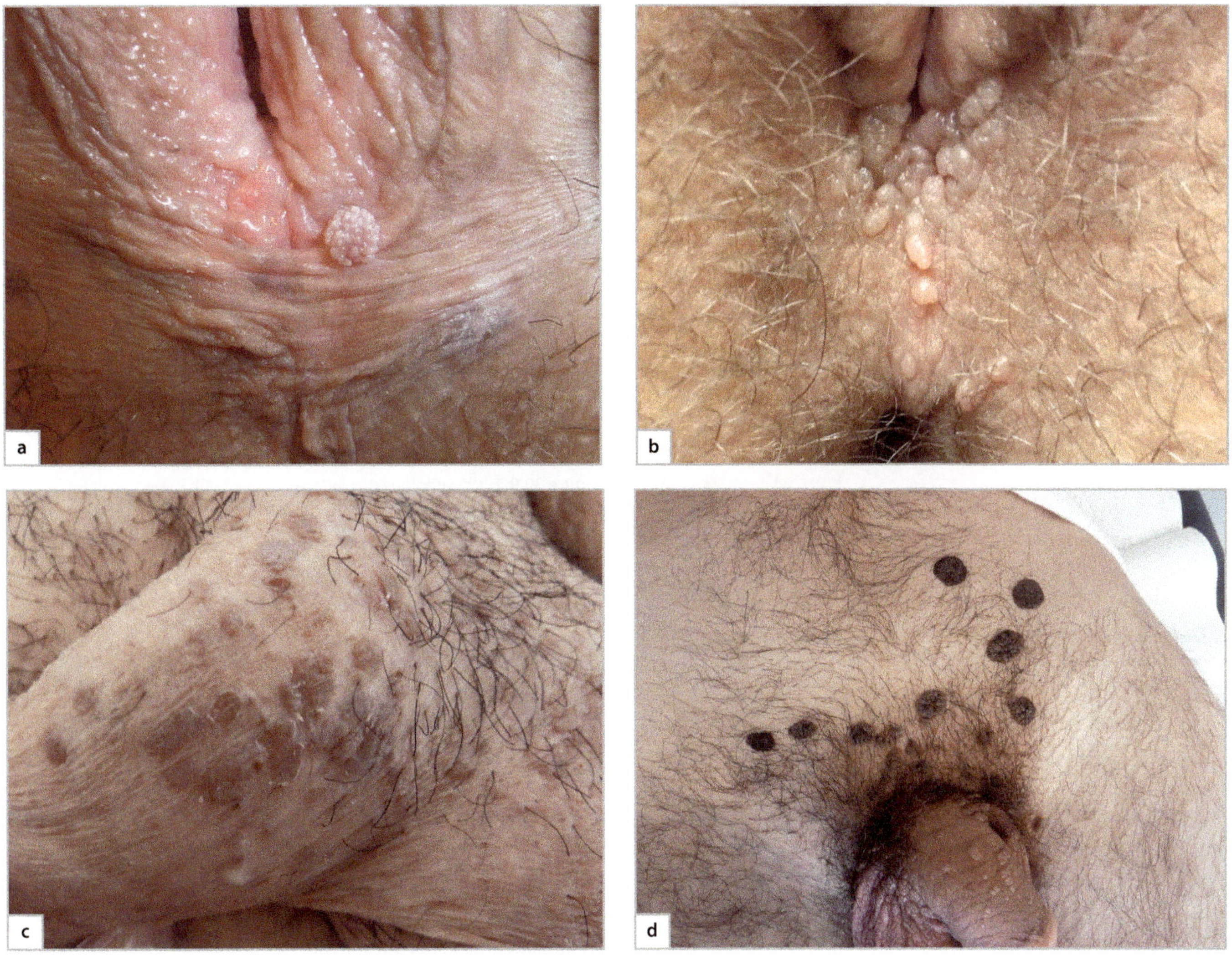

Figure 30.6 Clinical variants of genital warts. (a) Single papillary wart on the posterior fourchette. (b) Numerous HPV6-associated non-pigmented papules with smooth surface. (c) HPV6-associated pigmented papules indistinguishable from papules of intraepithelial neoplasia. (d) Seborrheic wart-like genital HPV6-associated lesions on pilose skin.

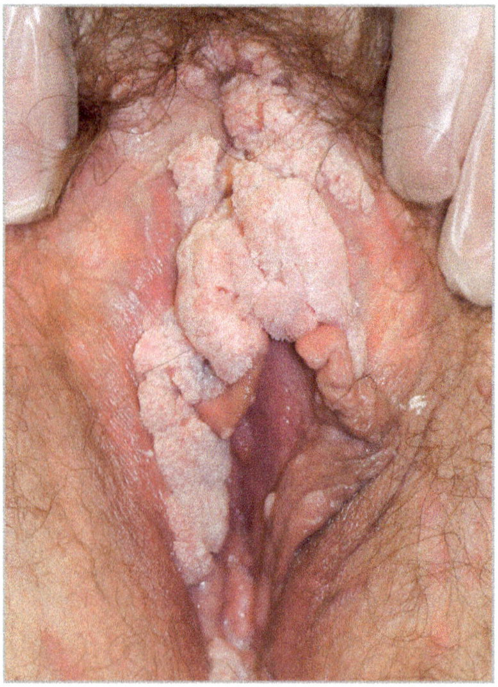

Figure 30.7 Warts proliferating in the form of cauliflower-like clusters invading extensive vulvar surfaces.

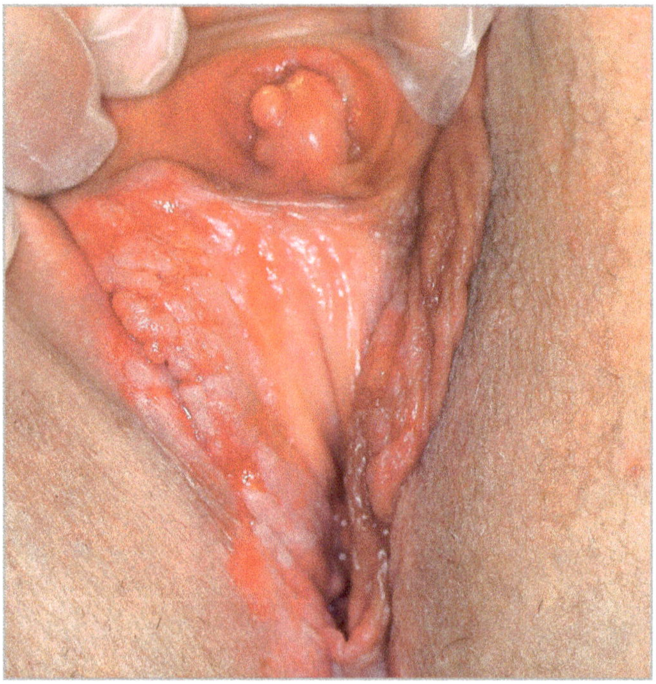

Figure 30.8 Vulvar warts associated with vulvar intraepithelial neoplasia (VIN3) (High-grade squamous intraepithelial lesion, new WHO & ISSVD terminology 2015).

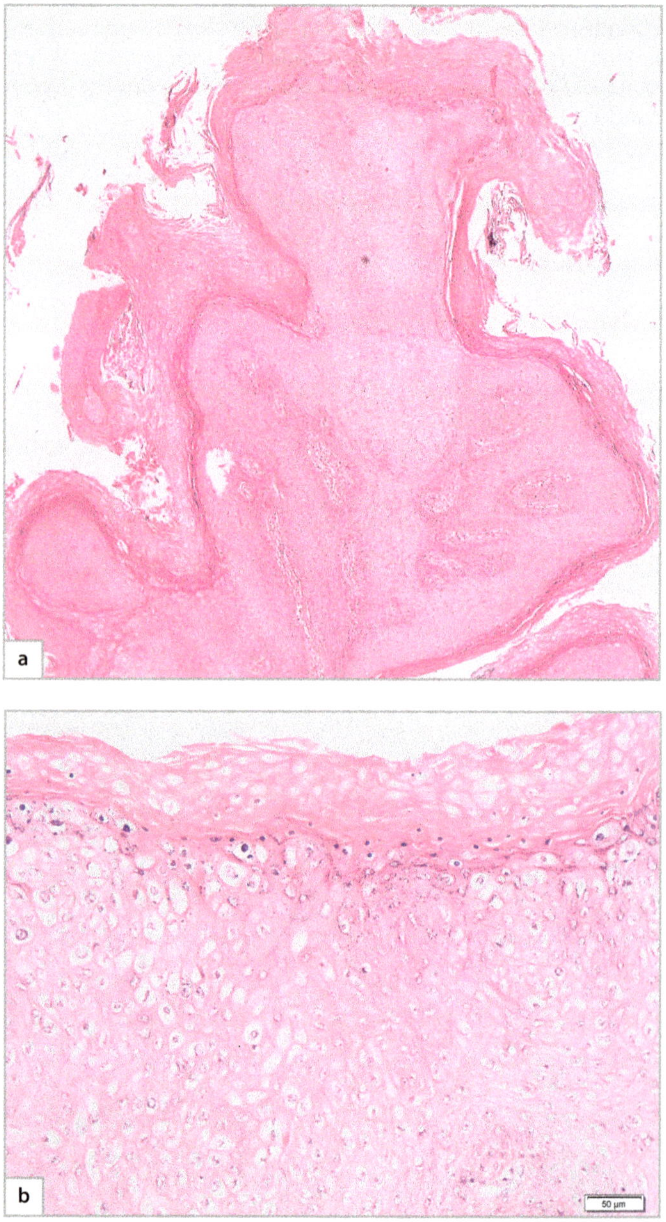

Figure 30.9 Histopathology of vulvar warts. (a) (× 40): The epidermis is thickened showing hyperkeratosis with focal parakeratosis, acanthosis, and papillomatosis. (b) (× 200): In the upper layers of the epithelium, the infected keratinocytes are transformed in koïlocytes. In the granular layer, koïlocytotic changes include clear cytoplasm (perinuclear vacuoles) and condensed nuclei. By courtesy of JC Noël, MD, PhD, Hôpital Erasme, Brussels, Belgium.

Biopsy is necessary if:

- Diagnosis is doubtful, especially in immunocompromised females
- Lesions are resistant to treatment
- AGW are atypical and similar to other clinical forms of HPV infection (high-grade squamous intraepithelial lesions of the vulva invasive carcinoma, etc.)
- AGW occur in children

Differential diagnosis

The main differential diagnosis is MC; other differential diagnoses are outlined in **Table 30.3**.

Principles of management

Prevention

The quadrivalent HPV vaccine provides protection against AGW, resulting from HPV 6/11 infections and HPV16/18. It has no therapeutic effect and is therefore not prescribed for women previously infected. Its safety and efficiency are now demonstrated. It can be given to immunocompromised patients. As a precaution, it is not used during pregnancy. Current evidence shows that administration of two doses of vaccine (0 and 6 months) may result in equivalent antibody levels as the administration of three doses of vaccine (0 and 1 or 2 months and 6 months) in young girls. After vaccination, the duration of efficient immunity is estimated as lasting at least 10 years (Brotherton 2014).

Table 30.3 Anogenital warts: differential diagnosis

	Differential diagnoses	Diagnostic test
Physiological variants	Sebaceous glands: Fordyce spots	Clinical
	Micropapillomatous labialis, Vestibular papillomatosis	History, clinical, biopsy
Pathological conditions	Mollusca contagiosa	Clinical, biopsy
	In situ or invasive vulvar squamous cell carcinoma	Biopsy
	Fibroepithelial polyps, common skin tags, intradermal nevus	History, biopsy
	Condylomata lata (secondary syphilis)	Serology
	Seborrheic keratosis	Clinical
	Lichen planus (cutaneous skin papules)	Clinical, biopsy
	Angiokeratoma	Clinical
	Lymphangiectasia	Clinical (do not biopsy)

Therapeutic options

Table 30.4 outlines the therapeutic options for AGW (Lacey et al. 2013, Thornsberry & English 2012).

Course of disease

Most HPV infections are subclinical and treatment is not recommended. The incubation period lasts from about 3 weeks up to 8 months. The AGW grow actively during 3-6 months while the host's immune response is developing. The host-virus-interactions result either in HPV clearance or in a balance between virus proliferation and human defenses. Reported spontaneous rates of remission vary from 0% to 50%. If HPV infection is controlled by immune mechanisms, sustained clinical remission is observed. If the immune system is not sufficiently competent, AGW persist or recur, sometimes for months or even years. Recurrences of AGW occur in 9-80% of the patients (Frazer 2009, Patel et al. 2013). Genital warts never turn into cancer but a coinfection with high-risk oncogenic HPV (especially 16 and 18) may result in concomitant intraepithelial or invasive squamous cell carcinoma. This risk is higher in immunocompromised patients (Garland et al. 2009).

Table 30.4 Therapeutic options in the treatment of vulvar (anogenital) warts (Lacey et al. 2013)

	Therapy	Posology	Location of therapy	Local side effects
Physical destruction	Electrosurgery (Ib,A) Scissors excision (Ib,A) Curettage (IIa,B) Laser surgery (IIa,B) Formal surgery (IV,C)	Anesthesia once	Office	Pain, bleeding, ulceration, superinfection, scars
	Liquid nitrogen (Ib,A) • spray gun device • closed cryoprobe system	Weekly Freezing for 10–20 seconds	Office	Pain, redness, blisters, ulcerations, depigmentation
Cytotoxic drugs (applied with a cotton swab)	Podophyllotoxin (Ib,A) * 0.5% solution, 0.15% cream	Twice daily inflammation/ulceration	Home	Irritation, erythema, depigmentation
	Trichloroacetic acid solution 80–90%	Two applications with an interval of 2 weeks	Office	
	Podophyllin * 20–25 %	Not recommended		
Immunomodulators	Imiquimod 5% cream†	Three times a week (up to 16 weeks) overnight (8 hours) then wash off	Home	Slight to severe inflammation, burning, pain, erosions, ulcerations
	Sinecatechins (Ib,A) * 10% or 15% ointment	Three times a day (up to 16 weeks)	Home	Stinging, burning or itching, swelling, erythema, blisters
	α- and β-interferons *	Not recommended		

*Cannot be used in pregnancy

†More data is needed before using imiquimod in pregnancy

Treatment modalities are the same for immunocompromised patients including HIV-infected individuals

In extended or recurrent lesions, the combination of treatments can be helpful

Consider follow up every 4 weeks until healing

Levels of evidence and grading of recommendations are given in Lacey et al. 2013

HUMAN HERPES VIRUS INFECTIONS/α-SUBFAMILY

HSV-1, HSV-2, and VZV belong to the α-subfamily of the human herpes viruses group and induce infections in anogenital regions.

Key features

- Lifelong infections affecting skin and mucous membranes
- Primary infection occurs after the virus initially enters the body through the skin or mucous membranes
- The virus remains latent in the sensory nerve ganglia corresponding to the infected cutaneous region
- Periodical viral reactivation induces viral shedding with or without localized lesions
- Immunocompromised patients have worsened clinical manifestations and a poorer prognosis
- The diagnosis is commonly clinical, confirmed by laboratory tests if necessary
- Morphological tests (histology, cytology) are not able to distinguish between the different herpes viruses
- The risk of vertical transmission is highest during primary infection
- Neonatal infection often has a poor prognosis
- The nucleoside analogs are the first and almost unique treatment choice

Genital herpes

Synonym

Herpes progenitalis

Introduction

Genital herpes is the most frequent cause of vulvar ulceration. In women, clinical manifestations of primary infection are severe and very painful. In young females, contamination often occurs at the start of the sexual life. Other STI are likely to be transmitted at the same time. In these cases, psychological support should be offered. Genital herpes should be explained to all infected women and especially to those of childbearing potential.

Epidemiology/transmission

Genital herpes is usually caused by HSV-2. Serology is the only data suitable for studying epidemiology. The prevalence of the HSV2 serology ranges from 10% to 60%. The increase in the practice of oral sex has resulted in an increased proportion of genital herpes caused by HSV-1. It is estimated that HSV-1 is responsible for at least 50% of the new genital primary infections (Gupta et al. 2007).

HSV infections are transmitted by direct contact with lesions or secretions of an infected individual.

Many people are unaware they are infected because most primary infections and reactivations are subclinical. The asymptomatic viral shedding is particularly common 6-12 months after contamination and is infectious (Patel et al. 2011).

Pathogenesis

HSV penetrates at the site of transmission and replicates in keratinocytes that coalesce and form multinucleated syncytial giant cells. The virions are gathered in nuclear inclusions. Keratinocytes detach from each other and an acantholytic vesicle results. Lymphatic dissemination is usual.

Afterwards, HSV penetrates the periphery sensory nerves. It remains latent in the corresponding ganglia and escapes from the host's immune defenses. Periodically, it is reactivated and is transported retrogradely towards the epithelial surfaces. There it replicates and ensures an effective transmission (Gupta et al. 2007).

Histopathology

The histopathology is illustrated in **Figure 30.10**.

Key features

- Intraepithelial vesicles with acantholysis and ballooning cellular degeneration
- Multinucleate syncytial giant keratinocytes
- Mixed inflammatory infiltrate in superficial and deep dermis

Pregnancy

Vertical transmission is rare and may occur in utero or during delivery. The risk of transmission is much higher for a primary infection, especially if it occurs within 6 weeks before delivery. It is low if recurrent herpes lesions are present at childbirth. The risk of infection to the baby depends on the severity and timing of the mother's infection and the prematurity of the newborn. Complications of neonatal infection are severe and can involve skin, eyes, and brain (Fatahzadeh & Schwartz 2007).

Risk factors

The same risk factors for STI (see box STI) apply for genital herpes. The main triggering factors are stress, menstruation, and sexual intercourse. Local or systemic immunosuppression also favors recurrence.

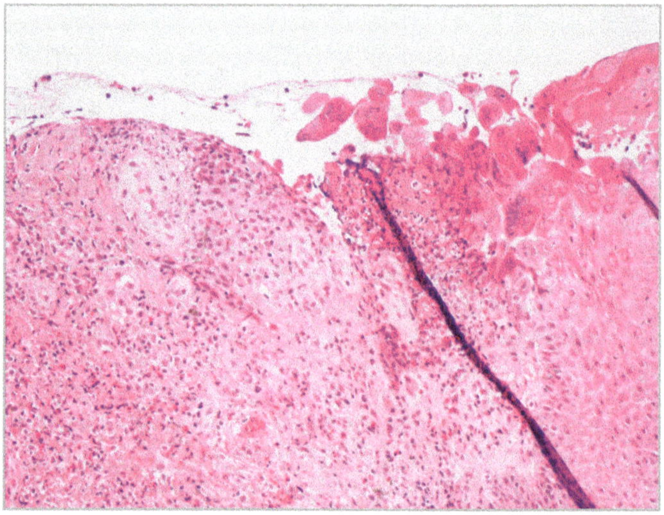

Figure 30.10 Histopathologically, the intraepidermal vesicles from herpes simplex virus and from herpes zoster virus infections are generally indistinguishable. Ballooning degeneration of the keratinocytes occurs that may lead to reticular degeneration. Acantholysis, and multinucleate syncytial giant keratinocytes are observed. The keratinocyte nuclei may contain basophilic or ground glass inclusions. Superficial and deep mixed inflammatory infiltrate is observed. By courtesy of J André, MD, Hôpital St Pierre, Brussels, Belgium.

Immunology

The penetration of HSV in the epithelium induces a local inflammation. In order to establish latency, herpes viruses are able to manipulate the immune system of the host. Accordingly, a decrease in immune surveillance of the virus allows its reactivation. Indeed, in immunocompromised patients, herpes activity is dramatically increased (Grinde 2013). A pre-existing HSV1 immunity protects from HSV-2 infection by diminishing the severity of the clinical manifestations (Gupta et al. 2007).

Clinical presentation

Development of the elementary lesion

Incubation period lasts 2–7 days. A painful or pruriginous prodrome is followed, 24–48 hours later, by breakable superficial vesicles that can coalesce into blisters. If the lesions are situated on moist mucosal surface, the vesicles are deroofed, and become erosions or ulcerations. If they are on skin, they dry into crusts. In healthy individuals, healing occurs within a few days, without scarring. In immunocompromised women, deep ulcerations are frequent with slow healing and scarring.

Primary infection

Most primary episodes are asymptomatic. When a primary genital infection is symptomatic, systemic symptoms such as fever, headache, arthralgia, and lymphadenopathy are common. In women, vesicles disseminate on the vulvar skin, the vaginal walls, and on the exocervix (**Figure 30.11**). The buttocks and the anal region can also be involved. Afterwards, the necrosis of vaginal mucous membranes induces leucorrhea. Pain is severe and induces dysuria and urinary retention. Accordingly, the patient often stops drinking and risks dehydration. Neurogenic bladder and aseptic meningitis are uncommon but serious complications requiring hospitalization (Fatahzadeh & Schwartz 2007, Gupta et al. 2007).

Initial non-primary infection

It is a symptomatic infection in a person who has already produced antibodies against the other type of herpes virus, e.g. a symptomatic HSV2 infection in a patient with pre-existing immunity against HSV1.

Recurrence

A recurrence is limited in extension and in severity. Generally, after 24–48 hours of prodrome, one or more groups of painful vesicles appear (**Figure 30.12**). Their evolution lasts on average 5–7 days, before healing. All recurrences usually occur at the same site. Infections caused by HSV-2 recur more frequently than those due to HSV-1. In woman, genital recurrences can be very frequent (monthly) without any detectable immunosuppression (Gupta et al. 2007).

Immunocompromised patients

In immunocompromised patients, regardless of the origin of the cell-mediated immunodeficiency, the vulvovaginal recurrences are more severe and look like herpetic primary infection (**Figure 30.13**).

Diagnosis

Confirmation of diagnosis by laboratory tests is useful when the lesions are atypical or the patient immunocompromised. Biopsy is not recommended.

HSV detection

Samples should be taken with swabs on the surface of the deroofed vesicles.

Virus culture and nucleic acid amplification with polymerase chain reaction technique (PCR) have high specificity and sensitivity, and allow virus typing. Both are expensive. PCR is more rapid. The culture results depend on the sampling method and on the transport conditions. PCR results depend on testing methodology. Antigen detection by direct immunofluorescence assay or by enzyme immunoassay is highly specific but less sensitive, rapid, and cheaper. Cytological examination is no longer recommended (Patel et al. 2011).

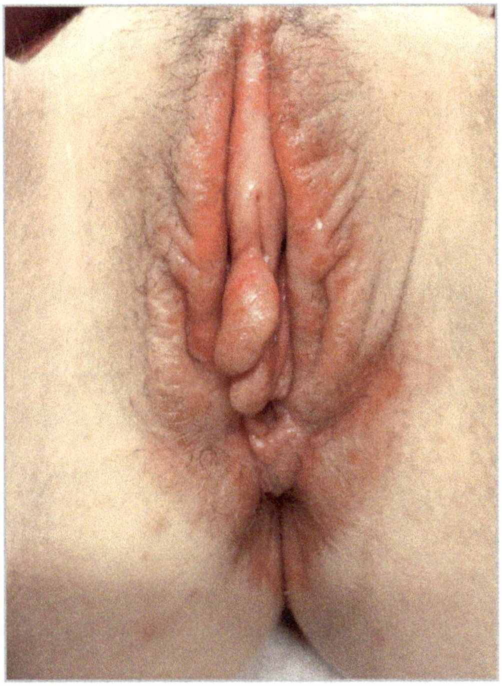

Figure 30.11 A HSV1 primary infection showing extensive redness, edema, and erosions on the anogenital region.

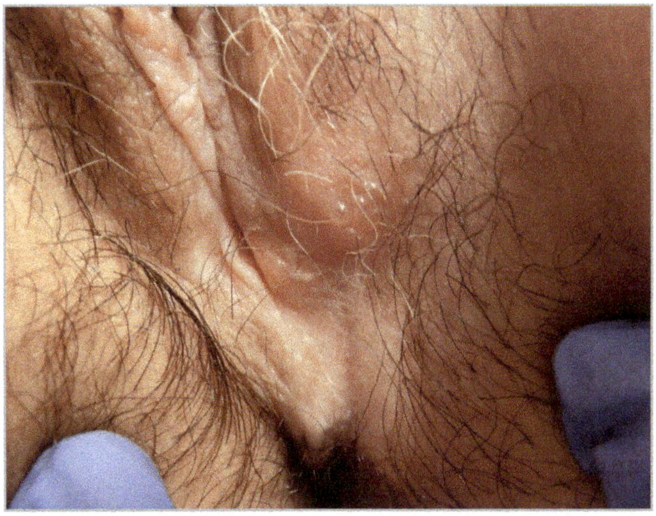

Figure 30.12 A herpetic recurrence showing the grouped vesicles on left labia majora.

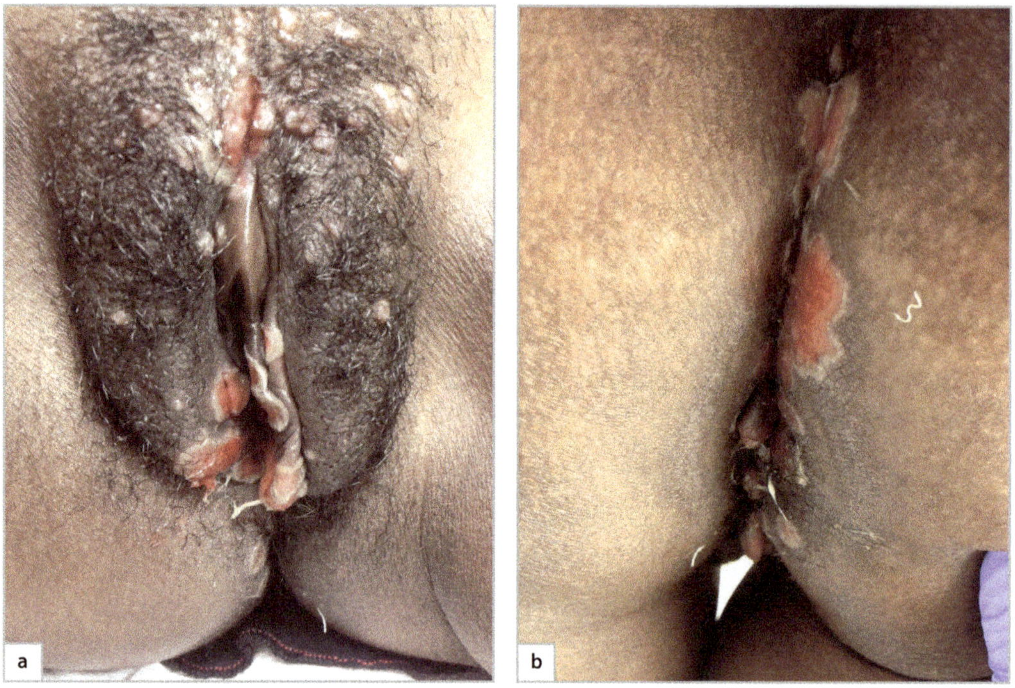

Figure 30.13 A non-primary initial infection in an HIV immunocompromised woman. (a) Chronic ulcerations are observed on vulva and introïtus. Numerous molluscum contagiosum are scattered on the pubis and on the labia majora. (b) Chronic ulcerations are also seen on gluteal folds and anal margin.

HSV serology

HSV serology is not recommended as a diagnostic tool but it is useful in some circumstances (Patel et al. 2011).

- Demonstration of seroconversion (wait for several weeks) when a primary infection is suspected
- Exclusion of 'herpes sine herpete' (painful viral reactivation without clinical lesions)
- Diagnosis of serodiscordant sexual partners in order to advise them

Differential diagnosis

In healthy patients, the differential diagnosis includes vesicular, erosive, or pustular diseases, in immunocompromised patients; it mainly concerns ulcerative disorders (**Table 30.5**).

Management and treatment

The nucleoside analogs are the only effective treatment on the severity and duration of a herpes manifestation. No treatment can eradicate the herpes virus and definitively cure the infection.

Table 30.5 Genital herpes simplex infection: differential diagnosis

	Differential diagnoses	Diagnostic test
Vulvar, vesicular, or pustular diseases	VZV infection (shingles)	Clinical History
	Folliculitis	Swabs
	Candidosis	Swabs
	Erythema multiforme (blisters)	Biopsy
	Lymphangiectasias	History
Vulvar ulcerative diseases	Syphilitic chancre	Serology
	Chancroid	History and swabs
	Donovanosis	Swabs and biopsy
	Sexual trauma	History
	Fixed drug eruption	Biopsy
	Behçet disease	Clinical: diagnostic criteria
	Vulvar aphthae: Lipschütz ulcers, HIV, CMV, EBV, etc.	Serology (HIV, EBV, CMV, etc.)
	Ulcerated granulomatous lesion or malignant tumor	Biopsy

Table 30.6 Therapeutic options in the treatment of genital herpes simplex infection (Patel et al. 2011)

	Type of herpetic infection	Drug	Dosage	Treatment duration
Non-immuno-compromised patients	Primary infection	Acyclovir	400 mg three times a day 200 mg five times a day	5 days
		Famciclovir	250 mg three times a day	5 days
		Valaciclovir	500 mg twice a day	5 days
	Recurrence Episodic therapy	Acyclovir	400 mg three times a day 200 mg five times a day	5 days
		Famciclovir	125 mg twice a day	5 days
		Valaciclovir	500 mg twice a day	5 days
	Recurrence Suppressive therapy*	Acyclovir	200 mg four times a day 400 mg twice a day	Suppressive effect is obtained after 5 days of treatment; check once a year the need of continued therapy
		Famciclovir	250 mg twice a day	
		Valaciclovir	500 mg once a day † 250 mg twice a day‡ 1 g once a day ‡	
HIV-infected patients and Immuno-compromised patients	Primary infection Twice the standard dosage for 10 days or until wound healing (no controlled trials)	Acyclovir	200 mg or 400 mg five times a day (IV,C)	10 days
		Famciclovir	250 mg or 500 mg three times a day (IV,C)	10 days
		Valaciclovir	500 mg or 1 g twice a day (IV,C)	10 days
	Recurrence Episodic therapy	Same schedule as for non-immunocompromised patients (Ib,A). For advanced disease: twice the standard dosage for more than 5 days (Ib,B).		
	Recurrence Suppressive therapy	Acyclovir	400 mg twice a day (Ib,A)	
		Famciclovir	500 mg twice a day (IIa,B)	
		Valaciclovir	500 mg twice a day (Ib,A)	
	Recalcitrant herpes	Topical trifluridine every 8 hours until complete healing: topical cidofovir gel (if available): foscarnet IV. 40 mg/kg/every 8 hours for 2 to 3 weeks or until complete healing (serious side effects)		
* >6 recurrences a year † <10 recurrences a year ‡ >10 recurrences a year				
Topical treatment is not recommended Oral administration is preferred to intravenous therapy that is reserved to patients unable to swallow				
Levels of evidence and grading of recommendations are given in Patel et al. 2011				

Table 30.7 Treatment of genital herpes simplex infection in pregnancy (Patel et al. 2011)

Pregnancy	Type of herpetic infection	Treatment with Acyclovir
First and second trimester	Primary infection	400 mg three times a day or 200 mg five times a day for 5 days + 400 mg three times a day from 36 weeks of pregnancy (Ib,B)
	Recurrence	Avoid treatment
Third trimester (IV,C)	Primary infection	As above for primary infection in early pregnancy * †
	Recurrence	400 mg three times a day from 36 weeks of pregnancy ‡ (Ia,A)
* Consider Caesarean section (Ib,B) † If vaginal delivery is unavoidable, acyclovir IV for the mother and the newborn is mandatory ‡ Vaginal delivery is indicated if there are no lesions at the time of childbirth		
Valaciclovir and acyclovir are recommended in pregnancy		

The recommended regimens are summarized in **Tables 30.6** and **30.7** (Patel et al. 2011).

Primary infection of genital herpes in women

- Hospitalization may be necessary
- Urinary catheter
- HSV detection and typing
- HSV serology
- *Candida* culture of vaginal secretions (vulvovaginal candidosis in 15% of the cases)
- Oral acyclovir better than intravenous route
- Oral effective analgesia
- Mild local antiseptics: (potassium permanganate lotion:dilution 1/10,000, 10 minutes, twice a day)
- STI screening

Varicella zoster virus

Introduction

Varicella infection in form of chicken pox also involves the anogenital skin and the vaginal mucous membrane. However, herpes zoster development on perineal dermatomes (S1 to S5 and L1, L2) is infrequent.

Epidemiology and transmission

About 98% of adults are seropositive for VZV. Transmission is due to contact with the saliva or with the vesicular fluid from chicken pox or herpes zoster. The initial contamination always results in chicken pox. Vaccination for chicken pox is not recommended for healthy children but is recommended for seronegative children undergoing solid organ transplantation.

Herpes zoster occurs in 20% of healthy adults and in 50% of immunocompromised individuals. It is a reactivation of latent virus. Its incidence increases with age (McCrary et al. 1999) or if immunocompromised.

Pathogenesis

VZV particles penetrate through mucosal/epithelial sites and infect regional lymphoid tissues. Infected T-lymphocytes enter into blood circulation and induce viraemia with viral dissemination into the skin and mucous membranes (chicken pox). Afterwards, the virions reach the sensory nerve ganglia and remain latent. The viral reactivation induces a migration towards the dermatome innervated by the infected neural ganglia (Zerboni et al. 2014).

Histopathology of HSV and VZV epithelial infection is comparable (**Figure 30.10**).

Course of disease

Chicken pox, the primary infection generally occurs in childhood. Herpes zoster occurs in older people as a clinical manifestation of a reactivation, spontaneously or favored by a triggering factor (Grinde 2013).

Clinical presentation

Primary infection: varicella, chicken pox

Incubation period lasts on average 14 days. Systemic symptoms and an itchy exanthema are typical. The red papules evolve into vesicles that then dry into crusts. A new eruption occurs every 4 days so that all kind of lesions are observed together.

Recurrence: herpes zoster, shingles

A localized prodromal phase precedes the occurrence of an erythematous unilateral plaque. Afterwards, a papular/vesicular eruption in a dermatomal distribution emerges. Systemic manifestations are rare. The healing period lasts about 3 weeks. The major complication is post-herpetic neuralgia (PHN).

Potential triggering factors (Weinberg 2007)

- Age greater than 50 years
- Immunocompromised patients
- Bone-marrow or solid organ transplantation
- Chronic steroid therapy
- Psychological stress
- Trauma

Diagnosis

The diagnosis is made clinically. The same type of laboratory tests used in HSV diagnosis is available for detecting VZV. Serology and histological examination are not recommended (Weinberg 2007).

Differential diagnosis

In the erythematous stage, herpes zoster may be confused with a contact dermatitis or erysipelas. Atypical herpetic recurrences may mimic herpes zoster. The PHN is part of the dysesthetic genital pain syndrome that includes herpes simplex neuralgia, spinal nerve compression, trauma, and other causes of vulvodynia.

Management and treatment

An early antiviral therapy (**Table 30.8**) decreases the severity and duration of the herpes zoster and reduces the occurrence of PHN. Therapeutic options for PHN are similar to those for neuropathic pain (Whitley et al. 2010).

The live attenuated VZV vaccine is recommended for people >60 years. It decreases the incidence of herpes zoster disease as well as PHN (Gershon 2013). In immunocompromised patients, VZV infections have high morbidity and mortality rates.

Table 30.8 Therapeutic options in the treatment of varicella zoster virus infections (Whitley et al. 2010)

Type of herpetic infection	Drug of choice	Dosage	Treatment duration
Primary infection = varicella	Acyclovir	20 mg/kg (maximum 800 mg) five times/day	5 days
Recurrence = shingles	Acyclovir	800 mg five times/day	7–10 days
	Famciclovir	500 mg three times/day	7 days
	Valaciclovir	1 g three times/day	7 days
Immunocompromised patients	Acyclovir	10 mg/kg every 8 hours	7–10 days

REFERENCES

Brotherton JML. Human papillomavirus vaccination: where are we now? J Paediatr Child Health 2014; 50:959–65.

Chen X, Anstey AV, Bugert JJ. Molluscum contagiosum virus infection. Lancet 2013; 13:877–888.

Fatahzadeh M and Schwartz RA. Human herpes simplex infections: epidemiology, pathogenesis, symptomatology, diagnosis and management. J Am Acad Dermatol 2007; 57:737–763.

Frazer IH. Interaction of human papilloma viruses with the host immune system: a well evolved relationship. Virology 2009; 384:410–414.

Garland SM, Steben M, Sings HL. Natural history of genital warts: analysis of the placebo arm of 2 randomized phase III trials of a quadrivalent human papillomavirus (types 6, 11, 16, 18) vaccine. J Infect Dis 2009; 199:805–814.
Gershon AA. Varicella zoster vaccines and their implications for development of HSV vaccines. Virology 2013; 435:29–36.
Grinde B. Herpes viruses: latency and reactivation¾viral strategies and host response. J Oral Microbiology 2013; 5:1–9.
Gupta R, Warren T, Wald A. Genital herpes. Lancet 2007; 370:2127–2137.
Lacey CJN, Woodhall SC, Wilkstrom A, et al. 2012 European guideline for the management of anogenital warts. J Eur Acad Dermatol Venereol 2013; 27:e263–e270.
Luke JD, Silverberg NB. Vertically transmitted molluscum contagiosum infection. Pediatrics 2010; 125:e423–425.
McCrary ML, Severson J, Tyring SK. Varicella zoster virus. J Am Acad Dermatol 1999; 41:1–14.
Ornstein A, Hatchette T. Human papillomavirus and anogenital warts in children. CMAJ 2012; 184:321.
Patel H, Wagner M, Singhal P, et al. Systematic review of the incidence and prevalence of genital warts. BMC Infect Dis 2013; 13:39–52.
Patel R, Alderson S, Geretti A, et al. European guideline for the management of genital herpes, 2010. Int J STD AIDS 2011; 22:1–10.
Scholz J, Rosen-Wolff A, Bugert J, et al. Epidemiology of molluscum contagiosum using genetic analysis of the viral DNA. J Med Virol 1989; 27:87–90.
Thornsberry L, English JC III. Evidence-based treatment and prevention of external genital warts in female pediatric and adolescent patients. J Pediatr Adolesc Gynecol 2012; 25:150–154.
Tyring SK. Molluscum contagiosum: the importance of early diagnosis and treatment. Am J Obstet Gynecol 2003; 189:S12–S16.
Van der Wouden JC, van der Sande R, van Suijlekom-Smit LW, et al. Interventions for cutaneous molluscum contagiosum (review). Cochrane Database Syst Rev 2009; 4:CD004767.
Weinberg JM. Herpes zoster: epidemiology, natural history, and common complications. J Am Acad Dermatol 2007; 57:S130–135.
Whitley RJ, Volpi A, McKendrick M, et al. Management of herpes zoster and post-herpetic neuralgia now and in the future. J Clin Virol 2010; 48:S20–S28.
Zerboni L, Sen N, Oliver SL, et al. Molecular mechanisms of varicella zoster virus pathogenesis. Nat Rev Microbiol 2014; 12:197–210.

FURTHER READING

Chan T, Barra NG, Lee AJ, et al Innate and adaptive immunity against herpes simplex virus type 2 in the genital mucosa. J Reprod Immunol 2011; 88:210–218.
Einstein MH, Schiller JT, Viscidi RP, et al. Clinician's guide to human papillomavirus immunology: knowns and unknowns. Lancet Infect Dis 2009; 9:347–356.
Ianhez M, Cestari SCP, Enokihara MY, Seize MBPM. Dermoscopic patterns of molluscum contagiosum: a study of 211 lesions confirmed by histopathology. An Bras Dermatol 2011; 86:74–79.

Chapter 31 Sexually transmitted diseases

Katherine Brown

INTRODUCTION

Sexually transmissible infections (STIs) are common and many, including HIV, have dermatological signs and symptoms (**Tables 31.1** and **31.2**). Some infections, such as syphilis, can mimic other conditions and should be kept in mind in the differential diagnosis of any unusual presentation. Infections that cause ulceration or mucosal inflammation increase the risk of acquisition or transmission of HIV (**Table 31.3**). Many STIs are notifiable to public health authorities and require contact tracing to reduce their spread. Check your local public health laws and guidelines if you are unsure about what applies in your jurisdiction. It is often advisable to retest those who have positive results 3 months after the initial infection as repeat infections are common (Guy et al. 2011), likewise negative results may need a later test as well as development of detectable antibodies takes time.

Table 31.1 Summary of STIs that may present in the vulvar clinic

STI	Symptoms	Skin signs	Tests	Treatment
Chlamydia trachomatis infection	Asymptomatic. May have vaginal discharge or pelvic pain	Psoriasis-like rash on palms and soles (see Chapter 22 for psoriasis)	PCR urine, vaginal swab, CT	Azithromycin 1 g one dose
LGV	Pain over site of buboes (groin, rectal)	Erythema buboes	PCR, CT	Doxycycline 100 mg bid for 21 days
Gonorrhea	May be asymptomatic. May have vaginal discharge or pelvic pain	Maculopapular rash if disseminated	Gonococcal PCR urine, vaginal swab and culture if positive	Ceftriaxone 500 mg + azithromycin 1 g stat
Syphilis	Usually painless	Painless ulcer, indurated margin, lymphadenopathy (compare Chapter 28 for other ulcers)	PCR from lesion and serology for syphilis	Penicillin (dose depends on stage)
Chancroid	Pain	Painful ulcers, lymphadenopathy	Culture for *Haemophilus ducreyi*	Azithromycin 1 g once only
Donovanosis	Limited discomfort initially	Non-tender exuberant ulcer with meaty appearance	Biopsy and stain for Donovan bodies	Azithromycin 1 g weekly for 4 weeks
Lice	Itch	Crab lice and nits in pubic hair	Clinical diagnosis aided by microscopy and dermoscopy	Topical permethrin
Scabies	Itch	Red papule or burrow	Clinical diagnosis	Topical permethrin
HIV infection	May be none until very immunosuppressed. Increased risk of CIN/HSIL/AIN	New dermatoses and worsening of existing ones	HIV antibody test, confirmatory Western Blot	Combination antiretroviral therapy
Herpes simplex (see Chapter 30)	Pain, dysuria	Multiple tiny vesicles or erosions, fine skin splits, tender lymph nodes	PCR	Episodic or suppressive oral antiviral acyclovir, valacyclovir, or famciclovir
Human papilloma virus infection (see Chapter 30)	Nil or mild itch	Warts HSIL/CIN/AIN	Clinical diagnosis	Cryotherapy, 5% imiquimod cream 3 times a week for 8–16 weeks, diathermy
Molluscum contagiosum (see Chapter 30)	Nil	1–2 mm pearly papules with central umbilication, navel to thigh	Clinical diagnosis aided by dermoscopy	Cryotherapy, hydrogen peroxide creams, mechanical techniques: squeezing the contents of the spots, curettage, no treatment

AIN, anal intraepithelial neoplasia; CIN, cervical intraepithelial neoplasia; CT, computed tomography; HIV, human immunodeficiency virus; HSIL, high-grade squamous intraepithelial lesions; LGV, lymphogranuloma venereum; PCR, polymerase chain reaction.

Table 31.2 HIV-related dermatological presentations (HIV may worsen symptoms of common diseases)

Disease	Timing	Symptoms	Skin manifestations	Diagnosis	Causative agent	Treatment
Seroconversion	Within weeks of infection	Fever, malaise, neutropenia, lymphadenopathy	Maculopapular truncal distribution	HIV antibody, Western Blot	HIV	Refer for full assessment
Seborrheic dermatitis (Chapter 16)	Any time, worsens with low CD4 count	Itch	Yellow to white, scaly eruption with erythematous base in central distribution over face, nose, trunk, or genitalia	Clinical diagnosis or biopsy		Topical ketoconazole
Psoriasis (Chapter 22)	Any time	Itch	Silver scale on extremities is not seen on genitals that usually have a shiny erythematous appearance	Biopsy	May have family history	Topical steroids, phototherapy, emollients, avoid soap
Ichthyosis (Chapter 8)	Increased problem in patients with low CD4 count	Itch	Generalized dryness especially lower limbs	Clinical diagnosis	HIV	Avoid soap, add emollients. Oral doxepin at night (titrate dose to symptom control)
Adverse cutaneous drug reactions (Chapter 17)	Any time, more common in immune suppressed	May have itch, fever, myalgia, headache	Red, maculopapular rash is most common	Clinical diagnosis	Sulfur Multiple antiretroviral drugs	Cease the causative agent
Aphthous ulcers (Chapter 28)	Any time, worse with low CD4 count	Pain	Large and/or multiple ulcers. May have oral ulceration as well as genital	Clinical and by exclusion of other causes of ulceration		Potent topical steroid, oral prednisone starting at 60–70 mg and tapering by 5 mg/day, thalidomide 50–200 mg
Lymphoma	Any level of CD4 count, more common in late disease	Weight loss, fever, night sweats	Lymphadenopathy	CT, MRI, biopsy of affected area	EBV for non-Hodgkin lymphoma	Refer to hematologist or oncologist
Kaposi sarcoma	Any level of CD4 count	Bleeding, anemia if gut involved. May involve respiratory tract. May have lymphedema	Vascular neoplasm, may be single or multiple purple/brown nodules of varying size. Not common in women	Biopsy–proliferation of spindle cells with extravasation of erythrocytes.	Human herpesvirus 8	Protease inhibitors as part of antiretroviral regime. May need chemotherapy or radiotherapy
Vulvar and perianal intraepithelial neoplasia and cancer (Chapter 34)	Diagnosis more likely with long-standing infection or immunosuppression	Itch, pain, bleeding	Squamous cell carcinoma–may have ulcerated center	Biopsy	HPV 16 and 18	Excision of HSIL and vulvar cancer, chemotherapy and radiotherapy for perianal and anal cancer
Candidosis (Chapter 29)	More common when immune suppressed	May have oral and esophageal involvement, moderate to severe genital itch	Recurrent infections with thick white discharge, erythema	Microscopy and culture. Check HIV Ab in recalcitrant candida cases	*Candida albicans*	Antiretroviral to raise CD4 count and oral azole as well as topical
Herpes simplex (Chapter 30)	Can occur any time but persistence for >1 month is an AIDS diagnosis. Active lesions increase risk of transmission of HIV	Pain at site of lesions, dysuria	Vesicles, erosions, may present as fine fissuring in genital skin	PCR from the lesions (serology is not useful in acute infection)	Herpes simplex virus 1 and 2	Antiviral therapy with acyclovir, valacyclovir or famciclovir in either episodic or suppressive regime
Herpes zoster (Chapter 30)	Any time but low CD4 associated with more widespread rash	Pain precedes the rash that has a dermatomal distribution	Bilateral or involving multiple dermatomes is indicative of immunosuppression	Varicella zoster virus antibody	Varicella zoster virus (herpes virus)	High-dose acyclovir, valacyclovir or famciclovir early to prevent neuropathic pain

Continued opposite...

Continued...

Disease	Timing	Symptoms	Skin manifestations	Diagnosis	Causative agent	Treatment
Epstein–Barr virus infection	Can occur at any time. Leukoplakia is more common in immune suppressed patients	Associated with non-Hodgkin lymphoma	Large painful ulceration in the genital region is rare Oral hairy leukoplakia (white plaques) on the side of the tongue	EBV IgM and IgG antibodies	EBV (herpes virus)	Topical analgesia for ulcerations until they resolve spontaneously
Cytomegalovirus infection	Reactivation of latent infection in immune suppressed patients	Retinitis (leading to blindness), colitis, cholangitis and pneumonia	Large painful ulceration	CMV IgM and IgG antibodies	CMV (herpes virus)	Ganciclovir IV for systemic disease plus topical analgesia for ulcers
Bacterial folliculitis	Any level of CD4	May have low grade itch or irritation	Multiple red pustules around hair follicles	Microscopy, culture and sensitivity	Most commonly *Staphylococcus aureus*. May be exacerbated by shaving	Antibiotics as indicated by sensitivity, antiseptic soap with triclosan 1%, topical mupirocin ointment
Eosinophilic folliculitis	Low CD4	Intense itch	Red papules around follicles, predominantly upper chest and arms	Biopsy if unsure of diagnosis	Unknown	Oral prednisone starting at 70 mg and tapering by 5 mg daily
Molluscum contagiosum (Chapter 30)	Any level of CD4 for minor lesions, low CD4 if widespread	Asymptomatic	May be larger and more widespread in immune suppressed, usually navel to thigh in adults	Clinical diagnosis	*Molluscum contagiosum* virus (pox virus)	Cryotherapy
Cryptococcal infection	May present early, usually low CD4 count	May have headache, nausea, vomiting if meningitis is also present	Subcutaneous nodule, cellulitis or ulcer	Biopsy, cryptococcal antigen	*Cryptococcus neoformans*	Refer to infectious diseases specialist
Tuberculosis	Any level of CD4 count	Check for pulmonary involvement	Enlarged lymph nodes, may have caseating skin lesions	Acid fast bacilli on biopsy	*Mycobacterium tuberculosis*	Refer for specialist TB treatment

CMV, cytomegalovirus; CT, computed tomography; EBV, Epstein–Barr virus; HIV, human immunodeficiency virus; HPV, human papilloma virus; HSIL, high-grade squamous intraepithelial lesion; MRI, magnetic resonance imaging; PCR, polymerase chain reaction; TB, tuberculosis.

Table 31.3 Infective causes of vaginal discharge

Pathogen	Discharge	Signs / Symptoms	Diagnosis	Treatment
Chlamydia	Nil or clear to white cervical discharge	Nil or pelvic pain on palpation	Polymerase chain reaction (PCR) urine, vaginal or cervical swab	Azithromycin 1 g stat
Neisseria gonorrhoeae	Mucopurulent cervical discharge	Nil or pelvic pain on palpation	PCR urine, vaginal, or cervical swab. Culture and sensitivity if positive	Ceftriaxone 500 mg i.m. + azithromycin 1 g stat
Trichomonas vaginalis	Green, frothy vaginal discharge, odor	Strawberry cervix, erythema	PCR or culture vaginal swab	Tinidazole 2 g stat relapsing cases need 400 mg metronidazole bid for 5 days
Mycoplasma genitalium	Nil or mucopurulent cervical discharge	Nil or pelvic pain on palpation	PCR or culture cervical swab	Doxycycline 100 mg bd for 14 days
Bacterial vaginosis (see Chapter 29)	Nil or gray-white vaginal discharge, odor	Nil	Culture vaginal swab	Metronidazole 400 mg bd for 7 days
Candida albicans (see Chapter 29)	White discharge	Erythema, itch	Culture vaginal swab	Fluconazole 150 mg oral once only +/– vaginal azole cream for 7 days
Candida glabrata (see Chapter 29)	Minimal discharge	Erythema, itch and pain	Culture vaginal swab	Nystatin vaginal cream 21 days or boric acid 600 mg vaginal pessaries 14–28 days
Group B *Streptococcus* usually not pathogenic (see Chapter 29)	Possibly thin green discharge	Erythema, may cause pain	Culture and sensitivity	Treatment is required in pregnancy to prevent neonatal infection. 2% Clindamycin vaginal cream 14 days or oral phenoxymethyl penicillin 500 mg bd for 10 days

Key features of STIs

- STIs require partners to be treated as well as the presenting patient
- STIs have public health as well as individual patient implications
- Re-testing patients who have previously had STIs is often useful

CHLAMYDIA

Key features

- Often asymptomatic
- Very common STI
- May cause pelvic inflammatory disease (PID) and tubal infertility
- Treat partners

Causative organism

Chlamydia trachomatis is one of the species in the genus *Chlamydia* that infects humans. *Chlamydia* species are unique because of their two part life cycle, alternating between extracellular and intracellular forms (the elementary body and the reticulate particle, respectively). They require host cells to provide ATP and other nutrients. Two distinct biovars (physiological variants) are associated with genital infection in humans. The trachoma biovar causes the eye infection, trachoma (serovars A, B, Ba, and C), and most anogenital and neonatal infections (serovars B and D-K). The lymphogranuloma venereum (LGV) biovar (serovars L1-L3) causes a much less common but often invasive anogenital infection. Chlamydia is one of the most common STIs worldwide and is particularly prevalent in sexually active men and women aged under 25 years (Franceschi et al. 2007; Walker et al. 2012).

Clinical presentation

Chlamydia trachomatis

Anogenital infections with *Chlamydia trachomatis* serovars D-K are commonly asymptomatic. In women, the sites of infection may initially include the cervix, endometrium, urethra, Bartholin glands, rectum, and pharynx. The patient may present with right upper quadrant pain caused by spread of the infection internally, resulting in perihepatitis. Spread of the infection from the cervix to the fallopian tubes may result in pelvic pain, leading to a diagnosis of PID that may be severe enough to warrant hospitalization. There may be a mucopurulent cervical discharge or cervical ectopy, and *Chlamydia* infection is a common cause of intermenstrual bleeding. The conjunctivae may be infected by contact with infectious material on the fingers, producing a pale cobblestoned appearance to the inner eyelid and a unilateral red eye with or without a mucopurulent discharge. Chlamydia is sometimes associated with a systemic inflammatory reaction (Reiter syndrome) that is more common in men than in women (Owlia & Eley 2010).

Lymphogranuloma venereum

LGV is an uncommon infection in Western countries but is endemic in some parts of the world. Recently, there have been an increased number of cases in men who have sex with other men (MSM), which may pose a risk for women with bisexual partners (White 2009). The primary lesion may be a small, non-indurated ulcer, or papule, although it is often asymptomatic in women, especially if it occurs inside the vagina or on the cervix rather than in the posterior fourchette or elsewhere on the vulva. The most common presenting symptom is the development of inflammation and swelling in the inguinal lymph nodes (known as a bubo) (**Figure 31.1**). This may occur up to 6 months after the initial infection. Sixty-six percent of these presentations are unilateral.

Dermatological signs

Chlamydia trachomatis

Reiter syndrome (arthritis, urethritis, and conjunctivitis) may be caused by *Chlamydia trachomatis*. The skin manifestations of this condition include keratoderma blenorrhagica (patchy thickened scales and pustules, primarily on the soles of the feet) (**Figure 31.2**). Other signs include scaly red patches similar to psoriasis on various parts of the body and mouth ulcers.

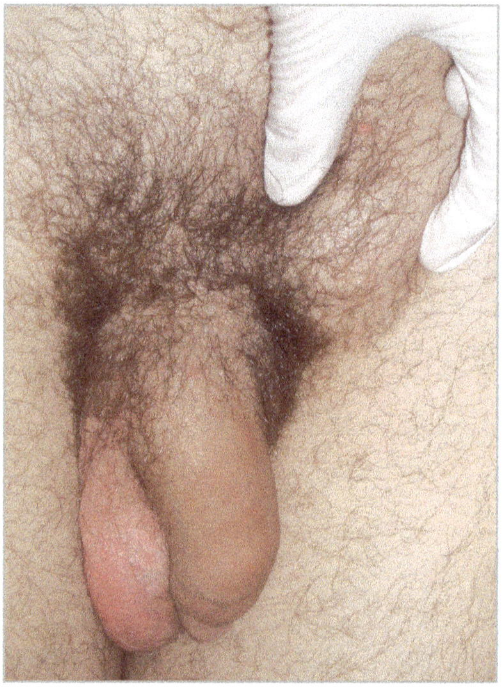

Figure 31.1 Lymphogranuloma venereum showing a bubo in left groin. By courtesy of Dr. Stuart Aitken, Gold Coast, Queensland, Australia.

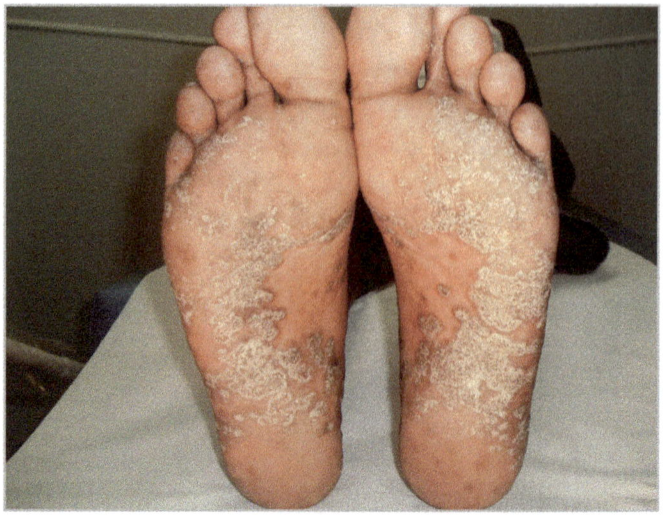

Figure 31.2 Chlamydia–keratoderma blenorrhagica. By courtesy of Dr Stuart Aitken, Gold Coast, Queensland, Australia.

Lymphogranuloma venereum

The skin over the bubo becomes red and adheres to the lymph node. This is associated with throbbing pain, fever, and lethargy. One-third of women develop inguinal signs. Others develop low abdominal or back pain associated with infection of the pelvic and lumbar lymph nodes. The rectal mucosa may be infected directly or following vaginal infection. The rectal mucosa becomes red and friable with multiple superficial erosions. Anal and perianal abscesses and fissures that mimic Crohn disease commonly appear. A rare complication is the development of sclerosing fibrosis in the vulva resulting in chronic ulceration in the labia majora, the groin, or the perineum.

Diagnosis

Chlamydia infections are currently diagnosed using nucleic acid amplification tests (NAATs). These are highly sensitive and specific. Positive tests should be confirmed using a different assay, particularly in populations with a low prevalence.

Management

Chlamydia trachomatis

Azithromycin (a macrolide antibiotic) is the current drug of choice. A single dose of 1 g orally is recommended for simple infections.

PID may be mild or severe. As the microbiological diagnosis is not known at the time of initial treatment, the regimen for outpatient management should include ceftriaxone 500 mg intramuscularly and azithromycin 1 g orally followed by 14 days of twice daily oral metronidazole 400 mg and either doxycycline 100 mg twice daily or a repeat dose of azithromycin at 1 week. Serious infections require hospitalization and intravenous therapy.

Rectal infection requires multiple dose treatment. A single dose of azithromycin should be followed with 10 days of doxycycline 100 mg twice daily or a second dose of azithromycin 7 days after the first.

Sexual contact should be avoided for 7 days after single dose treatment; condoms will provide some protection; however, any contact with body fluids places a risk of microbe transmission. In some countries, patient-delivered partner therapy has been used to increase the rate of partner treatment (Gift et al. 2011).

LGV

Doxycycline 100 mg twice daily for 21 days is recommended. Azithromycin 1 g orally every week for 3 weeks is an alternative treatment.

GONORRHEA

Key features

- Mucopurulent cervical discharge
- May cause PID and tubal infertility
- Undertake sensitivity testing for all positives as antimicrobial resistance is increasing worldwide
- Treat partners

Causative organism

Neisseria gonorrhea belongs to the genus *Neisseria* and is closely related to another human pathogen, *Neisseria meningitidis*. Humans are the only host for gonococci that are transmitted by close contact between two mucosal surfaces, usually sexual. Gonococci are gram-negative diplococci with very specific growth requirements and a variety of mechanisms for developing drug resistance. Gonorrhea is much less common than chlamydia in most countries but is usually more symptomatic.

Clinical presentation

The most common presentation is with a complaint of increased vaginal discharge emanating from the endocervical canal or the urethra, dysuria, or intermenstrual bleeding. Infection of the Bartholin or Skene glands may present as an abscess. Sometimes, the infection spreads to the endometrium and the fallopian tubes causing PID. These women present with pelvic pain and fever in addition to discharge. Rectal infection is often asymptomatic. Pharyngeal infection is usually asymptomatic but may be associated with increased risk of disseminated gonococcal infection (DGI). Conjunctivitis, presenting with bilateral purulent discharge, is uncommon in adults but more common in neonates.

Dermatological signs

DGI rarely occurs. It presents as a limited number of necrotic pustules or macules on the distal limbs (**Figure 31.3**) in addition to a painful joint or joints, most commonly wrists, metacarpals, ankles, or knees (Raychaudhuri et al. 2009). The rash is similar to that of *Neisseria meningitidis*.

Diagnosis

Gonorrhea can be diagnosed using NAATs but it is important to undertake antibiotic sensitivity tests if possible; so, any positive NAAT should be confirmed using culture. It is preferable to take a culture initially if there is a significant mucopurulent discharge. Blood cultures may be negative in DGI. Anogenital and pharyngeal tests should be undertaken in addition to blood culture if DGI is suspected.

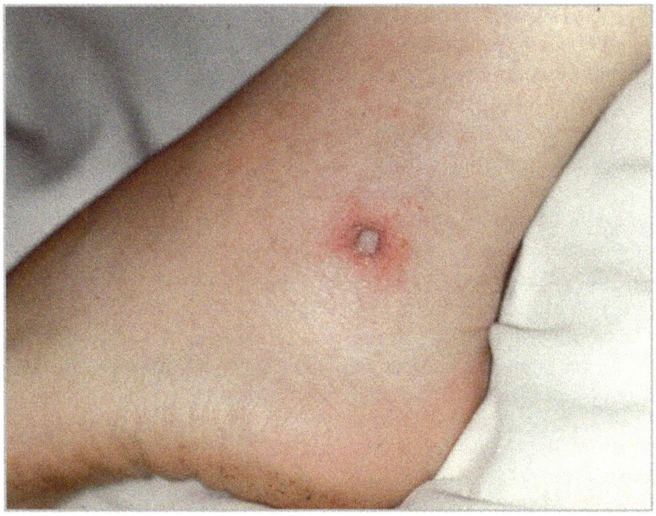

Figure 31.3 Typical pustule seen in disseminated gonococcal infection. By courtesy of Dr Lewis Marshall, Western Australia.

Management

There is an increasing problem with antibiotic resistance in gonorrhea. Penicillin, tetracycline, and fluoroquinolones have been used but now have high levels of resistance in many countries (Martin et al. 2012). Ceftriaxone 500 mg IM plus 1g azithromycin is now standard treatment for a simple gonococcal infection in many international guidelines. Management of PID is the same for chlamydia.

SYPHILIS

Synonym

Lues

Key features

- Often asymptomatic
- Vertical transmission up to 10 years, horizontal 1-2 years
- 10-30% risk of long-term complications if untreated
- Penicillin is the drug of choice
- Test and treat partners if positive

Causative organism

Syphilis is caused by the bacterium *Treponema pallidum*, closely related to the treponemes that cause yaws, bejel, and pinta. They have a characteristic spiral shape and corkscrew movements and are transmitted by skin-to-skin contact through microabrasions. The infection spreads rapidly through the bloodstream, infecting the central nervous system as well as multiple organs. The body usually recognizes pathogens because they have different compounds on their cell surfaces that trigger an immune response; however, *Treponema pallidum* initially manages to evade the immune system as it has few proteins and no liposaccharides in its outer membrane and therefore does not trigger that response. Without treatment, syphilis becomes a chronic (latent) infection with potential to cause serious disease decades after the initial infection.

Syphilis cannot be transmitted horizontally to a partner once it becomes latent (1-2 years) but it can be transmitted vertically (mother to child) for 8-10 years, which is one reason why syphilis testing forms part of the routine antenatal screen in many countries (Gomez et al. 2013). In pregnant women, the fetus is not affected until the mid-trimester when the immune system has developed sufficiently to produce an immune response following transplacental exposure.

The incubation period may be up to 90 days. The development of antibodies does not indicate immunity as an individual can have multiple episodes of infection with syphilis over a lifetime. In many developed countries, syphilis is now uncommon even though there is a recent increase in incidence again but it is still a problem in developing countries and in certain developed populations such as MSM, particularly those living with HIV. Syphilis is known as the great mimic and should be considered in the differential diagnosis of any genital ulceration.

Clinical presentation

Many people with syphilis do not notice any signs that they have this infection and only discover it when they have a blood test for another reason such as pregnancy, blood donation, or a sexual health screen. A patient with secondary syphilis may present with systemic symptoms such as fever, malaise, sore throat, headache, myalgia, and lymphadenopathy, but this stage may also be asymptomatic. Occasional patients experience bone pain associated with periosteal inflammation, hepatitis, iritis, anterior uveitis, or glomerulonephritis (Nguyen et al. 2013).

Untreated or undertreated, the patient then moves into the early latent (up to 1 year after infection) followed by the late latent phase. During latent phases of syphilis, the patient has no clinical symptoms. Up to 30% of people may develop tertiary syphilis over the next 20-30 years. Abnormalities in the cerebrospinal fluid may be found in primary and secondary syphilis but acute neurosyphilis is rare. Tertiary neurosyphilis may present as a complication of meningovascular infection with hemiparesis, aphasia, and seizures after 5-10 years or meningoencephalitis with psychiatric abnormalities, paresis, and optic atrophy after 15-20 years. Cardiovascular syphilis may be diagnosed after a latency of up to 30 years and is much less common in women than men. Aneurysm of the thoracic aorta, aortic regurgitation, and coronary artery disease may be found. Tertiary syphilis rarely presents with skin and bone involvement these days (Read & Donovan 2012).

Dermatological signs

Primary syphilis

In primary syphilis, the first sign is often a single (occasionally multiple) 1 cm painless ulcer with an indurated edge and a clear base that resolves untreated within 3-6 weeks (**Figure 31.4**). The ulcer is preceded by a smaller papule that is rarely noticed by the patient. The lesions in primary syphilis occur at the site of infection, usually genital, perianal or oral but occasionally on a finger or elsewhere if contact has occurred with an infected body part. As it is painless, women are more likely than men not to notice the primary lesion due to the hidden nature of their genital anatomy. The secondary stage usually occurs after the primary stage has resolved but occasionally occurs concurrently.

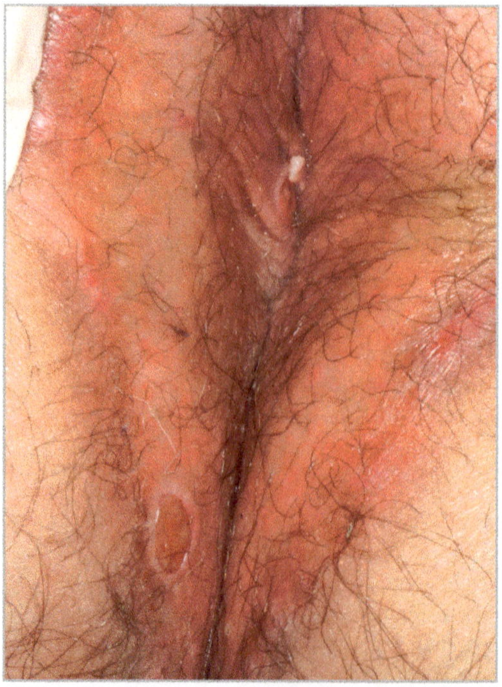

Figure 31.4 Painless ulcer of primary syphilis. By courtesy of Dr Chris Carmody, Sydney, Australia.

Secondary syphilis

Secondary syphilis is one of the few rashes to involve the palms of the hand and the soles of the feet and may have a number of other dermatological features including a generalized red-brown maculopapular rash (**Figure 31.5**), hypertrophic anogenital lesions resembling warts known as condylomata lata, and mucous patches resembling aphthous ulcers but without the pain. Some patients also develop patchy alopecia.

Early syphilis (primary, secondary, and latent syphilis of <2 years duration) is highly infectious.

Tertiary syphilis

Tertiary syphilis may present as a nodule or nodules, of varying size, with a necrotic centre. These are known as gummata. The face and limbs are most commonly affected.

Diagnosis

Treponemes cannot be seen using light microscopy. Dark field microscopy was used previously but this has been replaced by NAAT technology in developed countries. Serology is important for determining whether infection is acute or chronic. There is a 6-week window period; so, repeat tests if clinically suspicious. **Table 31.4** outlines the tests available and their place in diagnosis.

Management

Penicillin is the drug of choice. Primary, secondary, and early latent syphilis can be treated with a single dose of 1.8 g benzathine penicillin i.m. In penicillin allergy the alternative treatment is oral doxycycline 100 mg twice daily for 14 days.

Late latent syphilis requires three doses of 1.8 g benzathine penicillin i.m. at weekly intervals.

Pregnant women should be treated with penicillin. If they are allergic to penicillin, they should be referred for desensitization as tetracyclines are contraindicated in pregnancy, and erythromycin does not cure all fetal infections. Pregnant women may need hospitalization as a Jarisch-Herxheimer reaction may induce labor.

The uncommon Jarisch-Herxheimer reaction (chills, fever, arthralgia, and headache due to release of treponemal breakdown products) resolves within 24 hours and is managed with oral anti-inflammatory medication, typically systemic glucocorticosteroids. Prophylactic steroids are not helpful (Myles et al. 1998).

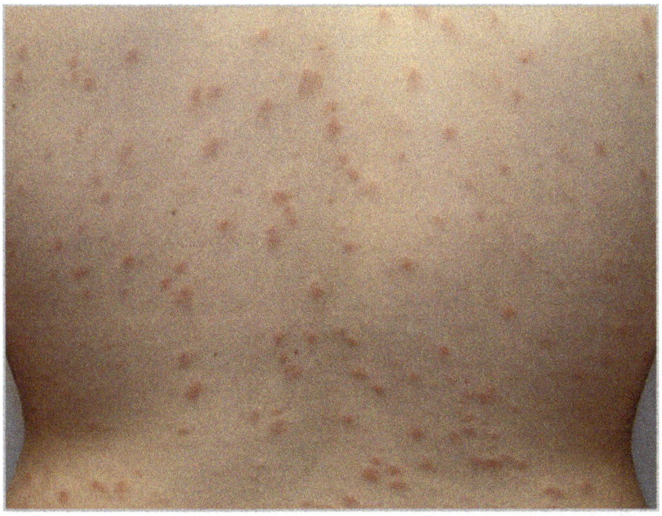

Figure 31.5 Typical widespread scaly red/brown macules and papules of secondary syphilis.

CHANCROID

Causative organism

Chancroid is caused by *Hemophilus ducreyi*. It is rare in the developed world but endemic in Africa, Asia, and Latin America. Humans are

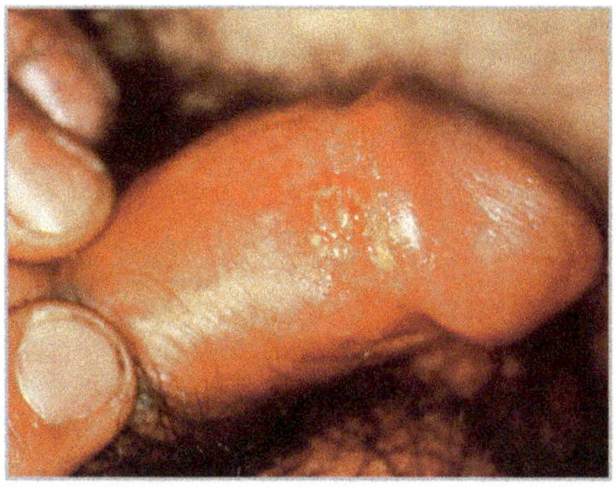

Figure 31.6 Chancroid. A patient presented with painful ulceration. By courtesy of Dr Gordon White, Canberra, Australia.

Table 31.4 Serological tests for syphilis

Test	Type	Usefulness	Acute infection	Chronic infection
TPEIA	Enzyme immunoassay	Screen	Positive	Positive
TP IgM EIA		Congenital or early acquired		Not useful
RPR	Non-treponemal	Acute infection, false positives may occur	Any dilution if no previous infection >fourfold increase if previous infection	Usually <4 May be negative if treated or untreated old disease
VDRL	Non-treponemal	Most useful in CSF	Positive	May be negative
TPPA or TPHA	Treponemal agglutination assays. React to any treponeme	Early syphilis Confirmatory	Positive. May all be negative in very early infection	Remain reactive indefinitely. Occasionally revert to negative if treated very early
FTA-Abs	Treponemal			
PCR	Nucleic acid amplification test	In cases where serology has not yet evolved	Primary chancre or secondary mouth ulcer or rash	Not useful

CSF, cerebrospinal fluid; FTA-Abs, fluorescent treponemal antibody absorption; RPR, rapid plasma regain; TPEIA, treponema pallidum enzyme immunoassay; TPHA, treponema pallidum hemagglutination assay; TPPA, treponema pallidum particle agglutination assay; VDRL, Venereal Disease Research Laboratory.

the only host. The gram-negative coccobacilli enter non-intact skin through areas of microtrauma.

Clinical presentation

The patient usually presents with painful ulcerations without noticing the papules or pustules that precede them (**Figure 31.6**) The most common site in women is the vaginal opening but they may also develop cervical, anal, and extragenital skin ulcers. Involvement of the inguinal lymph nodes may result in buboes similar to LGV.

Dermatological signs

Hemophilus ducreyi can infect both mucosal and keratinized squamous epithelium. Initially, it causes painless papules and pustules that develop into painful ulcerations over 7-14 days. Unlike syphilis, the edge of the ulcer is not indurated. The base may be covered with a necrotic, purulent yellow-gray exudate. The surface often bleeds when touched. Ulcers usually heal within 2 weeks after treatment. If untreated, they will not heal, in contrast to syphilis.

Diagnosis

Culture of *Hemophilus ducreyi* is complex and should be discussed with a microbiologist. Polymerase chain reaction (PCR) testing is not yet readily available but is more sensitive and specific than culture in research settings.

Management

Azithromycin 1 g orally as a single dose is the drug of choice. Alternative treatments include one dose of ceftriaxone 500 mg i.m. and ciprofloxacin 500 mg twice daily orally for 3 days. Buboes, if present, require incision and drainage (Kemp et al. 2011).

DONOVANOSIS

Causative organism

Donovanosis is caused by *Klebsiella granulomatis*. It has now become rare in developed countries but is still found in many developing countries.

Clinical presentation

The first sign of Donovanosis is a small nodule in the genital skin usually in association with some trauma. On the cervix, the lesion may be difficult to distinguish clinically from squamous carcinoma. Dissemination of infection and involvement of extragenital sites are rare.

Dermatological signs

The classical appearance of Donovanosis is a non-tender exuberant red ulcer with a meaty appearance that bleeds on touch (**Figure 31.7**). Less commonly the ulcer may be hypertrophic with an irregular edge or deep, necrotic, and malodourous.

Diagnosis

Biopsy specimens are required for a tissue smear looking for Donovan bodies. Diagnosis can also be made using NAATs.

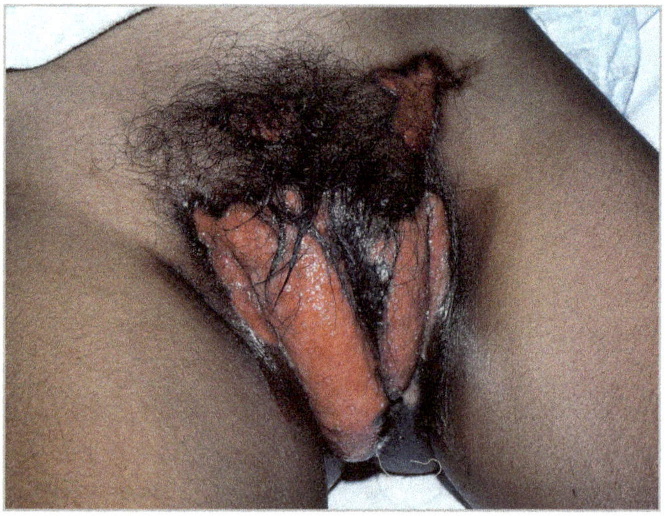

Figure 31.7 Donovanosis showing extensive typical ulceration with red friable base. By courtesy of Professor Basil Donovan, Sydney, Australia.

Management

Azithromycin 1 g orally taken weekly or doxycycline 100 mg twice daily for at least 4 weeks until the ulcer heals (O'Farrell & Moi 2010).

LICE

Causative organism

Infection with the pubic louse, *Pthirus pubis* is commonly known as crabs because the shape of this louse resembles a crab, unlike the linear appearance of head and body lice. The egg (nit) is laid on the hair and hatches within 5-10 days. After hatching the louse requires regular blood meals until maturity and deposits red feces onto the skin. Adult pubic lice can survive up to 24 hours off the body.

Clinical presentation

Itching, related to sensitization of the skin to salivary antigens, is the presenting symptom.

Dermatological signs

Pubic lice may infect the eyelashes, eyebrows, axilla, beard, and trunk as well as pubic hair (**Figure 31.8**) (Manjunatha et al. 2006). The current fashion for shaving pubic hair in some countries

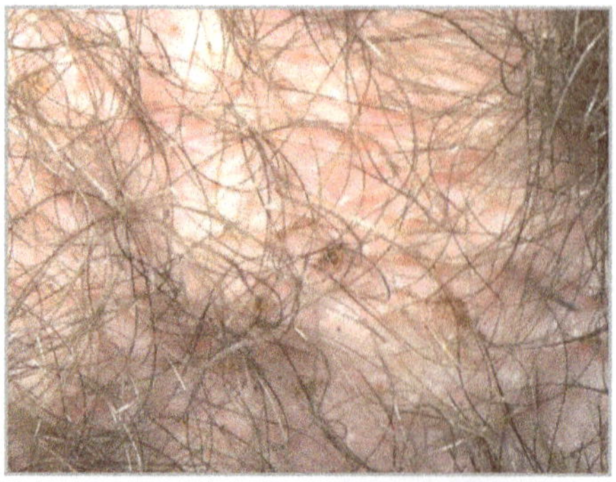

Figure 31.8 Pubic louse and nits. By courtesy of Associate Professor Richard Hillman, Sydney, Australia.

has resulted in a reduction in cases as the lice have no place to lay eggs!

Diagnosis

No tests are required for this diagnosis. It is done by visual inspection of the affected region. Mature lice can be seen moving on the skin and nits attached to the shaft of the hair.

Management

Permethrin 1% solution is used to eradicate lice. One treatment is usually enough but a second application may be required after 7 days. Infestation of the eyelashes responds to treatment with petroleum jelly applied twice daily for 10 days. Itching, due to allergic reaction, may continue after removal of the lice and eggs. This may need treatment with a topical steroid.

As well as treating the infestation all clothes, towels, and bedding must be washed in hot water.

The person should avoid sexual contact until the partner has been treated.

SCABIES

Causative organism

Scabies is caused by the mite, *Sarcoptes scabiei*. Transmission occurs following prolonged skin-to-skin contact or sharing clothes, towels, or bedding. The adult mite penetrates the skin and forms a linear burrow over the next few weeks. Scabies is an ancient disease with cyclical epidemics; it is not by definition a sexually transmitted disease. Close contact, e.g. in kindergartens or nursing homes, may cause endemic scabies outbreaks.

Clinical presentation

Common sites of infection include the finger webs, wrists, areolae, umbilical area, penis, and scrotum. Female labia are rarely infected. Following penetration the person is initially asymptomatic, but later develops intense itching. Reinfection leads to itching much earlier due to an immediate hypersensitivity reaction.

Dermatological signs

Scabies infection initially appears as a red papule, but in the finger webs and on the wrist this is later seen as a linear burrow. In genital skin, the area around each papule may become red and edematous. Crusted scabies may occur in immunosuppressed individuals. In crusted scabies, lesions have a markedly thickened scale teeming with mites.

Diagnosis

The diagnosis is made by observing the typical burrows or searching for the mite by scraping a burrow and looking at the scraping under microscopy. Dermoscopy is a helpful technique.

Management

Permethrin 5% cream is used to eradicate scabies and is safe in pregnancy. One treatment applied from the neck to the toes, left on for about 12 hours, is usually enough but a second application may be required after 7 days. Taking a shower before treatment is not recommended. Persistent itch after appropriate treatment may be related to treatment failure, re-infection or an allergic response to the mite (Norlund 2009). Severe post-treatment reactions may require anti-inflammatory treatment with, e.g. topical steroids for a week. Benzyl benzoate, malathion, and crotamiton seem less effective. Ivermectin may be used if permethrin is ineffective.

As well as treating the infestation, all worn clothes, towels, and bedding must be washed in hot water. Household and sexual contacts need treatment at the same time as the index case. The person should avoid close contact until treatment is completed.

HIV INFECTION

Key features

- HIV is relatively hard to catch compared with other STIs, and is most common in MSM and injecting drug users in developed countries. Some developing countries have a prevalence of 35% across the younger population.
- Seroconversion illness resembles many other acute viral infections The HIV antibody test may take up to 12 weeks but can often be positive within 4–6 weeks. Test partners and offer post-exposure prophylaxis if high risk and <72 hours since exposure.
- Frequent testing is advisable for high-risk clients in high prevalence settings.
- HIV is now managed as a chronic illness in countries with access to antiretroviral medications

Causative organism

Illness related to HIV infection was first recognized in 1981 and HIV is now known to infect millions of people throughout the world. HIV 1 is the most common type, with HIV 2 being found in West Africa and rarely elsewhere. HIV is a retrovirus. The prevalence is very high in sub-Saharan Africa and parts of south and South-East Asia.

HIV can be transmitted from person to person by sexual contact, from mother to child and through exposure to infected blood by transfusion, sharps injury, or shared injecting drug equipment. Receptive anal intercourse with ejaculation and without condoms poses the highest risk (1/70) with unprotected vaginal sex being much lower risk (1/1200). In developed countries, MSM and injecting drug users are the populations most affected. In developing countries, heterosexual transmission is more common and there is a higher risk of children being born with HIV if mothers do not have access to antiretroviral therapy during pregnancy and labor and children cannot access prophylaxis after birth. The risk of transmission also relates to the person's viral load, i.e. how much virus is circulating in their blood and body fluids.

Clinical presentation

There may or may not be a clinically obvious seroconversion illness. The symptoms and signs of seroconversion include fever, malaise, sore throat, generalized maculopapular rash, and lymphadenopathy. If undiagnosed, the patient will become immunosuppressed and may present with uncommon infections such as *Pneumocystis jiroveci* pneumonia (formerly *Pneumocystis carinii*), toxoplasma, or crypotococcal meningitis. Any patient with tuberculosis should also be tested for HIV.

Dermatological signs

Dermatological signs may be found at any time during the course of the infection. Common skin problems like eczema, seborrheic dermatitis, or psoriasis may worsen if the patient is immunosuppressed and unusual presentations occur with advanced disease such as prolonged infection with herpes simplex virus or candida, Kaposi sarcoma, or multidermatome herpes zoster (**Table 31.2**).

Diagnosis

HIV is diagnosed by taking a blood sample to test for HIV antigens and antibodies using an enzyme linked immunosorbant assay. A positive screening test is confirmed with a Western Blot to detect a series of antibodies to a range of HIV proteins, which may take a number of weeks to evolve into a fully positive result. In some locations, rapid tests taking 20–40 minutes and using saliva or finger prick blood samples can provide an earlier result. Any reactive test must be confirmed using a Western Blot.

Management

HIV infection is now managed as a chronic disease in countries that have access to the wide range of antiretroviral medications available and patients have a life span approaching that of the HIV negative population. In developing countries, these drugs may only be available for pregnant women. Antiretroviral therapy is very effective if taken regularly. Progress is monitored by checking the CD4 count and the viral load. As the drugs can have side effects, a number of other blood samples are required every 3-6 months to look for anemia, renal, or liver disease. People with HIV can undertake most forms of employment, have normal pregnancies and uninfected children and generally live a full and healthy life. In some locations, antiretroviral drugs can be taken for 28 days as prophylaxis if a high-risk exposure has occurred.

REFERENCES FOR TREATMENT

www.bashh.org/BASHH/Guidelines/Guidelines.aspx (accessed 8 December 2015)

www.bhiva.org/clinicalguidelines.aspx (accessed 8 December 2015)

www.cdc.gov/hiv/guidelines/index.html (accessed 8 December 2015)

www.sti.guidelines.org.au (accessed 8 December 2015)

REFERENCES

Francheschi S, Smith JS, Van Den Brule A, et al. Cervical infection with *Chlamydia trachomatis* and *Neisseria gonorrhoea* in women from ten areas in four continents. Sex Transm Dis 2007; 34: 563–569.

Gift TL, Kissinger P, Mohammed H, et al. The cost and cost effectiveness of expedited partner therapy compared with standard partner referral for the treatment of chlamydia and gonorrhoea. Sex Transm Dis 2011; 38:1067–1073.

Gomez GB, Kamb ML, Newman LM, et al. Untreated maternal syphilis and adverse outcomes of pregnancy: a systematic review and meta-analysis. Bull World Health Organ 2013; 91:217–226.

Guy R, Wand H, Franklin N, et al. Re-testing for *Chlamydia* at sexual health services in Australia 2004-08. Sex Health 2011; 8:242–247.

Kemp M, Christensen JJ, Lautenschlager S, et al. European guideline for the management of chancroid, 2011. Int J STD AIDS 2011; 22:241–244.

Manjunatha NP, Jayamanne GR, Desai SP, et al. Pediculosis pubis: presentation to ophthalmologist as pthiriasis palpebrarum associated with corneal epithelial keratitis. Int J STD AIDS 2006: 17:424–426.

Martin I, Sawatzky P, Allen V, et al. Emergence and characterisation of Neisseria gonorrhoea isolates with decreased susceptibilities to ceftriaxone and cefixime in Canada: 2001-2010. Sex Transm Dis 2012; 39:316–323.

Myles TD, Elam G, Park-Hwang E, et al. The Jarisch–Herxheimer reaction and fetal monitoring changes in pregnant women treated for syphilis. Obstet Gynecol 1998; 92:859–864.

Nguyen RH, Nuara AA, Suwattee P, et al. Uveitis and desquamating rash of the palms and soles. Am J Dermatopathol 2013; 35:494–495.

Norlund JJ. Cutaneous ectoparasites. Dermatol Ther 2009; 22:503–517.

O'Farrell N, Moi H. European guideline for the management of donovanosis, 2010. Int J STD AIDS 2010; 21:609–610.

Owlia MB, Eley AR. Is the role of *Chlamydia trachomatis* underestimated in patients with suspected reactive arthritis? Int J Rheum Dis 2010; 13:27–38.

Raychaudhuri M, Peall A, Page C, et al. A case of duplicitous diplococcic. Sex Transm Infect 2009; 85:441–442.

Read PJ, Donovan B. Clinical aspects of adult syphilis. Intern Med J 2012; 42:614–620.

Walker J, Tabrizi SN, Fairley CK, et al. *Chlamydia trachomatis* incidence and re-infection among young women–behavioural and microbiological characteristics. PlosOne 2012; 7:e377778: 1–9.

White J. Manifestations and management of lymphogranuloma venereum. Curr Opin Infect Dis 2009; 22:57–66.

FURTHER READING

Australasian Society for HIV Medicine, Australasian Contact Tracing Manual, 4th edition, 2010 (www.ashm.org.au/ctm).

Holmes KK, Sparling PF, Stamm WE, et al (eds), Sexually transmitted diseases, 4th edn. New York, NY: The McGraw-Hill Companies, 2008.

Russell D, Bradford D, Fairley C (eds), Sexual health medicine, 2nd edn. Melbourne, Australia: IP Communications, 2011.

Chapter 32 Cysts and diseases of the glands

George Meligonis

CYSTS

A cyst is an epithelium-lined cavity or sac usually containing liquid or semisolid material. Vulvar epithelial cysts are the third most common type of benign vulvar adnexal lesions (Baker et al. 2013). Cysts can be classified on the basis of embryological derivation, appendageal structure of origin, or type of epithelial lining (Jenkins & Morgan 2007). Integration of all of these features is required for accurate diagnosis but for a simplified practical approach, division into developmental and appendageal cysts follows (**Table 32.1**).

A schematic diagram demonstrating an outline of the vulvar anatomy (**Figure 32.1**) is used to indicate the most common locations of each cyst.

Developmental cysts

Developmental cysts in the genital area are of mesonephric, paramesonephric (Müllerian), or urogenital sinus origin and may arise from sequestered tissue that has failed to migrate completely during embryogenesis.

Bartholin gland cyst

Origin

Urogenital sinus: cystic dilatation is due to obstruction of Bartholin gland duct.

Site

Major vestibular (Bartholin) glands are bilateral pea-sized glands at the posterior introitus with ducts that empty into the posterolateral vestibule (**Figure 32.2**).

Clinical presentation

- Women of reproductive age
- Size: 1 cm to several centimeters in diameter
- Soft, cystic or nodular lesion (**Figure 32.3**)
- Usually asymptomatic but the development of an abscess is a relatively common complication as the retained glandular secretions become infected

Histopathology

The epithelium is most commonly transitional but squamous, ciliated, mucinous, or a combination of any of these can be found (**Figure 32.4**). Pre-existing glandular acini may be present in the wall of the cyst. Inflammation can result in partial or complete destruction of the cyst lining with abundant neutrophils in the lumen and macrophages in the stroma.

Management

Procedures include insertion of a Word catheter for a cyst or abscess, and marsupialization of a cyst. Cultures for *N. gonorrheae and C. trachomatis* may be obtained; however, abscesses tend to be polymicrobial, and empiric broad-spectrum antibiotic therapy should be used (Omole et al. 2003).

Excisional biopsy is recommended to exclude adenocarcinoma in menopausal or perimenopausal women.

Mucinous and ciliated cyst

Synonyms

Mucous cyst of the vestibule, dysontogenic cyst

Origin

Urogenital sinus

Site

Minor vestibular glands, superior aspect of the labium minus, vestibule or periclitoral area (**Figure 32.5**).

Clinical presentation

- Multiparous women in the third and fourth decades of life
- Smooth surface, superficial, solitary or multiple (**Figure 32.6**)
- Size: 0.5–3 cm
- Usually asymptomatic
- May be related to pregnancy or the use of exogenous hormones

Histopathology

The lining is ciliated columnar/cuboidal epithelium and/or mucinous epithelium (**Figure 32.7**). Mucin is often abundant in the apical cytoplasm of columnar cells and accumulates in the lumen. Many regard them as the minor vestibular gland counterpart of Bartholin gland cyst (Robboy et al. 1978).

Müllerian cyst

Synonym

Paramesonephric cyst

Origin

Müllerian duct remnants

Site

Any part of the upper vagina, commonly the anterolateral wall or areas of vaginal adenosis (**Figure 32.8**).

Clinical presentation

- Symptomatic only if large or secondarily infected
- Size: 1–7 cm

Histopathology

The cyst is lined by epithelium from any part of the female genital tract-endocervical, endometrial, tubal, or a combination of these.

Table 32.1 Differential diagnosis of common cysts

Developmental cysts			
Lesion	**Site**	**Epithelial lining**	**Other findings**
Bartholin gland cyst	Major vestibular gland/duct, posterolateral vestibule	Transitional, squamous, mucinous or combination of these	Usually unilateral Abscess: tender, purulent discharge Luminal contents: mucoid fluid Tissues in wall: small glandular acini
Mucinous and ciliated cyst	Labia minora, minor vestibular glands, periclitoral area	Mucinous and/or ciliated, cuboidal/ columnar	Luminal contents: mucoid fluid Tissues in wall: absence of endometrial stroma
Müllerian cyst	Anterolateral upper vagina	Any upper female genital tract epithelial lining (endocervical, endometrial, tubal)	Luminal contents: mucoid fluid Tissues in wall: absence of endometrial stroma
Mesonephric cyst	Lateral vestibule	Non-mucinous, non-ciliated, cuboidal/ columnar	Luminal contents: clear fluid Tissues in wall: smooth muscle
Mesothelial cyst	Labia majora, mons pubis, groin	Mesothelium	Luminal contents: clear fluid Tissues in wall: smooth muscle
Periurethral cyst	Adjacent to urethral meatus in vestibule	Urothelium	Luminal contents: small calculi (rare) Tissues in wall: nil
Dermoid cyst	Located near skeletal embryonic suture closure lines, especially of skull	Stratified squamous with granular layer	Luminal contents: laminated keratin, hair Tissues in wall: sebaceous glands, hair follicles, sweat glands
Appendageal cysts			
Lesion	**Site**	**Epithelial lining**	**Other findings**
Epidermoid cyst	Labia majora	Stratified squamous with granular layer	Luminal contents: Laminated keratin. Tissues in wall: Foreign body granulomatous inflammation if ruptured
Human papilloma virus-related cyst	Palms and soles	Stratified squamous with viral inclusions/vacuolated 'koilocytic' keratinocytes	Luminal contents: laminated keratin Tissues in wall: nil
Pilar/Trichilemmal cyst	Scalp, labia majora	Stratified squamous without granular layer	Solitary—sporadic Multiple—may be inherited (autosomal dominant) Luminal contents: Compact keratin, cholesterol clefts, calcification Tissues in wall: nil
Hidrocystoma	Periorbital areas, cheek, labia majora	Two cell layers—inner columnar epithelium with eosinophilic decapitation secretion (apical apocrine snouts) and an outer myoepithelial layer. Papillary projections result in overlap with apocrine cystadenoma	Derived from cutaneous apocrine glands, eccrine ducts, or anogenital mammary-like glands; associated hereditary conditions: Schopf-Schultz-Passarge syndrome and Goltz syndrome. Luminal contents: clear fluid Tissues in wall: nil
Steatocystoma	Sternum, axillae, labia majora, abdomen	Stratified squamous with undulating abluminal eosinophilic cuticle	Luminal contents: oily fluid Tissues in wall: sebaceous lobules
Vellus hair cyst	Sternum, axillae, head and neck, extremities	Stratified squamous with or without granular layer	Overlap with steatocystoma but with small vellus hair shafts in lumen
Cutaneous ciliated cyst	Lower legs, buttocks, scalp, trunk, perineum	Ciliated, cuboidal/ columnar, simple or pseudostratified, non-mucinous	Adolescent and young adult women Origin: ectopic Müllerian rests or ciliated metaplasia Luminal contents: clear fluid Tissues in wall: absence of endometrial stroma

Mesonephric cyst

Synonyms

Wolffian cyst, Gartner duct cyst

Origin

Mesonephric duct remnants

Site

Lateral aspect of vulva or vagina (**Figure 32.9**).

Clinical presentation

- Blue-red, thin-walled, translucent cyst containing clear fluid (**Figure 32.10**)
- Size: 1–3 cm
- Usually asymptomatic

Histopathology

Non-mucinous, non-ciliated cuboidal, or columnar epithelium lines the cyst with a layer of smooth muscle in the wall.

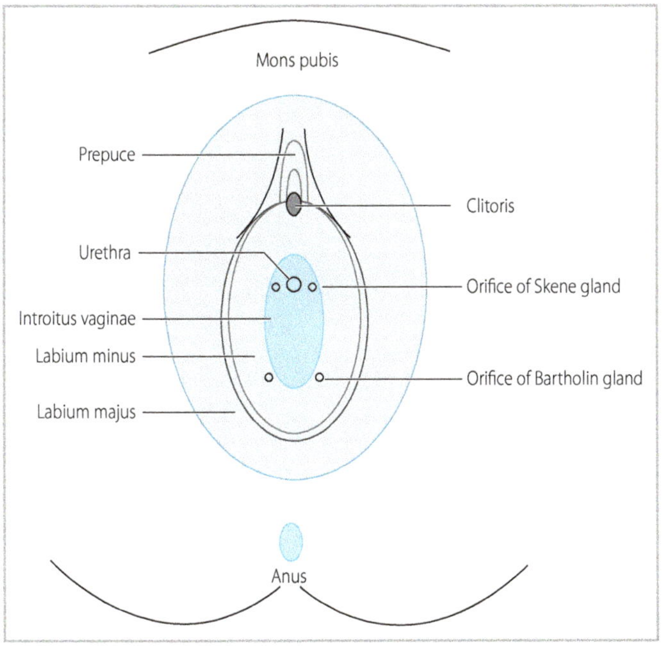

Figure 32.1 Sketch of anatomical structures of the vulva.

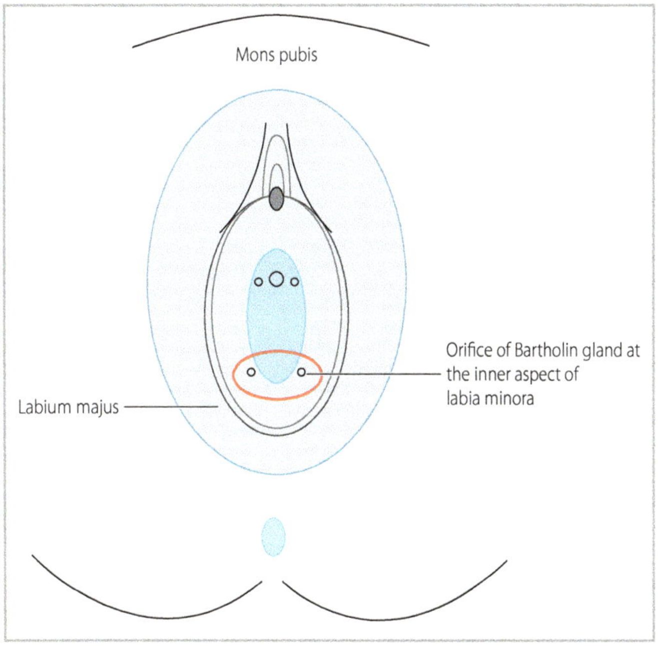

Figure 32.2 Site of presentation of Bartholin gland cysts.

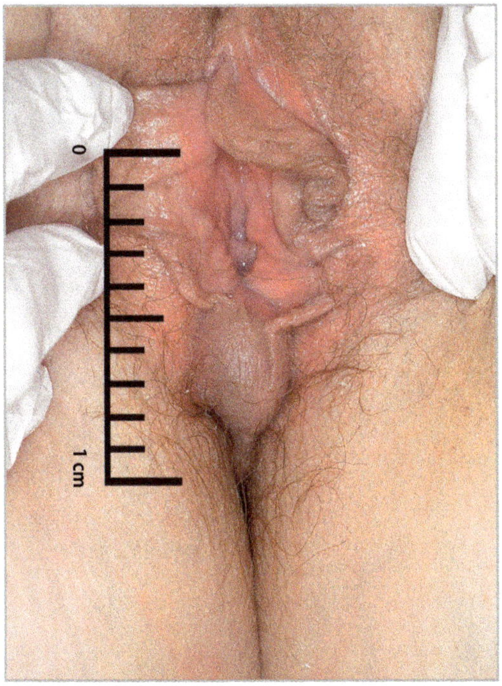

Figure 32.3 Bartholin gland cyst.

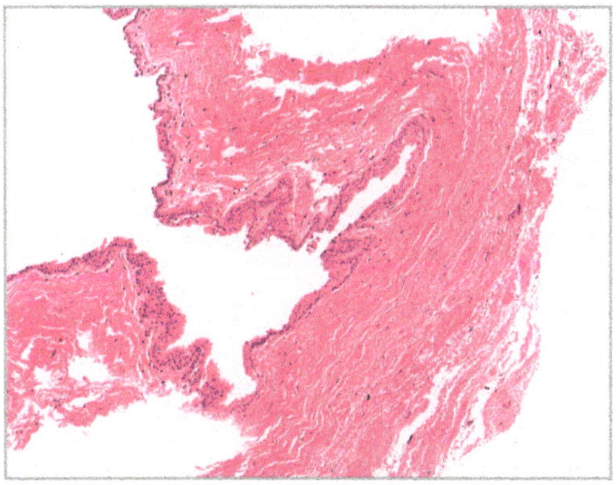

Figure 32.4 Bartholin gland cyst: the cyst has a transitional epithelial lining.

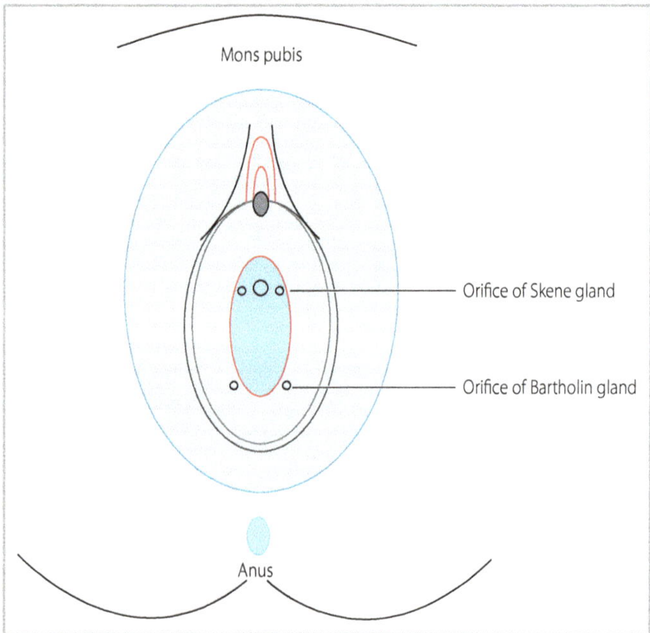

Figure 32.5 Site of presentation of mucinous and ciliated cysts.

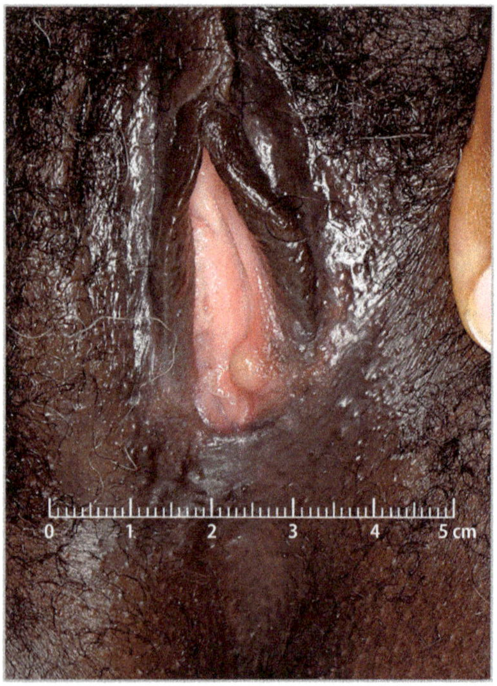

Figure 32.6 Mucinous and ciliated cyst.

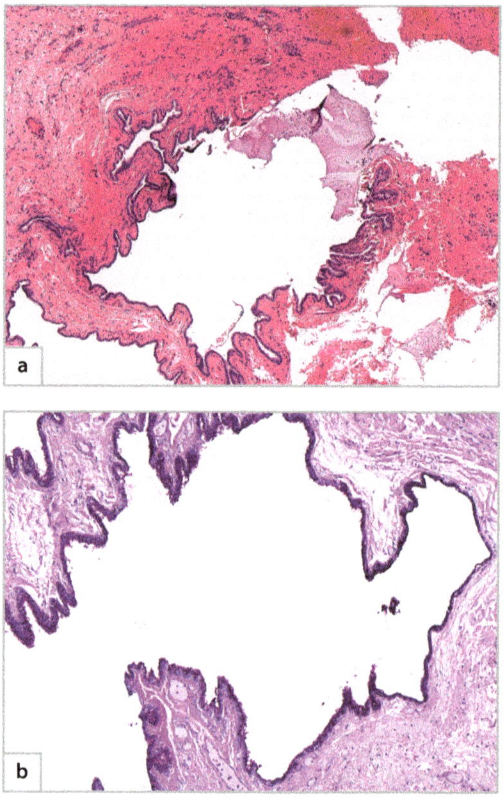

Figure 32.7 Mucinous and ciliated cyst: a single cuboidal layer of mucinous epithelium lines the cyst (a). Diastase Periodic acid–Schiff (PAS) staining highlights the cytoplasmic mucin in the epithelial cells (b).

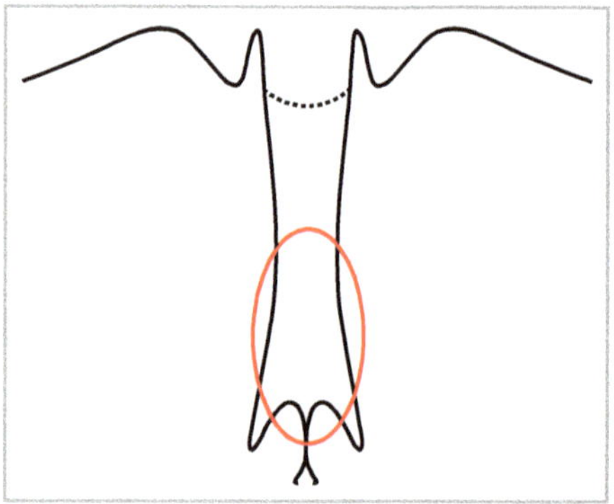

Figure 32.8 Site of presentation of Müllerian cysts.

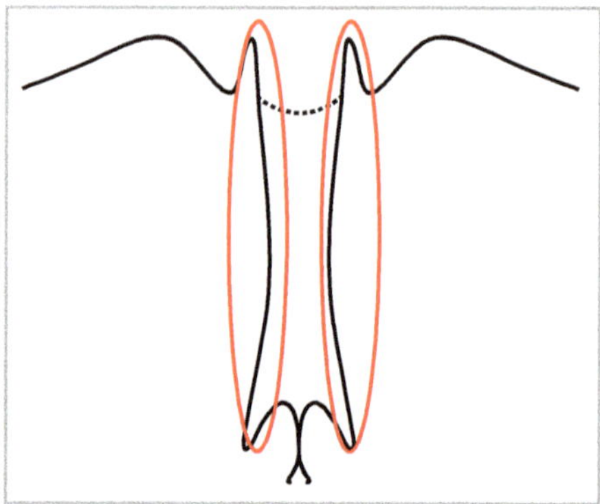

Figure 32.9 Site of presentation of Mesonephric cysts.

Mesothelial cyst

Synonyms

Cyst of canal of Nuck, female hydrocele

Origin

Failure of obliteration of the processus vaginalis peritonei that represents a rudimentary sac of peritoneal mesothelium carried down by the round ligament as it passes through the inguinal canal and inserts into the labium majus.

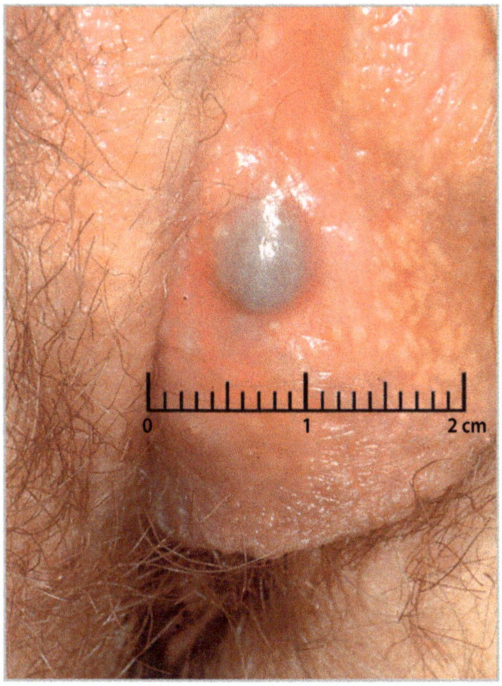

Figure 32.10 Mesonephric cyst.

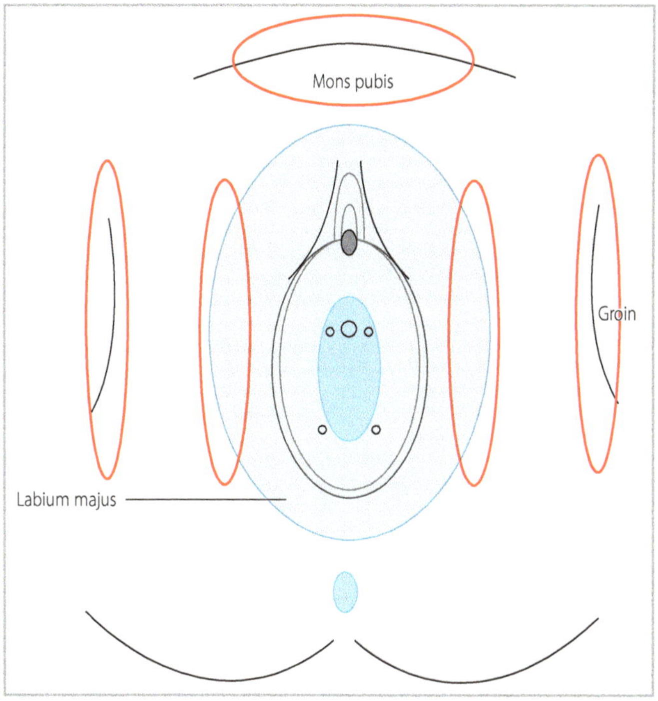

Figure 32.11 Site of presentation of mesothelial cysts.

Site

Inguinal canal, mons pubis, upper, and lateral labium majus (**Figure 32.11**).

Clinical presentation

- Young females
- Non-tender, soft, compressible
- Size: 1–7 cm
- May mimic or occur in association with an inguinal hernia and require herniorrhaphy

Histopathology

There is a single layer of mesothelium—cuboidal/columnar, non-ciliated cells surrounded by a layer of smooth muscle (**Figure 32.12**).

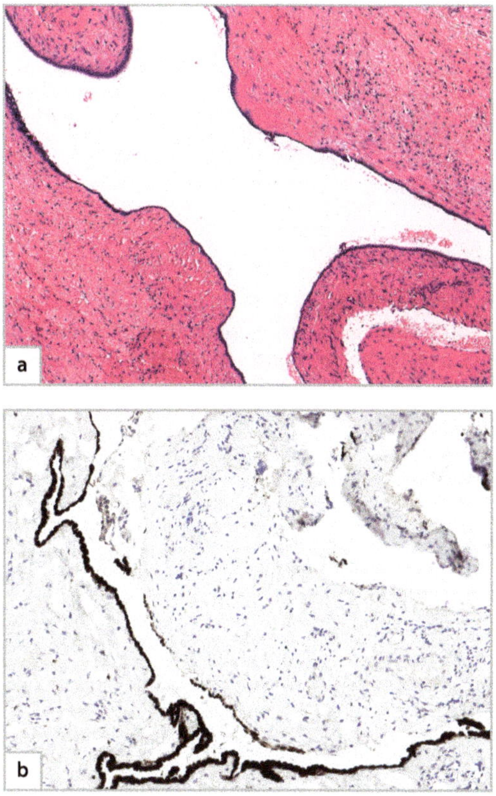

Figure 32.12 Mesothelial cyst: a single layer of mesothelium lines the cyst with smooth muscle in the wall (a). The mesothelial cells can be confirmed immunohistochemically with nuclear calretinin staining (b).

Periurethral cyst

Synonyms

Skene cyst, paraurethral cyst, urothelial cyst

Origin

Urogenital sinus. Skene gland is a paired organ located on either side of the urethral meatus and represents the female homologue of the male prostate.

Site

Upper lateral introitus adjacent to urethral meatus (**Figure 32.13**).

Clinical presentation

- Common in newborns and infants
- Asymptomatic, but if large, may cause urethral obstruction and urinary retention
- Size: 1–2 cm
- Ductal occlusion is thought to be secondary to infection

Histopathology

The lining is transitional epithelium (urothelium).

Appendageal cysts

Appendageal cysts are those derived from the overlying epidermis, pilosebaceous units (hair follicles and apocrine glands) or eccrine ducts.

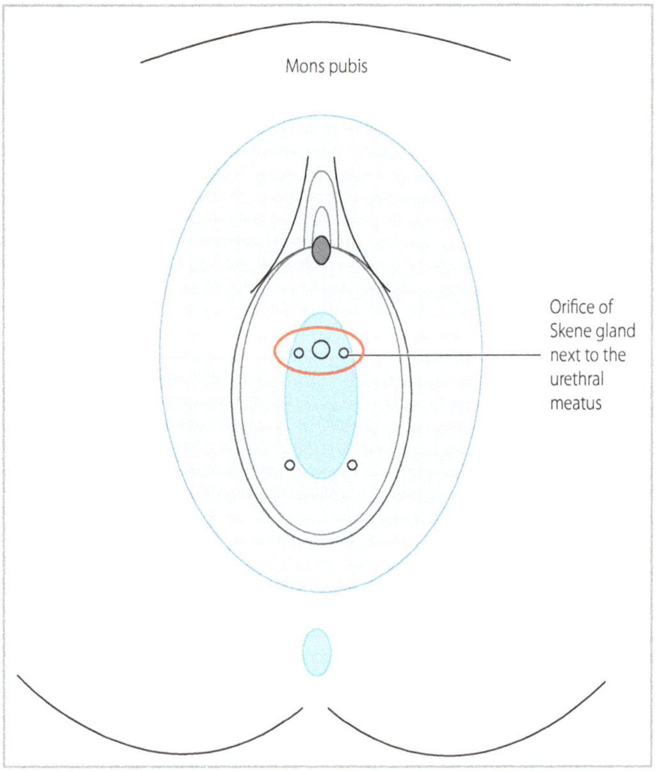

Figure 32.13 Site of presentation of periurethral cysts.

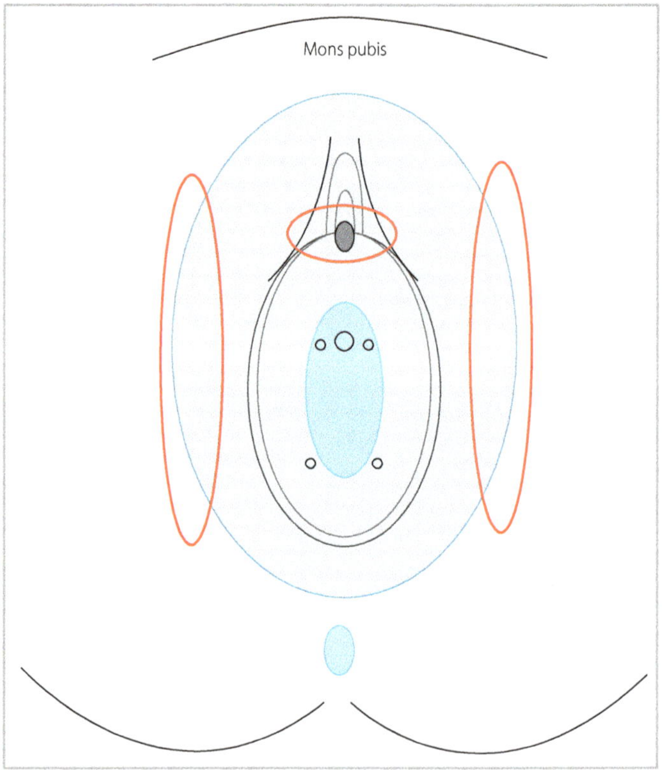

Figure 32.14 Site of presentation of epidermoid cysts.

Epidermoid cyst

Synonyms

Epithelial inclusion cyst, 'sebaceous cyst,' follicular infundibular cyst, keratinous cyst

Origin

Obstruction of hair follicles results in cyst dilatation. Alternatively, penetrating trauma to the skin causes implantation of squamous epithelium into the dermis. Lesions may rarely develop after female genital mutilation.

Sites

Labia majora, clitoris (**Figure 32.14**).

Clinical presentation

- Skin-colored, dome-shaped nodule with rubbery texture sometimes with an overlying punctum
- Size: A few millimeters up to several centimeters
- Foul-smelling cheesy contents can be expressed
- Usually solitary, but if multiple can be a feature of Gardner syndrome (polyposis coli, fibromatosis, jaw osteomas)
- Comedones may enlarge to form multiple small epidermoid inclusion cysts—Comedonal cysts (**Figure 32.15**)

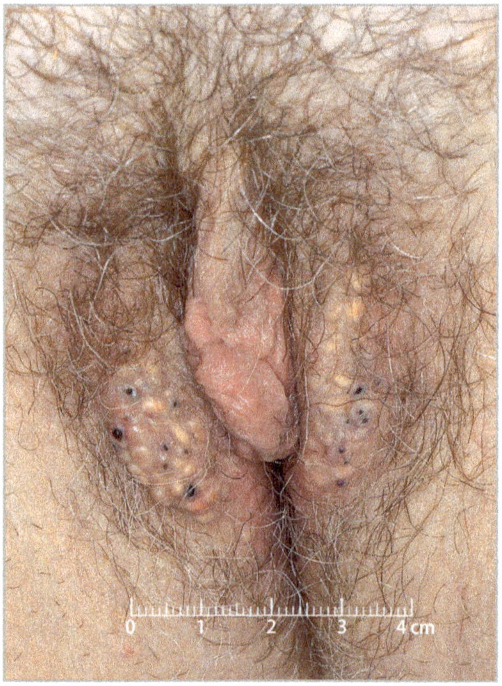

Figure 32.15 Comedonal cysts.

Histopathology

The cyst is lined by an epidermis-like epithelium including a granular cell layer with central lamellar keratinization (**Figure 32.16**). Inflammation may result in rupture of the cyst wall with a subsequent foreign body giant cell reaction that may obscure the cyst and leave behind only keratinaceous debris. Occasional areas of acanthosis or proliferation of the epithelium may result in a so-called proliferating epidermoid cyst. Some cysts demonstrate a lining with verrucous appearance attributed to human papillomavirus infection (verrucous cyst). In Gardner syndrome, part of the cyst lining may resemble a pilomatrixoma (hybrid cyst).

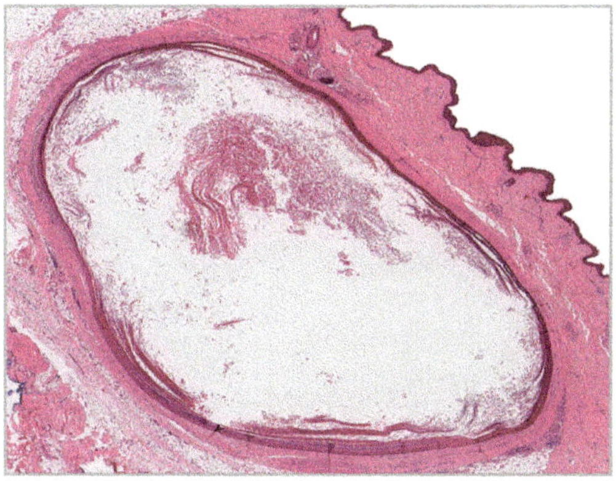

Figure 32.16 Epidermoid cyst: a unilocular cyst with a stratified squamous lining and laminated keratin debris in the lumen.

Steatocystoma

Synonyms

Steatocystoma simplex (solitary) or steatocystoma multiplex (multiple)

Origin

Most cases of the simplex variant are sporadic whereas the multiplex variant may be inherited in an autosomal dominant fashion and associated with mutations in the KRT17 or KRT6B genes, also found in pachyonychia congenita type 2 (Kazakov et al. 2012).

Sites

Chest, neck, scalp, face, axillae, back, vulva and groin (**Figure 32.17**).

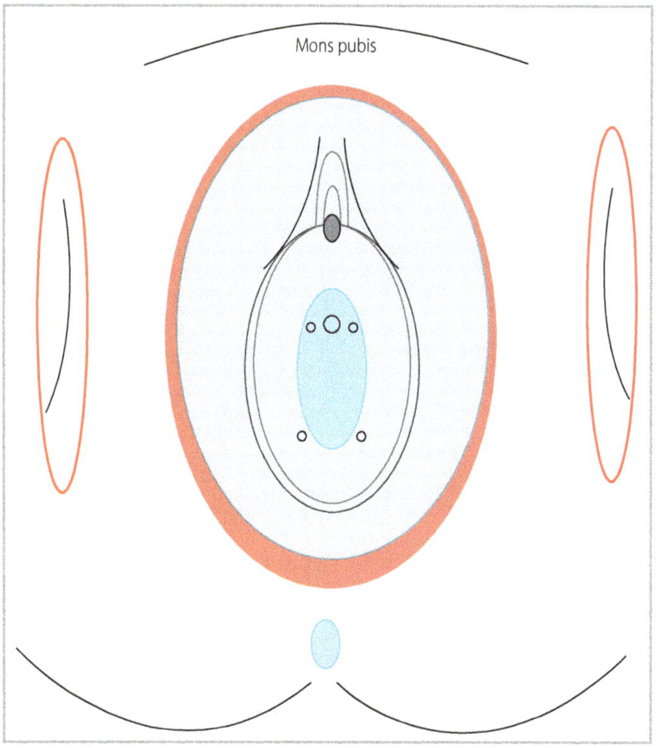

Figure 32.17 Site of presentation of steatocystomas.

Clinical presentation

- Commonly appear in adolescence
- Size: 0.2–3.0 cm
- Yellow to skin-colored cysts and papules

Histopathology

There is a thin lining of squamous epithelium often without a granular cell layer.

An eosinophilic corrugated cuticle on the inner surface of the cyst is characteristic and the wall has variably sized sebaceous lobules (**Figure 32.18**). The lumen is usually empty, but some cases contain small caliber hairs similar to those seen in vellus hair cysts.

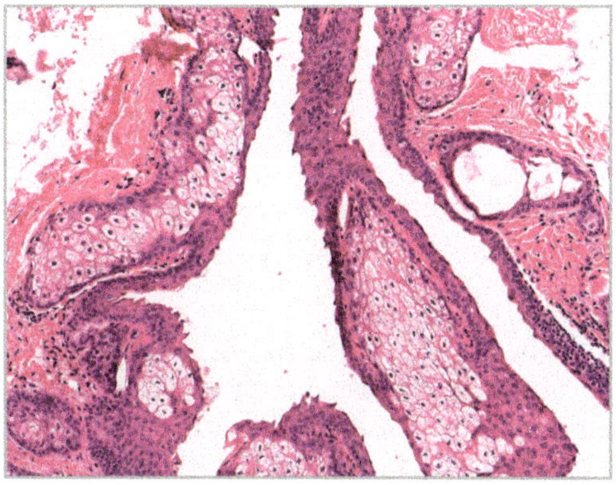

Figure 32.18 Steatocystoma: the cyst lining shows an undulating eosinophilic cuticle with a stratified squamous epithelium and numerous sebaceous lobules in the wall.

Pilonidal sinus

Synonym

Jeep disease

Origin

Inflammatory reaction to hair embedded in the dermis.

Sites

Intergluteal cleft, perineum, vulva, and anal canal (**Figure 32.19**).

Clinical presentation

- Chronic painful draining sinus
- Is a nidus for secondary infection and abscess formation
- Rarely, may be complicated by malignant transformation (usually squamous or basal cell carcinoma)

Histopathology

The sinus is lined by stratified squamous epithelium superficially with abscesses, granulation and scar tissue in the deeper surrounding dermis. One or more hair shaft fragments may occasionally be identified.

Management of cysts

The clinical appearance of cysts is not always specific and can overlap with malignant cystic tumors as well as non-cystic lesions; therefore, simple excision followed by routine histologic examination to render a definitive diagnosis is usually recommended. Once a histologic diagnosis of a benign cyst is made, no further treatment is necessary except for cosmetic reasons or because of irritation from rupture or superinfection.

GLANDULAR DISEASES

Endometriosis

Endometriosis denotes ectopic endometrial tissue. Cutaneous lesions are either scar-related (commonly after hysterotomy, Caesarean section or episiotomy), or the rarer spontaneous endometriosis mostly affecting the umbilicus (**Figure 32.20**).

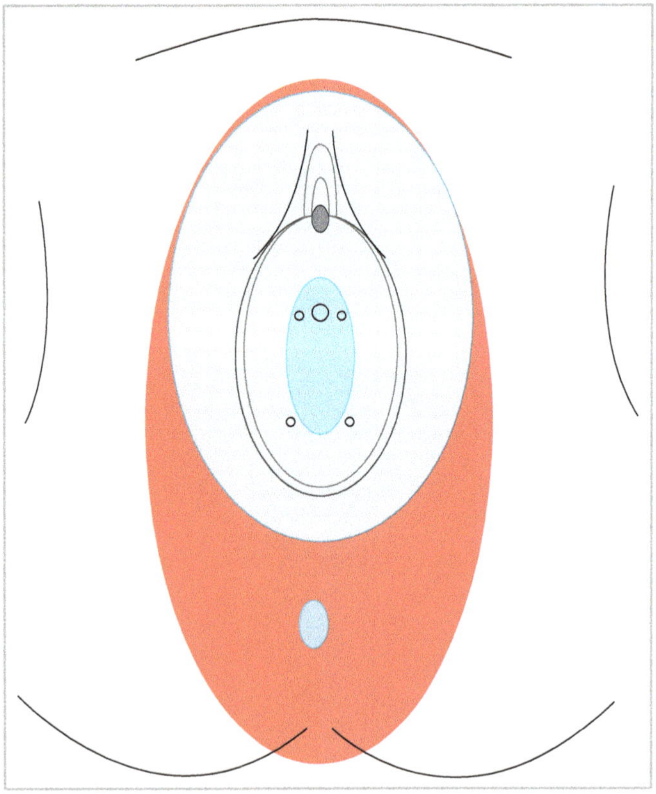

Figure 32.19 Site of presentation of pilonidal sinus.

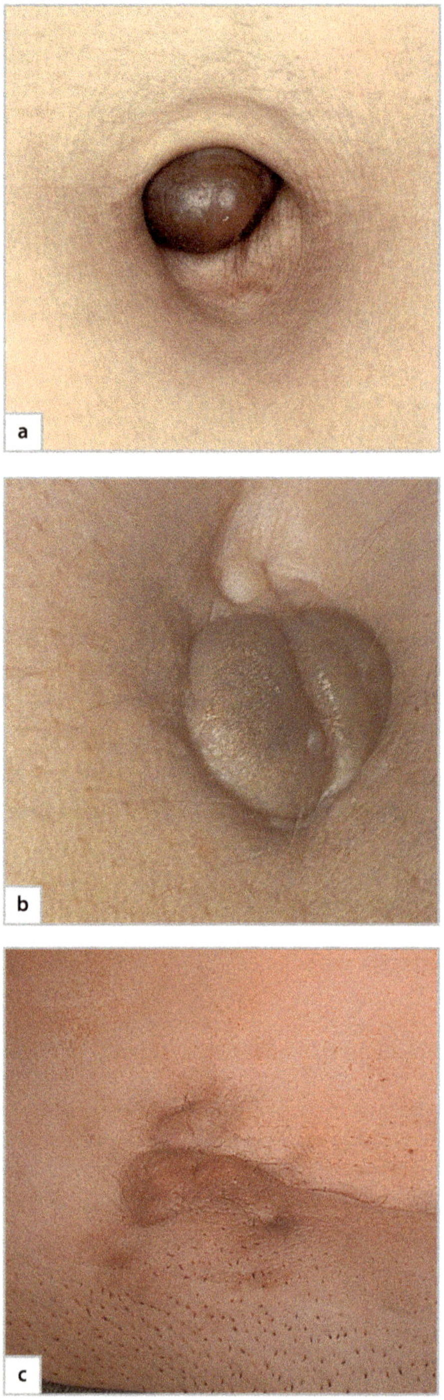

Figure 32.20 (a–c) Endometriosis of the navel and in a scar after a caesarean section. By courtesy of Dr Velja Mijatovic, VUmc Amsterdam and Professor J Keckstein, Villach, Austria.

Clinical presentation

- Young females with a mean age of approximately 35 years
- Usually 3–6 years following surgical procedure in scar-related cases
- Pink to brown superficial cystic mass or deep firm nodules
- May display cyclic enlargement and regression

Histopathology

Both endometrial glands and surrounding stroma are present often accompanied by hemosiderin deposition and variable chronic inflammation (**Figure 32.21**). Accumulation of blood may cause cystic degeneration (endometriotic cyst).

Endosalpingiosis refers to the rare aberrant growth of fallopian tube epithelium only outside its normal location and is also thought to be related to post-surgical implantation (Weedon 2009).

Management

There is no curative treatment for endometriosis. Hormonal treatment with the oral contraceptive pill or gonadotropin-releasing hormone agonists may suppress cyclic changes. Surgical intervention may be needed in troublesome lesions of the skin and elsewhere that may lead to quite extensive surgery, cystectomy in endometrioma of ovaries or possibly laser treatment of peritoneal infiltration.

Fox-Fordyce disease

Synonyms

Apocrine miliaria, chronic itching papular eruption of the axillae and pubic region

Origin

The exact cause is unknown but a hormonal link has been postulated.

Sites

In areas containing apocrine sweat glands—mons pubis, labia majora, perineum (**Figure 32.22**) the axillae, and areola.

Clinical presentation

- Multiple, firm, flesh-colored or pigmented folliculocentric papules (**Figure 32.23**)
- Size: 2–5 mm
- 90% occur in women of reproductive age
- Sometimes progress during pregnancy and may subside after menopause

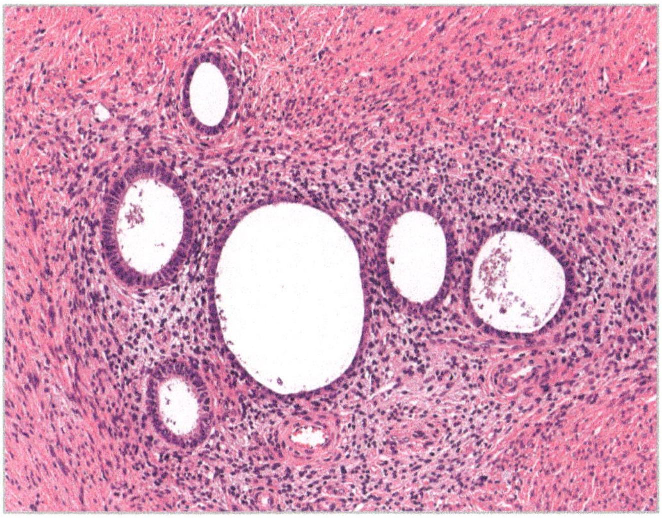

Figure 32.21 Endometriosis: ectopic endometrial glands surrounded by endometrial stroma.

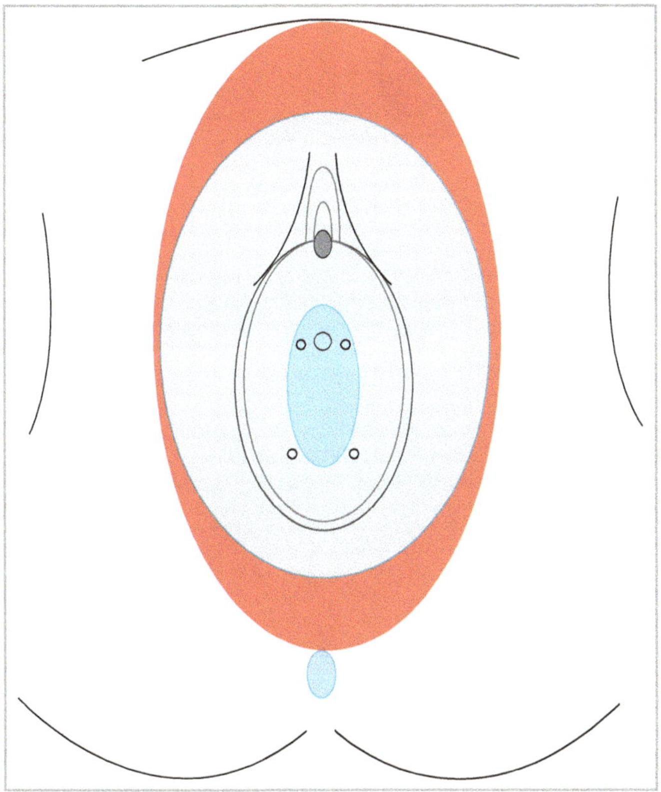

Figure 32.22 Typical genital sites for Fox–Fordyce disease.

Histopathology

There is dilatation with acanthosis and spongiosis of the follicular infundibulum with plugging and occasionally cornoid lamellation. Foamy histiocytes and a lymphocyte infiltrate are often present around infundibula and apocrine ducts.

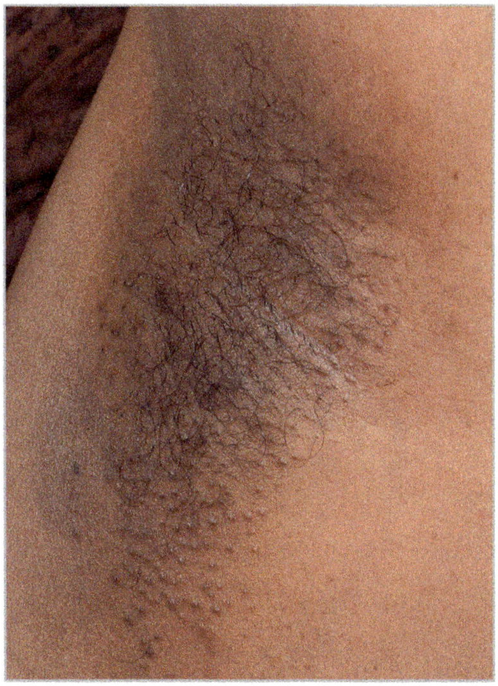

Figure 32.23 Fox–Fordyce disease.

Management

Definitive therapy is not established, although relief of symptoms may be achieved with the use of oral contraceptives, antibiotics (e.g. topical clindamycin), antipruritics, topical steroids, and isotretinoin (Kurman et al. 2011); surgery including CO_2 laser treatment is used successfully too.

Benign mucinous metaplasia

Mucinous metaplasia of the vulva is a rare phenomenon of the genital area of elderly females. It is clinically non-distinctive and occurs in conjunction with an inflammatory process, usually lichen sclerosus or Zoon vulvitis (Kazakov et al. 2012). The lesions may be quite extensive, involving both labia minora, the clitoral hood, and part of the introitus.

It needs to be distinguished from mucinous syringometaplasia, extramammary Paget disease, cutaneous squamous cell carcinoma in situ with mucinous metaplasia, superficial spreading malignant melanoma, and epidermotropic metastasis.

Histopathology

The normal or inflamed squamous epithelium is focally replaced by columnar cells that contain cytoplasmic mucin (**Figure 32.24**). Immunohistochemically, the cells stain for CK7, CEA, EMA, and CAM5.2. The important distinction from extramammary Paget disease is based on the lack of nuclear atypia in metaplastic epithelium and infiltration of the epidermis in the latter (Böer-Auer et al. 2011).

Management

The underlying inflammatory disease needs to be treated.

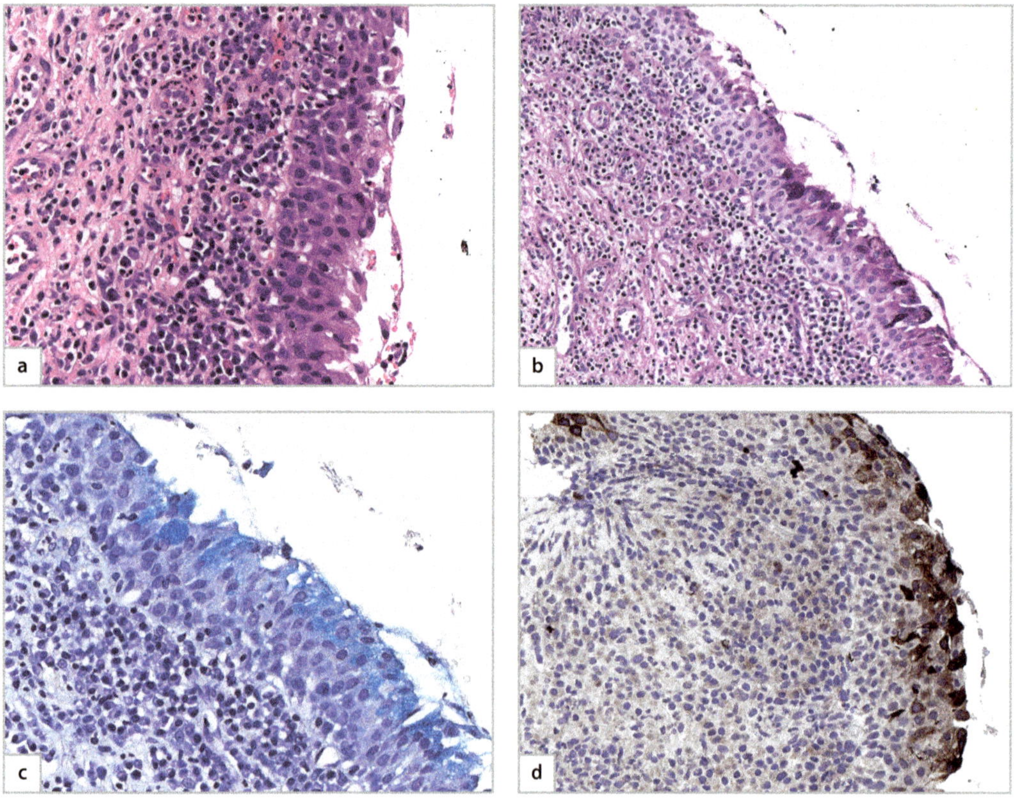

Figure 32.24 Benign mucinous metaplasia: a biopsy from the labia minora in a case of Zoon vulvitis showing mucinous metaplasia of the surface layer of the epithelium (a). Cytoplasmic mucin is highlighted with diastase PAS (b) and alcian blue (c). The mucinous cells are immunoreactive with CK7 (d).

REFERENCES

Baker GM, Selim MA, Hoang MP. Vulvar adnexal lesions: a 32-year, single-institution review from Massachusetts General Hospital. Arch Pathol Lab Med 2013; 137:1237–1246.

Böer-Auer A, August C, Falk TM, et al. Benign mucinous metaplasia of the genital mucosa: histomorphological and immunohistochemical features and criteria for differentiation from extramammary Paget disease. Br J Dermatol 2011; 165:1263–1272.

Jenkins JR, Morgan MB. Dermal cysts: a dermatopathological perspective and histological reappraisal. J Cutan Pathol 2007; 34:815–829.

Kazakov DV, McKee PH, Michal M, et al. Cutaneous adnexal tumors, 1st edn. Philadelphia, PA: Lippincott Williams & Wilkins, 2012

Kurman RJ, Ellenson LH, Ronnett BM. Blaustein's Pathology of the female genital tract, 6th edn. New York, NY: Springer, 2011.

Omole F, Simmons BJ, Hacker Y. Management of Bartholin's duct cyst and gland abscess. Am Fam Physician 2003; 68:135–140.

Robboy SJ, Ross JS, Prat J, et al. Urogenital sinus origin of mucinous and ciliated cysts of the vulva. Obstet Gynecol 1978; 51:347–351.

Weedon D. Weedon's Skin pathology, 3rd edn. New York: Churchill Livingstone, Elsevier, 2009.

Chapter 33 Solid benign tumors

Iskander H Chaudhry, William James Merchant

INTRODUCTION

This chapter covers commonly encountered entities, as well as highlighting some less well-known mesenchymal tumors that can be locally aggressive (**Table 33.1**).

Key features

- Solid benign tumors may be divided into three categories:
  - Surface epithelial tumors
  - Adnexal or glandular tumors
  - Mesenchymal tumors
- Many present as a solitary lump and may only be diagnosed by histological evaluation
- Rarely benign tumors may be a feature of a syndrome such as Birt–Hogg–Dubé; Cowden or Muir–Torre syndrome

Solid benign tumors

These derive from various tissues and are categorized accordingly:

- Surface epithelium
- Adnexal or glandular structures
- Soft tissue or mesenchyme

While surface epithelial tumors may show scaling, assisting with the clinical diagnosis, most neoplasms discussed in this chapter have fairly nondescript clinical appearances and require histological evaluation. Many are difficult to diagnose from clinical appearances alone. These entities should be considered in the light of chapter 34 (*Benign and malignant pigmented lesions of the vulva*), as it is important to exclude malignancy when evaluating solid cutaneous tumors.

Table 33.1 Most frequent types of benign solid tumors found in the vulva

	Benign Tumor	Single or multiple	Distribution	Associations
Surface epithelial	Seborrheic keratosis	Usually multiple	Found all over the body	Usually none but sudden eruption of multiple lesions in young patients may be paraneoplastic
With adnexal or glandular differentiation	Syringoma	Usually multiple	Frequently found on the eyelids	Increased in Down syndrome; rarely part of Brooke–Spiegler syndrome
	Nodular hidradenoma	Usually solitary	Any site	
	Benign mixed tumor	Usually solitary	Any site	
	Papillary hidradenoma (hidradenoma papilliferum)	Solitary	Vulva most frequent site	
	Trichoblastoma	Usually solitary, may be multiple	Any site	
	Fibrofolliculoma	Marker for a syndrome if multiple	Face and upper trunk	Multiple in Birt–Hogg–Dubé–syndrome
Mammary-type	Hamartomas	Solitary	Any site along the milk line	
Mesenchymal	Fibroma molle (skin tag) (**Figure 33.1**)	May be solitary or multiple	Flexural sites including axillae, groins and neck	
	Leiomyoma	Usually solitary in vulva, may be multiple elsewhere	Any site	Multiple with uterine fibroids may be associated with renal cell cancer or Alport syndrome
	Aggressive angiomyxoma	Solitary, may be pedunculated	Almost exclusively present in vulva region	
	Cellular angiofibroma	Solitary	Vulva	
	Angiomyofibroblastoma	Solitary	Almost exclusively occur in vulva region	

SURFACE EPITHELIAL TUMORS

Seborrheic keratosis

Clinical presentation

Seborrheic keratoses typically occur on the labia majora of middle-aged or elderly women. The lesions range from light tan to dark brown in color and are well demarcated and often slightly raised (**Figure 33.2a**). Horn pseudocysts may be visible in the structure of the lesion. In the flexures, the warty surface may be lost. Dermoscopy reveals milia-like cysts. Solitary lesions need to be differentiated from malignant melanoma. Rare neoplasms such as myoepithelioma of the vulva should be distinguished from more common epithelial and mesenchymal neoplasms (Fukunaga 2003).

Histopathology

There is a proliferation of bland keratinocytes (**Figure 33.2b**) that can lead to acanthosis and anastomotic cords, with characteristic 'squamous eddies' (defined as eosinophilic flattened squamous cells arranged in an onion-like pattern). No cytological atypia is seen, however. The role of human papillomavirus in seborrheic keratosis is unclear with conflicting results in the literature (Hai et al. 2003, Zhang et al. 2005). The main differentials to consider are viral warts (Chapter 30) and possibly melanoma (Chapter 34). Viral warts demonstrate hypergranulosis, papillomatosis, and 'church spire' parakeratosis. Viral inclusions may be seen on histology.

Management

No treatment is necessary but lesions may be shave-excised or treated with cryotherapy if symptomatic.

TUMORS SHOWING ADNEXAL DIFFERENTIATION (ECCRINE/APOCRINE TUMORS) AND GLANDULAR DIFFERENTIATION

Solid tumors of the sweat glands can arise from dermal constituents: syringomas, hidradenomas (clear cell and poroid types), mixed tumors. Mixed tumors may also arise from Bartholin glands, ectopic breast tissue, or mammary-type glands (Scurry et al. 2009).

Syringoma

Syringomas are benign adnexal tumors of the sweat glands (Huang et al. 2003). They may be solitary but are usually multiple, presenting as skin-colored dermal papules. Giant lesions, in plaque form, may occur. They are asymptomatic but are sometimes itchy. Often a clinical diagnosis is possible (**Figure 33.3**).

Histopathology

Syringomas comprise small ducts lined by cuboidal epithelium, some of which contain eosinophilic material (**Figure 33.4a**). These ducts have a 'comma-like' tail (**Figure 33.4b**).

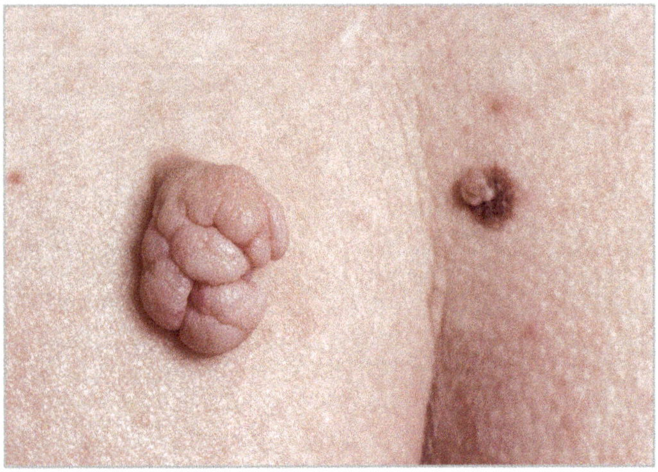

Figure 33.1 Soft fibroma/skin tags are common and frequently appear at flexural sites such as axillae and groins. By courtesy of Prof. Theo Starink, Amsterdam, the Netherlands.

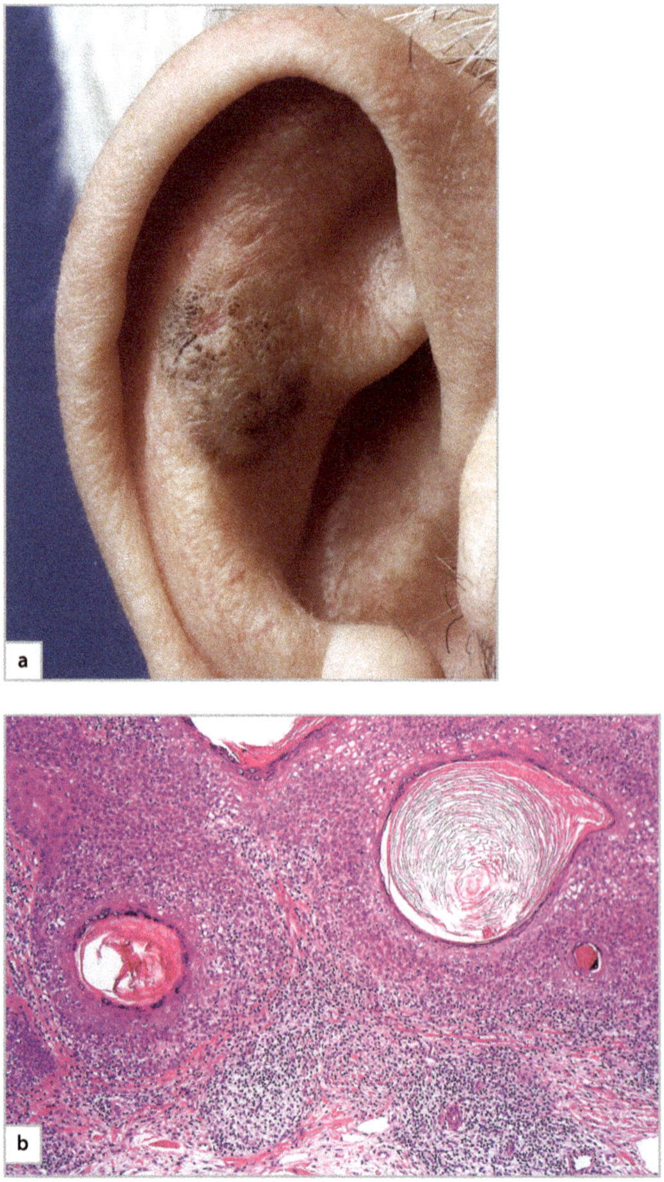

Figure 33.2 Seborrheic keratosis on the ear, with typical waxy surface, different colors and keratotic plugging (a). By courtesy of Prof. Theo Starink, Amsterdam; a proliferation of bland keratinocytes with acanthosis and horn pseudocysts on histology (b).

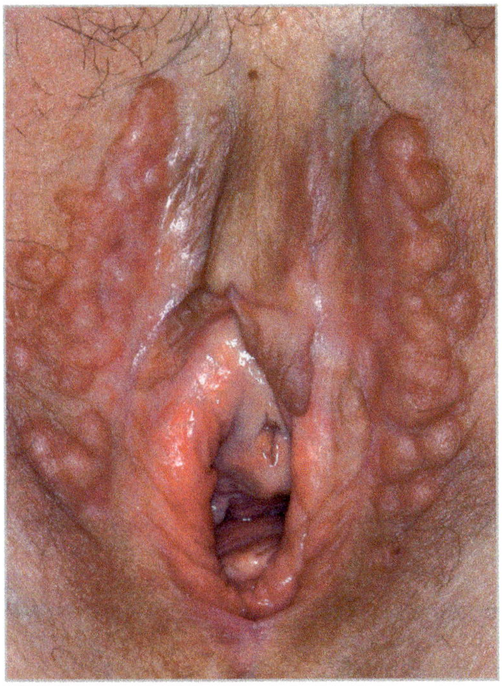

Figure 33.3 Multiple skin-colored papules of syringoma. By courtesy of Dr Gudula Kirtschig, Tübingen.

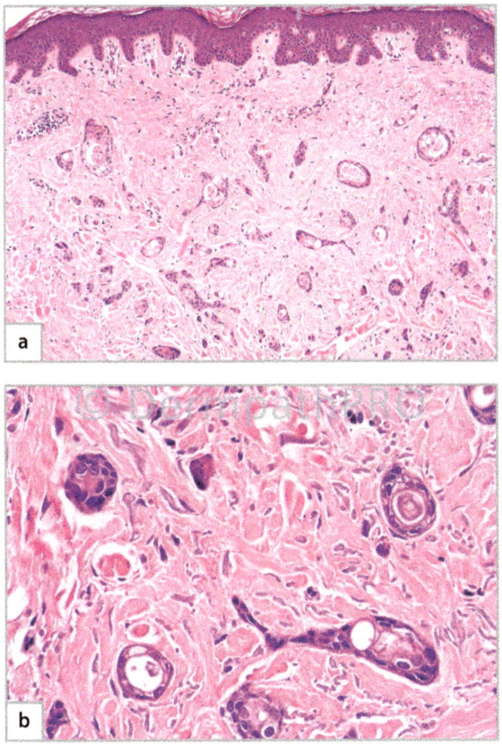

Figure 33.4 An ill-defined superficial tumor composed of small ducts lined by cuboidal epithelium, some of which contain eosinophilic material (a). Some ducts have a 'comma-like' tails (b).

Management

No treatment is necessary.

Nodular hidradenoma

Nodular hidradenomas may be eccrine or apocrine in origin (El Demellawy et al. 2008). They form solitary nodules that are often partly solid, partly cystic. Histologically, there is ductal differentiation and intracytoplasmic lumina. Two types of cells are visible, one polyhedral with a rounded nucleus and a basophilic cytoplasm, the other round with a clear cytoplasm. Clear cell change may be prominent giving the designation clear cell hidradenoma. Mitotic figures are often present, although this is of little prognostic significance.

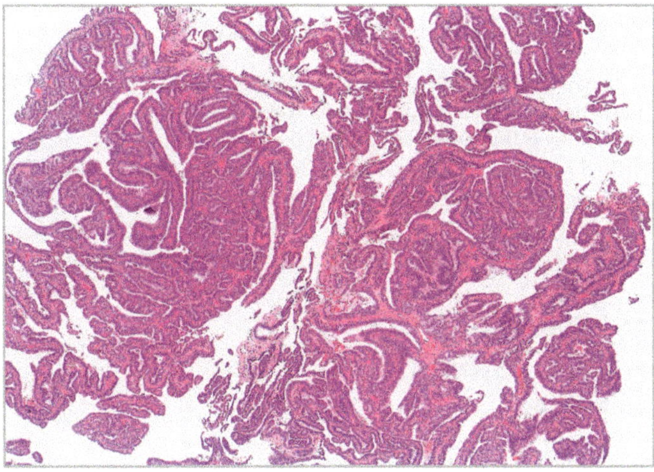

Figure 33.5 Papillary hidradenoma shows a villoglandular growth pattern with complex papillary structures.

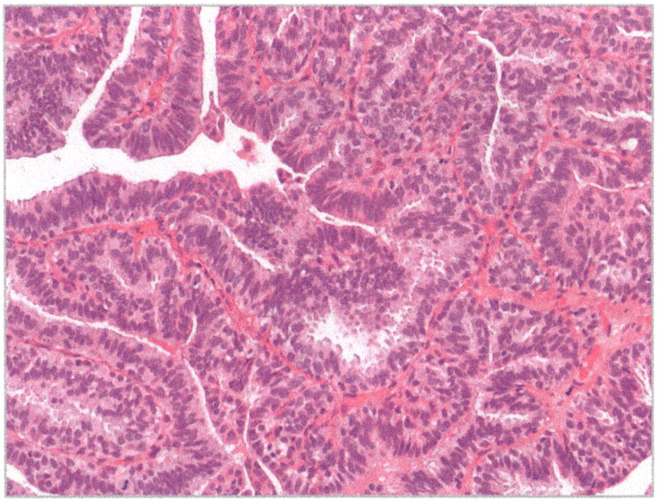

Figure 33.6 Papillary hidradenomais typically lined by columnar cells with no cytological atypia.

Papillary hidradenoma (hidradenoma papilliferum)

Papillary hidradenoma, arising from apocrine glands in reproductive age and postmenopausal patients, can occur at any site but are typically found on the labia (Woodworth et al. 1971). They arise as small skin-colored papules but are almost never diagnosed from clinical appearances alone. They are histologically well circumscribed, and demonstrate a villoglandular growth pattern with complex papillary structures (**Figures 33.5** and **33.6**). Very rarely malignant transformation occurs into apocrine carcinoma. Intraductal papilloma arising in ectopic breast tissue should be considered in the differential diagnosis.

BENIGN MIXED TUMORS

Benign mixed tumors are the cutaneous counterpart of mixed tumors (pleomorphic adenoma) of the salivary gland, and are therefore sometimes called 'mixed tumors of the skin'. They are well circumscribed tumors located in the dermis and subcutaneous tissue and typically occur in middle-aged and elderly patients. These tumors consist of epithelial components (nests, islands, ducts, and tubular structures) set in a chondroid, myxoid, and/or fibrous stroma.

Follicular tumors

Trichoblastoma

Synonyms

Trichoepithelioma, trichoblastic fibroma

Trichoblastomas are well circumscribed, dermal symmetrical tumors composed of basaloid islands with peripheral palisading (**Figure 33.7**). Follicular differentiation is apparent, but they typically lack high grade atypia, mitoses, and retraction artifact. Specific to vulva is the giant variant of trichoepithelioma (Regauer & Nogales 2005).

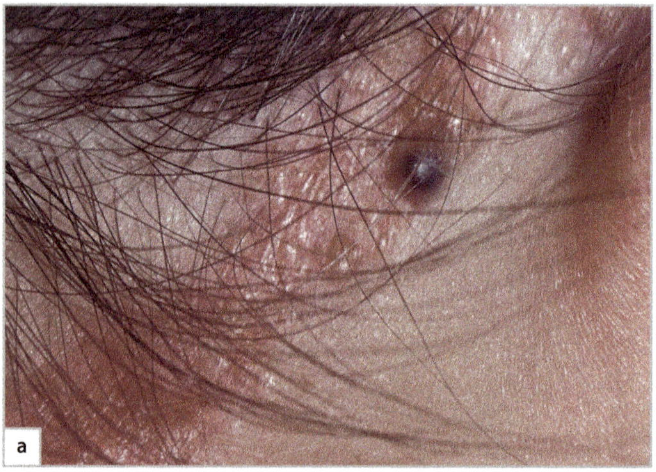

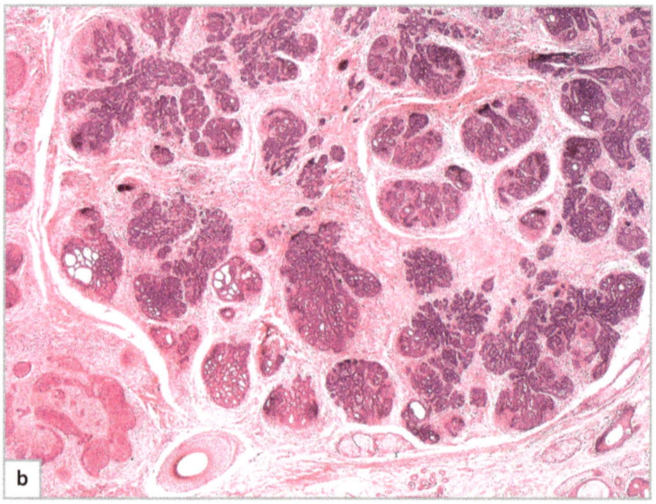

Figure 33.7 Well circumscribed, slightly pigmented papule behind the ear (a). By courtesy of Prof. Theo Starink, Amsterdam, the Netherlands. Trichoblastoma is a well circumscribed, dermal symmetrical tumor composed of basaloid islands with peripheral palisading. Follicular differentiation is apparent (b)

The main differential here is basal cell carcinoma. Basal cell carcinomas tend to be ulcerated, show artificial clefting, and lack advanced trichogenic differentiation and show nuclear atypia. Other follicular tumors that can arise are fibrofolliculoma (seen in Birt-Hogg-Dubé, **Figure 33.8**), inverted follicular keratosis, and pilar tumors.

SOFT TISSUE/MESENCHYMAL TUMORS

A wide spectrum of mesenchymal tumors can arise in the vulva, with overlapping clinical, and immunohistochemical features making for a challenging diagnosis (McCluggage 2005).

Leiomyomas

Genital leiomyomas arise from dartos and vulvar smooth muscles and are similar to pilar leiomyomas. They are usually solitary in the vulva area and present as small red/brown flesh-colored papules. They are histologically ill-defined with interlacing fascicles of smooth muscle (**Figure 33.9**). Rarely, they are familial and associated with multiple lesions (**Figure 33.10**), uterine fibroids, and renal cell carcinoma. No treatment for individual lesions is required, but they are usually excised in the vulvar site.

Angioleiomyomas

Angioleiomyomas arise from muscles of veins and are well circumscribed and contain numerous vessels interspersed with smooth muscle fibers.

Aggressive angiomyxoma

Aggressive angiomyxoma occurs in women of reproductive age; vulvar masses may be considered clinically for Bartholin cysts or a hernia. Although they are typically indolent in behavior, they have a tendency to recur after incomplete excision. Lesions may become very large and pedunculated.

Histological appearance is of a hypocellular spindle cell tumor set in a loose myxoid stroma, with scattered blood vessels. Unlike other vulvar mesenchymal tumors, 50% express HMGA2.

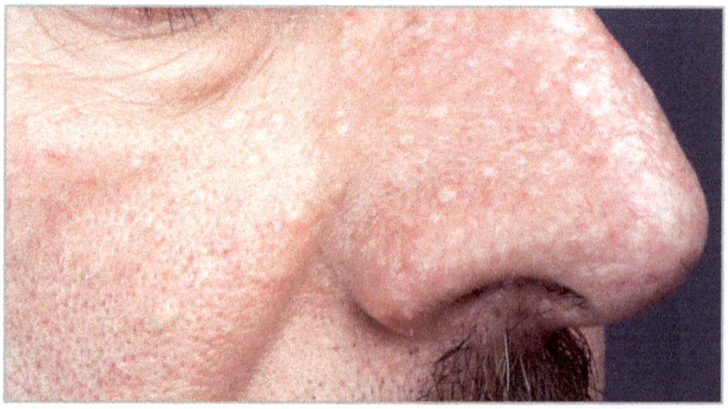

Figure 33.8 Fibrofolliculoma in Birt–Hogg–Dubé syndrome usually appears on the face and upper trunk. This syndrome is a autosomal dominant genetic disorder and may cause susceptibility to kidney cancer, renal, and pulmonary cysts, and non-cancerous tumors of the hair follicles, called fibrofolliculomas. By courtesy of Prof. Theo Starink, Amsterdam, the Netherlands.

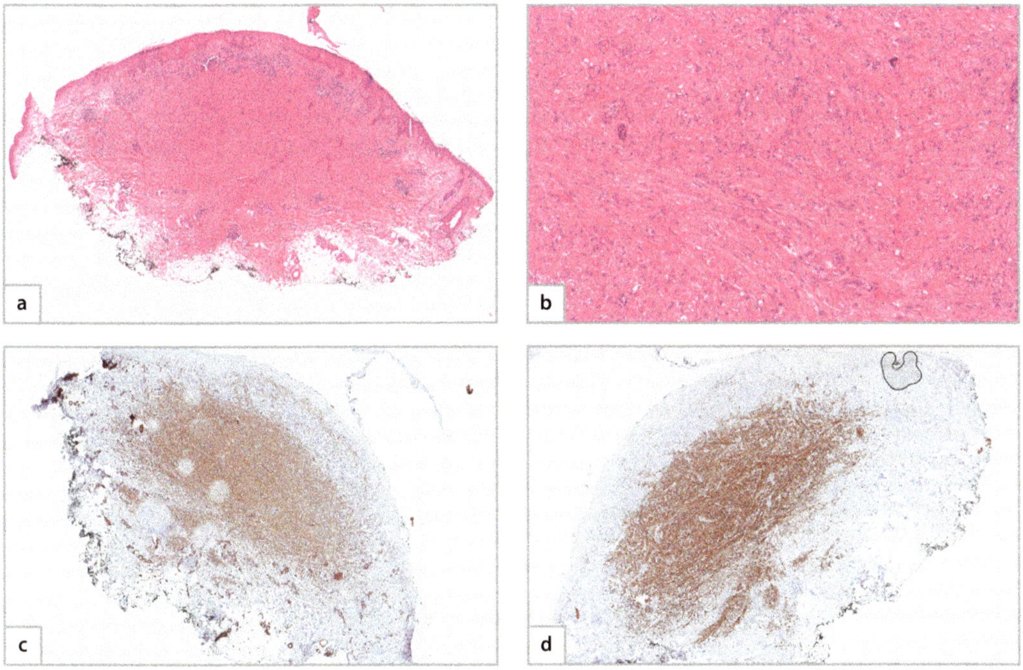

Figure 33.9 (a) Cutaneous leiomyoma: histology shows an ill-defined smooth muscle tumor arising in the dermis. (b) The tumor cells form fascicles and show no nuclear atypia. (c, d) The tumor is positive for smooth muscle immunohistochemical markers (c, SMA stain; d, desmin stain).

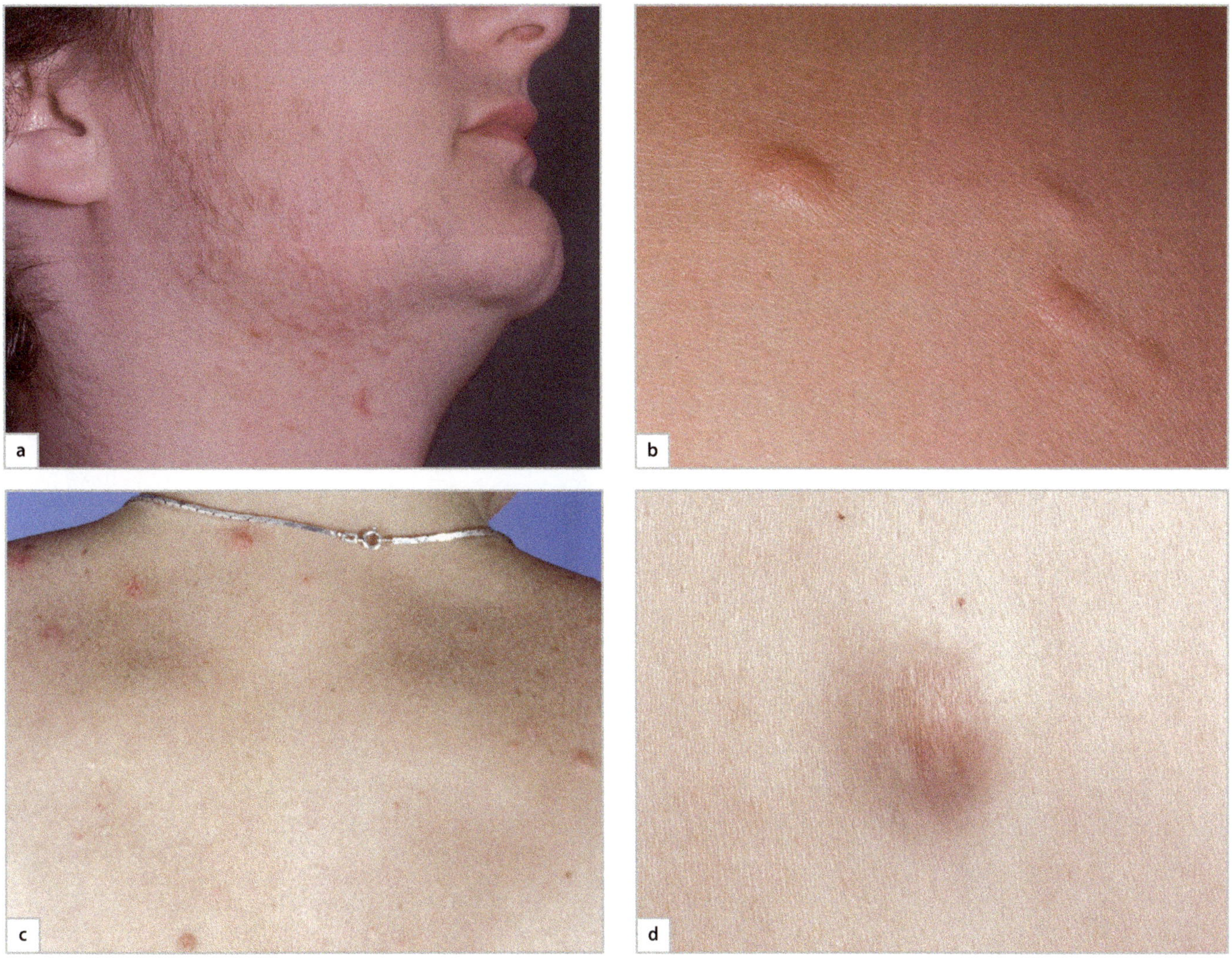

Figure 33.10 Multiple leiomyomas on the face and neck (a, b) and back (c, d). By courtesy of Prof. Theo Starink, Amsterdam, the Netherlands.

Cellular angiofibroma

Cellular angiofibromas are well circumscribed tumors arising in reproductive age and postmenopausal patients. They are unlikely to be diagnosed until after excision. Median size is 2.8 cm, but some lesions can reach 12 cm in size. As the name suggests, the histology shows cellular proliferation of spindle cells in interlacing fascicles. Mitoses are not commonly seen.

Angiomyofibroblastoma

Angiomyofibroblastoma presents as a painless vulvar mass in adult women. Histology shows hypercellular and hypocellular areas with thin walled arborizing vessels. Although benign, angiomyofibroblastoma may recur after excision.

Other

Prepubertal vulvar fibroma, superficial myofibroblastoma, rhabdomyomas, superficial angiomyxoma, and granular cell tumors can arise at this site. Fibrous, neural, vascular, and adipocytic tumors may also occur.

MALIGNANT COUNTERPARTS

Rare malignant examples of adnexal and glandular tumors can arise at this site such as adenocarcinoma of Skene gland origin, hidradenocarcinomas, and adenoid cystic carcinomas. Malignancy must always be considered and histopathological examination of any new mass is recommended.

REFERENCES

El Demellawy D, Daya D, Alowami S. Clear cell hidradenoma: an unusual vulvar tumor. Int J Gynecol Pathol 2008; 27:457–460.

Fukunaga M. Myoepithelioma of the vulva. APMIS 2003; 111:416–420.

Hai H, Cviko A, Granter S, et al. Immunophenotypic and viral (human papillomavirus) correlates of vulvar seborrheic keratosis. Hum Pathol 2003; 34:559–564.

Huang Y, Chuang Y, Kuo T, et al. Vulvar syringoma: a clinicopathologic and immunohistologic study of 18 patients and results of treatment. J Am Acad Dermatol 2003; 48:735–739.

McCluggage WG. A review and update of morphologically bland vulvovaginal mesenchymal lesions. Int J Gynecol Pathol 2005; 24:26–38.

Regauer S, Nogales FF. Vulvar trichogenic tumors. A comparative study with vulvar basal cell carcinoma. Am J Surg Pathol 2005; 29:479–484.

Scurry J, van der Putte SC, Pyman J, et al. Mammary-like gland adenoma of the vulva: review of 46 cases. Pathology 2009; 41:372–378.

Woodworth H Jr, Dockerty MB, Wilson RB, et al. Papillary hidradenoma of the vulva: a clinicopathologic study of 69 cases. Am J Obstet Gynecol 1971; 110:501–508.

Zhang H, Storthz K, Malpica A. Vulvar seborrheic keratosis, is it indeed related to HPV infection? [Abstract] Mod Pathol 2005; 18:209A.

Chapter 34 Benign and malignant pigmented lesions of the vulva

Sigrid Regauer

INTRODUCTION

An estimated 1 in 10 women has a pigmented lesion on their vulva. Melanin accounts for the vast majority of vulvar pigmentation, although hemosiderin and tattoo pigment may also result in pigmentation. The number and distribution of melanocytes in the female genital area do not vary between the different parts (labia majora, minora, introitus), but the melanocytes in modified mucosa produce and transfer more pigment to keratinocytes and in glycogenated mucosa contain immature melanosomes with scant mature pigment.

Etiology

Melanocytic lesions may be divided according to etiology into three main groups:

- Pigmentary changes associated with inflammatory disease
- Hyperpigmentation without melanocytic proliferation
- Melanocytic proliferations (benign or malignant)

Further classification

- Post-inflammatory pigmentary disorders of the vulva
  - Related to underlying disease
  - As a treatment reaction
- Hyperpigmentation due to increased melanin production without proliferation of melanocytes
  - Pigmented epithelial neoplasms
  - Melanosis
- Melanocytic proliferations
  - Benign melanocytic proliferation
    - Lentigo simplex
    - Melanocytic nevi
      - Congenital nevus
      - Atypical melanocytic nevus of genital type (AMNGT)
      - Blue nevus cell nevus
      - Spitz nevus
      - Common acquired nevus
  - Malignant melanoma of the vulva
    - Cutaneous malignant melanoma
    - Mucosal malignant melanoma

The clinical terminology of localized hyperpigmentations is not uniform. In particular, the terms melanosis and lentigo are used interchangeably in clinical settings, contributing to considerable confusion in the published literature and interdisciplinary communication.

POST-INFLAMMATORY PIGMENTARY DISORDERS OF THE VULVA

Introduction

Post-inflammatory hyperpigmentation is due to:

- An underlying disease
- As a treatment reaction

Lichen planus and lichen sclerosus as prototypes of lichenoid and vacuolar interface dermatoses are typically associated with post-inflammatory pigmentary changes. Infections, e.g. tinea and herpes virus infection, may also result in pigmentation; fixed drug reactions are an important cause of asymmetrical genital pigmentation. Treatment-induced inflammatory reaction, e.g. after therapy with tacrolimus (Kim & Kang 2007), imiquimod (O'Mahony et al. 2010), and laser ablation are common.

Pathogenesis and histopathology

The lymphocytic infiltrate disrupts the basement membrane and injures cell membranes of basal keratinocytes and melanocytes. Melanin granules are released from the cytoplasm into the subepithelial tissues and are phagocytosed by dermal and submucosal macrophages. Clusters of dermal melanophages cause patchy and irregular hyperpigmentation. Destruction of melanocytes leads to a (temporary) loss of melanin production and patches of hypopigmentation (O'Mahony et al. 2010).

Clinical features and management

An underlying skin disease is usually recognizable, e.g. lichen planus (**Figure 34.1a** and **b**). The alternating hypo- and hyperpigmented areas are macular changes with no induration or tumorous impression. Fixed drug reactions (see Chapter 17) result in patches of asymmetrical pigmentation with episodic inflammation related to the causative drug.

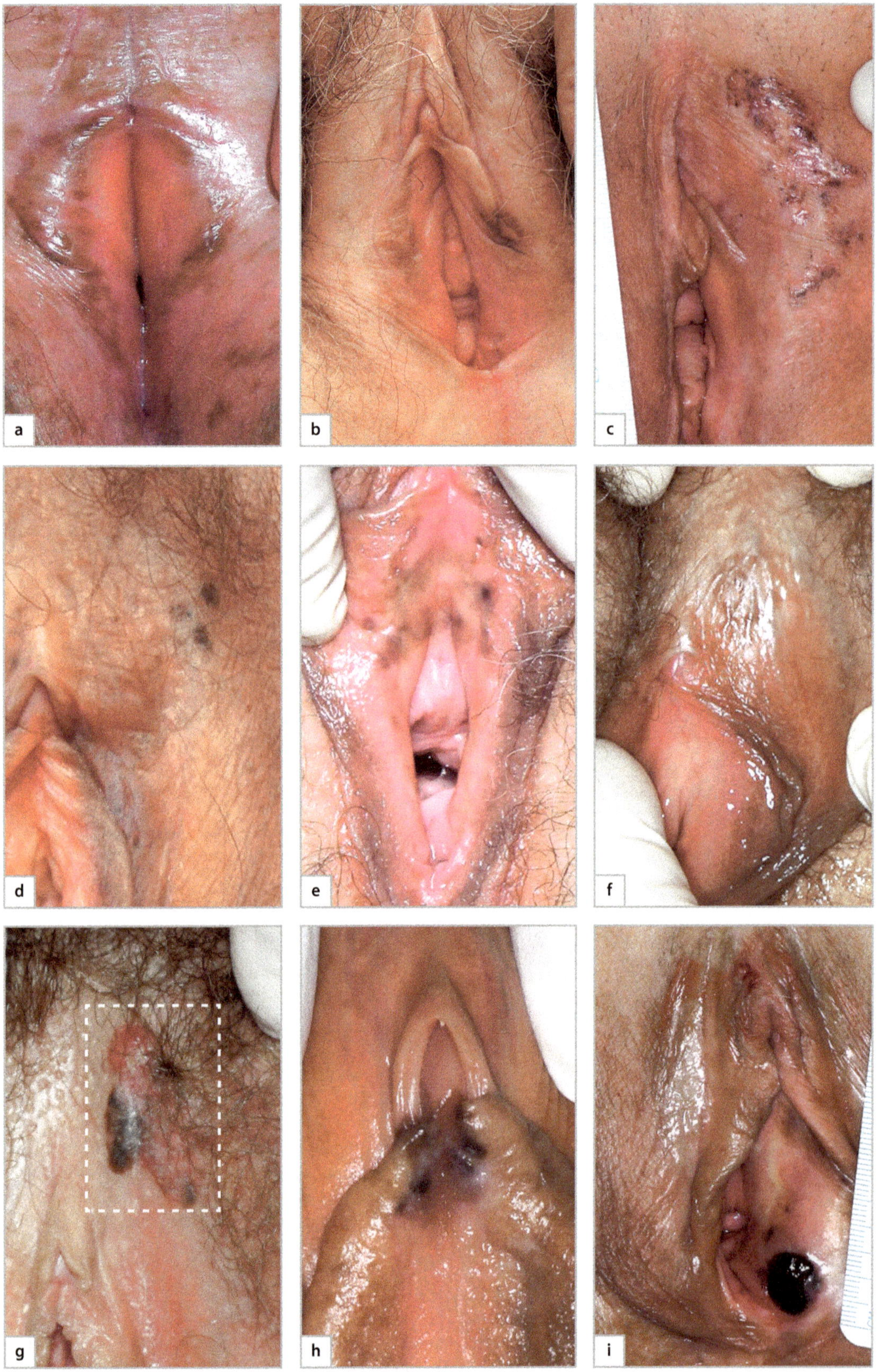

Figure 34.1 Pigmented vulvar lesions. (a–c) Pigmentary changes associated with dermatoses and epithelial neoplasms. (a) Diffuse pigmentary changes in a 78-year-old woman with advanced long-standing vulvar lichen planus with alternating hypo- and hyperpigmented macules (courtesy of Dr Barbara Eberz, Mürzzuschlag, Austria). (b) Localized hyperpigmentation of the posterior labium minus in a patient with lichen planus (courtesy of Dr Barbara Eberz, Mürzzuschlag, Austria). (c) A trichoepithelioma presenting as pigmented indurated plaque with irregular surface and pigmentation (courtesy of the Gynecology Department, Medical University Graz, Austria). (d–f) Clinical variations of lentigo simplex. (d) Three grouped, slightly depressed, well-circumscribed macules and plaques of lentigo simplex in a 51-year-old woman (courtesy of Dr Barbara Eberz, Mürzzuschlag, Austria) (e) Multiple irregular macular lesions in the anterior vestibulum of a 52-year-old woman (courtesy of Gynecology Department, Medical University Graz, Austria). (f) A lentigo simplex with numerous yellow nodules corresponding to sebaceous glands in a 37-year-old woman (courtesy of the Gynecology Department, Medical University Graz, Austria; see histology in Figure 34.2f). (g–i) Malignant melanoma of vulva. (g) Cutaneous pT3b malignant melanoma of a 36-year-old woman with regional lymph node metastasis (courtesy of Gynecology Department, Medical University Graz, Austria) and a b-raf mutation (V600E) presenting as asymmetrical plaque with poor circumscription toward hair-bearing skin (box), variegated color and shades, a diameter of >1 cm and recent growth. This patient died of disseminated metastases at age 42 years, 6 years after initial diagnosis. (h) pT1a malignant melanoma of a 49-year-old woman arising in periclitoral modified mucosa featuring asymmetry, poor circumscription, variegated color, and central regression/ulceration (courtesy of the Gynecology Department, Medical University Graz, Austria). This patient developed liver metastases 6 years later and died of disease. (i) pT4 nodular malignant melanoma in glycogenated vestibular mucosa of introitus vaginae of a 85-year-old-woman (courtesy of the Gynecology Department, Medical University Graz, Austria). Note at least two additional dark pigmentations toward vagina and an adjacent vaginal discoloration. She died of widespread metastatic disease within 1 year after diagnosis.

Patients should be made aware of the possibility of post-inflammatory hyperpigmentation after treatments associated with inflammation. Due to the characteristic clinical presentation, a correct diagnosis on clinical grounds is possible. Therapy is not necessary or possible and it may be advised that hyperpigmentation may resolve spontaneously with time (months to years).

Differential diagnosis

Precancerous epithelial lesions or melanocytic proliferations need to be excluded and a biopsy performed if there is diagnostic doubt.

HYPERPIGMENTATION DUE TO INCREASED MELANIN PRODUCTION WITHOUT PROLIFERATION OF MELANOCYTES

- Pigmented epithelial neoplasms
- Melanosis

Introduction

Acquired hyperpigmentation without melanocytic proliferation may occur in association with an epithelial neoplasm or as macular hyperpigmentation without neoplasia.

Pigmented epithelial neoplasms

• Benign:	Seborrheic keratosis, hidrocystoma and trichoepithelioma/trichoblastoma
• Premalignant:	Vulvar intraepithelial neoplasia (VIN) (human papillomavirus [HPV]-induced squamous epithelial lesions >> HPV-negative dVIN)
• Malignant:	Basal cell carcinoma, Paget disease

In the vulvar skin and modified mucosa, precursor lesions of invasive squamous cell carcinoma may be pigmented (or whitish when hyperkeratotic), in particular the HPV-induced high-grade squamous intraepithelial lesions (HSIL), old terms are usual VIN (vulvar intraepithelial neoplasia), Bowen disease and Bowenoid papulosis (Crum et al. 2014). Plaques of HPV-negative differentiated VIN (dVIN) typically occurring in the background of lichen planus and lichen sclerosus can also be pigmented.

Clinical features

HPV-induced vulvar HSIL is usually asymptomatic, but can be itchy and sore, rarely painful and give rise to pigmented asymmetrical papules and plaques that are often well demarcated. In mucosal sites, they are more discrete and may be visualized with application of 3-5% acetic acid. Pigmented Paget disease is unusual, but may present as slowly expanding asymmetrical plaque or spread in a diffuse papular pattern (Chapter 36).

Differential diagnoses

Pigmented plaques of hypertrophic lichen planus/sclerosus and seborrheic keratoses are the main differential diagnoses. Hidrocystoma or trichoepithelioma (**Figure 34.1c**) in vulvar skin and modified mucosa may be confused with a pigmented basal cell carcinoma that presents as an isolated nodular and pearly lesion or patches (Regauer & Nogales 2005).

Melanosis

Melanosis is an acquired localized macular hyperpigmentation in vulvar modified mucosa without associated epithelial and melanocytic proliferation. Many clinicians refer to any circumscribed macular hyperpigmentation in the vulva as 'melanosis' independent of the clinical presentation.

Clinical presentation ranges from diffuse symmetrical hyperpigmentation of both labia minora, to numerous brown or dark macules with irregular outlines involving labia minora, interlabial sulcus, and the vestibule, or small grouped macules. Due to the lack of proliferative activity, there should be no induration, plaque, or tumor (Rudolph 1990).

Pathogenesis and histopathology

The stimulus for increased melanin production and transfer to (basal) keratinocytes remains elusive. Melanosis may be related to hormonal stimuli (e.g. pregnancy). Histologically, melanosis shows darkly pigmented basal keratinocytes without melanocytic proliferation, inflammatory infiltrate, loss of pigment, and subepithelial melanophages, and most importantly, a regular melanocyte/keratinocyte ratio. Since melanocytes cannot be reliably identified in hematoxylin and eosin (HE)-stained sections, their demonstration requires immunohistochemical analysis with melanocytic markers.

Differential diagnosis

A pigmented epithelial proliferation may raise the differential diagnosis of melanocytic neoplasia. Melanosis may be indistinguishable from macular lentigo simplex, or rarely an in situ malignant melanoma. A biopsy may be helpful to distinguish them.

Management and prognosis

When in doubt, pigmented lesions should be biopsied or excised. Malignant epithelial and melanocytic tumors and precursor lesions need to be treated. Melanosis has no malignant potential.

MELANOCYTIC PROLIFERATIONS

Introduction

Melanocytic neoplasia can be divided into benign and malignant proliferations, and the ABCDE rule (**Table 34.1**) can assist in this separation. Photographic documentation allows an objective evaluation of changes over time. If a pigmented lesion is suspicious and clinically not unequivocally identifiable as benign or malignant, a biopsy or excision is advised. In contrast to earlier belief, biopsies of pigmented lesions are not harmful or associated with worse prognosis.

Benign melanocytic proliferations

Subtypes of benign melanocytic proliferations

- Lentigo simplex
- Melanocytic naevi

Table 34.1 Clinical evaluation of melanocytic lesions: ABCDE rule

Nevus cell navus	Malignant melanoma
A Symmetrical lesion	A Asymmetry
B Sharp borders	B Poorly circumscribed borders
C Uniform color	C Variegated color
D Small diameter, usually <4 mm	D Large diameter, usually >6 mm
E Evolution: no change	E Evolution: recent change, e.g. growth, itch, ulceration

Lentigo simplex

Synonyms

Lentigines, melanotic macules

Introduction

Clinically, the terms melanosis and lentigo simplex often are used synonymously. Lentigo simplex results from proliferation of single melanocytes within basal keratinocytes, resulting in an increased melanocyte/keratinocyte ratio (Barnhill et al. 1990). With the exception of the rare congenital syndromes (LEOPARD syndrome, LAMB syndrome, Peutz-Jeghers syndrome, Bannayan–Riley–Ruvalcaba syndrome, and the Carney complex), vulvar lentigo simplex is an acquired lesion in adult/older women with unclear etiology. A lentigo simplex has no malignant potential (Rhodes et al. 1984).

Clinical features

Lentigo simplex presents with small, round, or oval-shaped macules with a smooth or jagged outline and may range in color from light brown to black. They may occur anywhere on the genital skin including mucous membranes, may be multiple and are asymptomatic. Occasional small, slightly lighter nodules (sebaceous glands) can be appreciated within the pigmented areas (**Figure 34.2a**).

Histopathology

There are increased melanocytes within the basal layer of the epithelium that typically shows an increase in epithelial thickness (acanthosis). The small yellow nodules within the pigmented areas correspond to hyperplastic sebaceous glands. A flat and depressed lentigo simplex reveals subepithelial fibrosis. The reason for the proliferative stimulus on epithelial cells and sebaceous glands is unclear (**Figure 34.1d,e** and **34.2e**).

Differential diagnosis

The differential diagnosis of a solitary lentigo simplex is melanosis or an early malignant melanoma and a biopsy may be needed for correct diagnosis. Unequivocal distinction of melanosis and lentigo simplex is achieved immunohistochemically via demonstration of increased melanocytes within the basal layer of the epithelium. Dendrites may be rather prominent. In a lentiginous melanoma, the proliferating melanoma cells are individual cells no longer restricted to the basal keratinocyte cell layer, but extending through all layers of the epidermis. Dermatoscopy may be helpful for this distinction; however, this may be difficult to apply at the vulva (Mannone et al. 2004, Ronger-Savle et al. 2011).

Management and prognosis

Having no malignant potential, a lentigo simplex can be followed expectantly without further therapy.

Melanocytic nevi

Synonym

Nevus cell nevi

Introduction

Congenital melanocytic nevi develop from a premature cessation of melanocyte migration along their migration from the neural crest to their final destination in pigmented tissues during fetal development. They are present at birth. Acquired nevi develop in young women from melanocytes that have reached their final destination within the epidermis.

Subtypes of melanocytic nevi

- Congenital nevi
- Atypical melanocytic nevus of genital type (AMNGT)
- Blue nevus cell nevi
- Spitz nevi
- Common acquired nevi

Clinical features and histology

Congenital nevi

Congenital nevi are flat or elevated pigmented plaques or nodules. They occur mostly at cornified sites of the vulva. They are composed of nests or sheets of melanocytes in epidermis, dermis, skin appendages, muscle, lymphatic vessels, and/or fatty tissue. Hairy congenital nevi are rare in the vulva.

Atypical melanocytic nevus of genital type

Synonyms

Flexural nevus, milk line nevus, nevus of special site

AMNGT (**Figure 34.3**) are asymptomatic and often incidentally discovered pigmentations on the labia minora and clitoris of children and young women (e.g. during pregnancy). They are dark brown or black macules or papules with warty architecture and a diameter between 2 mm and 20 mm (typically >10 mm). The black color may raise the concern of a melanoma clinically.

On histology, presence of cytologic atypia in the large epidermal and dermal nests of epithelioid uniform cells that contain large course melanin granules and prominent nucleoli, pagetoid intraepithelial spread and dermal mitoses may be worrisome. Some publications/pathologists refer to these nevi erroneously as dysplastic nevi, but they lack eosinophilic and lamellar fibroplasia. A close interdisciplinary interaction and clinico-pathological exchange will ensure a correct diagnosis (Brenn 2011, Clark et al. 1998, Gleason et al. 2008).

Blue nevus cell nevi

Synonyms

Nevus coeruleus, related lesions such as nevus of Ota/nevus of Ito

Clinically, they present as well-circumscribed, small macules, or nodules of very dark color. The cell of origin is unknown, but believed to arise from a melanocytic precursor cell of which migration was arrested in the dermis. In syndromes, they are multiple, can be seen at any site, and are typically present at birth or very young age. They occur together with hyperpigmentations in the Carney complex. The vast majority, however, occur as acquired sporadic blue nevi, in children or young adults of any age in keratinized skin and in mucosa.

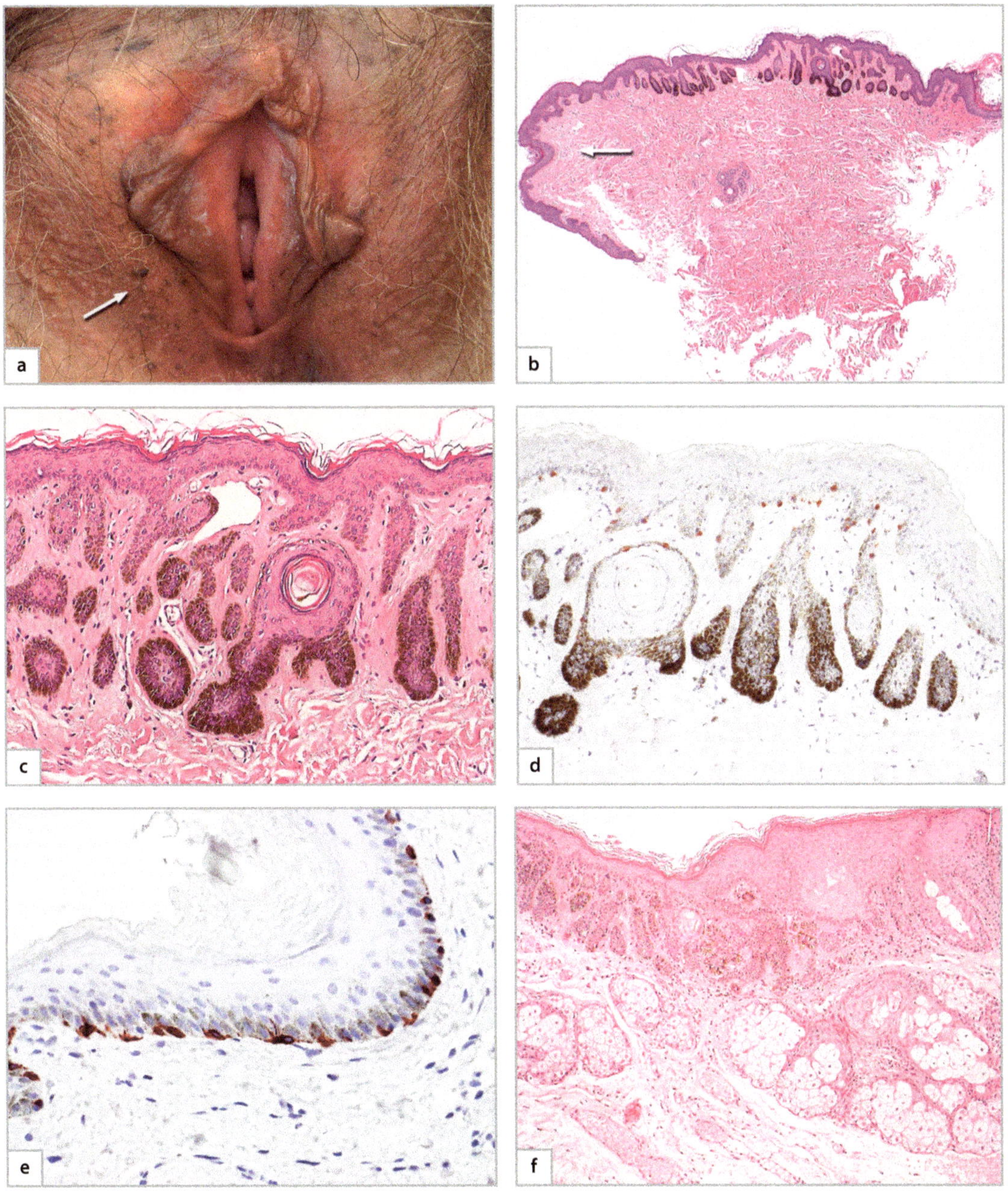

Figure 34.2 Lentigo simplex. (a) A 78-year-old woman with numerous, grouped, darkly pigmented macules, small papules, and plaques on the entire vulva. One papule (arrow) was resected (by courtesy of Dr. Barbara Eberz, Mürzzuschlag, Austria. (b) The excisional biopsy revealed a well-circumscribed pigmented lesion. The area at the arrow tip is shown in (e). (c) In the central portion of the lesion, the epidermis reveals elongated rete with hyperpigmentation of basal keratinocytes. The subepithelial connective tissue is fibrotic with wide vessels. No mitotic activity is seen. (d) An immunohistochemical stain with antibody to Mel-A reveals a mild increase of melanocytes (immunohistochemistry with antibody to MEL-A) within the hyperplastic epidermis. (e) 'Normal' appearing epidermis adjacent to the papule reveals significantly increased melanocytes with prominent dendrites in the basal keratinocyte layer [area of arrow in (b)], (f) Histology of lentigo simplex shown in Figure 34.1f. Hyperplastic sebaceous glands correspond to yellow nodules.

Histologically, blue nevus cell nevi are either composed of spindled cells with dark and course cytoplasmic pigment located in fibrosed subepithelial tissues/dermis without an epidermal component. This type is referred to as desmoplastic blue nevus cell nevus. The dark pigmentation and deep dermal position of nevus cells give these nevi a blue hue and hence its name. Another variant is the cellular blue nevus with large epithelioid pigmented nevus cells arranged in a 'tear drop' configuration in addition to the spindled component, e.g. the base of the lesion is located deep in the dermis/subcutaneous fat.

Spitz nevi

Synonyms

Spindled and epithelioid nevus cell nevus

Spindled and epithelioid nevi cell nevi occur in children, but are rare in the vulva (**Figure 34.4**). They are papular, well-circumscribed, homogenously pigmented tumors composed of spindle and epithelioid melanocytes similar to extragenital sites (Polat et al. 2009).

Histologically, they are composed of large intraepithelial and dermal nest of partly darkly pigmented spindled and epithelioid nevus cells. Nest in the epidermis may be large, and an occasional mitosis in epidermal nests can be recognized.

Common acquired nevi

Subtypes of common acquired nevi

- Junctional
- Compound
- Dermal

Common acquired nevi occur in vulvar skin and modified mucosa.

- The first developmental stage is the junctional nevus, a light brown macule, or a thin plaque. On histology, they show regular small intraepithelial nests of nevus cells along the basement membrane (junction) zone.

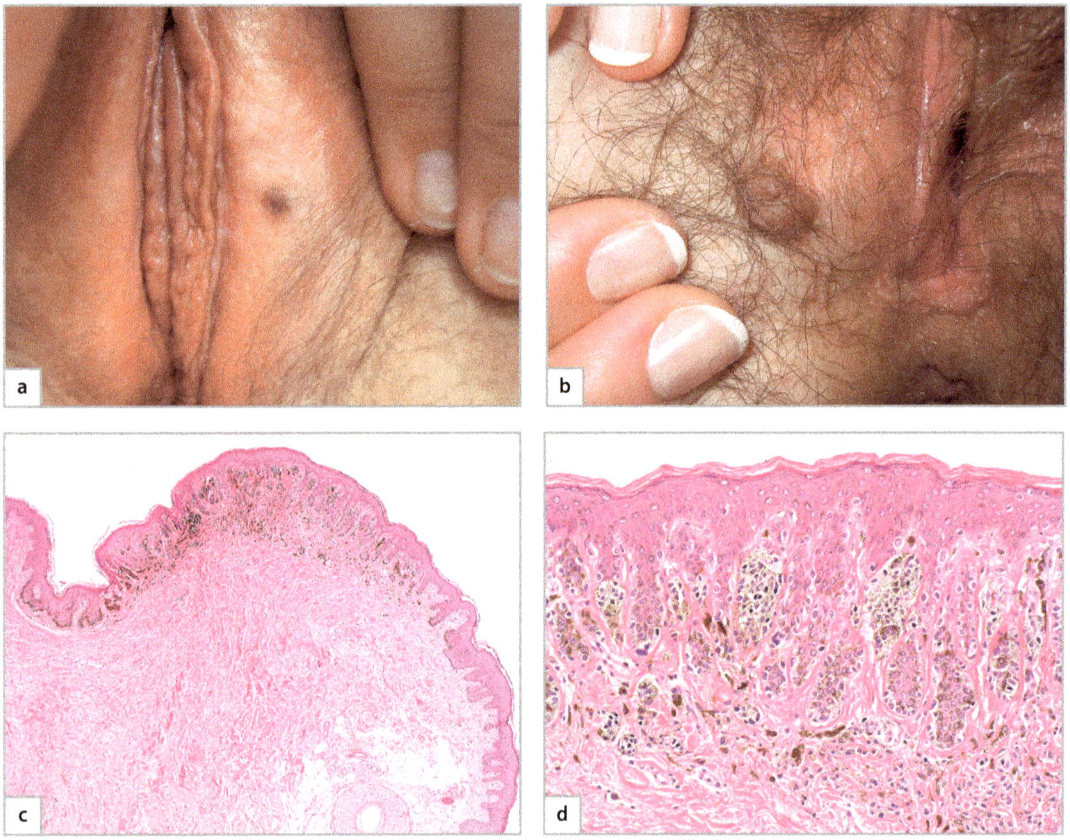

Figure 34.3 Atypical melanocytic nevi of genital type. (a) An inhomogenously pigmented papule and (b) a raised polypoid brown pigmented lesions located on the labia majora (clinical pictures by courtesy of Dr Barbara Eberz, Mürzzuschlag, Austria). (c) Histology shows a circumscribed darkly pigmented proliferation with large nests with pigmented uniform nevus cells. (d) Cellular atypia seen within the intraepithelial melanocytic nests with hyperchromasia of enlarged nuclei. Subepithelial fibrosis is present but not as pronounced as in dysplastic nevi.

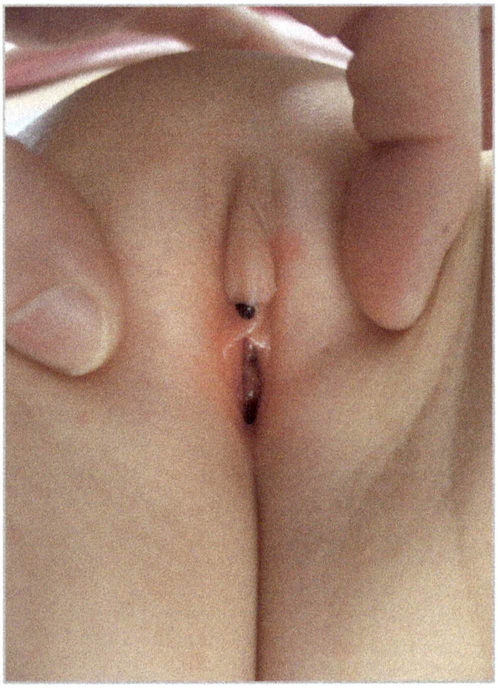

Figure 34.4 Spitz nevus in a prepubertal child. The lesion was not excised but follow-up was offered. The lesion did not change after 1 year. By courtesy of Dr G. Kirtschig, Tübingen, Germany.

- A compound nevus develops when the nevus cells migrate from the epidermis into the dermis, clinically visible as a plaque or nodule with a homogenous uniform pigmentation.
- The third stage of a dermal nevus features nests in the dermis only and presents as a slightly indurated plaque or nodule.

Treatment

None of these nevi needs to be excised; however, if the diagnosis is not clear and malignant melanoma cannot be excluded, they should be excised. Nevi may regress completely or be destroyed by a lymphocytic immune reaction. When lymphocytes destroy nevus cells patients may complain about itching and a developing red halo around the original nevus, which later turns white (so-called *halo nevus*).

Malignant melanoma of the vulva

Introduction

Melanomas are extremely rare and are divided according to location into cutaneous and mucosal melanomas. Unlike cutaneous vulvar melanomas, mucosal melanomas of the vagina and vestibule are equally common in white and black people. They can occur at any age, although typically arise in elderly women (Verschraegen et al. 2001).

Pathogenesis

UV-light and b-raf mutations demonstrated in sun-exposed cutaneous melanoma do not play a significant role in the etiology of vulvar malignant melanomas. C-kit mutations have been demonstrated in non-sun-induced vulvar and anorectal malignant melanomas. Mucosal vaginal melanomas reveal a high degree of n-ras mutations (Curtin et al. 2005, Micci et al. 2003, Omholt et al. 2011).

Cutaneous malignant melanoma of the vulva

The cutaneous vulvar melanoma is a tumor with lymphatic metastasis, classified according to TNM Classification of Malignant Tumours

(Sobin et al. 2009) and American Joint Committee on Cancer (AJJC) (see below). It arises in hair-bearing skin and modified mucosa (see below).

Clinical features

The typically solitary tumors arise in hair-bearing skin and modified mucosa, both of ectodermal origin. In areas of modified mucosa bordering mucosal sited with glycogenated mucosa, they may show overlap with mucosal melanoma. Melanomas can be evaluated with the ABCDE rule (**Table 34.1**). Vulvar cutaneous melanomas are classified in the TNM classification system that is the sum of Clark level, Breslow index, and presence/absence of ulceration (Sobin et al. 2009) and the AJCC staging system, which additionally includes mitotic count (**Table 34.2**).

Subtypes of cutaneous MM of the vulva

- Superficial spreading malignant melanoma
- Nodular melanoma
- Lentiginous malignant melanoma

Superficial spreading malignant melanoma

The most common type is the superficial spreading malignant melanoma (SSMM) (**Figure 34.1g** and **h**). Clinical presentation depends on the growth phase, e.g. invasion of the various anatomical skin levels referred to as Clark levels (**Table 34.2**). An SSMM begins as an intraepithelial proliferation that spreads laterally to produce an asymmetrical larger patch with poorly circumscribed borders and a homogeneous color. These in situ melanomas and early invasive melanomas in the papillary dermis are in the radial/horizontal growth phase, while the deeply invasive SSMM in the vertical growth phase are recognized as nodules within a pigmented patch. They elevate above skin surface and feel indurated and firm on touch. Depressed gray-white areas within a pigmented plaque (so-called 'regression') develop through an immunologic destruction of melanoma cells by lymphocytes.

Nodular melanoma

A nodular melanoma is a large, well-circumscribed, often ulcerated melanoma in vertical growth phase without an adjacent rim of malignant melanoma in radial growth phase. Nodular melanomas typically infiltrate the reticular dermis or adipose tissue at primary presentation, e.g. they present in vertical growth phase, often with presence of regional lymphatic metastases. There is still some debate or unresolved matter as to whether a nodular melanoma is an advanced SSMM, in which the radial growth phase is no longer present, or if it represents a separate entity.

Lentiginous malignant melanoma

Lentiginous melanomas are poorly circumscribed pigmented plaques. They present as extensive intraepithelial proliferation of single melanoma cells or as invasive melanoma.

Histopathology

Histologically, cutaneous superficial spreading and nodular malignant melanomas are composed of large epitheloid cells in nested pattern in both intraepidermal and invasive component. Lentiginous melanomas reveal extensive intraepithelial spread of individual single melanoma cells in all epithelial layers. The invasive component may reveal spindle cell differentiation. When in doubt, immunostaining with antibody to S-100, HMB45, and Mel-A can confirm the diagnosis.

Table 34.2 Classification of cutaneous vulvar melanomas

1. Clark levels		
Clark level I	MM in situ	**Radial / horizontal growth phase** Clinically: irregular patch or macule or plaque with variegate color
Clark level II	Early invasion of papillary dermis	
Clark level III	Expansion of papillary dermis	
Clark level IV	Invasion of reticular dermis	**Vertical growth phase** Clinically: nodule within or without surrounding pigmentation
Clark level V	Invasion of subcutaneous fat	
2. Measurements of invasion depth (Breslow index)		
Measurements of invasion depth from granular cell layer to deepest melanoma cell in millimeters with 2 decimal digits after period /comma (e.g. 1.25 mm or 1,25 mm)		
3. Ulceration		
Clark levels + invasion depth + presence / absence ulceration → **TNM classification**		
Tis :	Melanoma in situ	
T1a :	The melanoma is less than or equal to 1.0 mm thick without ulceration	
T1b :	The melanoma is less than or equal to 1.0 mm thick with ulceration	
T2a :	The melanoma is between 1.01 and 2.0 mm thick without ulceration	
T2b :	The melanoma is between 1.01 and 2.0 mm thick with ulceration	
T3a :	The melanoma is between 2.01 and 4.0 mm thick without ulceration	
T3b :	The melanoma is between 2.01 and 4.0 mm thick with ulceration	
T4a :	The melanoma is thicker than 4.0 mm without ulceration	
T4b :	The melanoma is thicker than 4.0 mm with ulceration	
4. Mitotic count		
TNM classification + mitotic count → **American Joint Committee on Cancer (AJCC) Staging**		
T1a :	The melanoma is less than or equal to 1.0 mm thick without ulceration and mitotic rate of less than $1/mm^2$	
T1b :	The melanoma is less than or equal to 1.0 mm thick with ulceration and/or the mitotic rate is $\geq 1/mm^2$	

Management and prognosis

Any lesion suspicious for melanoma needs to be excised completely and evaluated histologically. Usually, excision with a 1–2 mm margin around the visible border is recommended. Due to the complex vulvar anatomy, a primary complete excision of melanocytic lesions may not be possible. A diagnosis can be established by taking a biopsy: small lesions should be excised completely. However, complete excision with adequate surgical margins should follow quickly once the diagnosis and the stage of the melanoma are established. Cutaneous melanomas metastasize via lymph vessels to regional lymph nodes. Metastatic tumor deposits within 2 cm of the primary melanoma are called satellite nodules, at a distance >2 cm in-transit metastases. In principle, cutaneous vulvar melanomas are staged and treated similarly to cutaneous melanomas at extragenital sites. Wide surgical excision is not always possible in the vulva, but radical surgery does not seem to improve survival dramatically (Leitao 2014). Five-year-survival depends on size of primary melanoma, nodal status, and mutational status, but is typically <50% (Hodi et al. 2013). Palliative radiotherapy has been tried for extensive local disease. Immunotherapy (e.g. anti-CTLA4 antibodies or PD-1 inhibitors) may improve survival rates. Depending upon the presence of specific mutations, targeted c-KIT inhibitor or BRAF-inhibitor therapies can be considered and are offered in specialized centers.

In clinically node negative melanoma patients, sentinel node identification and resection are possible, but identification of metastatic tumor cells requires complete workup of the entire lymph node with HE-stained sections and immunohistochemical workup with antibodies to melanocytic markers, which is rather costly.

Mucosal malignant melanoma of the vulva

Mucosal vulvar malignant melanoma is an aggressive, often multifocal, patchy, inhomogenously pigmented, or amelanotic tumor with early hematogenous metastases. It arises in endodermally derived glycogenated mucosa of the vestibulum including periurethral mucosa and hymenal ring and vagina (**Figure 34 1i**).

Clinical features

Mucosal melanomas are often multifocal and poorly circumscribed darkly pigmented patches in the vulvar vestibulum including periurethral mucosa, hymenal ring, and lower vagina.

Dermoscopy

Dermoscopy can be applied to aid the diagnosis of pigmented skin lesions on the vulvar area. it can help to distinguish melanocytic neoplasms from other lesion types. Ultrasound gel can be used as an immersion liquid in concave anatomical areas. Different algorithms exist (de Giorgi et al. 2005, Ferrari et al. 2011, Ronger-Savle et al. 2011).

Histopathology

Mucosal melanocytes have an immature phenotype (e.g. immature melanosomes) that explains their amelanotic, or only scantly and inhomogenously pigmented clinical presentation. Most mucosal melanomas are highly vascularized diffuse proliferation of immature, round melanocytes with a prominent round nucleus, and a prominent nucleolus. Occasionally, the nucleus is eccentrically located and the melanoma cells assume plasmacytoid cytology. Mucosal melanoma cells react with antibody to HMB45 and Mel-A, but not or inconsistently with S-100.

Treatment and prognosis

Wide excision is the treatment of choice. However, as the lesions may be multifocal and lack well-defined borders due to lack of pigmentation, complete excision may be difficult. Late presentation, multifocality with incomplete resection explains the high rate of recurrences and residual mucosal melanoma. Invasion into the highly vascularized submucosal tissue leads to early distant hematogenous metastases. Survival is poor with <20% 5-year-survival, despite radical excision and adjuvant therapy. The benefit of lymph node dissection remains questionable.

REFERENCES

Barnhill RL, Albert LS, Shama SK, et al. Genital lentiginosis: a clinical and histopathologic study. J Am Acad Dermatol 1990; 22:453-460.

Brenn T. Atypical genital nevus. Arch Pathol Lab Med 2011; 135:317–320.

Clark WH, Jr, Hood AF, Tucker MA, et al. Atypical melanocytic nevi of the genital type with a discussion of reciprocal parenchymal-stromal interactions in the biology of neoplasia. Hum Pathol 1998; 29(Suppl):S1–S24.

Crum C, Herrington S, McCluggage WG, et al. Tumours of the vulva. Epithelial tumours. In: Kurman RJ, Carcangiu ML, Herrington CS, et al (eds), World Health Organisation Classification of Tumours of the Female Genital Tract. Lyon: IARC, 2014:232–236.

Curtin JA, Fridlyand J, Kageshita T, et al. Distinct sets of genetic alterations in melanoma. N Engl J Med 2005; 353;20:2135–2147.

de Giorgi V, Massi D, Salvini C, et al. Thin melanoma of the vulva: a clinical, dermoscopic-pathologic case study. Arch Dermatol 2005; 141:1046–1047.

Ferrari A, Zalaudek I, Argenziano G, et al. Dermoscopy of pigmented lesions of the vulva: a retrospective morphological study. Dermatology 2011; 222:157–166.

Gleason BC, Hirsch MS, Nucci MR, et al. Atypical genital nevi. A clinicopathologic analysis of 56 cases. Am J Surg Pathol 2008; 32:51-57.

Hodi FS, Corless CL, Giobbie-Hurder A, et al. Imatinib for melanomas harboring mutationally activated or amplified KIT arising on mucosal, acral, and chronically sun-damaged skin. J Clin Oncol 2013; 31:3182–3190.

Kim YJ, Kang HY. Pigmentation after using topical tacrolimus to treat lichen sclerosus: possible role of stem cell factor. J Am Acad Dermatol 2007; 57(Suppl):S125–S127.

Leitao MM, Jr. Management of vulvar and vaginal melanomas: current and future strategies. Am Soc Clin Oncol Educ Book 2014; e277–e281.

Mannone F, De Giorgi V, Cattaneo A, et al. Dermoscopic features of mucosal melanosis. Dermatol Surg 2004; 30:1118–1123.

Micci F, Teixeira MR, Scheistroen M, Abeler VM, Heim S. Cytogenetic characterization of tumors of the vulva and vagina. Genes Chromosomes Cancer 2003; 38:137–148.

O'Mahony C, Yesudian PD, Stanley M. Imiquimod use in the genital area and development of lichen sclerosus and lichen planus. Int J STD AIDS 2010; 21:219–221.

Omholt K, Grafstrom E, Kanter-Lewensohn L, et al. KIT pathway alterations in mucosal melanomas of the vulva and other sites. Clin Cancer Res 2011; 17:3933–3942.

Polat M, Topcuoglu MA, Tahtaci Y, et al. Spitz nevus of the genital mucosa. Indian J Dermatol Venereol Leprol 2009; 75:167–169.

Regauer S, Nogales FF. Vulvar trichogenic tumors: a comparative study with vulvar basal cell carcinoma. Am J Surg Pathol 2005; 29:479-484.

Rhodes AR, Silverman RA, Harrist TJ, et al. Mucocutaneous lentigines, cardiomucocutaneous myxomas, and multiple blue nevi: the "LAMB" syndrome. J Am Acad Dermatol 1984; 10:72-82.

Ronger-Savle S, Julien V, Duru G, et al. Features of pigmented vulval lesions on dermoscopy. Br J Dermatol 2011; 164:54-61.

Rudolph RI. Vulvar melanosis. J Am Acad Dermatol 1990; 23:982-984.

Sobin LH, Gospodarowicz MK, Wittekind C (eds). TNM classification of malignant tumours. UICC International Union Against Cancer, 7th edn. Chichester, UK: Wiley-Blackwell, 2009.

Verschraegen CF, Benjapibal M, Supakarapongkul W, et al. Vulvar melanoma at the M. D. Anderson Cancer Center: 25 years later. Int J Gynecol Cancer 2001; 11:359–364.

Chapter 35 Malignant and premalignant non-pigmented tumors

Joanne de Hullu, Irene A M van der Avoort, Hedwig van de Nieuwenhof

INTRODUCTION

Vulvar cancer is a rare disease and accounts for approximately 3–5% of all gynecological malignancies. About 85% of vulvar cancers are squamous cell carcinomas (SCC); the other 15% comprise a variety of tumors such as adenocarcinomas, melanomas, Paget disease, and basal cell carcinomas.

There are two different types of vulvar SCCs. The most common type occurs in elderly women and is related to lichen sclerosus (LS) and differentiated vulvar intraepithelial neoplasia (dVIN). There is an ongoing discussion about the role of vulvar lichen planus (LP) in the oncogenesis of vulvar SCC (Regauer et al. 2014). The second type primarily affects younger women and is caused by an infection with high-risk human papillomavirus (HPV) (mainly HPV 16 or 18) and develops on a background of high-grade squamous intraepithelial lesions of the vulva (HSIL) (van de Nieuwenhof et al. 2008) (see **Figure 35.1** for an overview of the oncogenesis of vulvar SCC).

NOMENCLATURE

In 2015, the International Society for the Study of Vulvovaginal Disease (ISSVD) decided to adopt the WHO modification of the Lower Anogenital Squamous Terminology (LAST), for the classification of vulvar squamous cell precursors. In LAST, HPV related vulvar squamous lesions are now classified in low-grade and high-grade squamous intraepithelial lesions. The WHO modification added VIN (differentiated type) to the classification as only HPV lesions were considered in LAST (Bornstein 2015). For an overview of the terminology see **Table 35.1**.

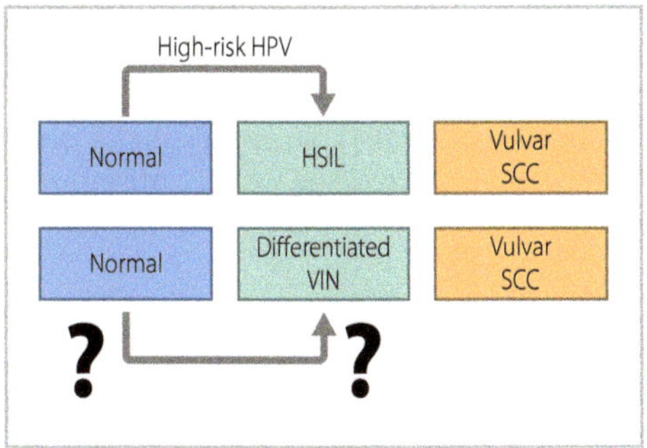

Figure 35.1 Etiology of vulvar squamous cell carcinoma. HPV, human papilloma virus; HSIL, high-grade squamous intraepithelial lesion; SCC, squamous cell carcinoma; VIN, vulvar intraepithelial neoplasia.

Table 35.1 'Old' and 'new' nomenclature of squamous intraepithelial lesions of the vulva

Old nomenclature	ISSVD 2004 nomenclature	ISSVD 2015 nomenclature (following WHO criteria)
VIN1	No cancer precursor	LSIL of the vulva
VIN2/VIN3	Usual VIN	HSIL of the vulva
(Well) differentiated VIN	Differentiated VIN	Differentiated VIN

HSIL, high grade squamous intraepithelial lesion; LSIL, low grade squamous intraepithelial lesion; VIN, vulvar intraepithelial neoplasia

VULVAR SQUAMOUS CELL CARCINOMA

The majority of SCCs are diagnosed in the seventh decade. Common symptoms are localized pruritus, palpable or visible mass, bleeding, pain, discharge, or urinary tract symptoms. Patient's and doctor's delay in diagnosis is frequent. Initial spread occurs to the inguinofemoral lymph nodes; therefore, the number of inguinofemoral lymph node metastases is the most important prognostic factor. Hematogenous spread and spread by direct extension are less frequent. The importance of the lymph node status is reflected in the surgicopathological staging that was revised in 2009 by The Fédération Internationale de Gynécologie et d'Obstétrique (FIGO) (**Table 35.2**) (Pecorelli 2009) (see **Figures 35.2** and **35.3** for examples of SCC of the vulva).

Treatment

The cornerstone for the treatment of vulvar SCC is surgery with a limited role for radio- and chemotherapy (de Hullu et al. 2006). For years, radical vulvectomy with bilateral inguinofemoral lymphadenectomy was the standard treatment. More and more efforts have been made to individualize treatment and define subgroups of patients who may be treated by less radical procedures. In case of microinvasive tumors (≤1 mm invasion and a maximum diameter of 2 cm), patients are treated with a wide local excision (WLE) only and treatment of the groins can be safely omitted. Currently, standard treatment of SCC with a depth of invasion >1 mm and diameter >4 cm and/or multifocal disease entails a WLE with uni- or bilateral inguinofemoral

Table 35.2 FIGO classification of VSCC (2009)

Stage	
Stage I	Confined to the vulva or perineum; no nodal metastasis
A	Lesions ≤2 cm in size with stromal invasion ≤1 mm*
B	Lesions >2 cm in size or stromal invasion >1 mm*
Stage II	Adjacent spread to the lower urethra, the vagina, or the anus; no nodal metastasis
Stage III	Tumor confined to vulva or adjacent spread to the lower urethra, the vagina, or the anus and positive inguinofemoral lymph nodes
A	One lymph node metastasis ≥5 mm or 1–2 lymph node metastases <5 mm
B	Three or more lymph nodes <5 mm or ≥2 lymph nodes ≥5 mm
C	Lymph nodes with extracapsular spread
Stage IV	
A	Tumor with fixed or ulcerated lymph nodes or tumor with spread into upper urethra/vagina, bladder, rectal mucosa, bone, or fixed to pelvic bone
B	Any distant metastasis, including pelvic lymph nodes

FIGO, International Federation of Gynecologists and Obstetrics; VSCC, vulvar squamous cell carcinoma

*The depth of invasion is defined as the measurement of the tumor from the epithelial–stromal junction of the adjacent most superficial dermal papilla to the deepest point of invasion

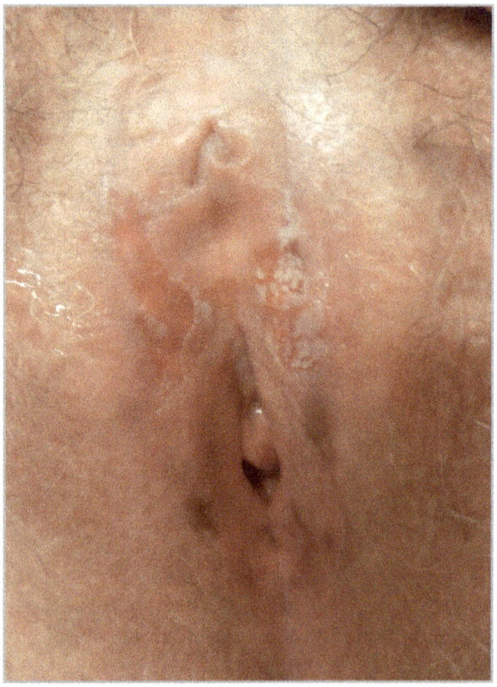

Figure 35.2 Squamous cell carcinoma of the vulva on the left side, differentiated vulvar intraepithelial neoplasia on the right side.

lympadenectomy via separate incisions. This change in treatment modality has significantly improved the quality of life because it has a less mutilating effect, but complication rates (wound breakdown, infection, erysipelas, and leg edema) are still high approaching 70% (de Hullu et al. 2006). In the case of more than one intranodal metastasis and/or extranodal growth, postoperative radiotherapy of the pelvis is recommended. In case of close margins, local re-excision, follow-up, or radiotherapy is advised.

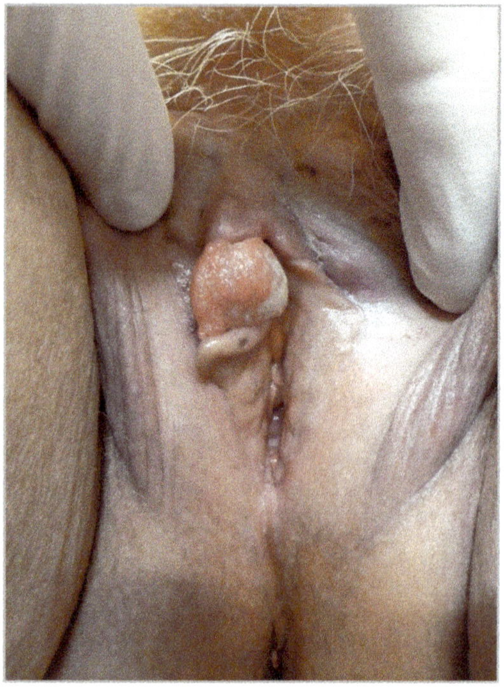

Figure 35.3 Squamous cell carcinoma of the vulva on the right side.

Early stage disease

Sentinel lymph node (SLN) dissection has been introduced in early stage SCC and has shown promising results with a very high-negative predictive value of a negative SLN as shown in GOG 170 (Levenback et al. 2012) and the GROningen INternational Study on Sentinel nodes in Vulvar cancer (GROINSS V-I) (van der Zee et al. 2008). Strict criteria (tumor <4 cm, only unifocal lesions) and enough experience of the multidisciplinary well-trained team (gynecologic oncologist, nuclear physician, and pathologist) are necessary to safely perform SLN procedures and to consider SLN procedure as standard treatment in these early stage patients (Van der Zee et al. 2008). In clinical settings where vulvar cancer is rare and surgeons' experience is limited, referral to a high-volume center is appropriate. Patients should be informed about the low risk of missing a positive SLN, and patients are preferably treated within the protection of a clinical study such as GROINSS-V-II under strict protocol and follow-up.

Advanced disease

When neighboring structures are involved and an exenteration and/or (partial) resection of affected bones or muscles would be necessary to remove the cancer tissue with clear resection margins, SCC is considered locally advanced. Positive (bulky) lymph nodes in the groin are found in 60% of these patients, making advanced-stage SCC difficult to treat. Primary chemoradiation is an option in order to reduce tumor volume and reduce the extent of surgery (de Hullu & van der Zee 2006). So far, results of small observational studies, in terms of survival and toxicity, are promising (Moore et al. 2012).

Prognosis

Inguinofemoral lymph node status at initial diagnosis is of critical prognostic importance for patients with vulvar SCC. Vulvar SCC relapses on the vulva in 26–37% of the cases: approximately 40–60% of treatment failures develop within 2 years of primary treatment and most of these are local, probably de novo SCCs. Groin recurrences are rare but nearly always fatal. Overall 5-year survival in vulvar SCC is around 70% (de Hullu et al. 2006, de Hullu & van der Zee 2006).

HIGH-GRADE SQUAMOUS INTRAEPITHELIAL LESIONS OF THE VULVA

Key features

- HSIL of the vulva is a premalignant condition
- It is caused by high-risk HPV types
- Despite treatment, it has a high recurrence rate
- It has a low conversion rate to malignant disease

Epidemiology

The incidence of vulvar HSIL is approximately five per 100,000 women per year and increasing worldwide, due to the increase in HPV prevalence (Joura 2002). HSIL of the vulva has a predilection for young women, often in their 30s and 40s. Cigarette smoking and vulvar condylomata are common in women with vulvar HSIL (Hart 2001). Moreover, the use of immunosuppressants to prevent rejection after transplantation or to treat a chronic autoimmune disease increases the risk of developing vulvar HSIL. Because of the recently introduced HPV vaccines, a decrease in incidence is to be expected.

Pathogenesis

High-risk HPV types, mainly 16 and 18, play a major role in the etiology of vulvar HSIL (mean HPV positivity is 89.9%) (van de Nieuwenhof et al. 2008). Due to this viral cause, the immune system plays an important role in clearance and persistence of the HPV infection and development of vulvar HSIL.

Clinical presentation

Key features

- Raised
- Well demarcated
- Asymmetrical lesions
- Often multicentric

The raised and well-demarcated lesions often produce large whitish, erythematous plaques, while some lesions are pigmented (**Figures 35.4** and **35.5**). Multifocal involvement of the vulva occurs in >40% of cases (Hart 2001). Because of a high percentage of women with multicentric disease (cervix, vagina, and anus), a cervical smear should be performed (van de Nieuwenhof et al. 2009). The most common presenting complaint is pruritus; other presenting symptoms can be pain, ulceration, and dysuria (McNally 2002).

Histopathology

The epidermis is thickened and is accompanied by a surface reaction of hyperkeratosis and/or parakeratosis of the most superficial cell layers.

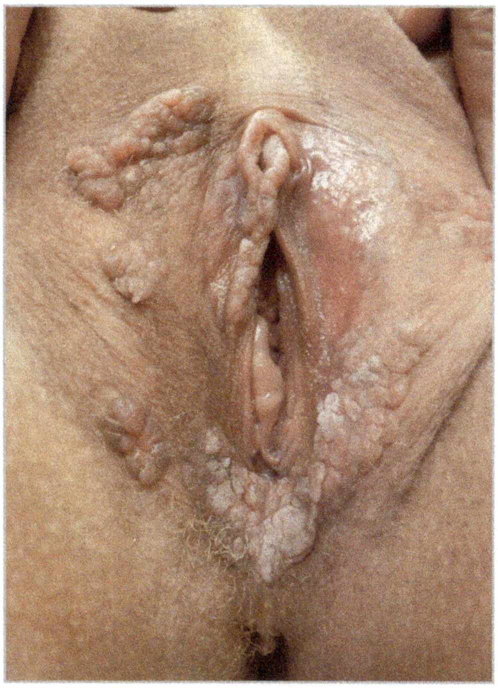

Figure 35.4 HSIL at different areas of the vulva.

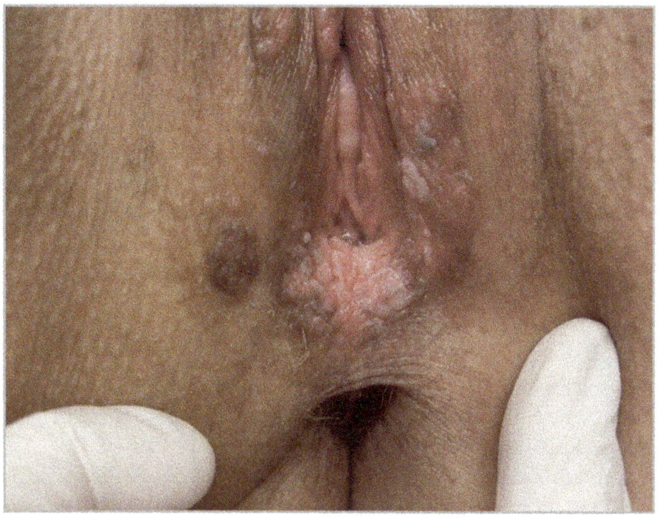

Figure 35.5 HSIL on the perineum showing the typical white 'warty' changes.

Microscopic features

The characteristic microscopic features include the following key features (Hart, Wilkinson 2002) (**Figure 35.6**):

- Wind-blown appearance of the epidermis
- High nuclear-to-cytoplasmic ratio
- Nuclear hyperchromasia
- Irregularities of the nuclear membranes
- Numerous mitotic figures at all levels of the epidermis

Differential diagnosis

The differential diagnosis of vulvar HSIL comprises benign processes like reactive epithelial changes and malignant ones including vulvar

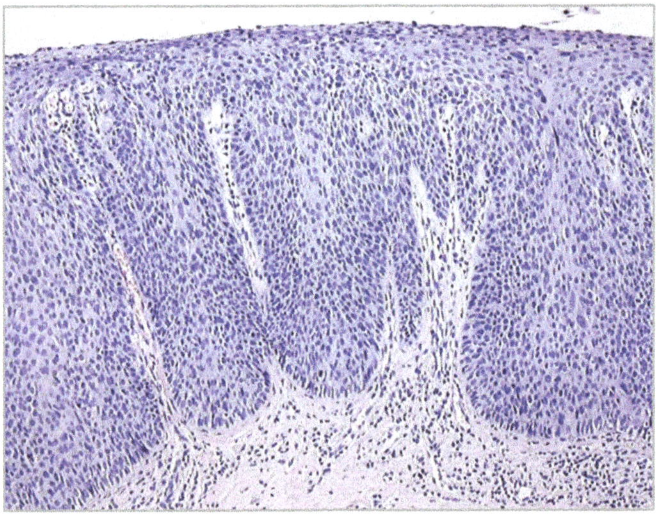

Figure 35.6 Histopathology of vulvar HSIL showing typical full thickness epidermal dysplasia.

Table 35.3 Alternative second-line medical treatment options for HSIL of the vulva

Type of medication	Action	Comments
5-Fluorouracil	Topical chemotherapeutic agent	Severe side effects Limited results
Interferon	Inhibits replication of viruses	Limited effects High costs Few side effects
Cidofovir	Potent antiviral activity against viruses such as HPV	Shown to be effective in a phase 2 RCT
Photodynamic therapy	Tumor localizing photosensitizing and light of appropriate wavelength	Well tolerated with excellent tissue preservation without scarring Optimal light dose has to be determined Equally effective to laser vaporization or local excision Shorter healing time Larger studies needed

HPV, human papillomavirus; RCT, randomized controlled trial

Paget disease and malignant melanoma. Also condylomata acuminata may mimic the signs of HSIL.

Principles of management

Surgery

Recent reports have shown that positive surgical margins rarely predict the development of invasive disease. Therefore, wide local excision, consisting of removal of all visible lesions, is the surgical technique of choice (van de Nieuwenhof et al. 2008). An alternative treatment may be laser excision or vaporization to prevent multiple surgeries/scarring in these relatively young women with high recurrence rates. Overall recurrence rates of different surgical techniques are around 20% (van Seters et al. 2005).

Medical

Medical treatments have been tried to avoid surgery in patients with HSIL of the vulva. Medical treatment does not provide a specimen for histological evaluation and occult invasion may be missed.

Imiquimod inhibits viral replication and focuses on the cause of HSIL and preserves the anatomy and function of the vulva. It has been shown to be effective in randomized controlled trials (Mathiesen et al. 2007, van Seters et al. 2008). Side effects (burning, itching, and/or ulcer development) are common, which make some patients stop the treatment. A complete response is not achieved in all women who will need additional therapy. When a complete response has been achieved with imiquimod, it has a 9% recurrence rate (Terlou 2011). In different studies, different regimens of application have been described. One example of a treatment regimen, used in the Radboud University Nijmegen Medical Centre, is as follows: We prescribe imiquimod 5% cream 6.25 mg ante noctem to be applied two or three times a week for about 16 weeks. We also prescribe emollients containing lidocaine 3% for application on the other days to diminish side effects. When patients experience severe side effects (soreness/ulceration of the skin), we advise to use imiquimod less frequently. In exceptional cases, the patient should stop imiquimod based on side effects. It may be helpful for patients to see them in 4–6 week intervals during treatment at the outpatient clinic. After treatment, biopsies are only necessary in case of residual disease for possible additional therapy. New agents such as epigallocatechin-3-gallate are under investigation. Follow-up after successful treatment is recommended once or twice per year for life (see **Table 35.3** for alternative, less frequently used treatment options). A recent RCT showed comparable efficacy of cidofovir and imiquimod in the treatment of HSIL (Tristram et al. 2014).

It is obvious that the current treatments of HSIL need to be improved. An individual strategy has to be made based on the extent of the disease and patient preferences.

Prevention

Two prophylactic vaccines have been introduced to prevent infections with high-risk HPV subtypes (HPV 16 and 18). The vaccine was 97% effective in preventing vulvar HSIL associated with HPV 16 and 18 in a population that was naive to these viruses at the time of first vaccination. The vaccine should be recommended for women in target populations (Munoz et al. 2010). In the Netherlands, all girls are invited to the vaccination program at the age of 13 years; however, some countries recommend the vaccination at 9 years of age. A vaccine containing nine subtypes will be available soon. Cigarette smoking is a known risk factor, cessation should be encouraged.

Course and prognosis; malignant potential

Recurrence

Recurrence rates of vulvar HSIL, even after extensive surgical procedures, are high (approximately 20%) (van Seters et al. 2005). Surgical margins are often positive, irrespective of the type of surgery (van de Nieuwenhof et al. 2008). Recurrences were found to be associated with smoking, larger lesion size, and positive margins (Wallbillich et al. 2012). The presence of positive surgical margins rarely predicts the development of invasive SCC.

Progression to invasive vulvar cancer

Generally, the malignant potential of vulvar HSIL is considered to be low. In two large studies, a percentage of 3.3–4.2 was found (Jones et al. 2005, van Seters et al. 2005). Advanced age, raised lesions, radiotherapy, and an immune compromised state are known risk factors for progression of HSIL (van de Nieuwenhof et al. 2008).

Spontaneous regression

Regression of vulvar HSIL has been described in a couple of women, mostly related to a change of the immune status after giving birth and/or of an improvement in the immune compromised state, e.g. by refraining from the use of immune suppressants or cessation of smoking (van de Nieuwenhof et al. 2008).

Follow-up

Because of the risk of recurrence and progression, patients should be monitored at 6 and 12 months after initial therapy and annually thereafter (ACOG Committee Opinion No. 509 2011).

DIFFERENTIATED VULVAR INTRAEPITHELIAL NEOPLASIA

Key features

- Differentiated VIN is a vulvar premalignancy of unknown etiology
- Often occurs on a background of LS
- Relatively high conversion rate for malignant disease
- Difficult diagnosis for clinician and pathologist

Epidemiology

The exact incidence of dVIN is unknown. Around 2–5% of all VIN lesions are of dVIN and of non-HPV-related origin (Preti et al. 2005, van de Nieuwenhof et al. 2009). Underdiagnosis is very likely, because of the difficult clinical and histological diagnosis. Differentiated VIN characteristically occurs in postmenopausal women (mean age 67 years) and is associated with LS (Hart 2001). In cases where dVIN is found without any sign of invasion, the patient has often been previously treated for vulvar SCC, and also suffers from LS (Scurry et al. 2006); however, also isolated dVIN lesions can occur in patients without a history of vulvar SCC.

Pathogenesis

The etiology of dVIN remains to be elucidated. HPV is very uncommon in dVIN and does not play a role in its pathogenesis (Pinto et al. 2000, Preti et al. 2005, van der Avoort et al. 2006). Because of its high concurrence with LS, a causative role for LS is likely, but other factors may play a role. Squamous cell hyperplasia with atypia may represent a step in the carcinogenesis (Pinto et al. 2000); however, it is still unclear whether it is a direct precursor of invasive vulvar SCC (Hart 2001). Also, LP has been suggested to be related to the development of dVIN and vulvar SCC in the non-hair-bearing vulvar mucosa (Regauer et al. 2014).

Clinical presentation

Key features

- Often associated with LS or LP
- Often unifocal
- Variable clinical presentation

Differentiated VIN is most often seen adjacent to LS and/or invasive SCC. However, also patients with dVIN who developed vulvar SCC without suffering from LS have been described (Roma & Hart 2007). Differentiated VIN has multiple forms of presentation, which are presented and described in **Figures 35.7** to **35.9**. We may see an area of grey-white discoloration with a roughened surface, an ulcerative red lesion, an erythematous red lesion, or as an ill-defined raised white plaque. It may be difficult to distinguish it from the often-present background of LS (Yang & Hart 2000). In most cases, dVIN forms smaller lesions than HSIL and more often the lesions are unifocal.

Apart from visible changes or progression of an ulcerative lesion despite increased dosage of steroid cream, most dVIN patients report

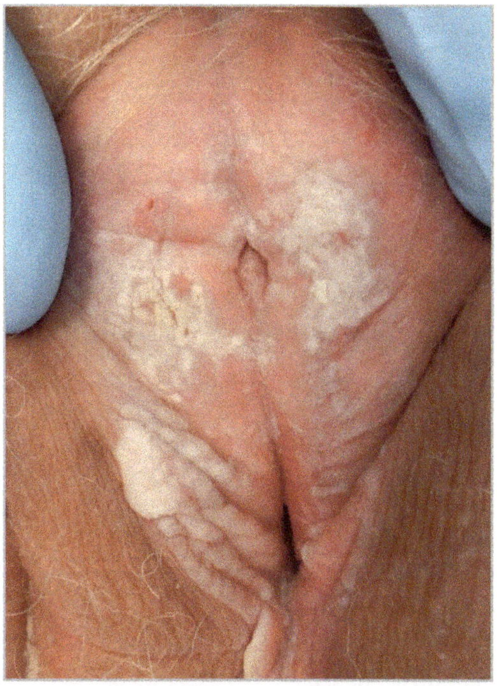

Figure 35.7 Differentiated vulvar intraepithelial neoplasia at biopsies of white areas.

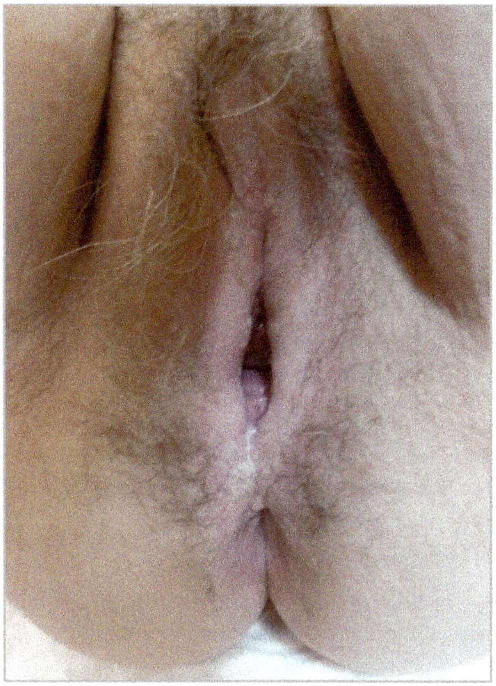

Figure 35.8 Extensive lichen sclerosus with differentiated vulvar intraepithelial neoplasia on biopsy of the perineum.

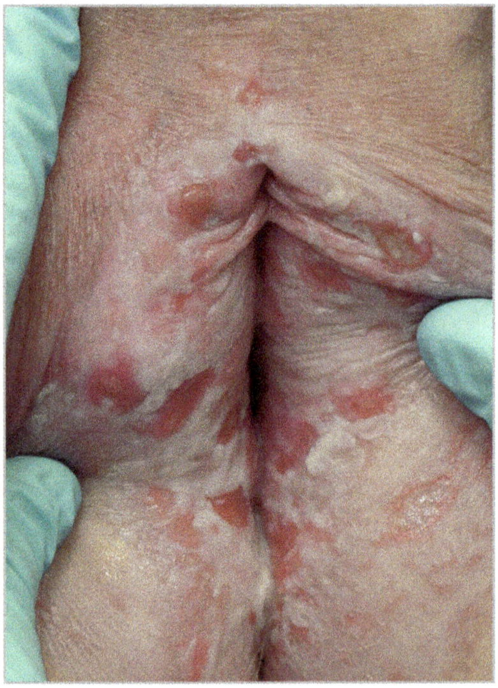

Figure 35.9 Differentiated vulvar intraepithelial neoplasia at different spots of the vulva.

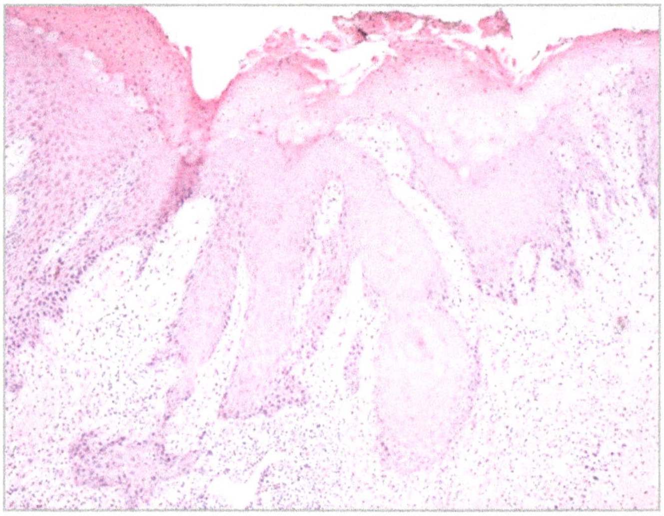

Figure 35.10 Histopathology of differentiated vulvar intraepithelial neoplasia. Atypical cells are confined to the basal and parabasal layer of the epidermis..

itching as their main symptom, probably due to the underlying LS (see also Chapter 19).

Histopathology

Key features

- May be difficult to recognize
- Cellular atypia confined to basal and parabasal epithelium
- MIB1 and p53 can be helpful biomarkers

Histopathologically, dVIN is difficult to recognize, mainly because of the high degree of cellular differentiation combined with an absence of widespread architectural disarray, nuclear pleomorphism, and diffuse nuclear atypia (Hart 2001). The atypia in dVIN lesions is strictly confined to the basal and parabasal layers of the epithelium, where the cells have abundant cytoplasm and form abortive pearls (Hart 2001, Wilkinson 2002). MIB1 and p53 can be helpful biomarkers to distinguish dVIN from normal epithelium, LS, or HSIL (van der Avoort et al. 2007). Scattered mitotic figures are common in the basal areas, but can extend into the upper levels of the epidermis (Yang & Hart 2000). Typically, the epidermis is thickened with parakeratosis (Hart 2001). In the underlying or adjacent papillary dermis, there is a chronic inflammatory cell infiltrate, consisting of predominantly lymphocytes, plasma cells, and occasionally eosinophils (Hart 2001).

When dVIN invades the dermis, nodules of enlarged eosinophilic keratinocytes appear to fall from the basilar epidermis or from elongated rete ridges. In superficial biopsies, the distinction of dVIN from early invasive vulvar SCC may be difficult (Hart 2001) (**Figure 35.10**).

Differential diagnosis

Clinically, dVIN can be difficult to distinguish from LS, vulvar SCC, HSIL, and sometimes condylomata or inflammation. Histopathologically, the distinction from normal epithelium, squamous cell hyperplasia, HSIL, LS, or (minimally invasive) vulvar SCC can be difficult.

Principles of management

Management of dVIN should aim at early detection and removal of the entire lesion. No follow-up schedules have been investigated for best outcome or earlier detection. Follow-up of patients previously treated for dVIN should occur at a specialized vulvar clinic or by a vulvar specialist (a consultant dermatologist or gynecologist who has had an additional training in managing vulvar disease) (Jones et al. 2008).

As dVIN is often unifocal, radical surgical excision is the preferred treatment. As cryotherapy and ablative/laser vaporization do not provide a pathological specimen, these options are considered less attractive. Vulvar reconstruction is often feasible as dVIN is usually confined to non-hair-bearing areas or the external sides of atrophic labia minora. Recurrent lesions are common, and so far, there is no place for medical therapy (Preti et al. 2005).

Course and prognosis/malignant potential

The exact pathway of carcinogenesis has not yet been established. It is suggested that dVIN is highly proliferative and therefore more likely to progress to an invasive SCC than LS and vulvar HSIL (Mulvany 2008, Roma & Hart 2007, Yang & Hart 2000) . The observation that most SCCs are dVIN-related and most high-grade intraepithelial vulvar lesions without concurrent invasion are HPV-positive, combined with the frequent finding of dVIN adjacent to rapidly growing invasive vulvar SCC, reinforces this presumption (van der Avoort et al. 2006, Yang & Hart 2000). Therefore, any suspicious area should be biopsied (Preti et al. 2005, Yang & Hart 2000). Regular follow-up of patients is recommended once or twice per year lifelong.

REFERENCES

Bornstein J. 2015 ISSVD Terminology Change. http://issvd.org/wp-content/uploads/2015/09/2015-ISSVD-VIN-terminology-for-the-website-v5.pdf (accessed 18 November 2015).

Committee on Gynecologic Practice of American College of Gynecologists. ACOG Committee Opinion No. 509: Management of vulvar intraepithelial neoplasia. Obstet Gynecol 2011; 118:1192–1194.

de Hullu JA, van der Avoort IA, Oonk MH, van der Zee AG. Management of vulvar cancers. European journal of surgical oncology : Eur J Soc Surg Oncol 2006; 32:825–831. (a)

de Hullu JA, van der Zee AG. Surgery and radiotherapy in vulvar cancer. Crit Rev Oncol Hematol 2006; 60:38–58. (b)

Hart WR. Vulvar intraepithelial neoplasia: historical aspects and current status. Int J Gynecol Pathol 2001; 20:16–30.

Jones RW, Rowan DM, Stewart AW. Vulvar intraepithelial neoplasia: aspects of the natural history and outcome in 405 women. Obstet Gynecol 2005; 106:1319–1326.

Jones RW, Scurry J, Neill S, MacLean AB. Guidelines for the follow-up of women with vulvar lichen sclerosus in specialist clinics. Am J Obstet Gynecol 2008; 198:496 e1–3.

Joura EA. Epidemiology, diagnosis and treatment of vulvar intraepithelial neoplasia. Curr Opin Obstet Gynecol 2002; 14:39–43.

Levenback CF, Ali S, Coleman RL, et al. Lymphatic mapping and sentinel lymph node biopsy in women with squamous cell carcinoma of the vulva: a gynecologic oncology group study. J Clin Oncol 2012; 30:3786–3791.

Mathiesen O, Buus SK, Cramers M. Topical imiquimod can reverse vulvar intraepithelial neoplasia: a randomised, double-blinded study. Gynecol Oncol 2007; 107:219–222.

McNally OM, Mulvany NJ, Pagano R, Quinn MA, Rome RM. VIN 3: a clinicopathologic review. Int J Gynecol Cancer 2002; 12:490–495.

Moore DH, Ali S, Koh WJ, et al. A phase II trial of radiation therapy and weekly cisplatin chemotherapy for the treatment of locally-advanced squamous cell carcinoma of the vulva: a gynecologic oncology group study. Gynecol Oncol 2012; 124:529–533.

Mulvany NJ, Allen DG. Differentiated intraepithelial neoplasia of the vulva. Int J Gynecol Pathol 2008; 27:125–135.

Munoz N, Kjaer SK, Sigurdsson K, et al. Impact of human papillomavirus (HPV)-6/11/16/18 vaccine on all HPV-associated genital diseases in young women. J Natl Cancer Inst 2010; 102:325–339.

Pecorelli S. Revised FIGO staging for carcinoma of the vulva, cervix, and endometrium. Int J Gynaecol Obstet 2009; 105:103–104.

Pinto AP, Lin MC, Sheets EE, et al. Allelic imbalance in lichen sclerosus, hyperplasia, and intraepithelial neoplasia of the vulva. Gynecol Oncol 2000; 77:171–176.

Preti M, Van Seters M, Sideri M, Van Beurden M. Squamous vulvar intraepithelial neoplasia. Clin Obstet Gynecol 2005; 48:845–861.

Regauer S, Reich O, Eberz B. Vulvar cancers in women with vulvar lichen planus: A clinicopathological study. J Am Acad Dermatol 2014; 71:698–707.

Roma AA, Hart WR. Progression of simplex (differentiated) vulvar intraepithelial neoplasia to invasive squamous cell carcinoma: a prospective case study confirming its precursor role in the pathogenesis of vulvar cancer. Int J Gynecol Pathol 2007; 26:248–253.

Scurry J, Campion M, Scurry B, Kim SN, Hacker N. Pathologic audit of 164 consecutive cases of vulvar intraepithelial neoplasia. Int J Gynecol Pathol 2006; 25:176–181.

Sideri M, Jones RW, Wilkinson EJ, et al. Squamous vulvar intraepithelial neoplasia: 2004 modified terminology, ISSVD Vulvar Oncology Subcommittee. J Reprod Med 2005; 50:807–810.

Terlou A, van Seters M, Ewing PC, et al. Treatment of vulvar intraepithelial neoplasia with topical imiquimod: seven years median follow-up of a randomized clinical trial. Gynecol Oncol 2011; 121:157–162.

Tristram A, Hurt CN, Madden T, et al. Activity, safety, and feasibility of cidofovir and imiquimod for treatment of vulval intraepithelial neoplasia (RT3VIN): a multicentre, open-label, randomised, phase 2 trial. Lancet Oncology 2014; 12:1361–1368.

van de Nieuwenhof HP, van der Avoort IA, de Hullu JA. Review of squamous premalignant vulvar lesions. Crit Rev Oncol Hematol 2008; 68:131–156.

van de Nieuwenhof HP, Massuger LF, van der Avoort IA, et al. Vulvar squamous cell carcinoma development after diagnosis of VIN increases with age. Eur J Cancer 2009; 45:851–856.

van der Avoort IA, Shirango H, Hoevenaars BM, et al. Vulvar squamous cell carcinoma is a multifactorial disease following two separate and independent pathways. Int J Gynecol Pathol 2006; 25:22–29.

van der Avoort IA, van der Laak JA, Paffen A, et al. MIB1 expression in basal cell layer: a diagnostic tool to identify premalignancies of the vulva. Mod Pathol 2007; 20:770–778.

van der Zee AG, Oonk MH, De Hullu JA, et al. Sentinel node dissection is safe in the treatment of early-stage vulvar cancer. J Clin Oncol 2008; 26:884–889.

van Seters M, van Beurden M, de Craen AJ. Is the assumed natural history of vulvar intraepithelial neoplasia III based on enough evidence? A systematic review of 3322 published patients. Gynecol Oncol 2005; 97:645–651.

van Seters M, van Beurden M, ten Kate FJ, et al. Treatment of vulvar intraepithelial neoplasia with topical imiquimod. N Engl J Med 2008; 358:1465–1473.

Wallbillich JJ, Rhodes HE, Milbourne AM, et al. Vulvar intraepithelial neoplasia (VIN 2/3): comparing clinical outcomes and evaluating risk factors for recurrence. Gynecol Oncol 2012; 127:312–315.

Wilkinson EJ. Premalignant and malignant tumors of the vulva. In: Kurman RJ (Ed), Blaustein's Pathology of the Female Genital Tract, 5th edn. New York: Springer-Verlag, 2002: 99–150.

Yang B, Hart WR. Vulvar intraepithelial neoplasia of the simplex (differentiated) type: a clinicopathologic study including analysis of HPV and p53 expression. Am J Surg Pathol 2000; 24:429–441.

Chapter 36 Extramammary Paget disease of the vulva

Laura T H Wang

Key points

- Rare intraepithelial neoplasm
- May be primary intraepithelial or secondary to other tumors
- Accounts for 1–2% of all vulvar cancers
- Typical clinical presentation: red, well demarcated, asymmetrical plaques with island of hyperkeratosis ('strawberries and cream'), may resemble eczema or psoriasis
- Diagnosis confirmed by histology and immunocytochemistry
- Frequent recurrences

INTRODUCTION

Paget disease is a cutaneous neoplasm of epithelial origin that favors apocrine-bearing skin of mammary (93%) and extramammary (7%) locations. Extramammary Paget disease (EMPD) is a rare cutaneous intraepithelial neoplasm with the vast majority presenting as a primary cutaneous intraepithelial adenocarcinoma; however, it may occur secondary to underlying neoplasms like urothelial or anorectal carcinoma; 40% of anorectal cases are associated with an underlying anorectal malignancy (Crum et al. 2014). The diagnosis, often delayed, is confirmed by histology and immunohistochemistry. Treatment has historically been chiefly surgical, although non-surgical modalities are gaining favor and may be equally efficacious. Recurrences are common, about one third. Prognosis is generally good, with disease-related mortality <10%.

EPIDEMIOLOGY

EMPD accounts for 1-2% of all vulvar malignancies. The exact incidence and prevalence are unknown. EMPD predominantly affects postmenopausal Caucasian women in the Western hemisphere (mean age 65 years, range 50s–80s). However, in recent years, more cases are reported from China and Japan, possibly with a male predilection (Delport 2013, Lam & Funaro 2010).

CLASSIFICATION

In 2002, Wilkinson and Brown classified vulvar EMPD based on the etiologic origin of Paget cells (**Table 36.1**).

Table 36.1 Wilkinson and Brown's classification of vulvar extramammary Paget disease 2002 (Wilkinson & Brown 2002)

Primary cutaneous origin
Intraepithelial neoplasm without invasion [carcinoma in situ (CIS)]
Intraepithelial neoplasm with invasion
Intraepithelial neoplasm as a manifestation of an underlying adenocarcinoma of skin appendage or a subcutaneous vulvar gland
Secondary non-cutaneous origin
Secondary to anorectal adenocarcinoma
Secondary to urothelial neoplasm
Secondary to adenocarcinoma of other sites

Primary cutaneous origin: >75%

- Intraepithelial neoplasm without invasion: The majority (60%) arises within the epidermis and remains in situ, often extending into the epithelium of contiguous skin appendages, but rarely invading the dermis. These tumors are slow growing, and have little potential for systemic metastasis and prognosis is excellent. In 10–18%, dermal invasion is noted (Fanning et al. 1999, Shaco-Levy et al. 2010, Wilkinson & Brown 2002), almost all are only diagnosed at initial surgery (Shaco-Levy et al. 2010), up to 30% having lymph node metastasis.
- Intraepithelial neoplasm with invasion: In microinvasion (defined as invasion of <1 mm), there is involvement of the papillary dermis. They are similar to intraepithelial in situ disease in recurrence risk and survival. In deep invasion (>1 mm), the reticular dermis or subcutaneous area is involved. Here there is an increased risk of lymphatic and systemic metastasis, resulting in decreased survival (Hatta et al. 2008).
- Intraepithelial neoplasm as a manifestation of an underlying adenocarcinoma of skin appendage or a subcutaneous vulvar gland (15–35%) (Lam & Funaro 2010): The underlying adenocarcinoma secondarily involves the overlying epidermis.

Secondary non-cutaneous origin: <25%

These non-cutaneous internal neoplasms arise from non-vulvar sites, but secondarily involve the vulva skin, possibly by contiguous extension or by epidermotropic metastasis. Location often provides a clue to its origin: anorectal adenocarcinoma involving the perianal tissue, as well as urothelial neoplasms involving the vestibule.

PATHOGENESIS

The pathogenesis is unknown but most agree that primary and secondary forms have distinct pathogenic mechanisms.

- In primary cutaneous EMPD, Paget cells are believed to arise either from pluripotent keratinocyte stem cells or from apocrine/eccrine glands. Another proposed precursor is the Toker cell (epidermal cell found in the same areas of skin as apocrine glands including nipple, lactiferous ducts, milk line/accessory nipples, and anogenital skin) (Delport 2013, Lam & Funaro 2010).

- In secondary non-cutaneous EPMD, Paget cells are believed to be neoplastic cells migrating from the underlying adeno- or urothelial carcinoma, through epidermotropic or contiguous spread.

CLINICAL PRESENTATION

Key clinical symptoms

- Pruritus 75%
- Pain and soreness
- Exudation
- Lesion/mass

Key clinical signs

- Erythematous plaque(s) with discrete white islands of hyperkeratosis/scales
- Asymmetrical and variable size
- Excoriation/erosion/exudation

The most common symptom is pruritus (75%). The typical lesion appears as a well-demarcated, slow growing erythematous plaque with superimposed discrete white islands of hyperkeratotic scales (**Figure 36.1**). Less frequently, an erythematous patch is the sole finding resembling eczema (**Figures 36.2** and **36.3**). Lesions may be single or multiple and unilateral in 54% and bilateral in 54% (Shaco-Levy et al. 2010). Nodules, when present, may indicate underlying adenocarcinoma. Excoriation, erosion, and exudation are common (**Figure 36.4**), possibly exacerbated by a superimposed fungal process.

Diagnostic delay is common, with an average of 20 months (2–84 months) between initial symptom and diagnosis (Shaco-Levy et al. 2010). Lesions are frequently mistaken for eczema or fungal infections, treated with corticosteroid topical regimens or antifungals with poor response. Although delay may lead to increased lesion size, it is not correlated with invasion, recurrence, or poor survival.

Location may provide a clue to origin as follows:

- Lateral labium majus or minus lesion indicates primary cutaneous Paget disease
- Perianal distribution is probably a cutaneous manifestation of an anorectal adenocarcinoma
- Involvement of the vestibule typically originates from a urothelial neoplasm.

Regional lymph node metastases occur in invasive disease.

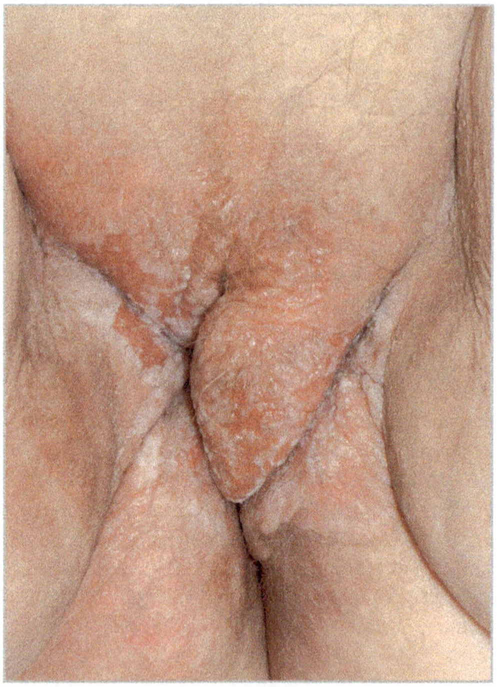

Figure 36.1 Paget disease of the vulva. Note the erythematous, eczematoid plaque with erosions and discrete white islands of hyperkeratotic scales. By courtesy of Prof. Hope Haefner Ann Arbor, USA.

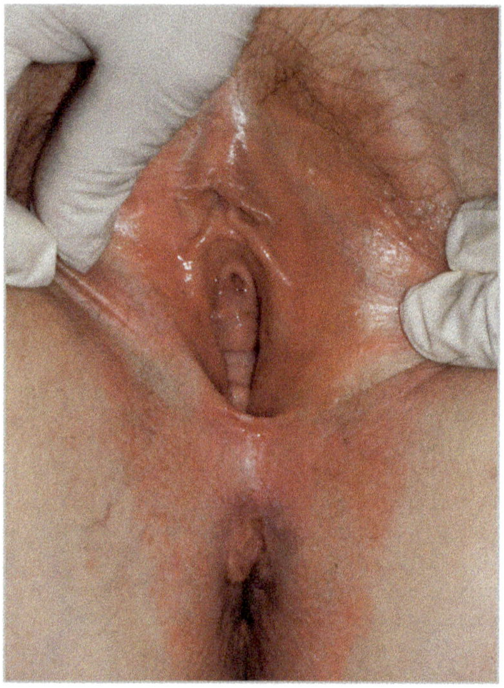

Figure 36.2 Paget disease of the vulva. Note the erythematous, eczematoid plaque. By courtesy of Prof. Hope Haefner Ann Arbor, USA.

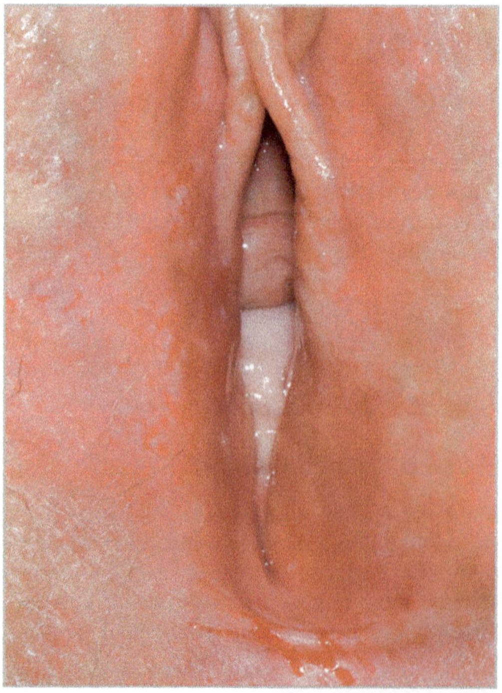

Figure 36.3 Paget disease of the vulva. Note the erythematous plaque with excoriations and lichenification. By courtesy of Prof. Hope Haefner Ann Arbor, USA.

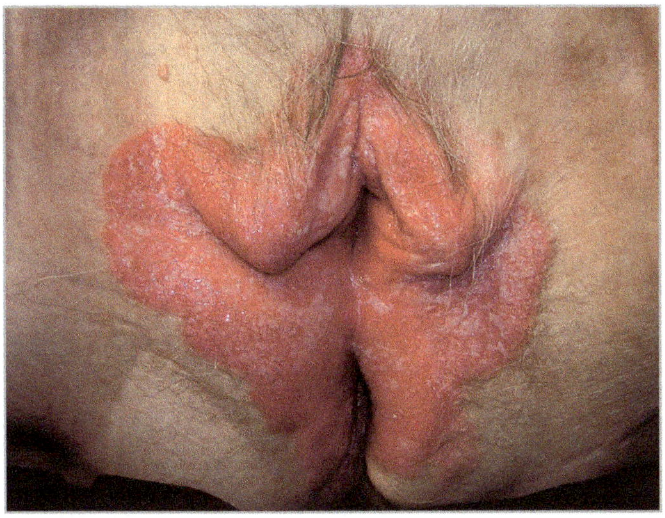

Figure 36.4 Extensive Paget disease.

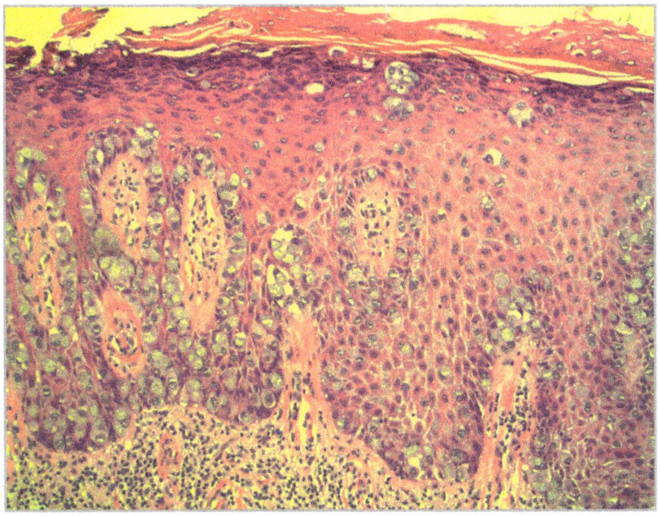

Figure 36.5 Paget disease (H&E ×100). Note the large cells with abundant, pale, vacuolated cytoplasm, large pleomorphic nuclei, and prominent nucleoli. They exist singly or in nests, mostly in the basal and parabasal layers, with a few scattered throughout, including in the superficial epithelium. By courtesy of Dr David Schammel, Greenville, USA.

Location in anogenital region (Shaco-Levy et al. 2010)

- Vulva 65%
  - Labium majus 68%
  - Labium minus 57%
  - Clitoris 20%
  - Perineum 18%
- Perianal 18–20%
- Other locations (also apocrine rich)
  - Groin
  - Thigh
  - Buttocks
  - Axilla
  - Eyelids
  - External ear canal

Association with malignancy

The secondary non-cutaneous form of EMPD is, by definition, associated with an underlying neoplasia.

It is controversial whether primary EMPD is associated with other non-vulvar malignancies. A literature review reported rates between 0% and 50% with no significant difference between the cancer rate in patients with Paget disease and an age and sex match cohort without Paget disease (Preti et al. 2003).

INVESTIGATIONS

The diagnosis must be confirmed histologically. Once the diagnosis has been made, the primary objective is to differentiate between primary cutaneous and secondary non-cutaneous forms of EMPD. The distinction is crucial, as their management and prognosis differ greatly. Their cutaneous and histological presentation on routine hematoxylin and eosin (H&E) stain is identical. Immunohistochemistry is essential in their differentiation. Adjunctive studies are necessary for diagnostic confirmation. For cases with dermal invasion, preoperative evaluation for nodal metastasis should be considered. This includes positron emission tomography (PET), sentinel node biopsy with or without single photon emission computed tomography (SPECT), and multidetector computed tomography (CT) (Delport 2013).

Histopathology

Hematoxylin and eosin

The histologic diagnosis of Paget disease requires the identification of Paget cells. These are large cells with abundant, pale, possibly vacuolated cytoplasm, large pleomorphic nuclei, and prominent nucleoli. They exist singly or in nests, mostly in the basal and parabasal layers, with a few scattered throughout the superficial epithelium (**Figures 36.5** and **36.6**); extension into adnexal structures is common. Hyperkeratosis, acanthosis, and parakeratosis are also frequent features.

Conditions that follow a 'pagetoid spread' distribution must be considered in the differential diagnosis. These include cells of epithelial, melanocytic, neuroendocrine, lymphoid, and histiocytic origins. However, clinically, these entities do not resemble EMPD; distinct immunochemistry profiles distinguish these entities.

In the presence of dermal invasion, the intraepithelial Paget cells contiguously extend into the underlying dermis, often in a 'spray-like' pattern. By contrast, Paget cell extension into the squamous epithelium of adjacent hair follicles and sweat glands does not constitute invasion.

When EMPD arises as a cutaneous manifestation of an underlying adenocarcinoma, Paget cells originate from a skin appendage (apocrine/eccrine gland), or a subcutaneous vulvar gland (Bartholin gland). Histologically, the Paget cell laden epithelium overlies and is contiguous with the glandular neoplasm.

Important: Primary cutaneous and secondary non-cutaneous EMPDs are usually indistinguishable on routine H&E staining.

Immunohistochemistry

Immunohistochemistry is important in ruling out the main histologic differentials of pagetoid cells in the epidermis, namely melanoma in situ and squamous cell carcinoma (SCC) in situ. In melanoma in

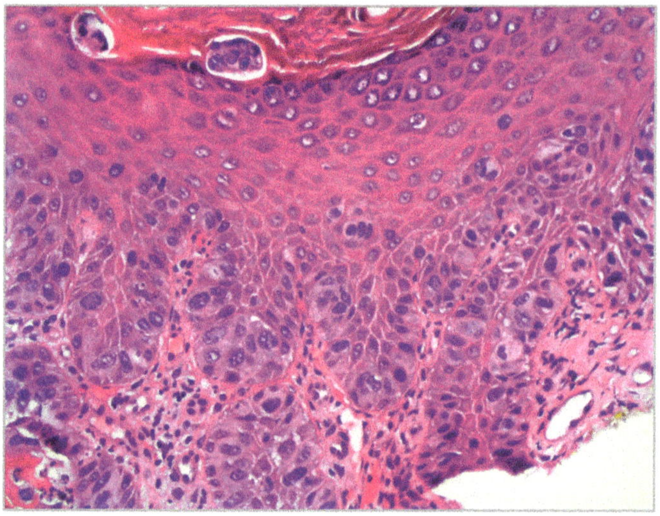

Figure 36.6 Paget cells with abundant, pale cytoplasm, and large pleomorphic nuclei (H&E ×100). By courtesy of Dr David Schammel Greenville, USA).

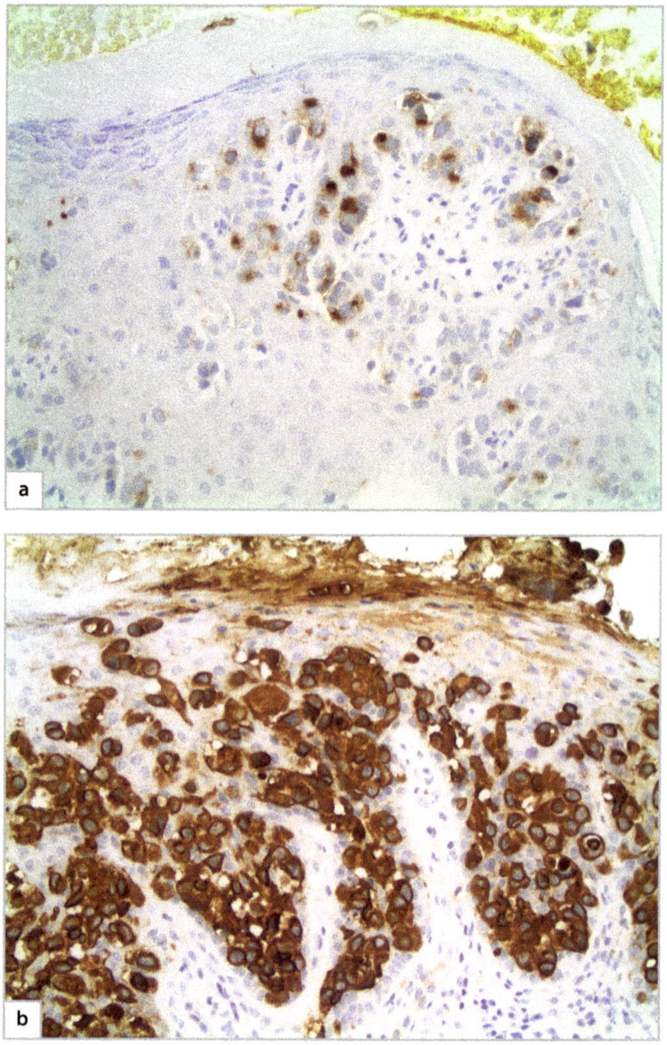

Figure 36.7 Primary cutaneous extramammary Paget disease. (a) Gross cystic disease fluid protein 15. (b) Cytokeratin 7 (CK7) immunoreactivity. By courtesy of Dr David Schammel, Greenville, USA).

situ, cells are MEL-A, S100, and human melanoma black (HMB45) positive. With SCC in situ, pankeratin markers are positive, whereas cytokeratin (CK7) is negative. Immunoreactivity is crucial in differentiating between the various EMPD subtypes, as each has a distinct immunoprofile (**Table 36.2**). Primary cutaneous Paget disease is uniquely immunoreactive to gross cystic disease fluid protein (GCDFP-15), but also to CK7 (**Figure 36.7a,b**). Paget disease secondary to anorectal adenocarcinoma is universally immunoreactive to CK20, but not to CK7 nor to GCDFP-15. Paget disease of urothelial origin is uniquely immunoreactive to uroplakin-III, but less consistently to CK7 and CK20.

SCREENING FOR MALIGNANCY

Given the uncertain association with distant malignancy, a protocol has not been defined; however, the investigations should be targeted depending on the immunohistochemical profile and site of origin. For

Table 36.2 Summary of immunoprofiles (Wilkinson & Brown 2002, Wilkinson Atlas 2012, Crum et al. 2014)

Immunostatins	1° EMPD	2° Anorectal	2° Urothelial	Melanoma in situ	SCC in situ
CK 7	+	–	–	–	–
CK 20	–	+	+/–	–	–
GCDFP-15	+	–	–	–	–
Uroplakin III	–	–	+	–	–
S100/Mel A/HMB45	–	–	–	+	–
Pankeratin	+	+	+	–	+
HER2/neu	+				
CDX2		+			
P53	+ (invasion)				

CK, cytokine; EMPD, extramammary Paget disease; GCDFP, gross cystic disease fluid protein; HMB, human melanoma black; SCC, squamous cell carcinoma example, EMPD affecting the vestibule with uroplakin III positivity should prompt a search for a urological tumor (cystoscopy). Perianal EMPD and CK20 positivity should prompt a search for bowel cancer (colonoscopy). There may be little value in screening EMPD affecting the lateral vulva and GCDFP-15 positivity as primary cutaneous disease is expected. It might be prudent to do a system's enquiry and a full body examination and target investigations if appropriate.

Adjunctive studies to consider

- Vaginal and cervical cytology
- Colposcopy
- Endometrial biopsy
- Hysteroscopy
- Pelvic sonography
- Bladder cytology
- Cystoscopy
- Intravenous pyelogram
- Colonoscopy
- Mammography

DIFFERENTIAL DIAGNOSIS

Clinically, conditions most commonly confused are psoriasis, eczema, candidosis, and high-grade squamous intraepithelial lesions of the vulva/differentiated vulvar intraepithelial neoplasia. Although the symptoms of candidosis are similar to that of EMPD, its cutaneous manifestations are symmetrical and less demarcated, with diagnosis readily confirmed on microscopy. Psoriasis is typically symmetrical. Eczema often presents with erythema, excoriation, and erosion, but is less associated with hyperkeratosis; it responds readily to corticosteroid regimen.

Main differential diagnoses of EMPD

- Psoriasis
- Eczema
- Candidosis
- Contact dermatitis
- Differentiated vulvar intraepithelial neoplasia
- High-grade squamous intraepithelial lesions of the vulva
- Lichen sclerosus, hyperplastic variety
- Lichen simplex chronicus
- Lichen planus
- Other neoplasms of the vulva
- Langerhans cell histiocytosis

TREATMENT

Many treatment modalities have been reported; however, due to the rarity of EPMD and lack of published prospective data, no specific treatment recommendations can be made from the currently available literature (Edey et al. 2013). For now, therapeutic decisions are based on clinical considerations, including anatomic involvement, dermal invasion, lesion size, patient's age, general condition, and preferences (Delport 2013). Treatment objectives are eradication of macroscopic and microscopic disease, while avoiding overtreatment and long-term sequelae. In secondary non-cutaneous EMPD, the focus is on treating the underlying malignancy.

Surgery

Surgery has historically been the most favored approach; however, surgery may be mutilating when disease is extensive or in difficult anatomical sites such as the clitoral hood and recurrence is common. Furthermore, it is difficult to define margins required for surgery. In intraepithelial neoplasm without invasion or microinvasion <1 mm, wide local excision of all clinically visible disease plus a 2–3 cm lateral margin is the most accepted approach. Resection of the subcutaneous tissue down to the level of the fascia to remove all skin appendages is essential to rule out invasion and underlying adnexal adenocarcinoma. However, despite the 2–3 cm lateral margin, 40–70% of specimens are positive on permanent section (Jones et al. 2011), but the positivity has no effect on recurrence rate or survival, especially with normal appearing skin. Frozen section margin assessment is of little value, as the risk of associated underlying adenocarcinoma peripheral to clinically evident disease is virtually non-existent (Wilkinson Atlas 2012). Defect closure may be primary or with a rotational versus split-thickness graft. Lymph node dissection is not indicated, as lymphatic metastasis is extremely rare. In intraepithelial neoplasms with invasion >1 mm or associated underlying adnexal adenocarcinoma due to increased risk of nodal involvement, both surgical excision of cutaneous lesion and lymphatic assessment are indicated. Preoperative PET may aid intraoperative planning (Delport 2013). For inguinofemoral lymphadenectomy, ipsilateral dissection is sufficient for laterally located disease, with bilateral dissection for centrally located disease. Alternatively, sentinel node biopsy carries a lower risk of infection and chronic lymphedema. Positive involvement may require complete dissection or radiotherapy.

Mohs micrographic surgery

Mohs micrographic surgery allows for mapping of microscopic tumor extent, enabling excision to include lesional tissue only. The mean margin to clear entire tumor is 2.5 cm, although a 5 cm margin is needed to remove all microscopic diseases in 97% of cases (Hendi et al. 2004).

CO_2 or Nd:YAG laser

This modality may be considered in those who are poor surgical candidates. However, no histologic assessment of margins is possible.

Imiquimod

Imiquimod is an immune modulator that enhances both innate and acquired immunity by stimulating the production and release of pro-inflammatory cytokines. The cytotoxic response leads to tumor cell destruction and apoptosis. Imiquimod may be used as monotherapy, as a neoadjuvant therapy before surgery to reduce disease burden, enabling a more conservative excision, or as an adjuvant therapy. Most clinicians treat clinically visible lesions plus a 2 cm margin of normal appearing skin, with varying dosage interval and treatment duration, ranging from -two to seven times a week, for 6–28 weeks; however, treating twice a week is better tolerated than daily treatment. Side effects are dose related, and include local irritation/erythema/pain, flu-like symptoms, nausea, and emesis. Treatment response rate may be up to 80%, with response relating to the length of treatment (Luyten et al. 2014). A typical regime used in vulvar clinics might be twice weekly application with an 8-week review. Patients require soothing emollients and mild topical corticosteroids to help with symptoms. However, treatment with imiquimod is used off label for this indication and long-term follow-up studies are required.

Photodynamic therapy

Photodynamic therapy (PDT) with methyl-5-aminolevulinic acid 20% may be used alone, combined with CO_2 laser, or as an adjuvant to surgery (Delport 2013, Lam & Funaro 2010). Dosage interval and treatment duration are not defined, and healing may be prolonged (Delport 2013, Lam & Funaro 2010). This is a promising treatment with the benefit of no scarring; however, it requires specialist treatment. Systemic PDT with porfimer sodium may be appropriate for deeper or resistant lesions.

Topical 5-fluouracil

Topical 5-fluorouracil cream may also serve as adjuvant therapy or in combination therapy, but is not used as monotherapy, as it cannot penetrate the full pathologic depth despite clearing visible disease. The optimal dosage interval and treatment duration are undefined (Lam & Funaro 2010).

Systemic chemotherapy

Systemic chemotherapy may be used in locally advanced disease or in metastasis. However, optimal drug combination, dosage interval, and treatment duration are not defined. Trastuzumab has been reported to be of use in resistant or metastatic EMPD, where the Paget cells were HER2 receptor positive (Karam et al. 2008).

Radiotherapy

Radiotherapy may serve as a neoadjuvant therapy before surgery, as adjuvant therapy after surgery for those with underlying adenocarcinoma or lymph node metastasis, or as monotherapy for the elderly, those with large lesions, or disease affecting functionally delicate anatomy. The optimal technique is undefined. Side effects may be acute or chronic, including vulvitis, vaginal stenosis, sexual dysfunction, cystitis, enteritis, and proctitis.

COURSE AND PROGNOSIS

Primary in situ disease

Primary in situ disease and those with microinvasion <1 mm have an indolent course, although diagnostic delay may allow for horizontal spread, resulting in a larger lesion that is more challenging to surgically excise. Dermal invasion, lymphatic, or distant metastasis is rare. Prognosis is excellent despite the diagnostic delay, and is independent of lesion size, treatment modality, and margin status, with no mortality attributable to EMPD.

Primary Paget disease

Primary Paget disease with invasion >1 mm and those with underlying adenocarcinoma have an intermediate course. Five-year mortality is 13–18% overall, but as high as 50% with lymphatic metastasis (Delport 2013, Lam & Funaro 2010). Clitoral involvement (Parker et al. 2000) and presence of a nodule suggesting invasive disease may be negative prognosticators.

Secondary non-cutaneous disease

Secondary non-cutaneous disease is typified by a more aggressive course. Its prognosis is guarded, dependent on its underlying malignancy. Mortality approaches 50%.

Local recurrences are common, ranging from 30% to 60% across all subtypes and treatment modalities. These are typically intraepithelial disease near the excision margin. They represent excision failures due to multifocal disease, irregular pattern of spread, and microscopic extension beyond clinically visible lesion. They are treated with repeat excisions. It is controversial whether margin status on permanent section correlates with recurrence rate (Black et al. 2007, Parker et al. 2000), further calling into question the utility of frozen section at the time of excision (Shaco-Levy et al. 2010). Local recurrences have little impact on prognosis. However, as they may occur as far out as 12 years after the initial diagnosis, long-term surveillance is imperative.

Distal recurrences occur remote from surgical margin, including nodal metastasis. They are secondary to the aggressiveness of the tumor. As expected, the prognosis is poor.

REFERENCES

Black D, Tornos C, Soslow R, et al. The outcome of patients with positive margin after excision for intraepithelial Paget's disease of the vulva. Gynecol Oncol 2007; 104:547–550.

Crum C, Herrington S, McCluggage WG, et al. Tumours of the vulva. Epithelial tumours. In: RJ Kurmar, ML Carcangiu, CS Herrington and RH Young (eds), World Health Organisation, Classification of Tumours of the Female Genital Tract. Lyon: IACR, 2014:232–240.

Delport ES. Extramammary Paget's disease of the vulva: an annotated review of the current literature. Australas J Dermatol 2013; 54:9–24.

Edey KA, Allan E, Murdoch JB, et al. Interventions for the treatment of Paget's disease of the vulva (review). The Cochrane Collaboration. Cochrane Library 2013; 10:1–26.

Fanning J, Lambert HCL, Hale TM, et al. Paget's disease of the vulva: prevalence of associated vulvar adenocarcinoma, invasive Paget's disease, and recurrence after surgical excision. Am J Obstet Gynecol 1999; 180:24–27.

Hatta N, Yamada M, Hirano A, et al. Extramammary Paget's disease: treatment, prognostic factors and outcome in 76 patients. Br J Dermatol 2008; 158:313–318.

Hendi A, Brodland D, Zitelli J. Extramammary Paget's disease: surgical treatment with Mohs micrographic surgery. J Am Acad Dermatol 2004; 51:767–773.

Jones ISC, Crandon A, Sanday K. Paget's disease of the vulva: diagnosis and follow-up key to management: a retrospective study of 50 cases from Queensland. Gyn Oncol 2011; 122:42–44.

Karam A, Berek JS, Stenson A, et al. HER/neu targeting for recurrent vulvar Paget's disease. A case report and literature review. Gyn Oncol 2008; 111:568–571.

Lam C, Funaro D. Extramammary Paget's disease: summary of current knowledge. Dermatol Clin 2010; 28:807–826.

Luyten A, Sorgel P, Clad Andreas, et al. Treatment of extramammary Paget disease of the vulva with imiquimod: a retrospective, multicenter study by

the German Colposcopy Network. J Am Acad Dermatol 2014; 70:644–650.
Parker LP, Parker JR, Bodurka-Bevers D, et al. Paget's disease of the vulva: pathology, pattern of involvement, and prognosis. Gyn Oncol 2000; 77:183–189.
Preti M, Micheletti L, Massobrio M, et al. Vulvar Paget disease: one century after first reported. J Low Genit Tract Dis 2003; 7:122–135.
Shaco-Levy R, Bean S, Vollmer R, et al. Paget disease of the vulva: a study of 56 cases. Eur J Obstet Gynecol Reprod Biol 2010; 149:86–91.
Wilkinson EJ, Brown HM. Vulvar Paget disease of urothelial origin: a report of three cases and a proposed classification of vulvar Paget disease. Human Pathol 2002; 33:549–554.

FURTHER READING

Kurman RJ, Ronnett BM, Sherman ME, Wilkinson EJ. Intraepithelial neoplasms: Paget disease and Paget-like lesions. AFIP Atlas of Tumor Pathology Series 4: Tumors of the Cervix, Vagina, and Vulva, 1st edn. Washington, DC: The American Registry of Pathology – Armed Forces Institute of Pathology, 2010: pp334–339.
Wilkinson EJ, Stone IK. Paget Disease. Atlas of Vulvar Disease, 3rd edn. Philadelphia, PA: Lippincott Williams & Wilkins, 2012: pp78–84.

Chapter 37 Vulvar vascular disease

Marianne G R De Maeseneer, Mirte Siemerink

Important vascular lesions of the vulva

- Varicose veins
- Vascular malformations
- Hemangioma of infancy
- Vulvar lymphedema

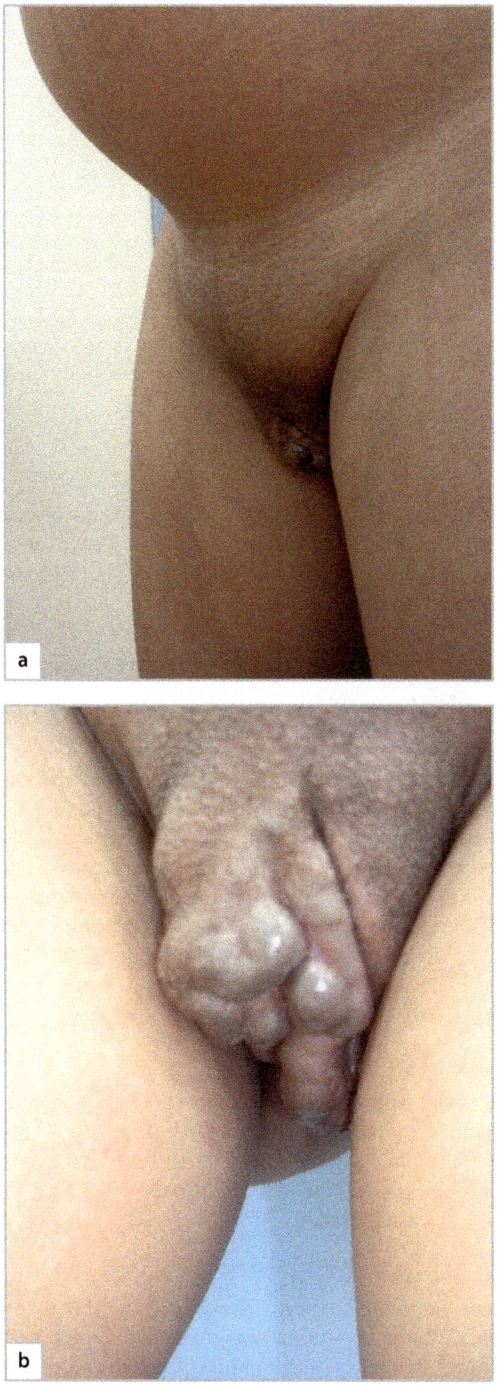

Figure 37.1 (a, b) Vulvar varices in pregnancy. Prominent vulvar varicose veins at 30 weeks of pregnancy.

VULVAR VARICOSE VEINS

Key points

- Vulvar varicose veins are related to pelvic vein incompetence in most cases
- If symptomatic, they can be treated by coil embolization and foam sclerotherapy
- In some patients, vulvar varices may be related to deep venous obstruction

Vulvar varices related to pelvic vein incompetence

Reflux in ovarian veins and/or internal iliac veins may cause dilatation of the veins of the vulvar region.

Clinical findings

Vulvar varicose veins are the most common vascular lesion of the vulva and are in particular precipitated by pregnancy (**Figure 37.1**). They occur in 10% of pregnant women, generally appearing during the 5th month of a second pregnancy, and subsequent pregnancies (van Cleef 2011). Vulvar varices are not an indication for a cesarean section delivery. Usually, vulvar varices disappear a month after delivery but sometimes they tend to persist after pregnancy, in particular in multiparous women. Vulvar varices usually are in direct connection with incompetent ovarian veins, and/or internal iliac veins. They may also connect with (recurrent) varicose veins in the great saphenous vein territory (**Figure 37.2**).

Women typically describe complaints of a heavy feeling in the vulvar region, pruritus, fatigue, and dyspareunia. Sometimes, vulvar varicose veins also can cause pain while sitting, walking, or cycling. Menstruation can worsen the symptoms in some women. Lying down may decrease symptoms, as in many other cases of chronic venous disease. The above mentioned complaints are often described as the 'pelvic congestion syndrome.' In addition to varicose veins of the vulva, these women may typically display varicose veins at the medial or posteromedial side of the thigh.

Diagnosis and management

Diagnosis is confirmed by duplex ultrasound (DUS) of the vulvar region, often combined with DUS of the lower limbs in case of varicose veins. In addition, transvaginal DUS may be helpful to confirm the pelvic origin of the varices. In most cases of symptomatic vulvar varicose veins, an additional venogram is needed to further analyze the pelvic veins (Castenmiller et al. 2013). If incompetent ovarian or internal iliac veins are found, these can immediately be treated by

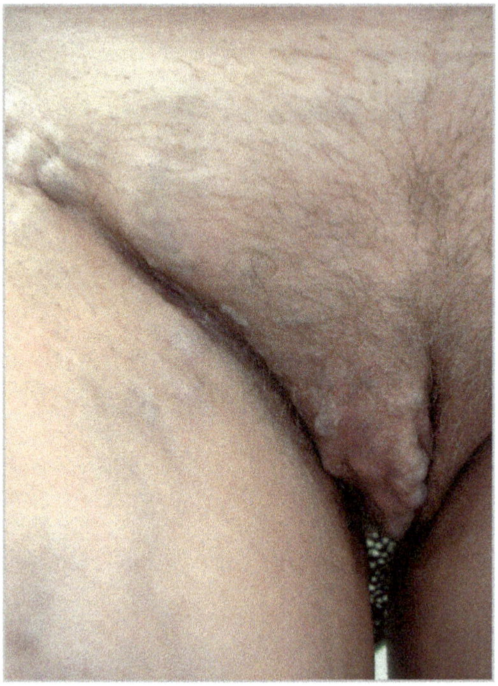

Figure 37.2 Recurrent varicose veins involving the vulva. Recurrent varicose veins at the right saphenofemoral junction 7 years after high ligation and stripping of the great saphenous vein, in connection with vulvar varicosities.

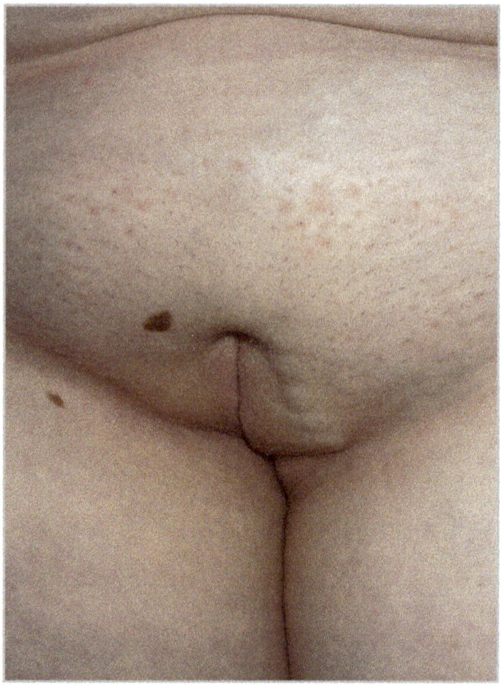

Figure 37.3 Vulvar varicose veins in post-thrombotic syndrome. Young woman (18 years) presenting with varix on the left labium, in connection with 'cross-over' pubic collateral veins. History of deep vein thrombosis of the left common iliac and external iliac vein 1 year earlier. Duplex ultrasound confirmed persistent left iliac obstruction.

the interventional radiologist in the same session, by means of coil embolization, often combined with foam sclerotherapy. If necessary, additional treatment of the vulvar veins is possible by (foam) sclerotherapy or, in rare occasions, by phlebectomy.

Vulvar varices related to deep venous obstruction

In some patients, varicose veins may develop in the (supra)pubic and vulvar region, secondary to an underlying iliac or iliocaval obstruction after deep vein thrombosis (DVT), or a non-thrombotic iliac vein lesion, such as in case of May-Thurner syndrome (compression of the left common iliac vein by the right common iliac artery), or even a nutcracker syndrome (compression of the left renal vein between the superior mesenteric artery and the aorta). In case of obstruction of the iliac veins, a cross-pubic collateral circulation may develop, deviating the venous flow from the affected leg to the contralateral deep venous system (Wittens et al. 2010).

Clinical findings

Typically, enlarged collateral veins can be seen (or palpated) passing over the pubic region, and even on the labia (**Figure 37.3**). These collaterals may dilate considerably after physical effort. Patients complain of symptoms of heaviness and increased tension in the pubic area, in addition to swelling of the affected leg.

Diagnosis and management

In particular when there is a history of previous (iliac) DVT, additional evaluation of the deep venous system above the groin and its collateral pathways, by means of abdominal DUS and computed tomography and/or venogram, is mandatory. If the vulvar 'varicose' veins are indeed part of the collateral circulation, they should not be treated. In certain patients with severe post-thrombotic syndrome due to residual obstruction after iliofemoral DVT, recanalization and stenting may be considered. After successful stent placement, pubic and vulvar collaterals may completely 'disappear.'

VASCULAR MALFORMATIONS

Vascular malformations are embryonic remnants derived from a very early, not yet differentiated stage of vascular tissue development. At the level of the vulva, they are rare. The exact incidence is unknown (Wang et al. 2009). They can be subcategorized by flow characteristics into high-flow (arterial or arteriovenous) and low-flow (capillary, venous, and lymphatic) malformations. Combinations of vascular malformations, e.g. capillary-venous malformation and capillary-lymphatic-venous malformation, are described as well.

Klippel-Trenaunay syndrome is a sporadic and complex malformation characterized by the clinical triad of (i) capillary malformation (nevus flammeus), (ii) soft tissue and bone hypertrophy, and (iii) atypical varicosities that may involve the vulvar region.

Vulvar vascular malformations

Clinical findings

In most cases, vulvar vascular malformations are obvious at birth. They mostly grow progressively after puberty. Rarely, they present in postmenopausal women (Wang et al. 2009). Clinical findings can range from small nodules to diffuse compressible swelling and may end up as a large (unilateral) vulvar mass (**Figure 37.4**). Some lesions remain asymptomatic but others cause tenderness or obvious discomfort and pain.

Diagnosis and management

Ultrasound can help to distinguish between low-flow and high-flow malformations, but in most cases T1- and T2-weighted MRI is needed to evaluate the extension of the vascular or lymphatic lesion. In older women, it is very important to rule out underlying malignancies (by imaging and/or a biopsy). Most cases do not need any specific treatment. However, in case of severe symptoms or complications, the patient should be referred to an experienced multidisciplinary team for further diagnosis and specialized treatment.

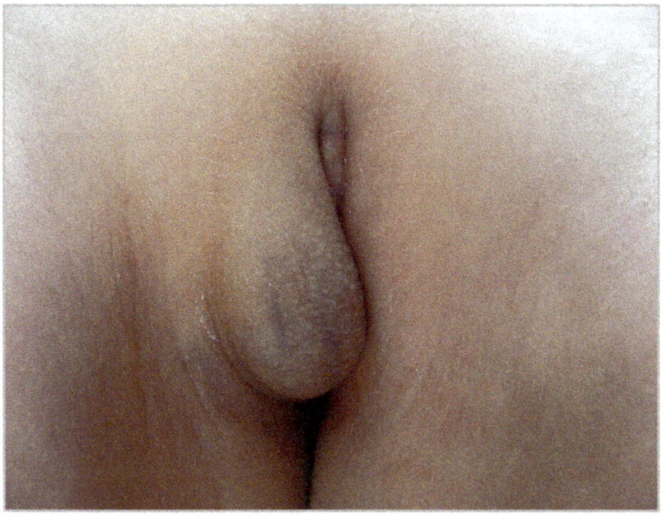

Figure 37.4 Venous malformation. Large venous malformation of the right labium in a 9-year-old girl.

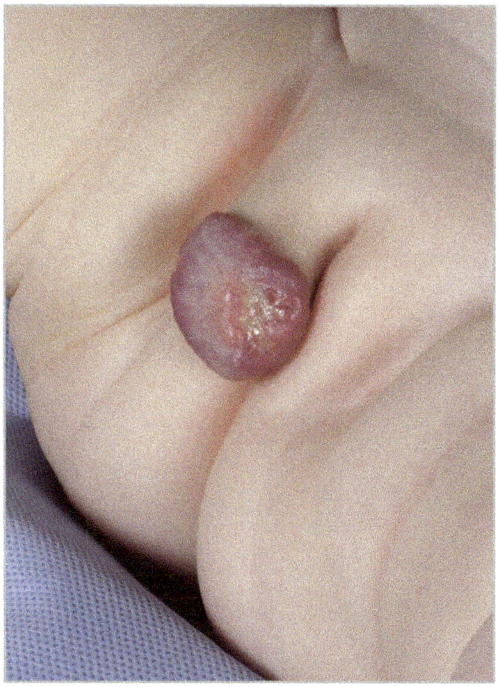

Figure 37.5 Infantile hemangioma of the right labium major in a 3-month-old baby.

VULVAR HEMANGIOMA OF INFANCY

This is the most common soft tissue tumor of infancy. It is not present at birth but appears soon after birth. It is a benign endothelial cell neoplasm that has a typical growth pattern, characterized by fast proliferation followed by gradual spontaneous involution. Clinical diagnosis is usually obvious (**Figure 37. 5**). Treatment is not always necessary, but local care may be difficult, as the lesion may ulcerate in the occluded nappy. In case of a large, obstructing, or ulcerating hemangioma treatment with systemic propranolol, prednisolone or atenolol should be considered, always in close collaboration with the pediatrician. Topical steroids, topical beta-blockers and ablative laser therapy may be indicated for smaller lesions or if beta-blocking therapy has failed.

Vulvar angiokeratomata

Angiokeratomata are well-circumscribed vascular lesions consisting of superficial vascular ectasia and hyperkeratosis. They can be single or multiple. Angiokeratoma results from dilation of pre-existing vessels in the papillary dermis. Etiology and pathogenesis remain unclear. In the vulvar region, angiokeratomata are also mentioned as 'angiokeratoma of Fordyce.' In some cases, the lesions may be associated with vulvar varicosities, hemorrhoids, or increased venous pressure during pregnancy (Terzakis et al. 2011).

When a patient has multiple angiokeratomata on the body, one has to consider 'angiokeratoma corporis diffusum,' also called Fabry disease. This is an X-linked inherited disorder caused by a deficiency of the lysosomal enzyme α-galactosidase.

Treatment of angiokeratomata is medically not necessary. Cosmetic removal can be achieved by surgical excision, electrocoagulation, or ablative laser therapy.

Vulvar lymphangioma circumscriptum

Lymphangioma circumscriptum is also mentioned as a superficial lymphatic malformation. Clinically it usually presents as papulovesicular lesions or cyst-like lesions. The condition is unpleasant but benign. Lymphangioma circumscriptum can be primary (present at birth or in early childhood) or secondary (acquired by impaired lymph flow due to, e.g. infections, trauma, surgery, radiation therapy, or lymphatic obstruction). Involvement of the vulva is quite rare. The differential diagnosis of lymphangioma circumscriptum of the vulva includes genital warts, molluscum contagiosum, tuberculosis verrucosa cutis, lymphogranuloma venereum, and filariasis (Shetty & Venkatesh 2012). Removal can be achieved by surgical excision or ablative laser therapy, but recurrence is frequent.

VULVAR LYMPHEDEMA

Vulvar lymphedema can be acute or chronic and can be caused by a broad range of underlying medical conditions resulting in lymphatic damage or dysfunction, which may be primary (e.g. Milroy disease) or secondary (e.g. due to trauma, surgery, obesity, malignancies, radiotherapy, and infections like erysipelas or filariasis in tropical countries).

Clinical findings can be diffuse enlargement with erythema and/or firm skin, papillomatous or verrucose plaques or even polyps or pedunculated masses, depending on the duration of lymphedema (Heller et al. 2014). Lymphangiectasia comprising small vesicles of lymphatic fluid may develop. These may leak fluid, which can be a distressing symptom. Vulvar lymphedema may become massive and interfere with normal walking in extreme cases (e.g. due to filariasis). Differential diagnosis of sarcomatous lesions or angiomyxoma should be considered (Papalas et al. 2013).

Treatment is that of the underlying condition. Massage and skin care advice is important. Compression hosiery/garments are difficult to use in the vulvar area. In case of recurrent erysipelas, long-term prophylactic antibiotics to prevent further damage to lymphatics due to recurring infections (often streptococcal) may be helpful. Difficult lymphangiectasia have been treated with the carbon dioxide laser but recurrence can be a problem.

REFERENCES

Castenmiller PH, de Leur K, de Jong TE, van der Laan L. Clinical results after coil embolization of the ovarian vein in patients with primary and recurrent lower-limb varices with respect to vulval varices. Phlebology 2013; 28:234–238.

Heller DS, Fitzhugh VA, Cracchiolo B, Barrett Jr T, Suidan RS. Massive localized lymphedema of the vulva: Report of a case and review of the literature. J Low Genit Tract Dis 2014; 18:46–49.

Papalas JA, Sangueza OP, Puri PK, Robboy SJ, Selim MA. Vulvar Vascular Tumors: A clinicopathologic study of 85 patients. Am J Dermatopathol 2013; 35:1–10.

Shetty V, Venkatesh S. Acquired lymphangioma circumscriptum of the vulva. Int J Gynaecol Obstet 2012; 117:190.

Terzakis E, Androutspoulos G, Zygouris D, et al. Angiokeratoma of the vulva. Eur J Gynaecol Oncol 2011; 32:597–598.

van Cleef JF. Treatment of vulval and perineal varicose veins. Phlebolymphology 2011; 18:38–42. Also available online from www.phlebolymphology.org/treatment-of-vulvar-and-perineal-varicose-veins/ (accessed 24 November 2015)

Wang S, Lang JH, Zhou HM. Venous malformations of the female lower genital tract. Eur J Obstet Gynecol Reprod Biol 2009; 145:205–208.

Wittens CH, Bukkems SF, Toonder IT. Abdominal wall venous collaterals: the latent clinical sign for central venous obstruction. Circulation 2010; 122:2089–2090.

Chapter 38 Vulvodynia

David Nunns

Key features

- Vulvodynia is a cause of chronic genital pain that has a variety of clinical presentations and treatment options
- Vulvodynia can be classified as provoked (vestibulodynia) or unprovoked, but many patients have both symptoms
- The history should be tailored to the presenting complaint and may include a pain and psychosexual history if appropriate
- A clinical examination is essential to exclude other overlooked causes of vulvar pain (e.g. fissures)
- The role of the generalist in secondary care is to make a diagnosis, counsel the patient, give written information, direct to patient support groups, and start basic treatment
- The current referral pattern of patients to secondary care may mean vulvodynia patients with chronic pain or psychosexual problems may need onward referral to a vulvar service where a multidisciplinary approach can be helpful. This will depend on the individual needs of the patient
- Good evidence for effective care is lacking

INTRODUCTION

Vulvodynia has been defined by the International Society for the Study of Vulvovaginal Disease as 'vulvar discomfort, most often described as a burning pain, occurring in the absence of relevant visible findings or a specific, clinically identifiable, neurologic disorder' (Haefner 2007) (see also Chapter 09). It is a neuropathic pain syndrome. The suffix 'dynia' refers to pain and vulvodynia is analogous to a variety of other neuropathic pain syndromes. Patients can be further classified by the anatomical site of the pain (e.g. generalized vulvodynia, hemivulvodynia, and clitorodynia) and also by whether pain is provoked or unprovoked. Patients with provoked pain usually complain of sexual pain and were formerly diagnosed as having 'vestibulitis.' This is incorrect as there is no evidence that vulvodynia is an inflammatory condition and patient with provoked pain should now be diagnosed as vestibulodynia. The clinician's perception is that these patients are difficult and chronic, but this is possibly as a result of late diagnosis, a lack of clinical recognition, and use of inappropriate treatments usually antifungals. Patients can lose confidence in health professionals and can become isolated in their condition through embarrassment and an unwillingness to discuss problems. This can lead to psychological upset. Some patients may have a combination of vulvodynia with another vulvar problem, e.g. irritant dermatitis or thrush, and both conditions may require treatment. If there is diagnostic uncertainty, a biopsy needs to be taken.

EPIDEMIOLOGY

No robust incidence or prevalence study has been carried out and misdiagnosis is common.

PAIN PATHOPHYSIOLOGY

Acute pain has an important protective function as it limits further harm and encourages healing. This pain is usually inflammatory, is associated with tissue damage or injury, and clinically exhibits sensory hypersensitivity, which is characterized by hyperalgesia and allodynia. Hyperalgesia is the exaggerated response to noxious substances through a general increase in the responsiveness of tissues. Allodynia is the production of pain by stimuli that do not usually cause pain by a reduction in the sensory threshold of neurons.

If pain persists beyond 3 to 6 months, in some patients a neuropathic pain cycle can become established as a result of both central and peripheral nervous systems sensitization. This neuropathic pain is not usually inflammatory and the phenomena of hyperalgesia and allodynia may or may not be present. It is important to note that some patients do not always identify the term 'pain' with neuropathic pain symptoms but can describe a variety of sensations that include burning, stabbing, shooting, aching, and electric shock sensations. Uncommonly, these can include genital arousal states (Pink et al. 2014).

The reasons why vulvodynia may develop remain unclear, but recurrent vulvar inflammation may be a factor. One laboratory study showed a neuronal proliferation and allodynia in the vulva following repeated attacks of thrush in mice (Farmer et al. 2011). Vestibular neuronal proliferation has also been demonstrated in patients with vestibulodynia so it is possible that vulvodynia is a chronic pain syndrome where there are an excess of dysfunctional vulvar skin nociceptors (Tympanidis et al. 2003).

CLINICAL PRESENTATION

History

A general history including a 'vulvar history' is essential. A pain history should include nature, severity, site, and aggravating or relieving factors. One differential diagnosis is pudendal neuralgia that is a nerve entrapment syndrome of the pudendal nerve. These patients usually experience pain on sitting, which is relieved by lying down or standing. They also might complain of a 'lump or egg' being present in the vagina. An assessment of the impact of pain on function is always revealing ('How does the pain affect you?' or 'What do you miss as a result of the pain?').

A psychosexual history should be explored if appropriate. For women with provoked pain, sexual pain is the main complaint and can often be missed in the initial referral. Not infrequently, vulvodynia can lead to secondary psychosexual problems such as avoidance, phobia of touch, loss of libido, and vaginismus (see 'Psychological and psychosexual therapy and support' below). Recognition of this as the main problem for the patient is crucial so that treatment can focus on sexual rehabilitation either through self-management (increasing communication with partners, use of lubricant, and vaginal dilators) or with a psychosexual counselor.

Examination

Clinical examination of the patient with vulvodynia is often unrevealing but important as other vulvar conditions that can produce pain, e.g. subtle vulvar fissures, inflammatory vulvar disease, and vulvar high-grade squamous intraepithelial lesions of the vulva (HSIL). Patients with vestibulodynia can have tenderness on light cotton-stick touch over the vestibule. Remember, a red appearance of the vulva/vestibule can be a normal finding in a healthy woman. Not uncommonly, in the presence of vulvar pain, patients and health professionals wrongly connect areas of neuropathic pain to these areas of redness that represent a normal appearance (see also Chapter 10). Patients can become fixated with appearances.

A holistic view is always important when examining pain in patients to look for clues of anxiety and apprehension. This may be relevant as many treatments may involve physical therapy to 'desensitize' the vulva.

VESTIBULODYNIA (PROVOKED PAIN)

Vestibulodynia (old term: vestibulitis) is a cause of superficial dyspareunia and is characterized by vestibular tenderness on light touch. This excessive sensitivity can be generalized throughout the vestibule or can be more focal, involving the opening of the ducts of the major vestibular glands or the posterior fourchette (Peckham 1986).

Clinical features

Women are usually Caucasian, aged between 20 and 40 years, and present with a history of provoked pain, such as superficial dyspareunia, tampon intolerance, and pain during gynecological examinations (Marinnoff & Turner 1991). There is often a delay between the onset of symptoms and receiving a diagnosis, which varies from months to years. With the increasing awareness of vulvar problems including vulvar pain, this is likely to be of shorter duration from onset of symptoms to diagnosis, but there still can be delays on accessing appropriate treatment. A 6-month period of time has been arbitrarily suggested from the onset of symptoms to making a diagnosis of vestibulodynia so as to exclude women recovering from acute vulvar inflammation from other causes (Peckham 1986).

There appears to be a subgroup of women with vulvar vestibulodynia who exhibit abnormal estrogen receptor-α expression (Eva et al. 2003). It is speculated that the risk of developing combined hormonal contraceptives-induced vestibulodynia may be due to lowered free testosterone combined with an inefficient androgen receptor (AR) that predisposes women to vestibular pain (Goldstein et al. 2014).

As the condition is frequently chronic, a high level of psychological morbidity is common. Some patients are prone to stress and anxiety, which may play a role in developing symptoms (Nunns & Mandal 1997). Sexual dysfunction is common and frequently reported. Reduced arousal, more negative sexual feelings, and less spontaneous interest in sex (not elicited by a partner) have all been described in vestibulodynia. These are all risk factors for significant psychosexual dysfunction, such as vaginismus and anorgasmia, the management of which usually requires self-management strategies or psychosexual therapy input (Schover et al. 1991).

A cotton-tip applicator gently applied can identify vestibular allodynia. A defining feature of vestibulodynia is that the labial skin is non-tender. Sometimes an erythema of variable degree at the vestibulum is described; however, overinterpretation of red skin at the vestibulum is common. The application of diluted acetic acid (used to demonstrate neoplastic changes turning white if touched with acetic acid, e.g. in HSIL) to the vulva does not assist in making a diagnosis.

UNPROVOKED VULVODYNIA

This is a cause of either localized or generalized vulvar pain. Unlike women with provoked pain, those with unprovoked vulvodynia have more constant neuropathic-type of pain in the vulva and occasionally the perianal area.

Clinical features

- Patients can be of all ages (rarely children) but are typically perimenopausal or postmenopausal and, like patients with vestibulodynia, can present with a long history of multiple, inappropriate use of topical agents (treatment attempts) prior to a diagnosis (McKay 1987). Superficial dyspareunia is not consistently reported, as many women are less sexually active. In addition, many experience rectal, perineal, and urethral discomfort and there may be an overlap with other perineal pain syndromes. Psychological morbidity is likely to be high as a consequence of chronic pain.
- The impact on function and the severity of pain can be severe and warrant pain management referral.
- Clinical examination of the vulva shows no pathological changes.

Treatment principles

- The outcomes of effective treatment should include (1) a reduction in pain level with improved function, (2) confidence in self-managing symptoms through education and self-empowerment, and if relevant, (3) a reduction in pain experienced with sex with an improvement in sexual function and satisfaction.
- Many patients respond to simple measures, many of which involve self-help and patient education.
- The current referral pattern of patients to secondary care may mean vulvodynia patients with chronic pain or psychosexual problems may need onward referral to a vulvar service where a multidisciplinary approach can be helpful. This will depend on the individual needs of the patient.
- The role of the general dermatologist or gynecologist in managing the vulvodynia patient is to make a diagnosis, counsel the patient, direct to patient support groups, and start basic treatment. Patients resistant to treatment will need referral on to the vulvar service.
- The MDT approach for patients with complex needs includes a variety of health professionals including physiotherapist, the pain management team, psychosexual therapists, gynecologists, and dermatologists. Combining treatment is likely to produce greater benefits.
- The evidence base is poor, but the British Society for the Study of Vulval Disease, a society representing health professionals who have an interest in vulvar diseases has produced national guidance on the management based on existing evidence (Nunns et al. 2010). This guidance focuses on stratifying patient care depending on needs with a focus on self-management and care within primary and secondary healthcare, and vulvar services.
- The current referral pathway in the United Kingdom for patients is often disjointed that can result in patient hitting 'bottle-necks' in care. Patients welcome a health professional who can lead and coordinate care.
- Think of the '4 Ps' when planning treatment as follows:

Patient education and reassurance

An explanation of the condition including the nature of the diagnosis, the role of chronic pain pathways, and acknowledge of painful sex is helpful as many patients will not have heard this from a health professional. In the absence of a diagnosis, a void in understanding of symptoms can lead to worry and a lack of confidence in health professionals, which can potentially impact on compliance with treatment. Reassurance is essential especially with regard to fertility in younger women. **Box 38.1** outlines communication tips for health professionals when counseling patients.

Informal patient support and information through patient organizations such as the Vulval Pain Society (www.vulvalpainsociety.org) and the National Vulvodynia Association (www.nva.org) can be helpful.

Sensible vulvar skin care should be practiced to reduce the chance of contact sensitivity.

Patient should be told to give the treatments time to work, address the pain holistically, combine treatments, and self-educate. Self-management should be encouraged.

Pain modification

Pain-modifying drugs (PMDs) play a role in pain management and are useful for moderate-to-severe unprovoked pain (>5/10 on a pain scale). They address the central and peripheral components of neuropathic pain and usually reduce pain level and flare-ups. Patients with lesser degree of pain may on balance decline PMD due to a balance of function without pain but side effect gain. The drugs are more likely to work when patients are motivated to start treatment.

PMDs include amitriptyline and/or gabapentin. For amitriptyline (an antidepressant if used in higher doses), a dose of 10 mg/day, increasing every week until the pain is controlled, has been suggested. The average dosage is 60 mg/day, although up to 100 mg/day can be used (Munday 2001). Side effects usually settle within 2 weeks. Patients intolerant to the side effects can try nortriptyline. The duration of treatment is debatable, but some patients continue long-term.

Patients who are intolerant to drugs and have severe pain or have a decline in function as a result of pain should be referred to the vulvar service, specifically pain management services. Subsequent management may include nerve blocks, intralesional injections, transcutaneous electrical nerve stimulation, and acupuncture as examples. The latter two treatments can be accessed at any time.

Local anesthetic gels/ointment prior to sex are worthy of mention as first-line treatment. Occasionally, contact dermatitis can develop so they should be used with caution.

Physical therapy

The pelvic floor muscles (levator muscles) are complex support muscles that encircle the vagina. Many studies demonstrate pelvic floor muscle hypertonicity that further exacerbates the pain cycle (Glazer 1995). Patients are not often aware of this and treatment aims to relax and desensitize ('make less sensitive') these muscles. Whether this is secondary effect of vulvar pain or a synchronous problem is not clear.

There are a variety of techniques evidenced in the literature including pelvic floor exercises, use of vaginal dilators, and digital pelvic floor trigger point therapy to name a few. Access to these treatments will depend on the skillset of the local physiotherapist. The original papers reported success with biofeedback therapy using surface electromyographic signals from the pelvic to help overcome pelvic floor muscle dysfunction in women with vestibulodynia (Glazer 1995).

Box 38.1 Communication tips for health professionals when speaking to vulvodynia patients (remember the 4 'P's will vary according to the needs of the patient).

Patient education and reassurance
'Skin contains nerve endings that detect a variety of sensations, e.g. hot, cold, vibration, and pain. The sensation of pain is important to protect and guard us from further injury. In vulvodynia, there is a malfunction in these nerve endings, which involves both the pain receptors in the skin and the 'pain center' that is located in the brain. A cycle of pain can develop (the chronic pain cycle) through excessive 'electrical' signal between the brain and the vulva. Stress and anxiety can increase the level of pain (increase the 'electrical' signal), whereas various treatments (outlined below) such as relaxation and exercise can reduce the level of pain (reduce the signal).'

Pain modification
'Pain modifying drugs (e.g. amitriptyline) do not usually cure pain but can reduce the pain intensity by reducing the level of 'electrical' signal in the pain cycle ('turning down the volume'). A reduction in pain can improve function, quality of life, and mood. It is important to give the treatment time to work over several weeks to months and increase the dosage according to your pain levels. Some drugs are antidepressants (usually much higher doses needed) but are used for the treatment of pain in vulvodynia and not depression. Side effects may occur within the first 2 weeks but usually subside.'

Physical treatments
'Your body's response to vulvar pain is to contract and protect. This can lead to a tightening (hypertonia) of the pelvic floor muscles, which are a large hammock of muscles sitting deep in the pelvis. This tightening can lead to further pain so retraining these muscles to encourage relaxation and less hypertonia can help reduce pain levels. There are a variety of ways of carrying this out including pelvic floor exercises or massage of the vulvar area with a finger. Sometimes this is overseen by a physiotherapist. These techniques are designed to 'desensitize,' i.e. make less sensitive to touch the vulvar area and are combined with your other treatments.'

Psychological and psychosexual therapy and support
'Understandably vulvodynia has a large impact on your ability to have penetrative sex. Vulvar pain produces a guarding or protective response and therefore, from a sexual function perspective, can lead to avoidance of intimacy, poor lubrication, loss of sex drive, and vaginismus. Vaginismus is the term we give to an involuntary tightening of the low pelvic floor muscles and is a guarding response. Tightening of these muscles on penetration leads to more pain (and more avoidance). With time, there can be a relationship breakdown usually because of a lack of understanding of the problem and poor communication. It is important to discuss these issues and your feelings with your partner as most problems can easily be resolved with simple measures including relaxation, the use of good lubricants, a greater focus on arousal, and using some of the desensitizing techniques (mentioned above). Vaginal dilators are small pieces of plastic to be inserted into the vagina by you, to build up confidence, and make you less phobic about touch and insertion. Either you can work through this with your partner (see www.vaginismus.com) or sessions with a trained psychosexual counselor can help to give you more of a focus and framework to work to.'

Effective treatment for vulvodynia involves combining many different treatment types (the '4Ps') to give an overall benefit.

Psychological and psychosexual therapy and support

Basic level psychological support should be given by all health professionals that includes reassurance that there is no underlying medical problem, challenge abnormal beliefs about symptoms, recognizing the 'body-mind' connection, and the role of stress and how it amplifies pain perception (stress can produce the 'flight-fight' response that increases the sensation of pain).

Some patients require more than basic support in a clinic consultation and mindfulness/cognitive-behavioral therapy (CBT). Self-management or formal referral to a clinical psychologist may be needed (Masheb et al. 2009). CBT can play an important role in addressing many issues that women with vulvodynia face. **Figure 38.1** outlines the 'hot-cross bun' connection that can exist between thoughts, emotions, physical sensations, and behavior.

Some women with vestibulodynia may require sexual therapy and this can be structured over several sessions with a psychosexual counselor, preferably with the woman's partner. Much of sexual therapists work, however, is basic education on the anatomy of the vulva and pelvis and sexual response cycle that could be outlined within the clinic consultation prior to referral. Psychosexual counselors can help improving physical non-coital sexual contact, overcome pelvic floor muscle hypertonia using sensate focus therapy (structured goal setting), and helping low libido and anorgasmia.

Surgery for provoked pain

Surgical removal of neuropathic painful skin from women with vestibulodynia is disputed; however, there are proponents of surgery who have produced favorable results. The clinical community remains divided on its value.

The modified vestibulectomy is the procedure of choice for patients with vestibulodynia. It involves excision of a horseshoe-shaped area of the vestibule followed by dissection of the posterior vaginal wall to cover the skin defect. In the largest series, the outcome was pain-free sex in 59% and the majority of patients had no regrets about surgery when followed up for long term (Eva et al. 2008).

In a randomized control trial, 78 women with vestibulodynia were randomized to one of three arms: (1) group CBT (12 weeks duration), (2) pelvic floor biofeedback therapy (12 weeks duration), and (3) vestibulectomy (Bergeron et al. 2001). At follow-up at 6 months, all patients reported significant improvements in pain scoring. Sexual functioning with surgery had the highest success rates; however, one concern was the high number of participants randomized to surgery who declined to be included in the study. The study did support both non-surgical treatments for vestibulodynia and suggested that patients prefer a behavioral approach to treatment than a surgical one.

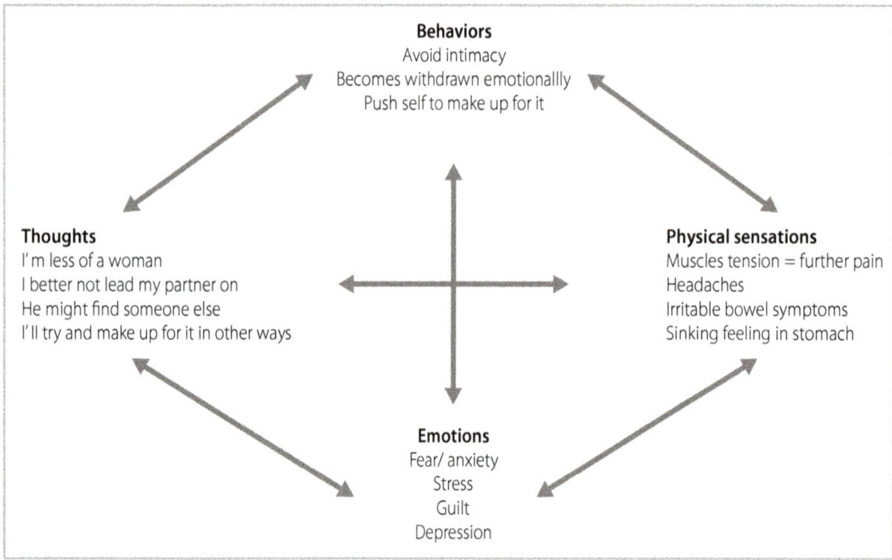

Figure 38.1 A 'hot-cross bun' diagram of how behaviors, thoughts, physical sensation, and emotions may be interlinked in patients with vulvodynia.

REFERENCES

Bergeron S, Bionic YM, Khalife S, et al. A randomised comparison of group cognitive–behavioural therapy, surface electromyographic biofeedback and vestibulectomy in the treatment of dyspareunia resulting from vulvar vestibulitis. Pain 2001; 91:297–306.

Eva LJ, Narain S, Orakwue CO, Luesley DM. Is modified vestibulectomy for localized provoked vulvodynia an effective long-term treatment? A follow-up study. J Reprod Med 2008; 53:435–440.

Eva LJ, MacLean AB, Reid WM, Rolfe KJ, Perrett CW. Estrogen receptor expression in vulvar vestibulitis syndrome. Am J Obstet Gynecol 2003; 189:458–461.

Farmer MA, Taylor AM, Bailey AL, et al. Repeated vulvovaginal fungal infections cause persistent pain in a mouse model of vulvodynia. Sci Transl Med 2011; 3:1–9

Glazer HI. Treatment of vulval vestibulitis syndrome with electromyographic biofeedback of pelvic floor musculature. J Reprod Med 1995;40:283–290.

Goldstein AT, Belkin ZR, Krapf JM, et al. Polymorphisms of the androgen receptor gene and hormonal contraceptive induced provoked vestibulodynia. J Sex Med 2014; 11:2764–2771.

Haefner HK. Report of the International Society for the Study of Vulvovaginal Disease terminology and classification of vulvodynia. J Low Genit Tract Dis 2007; 11:48–49.

Marinnoff SC, Turner MLC. Vulvar vestibulitis syndrome: an overview. Am J Obstet Gynecol 1991; 165:1228–1233.

Masheb RM, Kerns RD, Lozano C, et al. A randomized clinical trial for women with vulvodynia: Cognitive-behavioral therapy vs. supportive psychotherapy. Pain 2009; 141:31–40.

McKay M. Dysaesthetic vulvodynia. J Reprod Med 1993; 38:9–13.
McKay M. Subsets of vulvodynia. J Reprod Med 1987; 32:110–114.
Munday PE. Response to treatment in dysaesthetic vulvodynia. J Obstet Gynaecol 2001; 21:610–613.
Nunns D, Mandal D. Psychological and psychosexual aspects of vulval vestibulitis. Genitourinary Med 1997; 73:541–544.
Nunns D, Mandal D, Byrne M, et al. British Society for the Study of Vulval Disease (BSSVD) Guideline Group. Guidelines for the management of vulvodynia. Br J Dermatol 2010; 162:1180–1185.
Peckham BM, Mak DG, Patterson JJ. Focal vulvitis: a characteristic syndrome and a cause of dyspareunia. Am J Obstet Gynecol 1986; 154:855–864.
Pink L, Rancourt V, Gordon A. Persistent genital arousal in women with pelvic and genital pain. J Obstet Gynaecol Can 2014; 36:324–330.
Schover LR, Youngs DD, Cannata RN. Psychosexual aspects of the evaluation and management of vulval vestibulitis. Am J Obstet Gynecol 1991; 167:630–636.
Tympanidis P, Terenghi G, Dowd P. Increased innervation of the vulval vestibule in patients with vulvodynia. Br J Dermatol 2003; 148:1021–1027.

Chapter 39 Psychological and sexological aspects

Marjo J Ramakers

INTRODUCTION

The World Health Organization (WHO) defines sexual health 'as a state of physical, emotional, mental, and social well-being in relation to sexuality; it is not merely the absence of disease, dysfunction, or infirmity. Sexual health requires a positive and respectful approach to sexuality and sexual relationships, as well as having pleasurable and safe sex experiences, free of coercion, discrimination, and violence. For sexual health to be attained and maintained, the sexual rights of all persons must be respected, protected, and fulfilled' (WHO 2006). The WHO also champions the right of an individual to the 'highest attainable standard of sexual health' (WHO 2010). An integrative (biopsychosocial) approach focuses on sexual rights and availability of sexual healthcare. An international group recently proposed a new concept for defining health as 'the ability to adapt and to self-manage' (Huber et al. 2011). Following on from this, a new definition of sexual health has been proposed: 'the ability to sexually adapt and to self-manage with respect to the physical, emotional, and social challenges of life' (Leusink & Ramakers 2014).

Most patients do not spontaneously mention sexual problems, because they are afraid to bother their doctor with private issues or because of feelings of embarrassment, shame, or guilt.

Basic sexual history taking

- Do you have a partner?
- Are you sexually active? With this or another partner?
- Is your sexuality influenced by the problems/complaints/disease you visit me for?
  - What kind of sexual problem(s) do you have:
    - Is intercourse possible?
    - Without pain?
    - If painful intercourse:
      - Is the pain located at the introitus, deep in the vagina, or postcoital pain?
  - Is your (subjective feeling of) sexual desire/arousal diminished?
  - Is there vaginal dryness? Use of lubricants?
  - Aversive feelings? Did you have any negative sexual experiences?
    - As a child?
    - As an adult?
  - Do you have problem achieving orgasm?
- When did the sexual problem(s) start?
- How does your partner react to your (sexual or vulvovaginal) problem?
- Do you need any help (referral to sexologist or psychologist)?
- Have you ever had a genital examination before?
- Do you expect any problem concerning this examination?
- Do you expect any problem applying topical medication?
- Is there anything we didn't discuss, and I should know about?
- Do you have any (further) questions?

Sexual problems are common and may become more frequent with age. Doctors seeing patients with vulvar diseases should be able to take a sexual history (see opposite), to examine the patient carefully without causing distress and to offer treatment and/or appropriate referral if indicated.

SEXUAL HISTORY

Every patient with a vulvar problem should be asked about sexual partner(s) and sexuality; whether there are any problems with intercourse, sexual interest/arousal, and orgasm. This is especially important in case of vulvar pain, vulvar scarring, and/or after surgical procedures. Patients with sexual difficulties may need to give a more detailed history including any initiating factors, frequency and duration of symptoms, distress in the individual, and relational distress.

Be aware that older women and women without a regular partner may still be sexually active.

It needs to be established if the sex life was good before the onset of any problems and whether there has ever been any unwanted sexual attention. This needs to be asked sensitively. The examination of the patient may give important clues, including anxiety, response to being touched, etc.

Sexual dysfunctions

Using the biopsychosocial model, different factors affecting sexual function can be listed as follows:

- Somatic/medical
  - Age, hormonal changes
  - Somatic comorbidity, pain, and tiredness
  - Medication (side effects)
- Psychological/emotional
  - Stress, life events (e.g. giving birth), mourning (e.g. about infertility), anxiety, and depression
  - Negative thoughts (cognitions) and feelings such as guilt and shame
- Social/relational
  - Relational conflicts (dealing with sexual differences between patient and her partner)
  - Difficulties in being able to disclose own needs, desires, expectations, etc.
- Sexual
  - Inadequate sexual stimulation
  - Limited sexual repertoire
  - Performance-orientated sexual activity (performance anxiety)
  - Partner with a sexual problem
  - Irrational expectations

CLASSIFICATION OF SEXUAL DYSFUNCTION

Sexual dysfunction is classified in the diagnostic and statistical manual of mental disorders (DSM) and in the International Classification of Diseases (ICD). The most recent DSM-5 [American Psychological Association (APA) 2013] classifies female sexual dysfunction as:

1. Female sexual interest/arousal disorder
2. Female orgasmic disorder
3. Genitopelvic pain/penetration disorder
4. Substance/medication-induced sexual dysfunction

DSM-5 diagnosis

A DSM-5 diagnosis of sexual dysfunction requires:

- Symptoms experienced in ≥75% occasions of sexual activity
- Symptoms persist for a minimum duration of 6 months
- Symptoms cause clinically significant distress in the individual
- Sexual dysfunction is not better explained by a non-sexual mental disorder or as a consequence of severe relationship distress or other significant stressors and is not attributable to the effects of a substance/medication or another medical condition

DSM-5 subclassification

The DSM-5 further subclassifies sexual dysfunction as:

- Lifelong — Present since the individual became sexually active, *or*
- Acquired — Began after a period of relatively normal sexual function
- Generalized — Not limited to certain types of stimulation, or
- Situational — Only occurs with certain types of stimulation, situations, or partners
- Causing mild, moderate, or severe distress

Female sexual interest/arousal disorder (1)

This disorder is characterized by significantly reduced, sexual interest/arousal (APA 2013; see DSM-5 for further specification).

Key causes and points to consider

- **Somatic:** hormonal contraceptives, breastfeeding, prolactinoma, anorexia nervosa, kidney failure, antiestrogens, oophorectomy, chronic diseases/tiredness
- **Psychological/emotional:** life events [traumatic (sexual or obstetric) experience], midlife, postmenopause, depression, anxiety, guilt, shame
- **Social/relational:** major sexual differences between patient and partner
- **Sexual:** inadequate sexual (vaginal instead of clitoral) stimulation, limited sexual repertoire (intercourse orientated), anxiety to perform (orgasm), painful intercourse, partner with sexual problem (avoiding any sexual activity and intimacy), irrational expectations about sexual desire

Female orgasmic disorder (2)

This disorder is characterized by a marked delay in or infrequency of, or absence of orgasm and/or marked reduced intensity of orgasmic sensations (APA 2013; see DSM-5 for further specification).

Key causes and points to consider

- **Somatic:** none except, very rarely, bilateral traumatic/neurogenic destruction of pudendal nerve
- **Psychological/emotional:** unable to focus on own sexual excitement, more thinking/observing than doing/feeling, and afraid of letting go/losing control
- **Social/relational:** repressive upbringing, feelings of insecurity, guilt, and shame
- **Sexual:** inadequate sexual (vaginal instead of clitoral) stimulation, limited (intercourse orientated), anxiety to perform, partner having a sexual problem (erectile dysfunction), irrational expectations about orgasm (penetration necessary, not related to psychorelational aspects)

Genitopelvic pain/penetration disorder (3)

Pain (dyspareunia) and pelvic floor muscle contraction are closely related. This disorder is characterized by persistent or recurrent difficulties with one (or more) of the following:

- Vaginal penetration during intercourse
- Marked vulvovaginal or pelvic pain during vaginal intercourse or penetration attempts
- Marked fear or anxiety about vulvovaginal or pelvic pain in anticipation of, during, or as a result of vaginal penetration
- Marked tensing or tightening of the pelvic floor muscles during attempted vaginal penetration (vaginismus)

Substance/medication-induced sexual dysfunction (4)

This is an important consideration but beyond the scope of this chapter.

Treatment

In women, psychological, emotional, relationship, and sexual stimulation problems inhibit sexual desire/arousal far more frequently than somatic causes. These factors need to be assessed and addressed if necessary. Depression warrants referral to a psychiatrist/psychologist. Many therapists have a role to play including physiotherapists, psychotherapists, counselors, and couple therapists; however, the specialist skills of a sexologist may be required for further diagnosis and treatment. Rarely laboratory tests (testosterone and sex hormone-binding globulin) and hormonal treatment are indicated.

Many patients lack knowledge and therefore education is essential. This is particularly important with regard to orgasm as many women do not know that vaginal intercourse may not be sufficient to achieve orgasm. They may be unaware that adequate stimulation and swelling of the clitoral complex (including swelling of labia minora) is necessary to allow orgasm and that the brain can be 'emotionally blocked' by a number of factors such as anxiety and emotional problems.

There are a number of different causes of vulvar pain and therapy will depend on the cause (see Chapter 38 for details). Primary vaginismus, based on marked fear and avoidance of vaginal penetration (penis, fingers, tampons, and gynecological examination), usually prevents women from seeing a gynecologist. Referral to a sexologist is indicated, and eventually exercises will be performed that help to learn how to contract and relax the pelvic floor muscles. For other sexual and relational problems, sexologists will frequently give specific exercises for couples to communicate and complete focusing on specific areas of need. These may include learning to discover, communicate, and appreciate differences in the partners relating to needs, learning to relax, non-sexual touching techniques, and ways to increase sexual stimulation.

SEXUAL ABUSE

Both adults and children may be victims of sexual violence. Adults are more likely to present to acute services (usually police or emergency medical services) but may sometimes present to adult vulvar services with long lasting physical and emotional problems years after the incident. Children tend to present to health professionals through various routes. They will not necessarily talk about the abuse they have undergone and the signs of abuse may be hard to detect.

Child sexual abuse (CSA) covers a range of sexual activities including sexual touching of a child and penetrative sex. It also includes a failure to protect a child from seeing inappropriate images of a sexual nature and the taking or distribution of sexual images of children. Data from 55 studies (2001-2009) report prevalence estimates of child abuse between 8–31% in girls and 3–17% in boys (Barth et al. 2013). These children may present to health care professionals so it is important to be alert to the signs and symptoms of CSA, to know how to proceed and how to refer on to specialist services. A detailed review of the subject is beyond the remit of this chapter, the aim instead is to give advice on the management of CSA in the vulvar clinic.

Signs and symptoms of child sexual abuse

There may be physical and emotional signs of abuse (NICE 2009; WHO 2003). Some relatively common conditions such as lichen sclerosus, female genital mutilation, straddle injuries, streptococcal infection and large aphthous ulcers can be mistaken for CSA.

Genital and other physical signs of CSA include:

- Unexplained genital injury such as lacerations and bruising
- Anal dilatation, fissures, bleeding, pain
- Presence of sperm
- Sexually transmitted infections
- Urinary tract infections
- Vaginal discharge
- Pregnancy
- Foreign bodies in genital or anal cavities

Psychological and behavioral indicators of CSA include:

- Avoiding the abuser
- Sexually inappropriate behavior or language
- Regression in behavior
- Poor school performance
- Low self esteem
- Sleep disturbance

Assessment and examination

If CSA is suspected, the case should be referred to the relevant child protection services without delay. Hospitals will have a named health professional to give advice. Unnecessary examinations should be avoided, to limit the number of examinations that the child has to cope with. All findings must be accurately and contemporaneously recorded.

Adult manifestations of childhood sexual abuse

CSA may have lasting effects. In her book *Trauma and Recovery* Herman documents the struggle of survivors and discusses factors that determine psychological consequences of sexual abuse (Herman 1992).

Factors determining the psychological consequences of sexual abuse include:

- The type, seriousness, frequency and duration of abuse
- The age at which abuse started and ended
- The relationship between victim and perpetrator
- The reaction of friends and family

Emotional sequelae

Survivors of CSA may experience emotional problems such as guilt, shame and fear (ACOG 2011). They may develop symptoms of post-traumatic stress. The term psychological trauma is reserved for a serious, overruling, exhausting and life threatening experience from which there is no escape (Kleber & Brom 1992). Some individuals may experience flashbacks and intrusive thoughts. A common coping mechanism of CSA is dissociation and denial where the sense of self is separated from the physical body. Dissociation is an unconscious psychological process of 'physically being alive but emotionally blanking out.'

Physical sequelae

Physical symptoms such as chronic pelvic pain, eating disorders, obesity, substance abuse, smoking, alcohol abuse and self neglect are commoner in those who have suffered CSA.

Sexual sequelae

There may be a number of consequences including difficulties in desire, arousal and achieving orgasm. CSA survivors are more likely to engage in risk taking behaviour and also be at greater risk of sexually transmitted infections, unwanted pregnancy and prostitution.

Sexual history taking in cases of CSA

The goal of taking a sexual history is to sensitively gain relevant information, recognising that genital examinations can be frightening and painful. Try to make the questions as normal and natural as you can. If abuse is enquired about routinely the physician will become more comfortable asking these types of questions. The woman needs to feel she is in charge of the timing of any disclosure. Sometimes examinations may need to be postponed to another visit .

The goal of taking a sexual history in cases of CSA is to gather information on the following:

- If the patient has experienced sexual problems, such as:
  - aversive feelings to sexual activity (common in sexually abused women)
  - deep dyspareunia (common in sexually abused women)
  - any other sexual problems
- If, and under what conditions, the patient can undergo genital examination
- If she can tolerate prescribed topical medication (some women are aversive to their own genitals and unable to touch their vulva)
- If she needs further help or referral to, e.g., a psychiatrist, psychologist, psychotherapist or sexologist

Management

Specialist counselling, emotional support and mental health assessments may be necessary. The physician should be aware of locally available services.

FEMALE GENITAL MUTILATION

Female genital mutilation (FGM), also termed female circumcision or female genital cutting, is the removal of part of the female genitals for non-medical reasons. It is widely practiced in certain African countries as well as in Yemen, Iraqi Kurdistan, Indonesia and Malaysia (**Figure 39.1**). The highest prevalence is in Somalia where 98% of girls are estimated to have undergone FGM (UNICEF data 2014).

FGM is illegal in many countries of the world including some of those where the practice is widespread. There are complex cultural reasons why FGM is practiced, including ideas around the preservation of virginity, cleanliness and eligibility for marriage; however, the WHO considers FGM to be a serious violation of the human rights of women and children. There are no health benefits. FGM may be performed at any time from infancy to late teens.

FGM is commonly classified into four types:

Type I:	Clitoridectomy, removal of part or all of the clitoris
Type II:	Excision, removal of the clitoris and labia minora
Type III:	Infibulation or infundibulation, excision of part or all of the external genitalia followed by stitching with narrowing of the vaginal opening
Type IV:	Other, includes harmful procedures such as piercing, incising or scraping

Complications

FGM has serious implications for the medical and psychological health of women and children (**Table 39.1**). FGM procedures are carried out by physicians as well as by local practitioners using instruments such as razors, glass and scissors, in non-sterile conditions. Acute complications include infection and bleeding.

Sexological aspects

FGM may have a profound effect on sexual relations depending on the type and extent of the procedure. Dyspareunia and apareunia may occur. If there is some clitoral tissue retained orgasm may be reached; however, specialist help from a sexologist may be helpful.

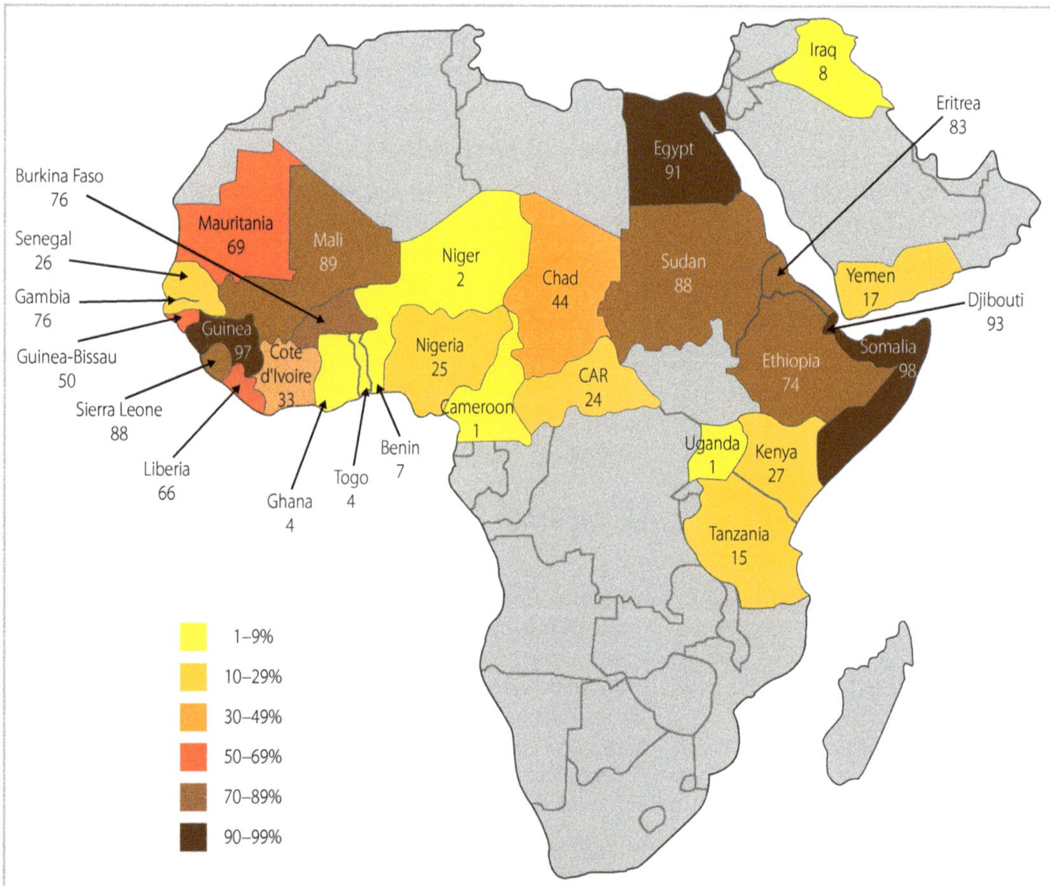

Figure 39.1 Prevalence (as a percentage) of female genital mutilation. With permission from UNICEF 2014. CAR, Central African Republic.

Table 39.1 Complications of FGM

Acute complications	Chronic complications
Psychological distress	Psychological distress
Severe pain	Impaired sexual function
Haemorrhage	Menstrual pain, haematocolpos
Infection	Recurrent urinary tract infections
	Chronic pelvic infection
Genital swelling	Increased blood borne infection such as hepatitis C and HIV
Urinary retention	Urethral stricture, fistula
	Vulvar cysts and neuromas
	Infertility
Death	Obstructed labour

In a systematic review of published sources on FGM between 1997 and 2005 the author concluded that sexual activity or the enjoyment of sexual relations may not always be precluded in females who have undergone FGM, however, a limitation of the study design is that complicated cultural and psychosocial aspects of sexuality may not have been taken fully into account (Makhlouf Obermeyer 2005).

Recognition and management

When a woman from a country where FGM is practiced presents with vulvar or urinary tract problems or pelvic pain, it is important to be alert to the possibility of FGM and enquire sensitively about the practice in a non-judgmental way. Individual countries will have different laws and regulations for reporting of cases. For example, in the UK there is an obligation for health professionals to register all cases and to refer all children who have undergone or are at risk of undergoing FGM to child protection services.

Referral to a specialist FGM service is required if there are complications or symptoms (RCOG 2015). De-infibulation to improve the size of the vaginal opening may be considered in cases where there has been infibulation with resultant narrowing of the opening to the vagina. There is no evidence that clitoral re-construction is effective and this should not be recommended.

Pregnancy and childbirth

There are particular problems associated with pregnancy and childbirth, for example an increased risk of perineal trauma, prolonged labor and post-partum haemorrhage. In pregnancy, the size of the vaginal opening must be assessed before labor to ensure safe vaginal delivery is possible. If it is not, arrangements should be made to perform a de-infibulation procedure before delivery. Occasionally, women will present in labor and the procedure needs to be carried out immediately to permit safe vaginal delivery.

REFERENCES

American College of Obstetricians and Gynecologists. Committee on Health Care for Underserved Women. Committee opinion no. 498: Adult manifestations of childhood sexual abuse. Obstet Gynecol 2011; 118(2 Pt1): 392–395.

American Psychiatric Association: Desk Reference to the Diagnostic Criteria from DSM-5. Arlington VA: American Psychiatric Association, 2013.

Barth J, Bermetz L, Heim E, Trelle S, Tonia T. The current prevalence of child sexual abuse worldwide: a systematic review and meta-analysis. Int J Public Health 2013; 58:469–483.

Finkelhor D. How widespread is child sexual abuse? Children Today 1984; 3:2.

Herman JL. Trauma and recovery. New York: Basic Books, 1992.

Huber M, Knottnerus JA, Green L, et al. How should we define health? BMJ 2011; 343:d4163.

Kleber RJ, Brom D. Coping with trauma. Theory, Prevention and Treatment. Amsterdam: Swets en Zetlinger, 1992.

Leusink P, Ramakers M. Inleiding. In: Leusink P and Ramakers M (eds), Handboek seksuele gezondheid. Assen: Koninklijke van Gorcum, 2014.

National Institute of Health and Care Excellence (NICE). Child maltreatment; when to suspect maltreatment in under 21's. CG 89. London: NICE, July 2009.

Obermeyer CM. The consequences of female circumcision for health and sexuality: An update on the evidence. Cult Health Sex 2005; 7:443–461.

Royal College of Obstetricians and Gynaecologists (RCOG). Female genital mutilation and its management (Green top guideline no 53). London: Royal College of Obstetricians and Gynaecologists, 2015.

UNICEF. Female Genital Mutilation/Cutting: A statistical overview and exploration of the dynamics of change. UNICEF, 2014. http://data.unicef.org/resources/female-genital-mutilation-cutting-a-statistical-overview-and-exploration-of-the-dynamics-of-change.html (accessed 8 December 2015).

World Health Organization (WHO). Guidelines for medico-legal care for victims of sexual violence WHO 2003. Chapter 7: Child sexual abuse. Geneva: World Health Organization, 2003.

World Health Organization (WHO). Sexual and reproductive health. WHO, 2006. http://www.who.int/reproductivehealth/topics/sexual_health/sh_definitions/en/ (accessed 24 November 2015)

World Health Organization. Standards for Sexuality Education in Europe. A framework for policy makers, educational and health authorities and specialists. Cologne: WHO Regional Office for Europe, 2010.

Chapter 40 Vulvar cosmetic surgery

Claudia E Marchitelli

INTRODUCTION

Key points

- The 'standard' or 'normal' vulva does not exist
- Women are increasingly aware of their vulvar anatomy and may seek the 'perfect' vulva or vagina
- Aesthetic vulvovaginal surgery is increasingly performed
- Preoperative counseling is vital before any procedure
- Therapeutic surgery may be valuable in selected cases of scarring disorders such as lichen sclerosus and mucosal lichen planus

Over the past decade, there has been a surge in aesthetic vulvovaginal surgery (ACOG Committee Opinion 2007) with media coverage placing these procedures firmly in the public eye (Bramwell et al. 2007). As a consequence, women observe their genitals in more detail and may compare them to other women, using online searches or magazines. This awareness has encouraged the concept of an 'adequate vaginal design' or a 'perfect vulva or vagina' (Renganathan 2009). Women now consult their gynecologist searching for a solution to a technically non-existent problem. Marketing of these practices is controversial, raising some ethical concerns.

There is no scientific evidence for the role of surgery to increase sexual pleasure. Some practitioners promote vulvar and vaginal aesthetic surgery as a way to gain better orgasms or greater sexual pleasure. These surgical procedures are strictly anatomical and are not oriented toward vulvar physiology, and therefore do not guarantee sexual improvement. However, for some women, a change in vulvar or vaginal anatomy may lead to increased self-confidence and comfort allowing enjoyment of sexual intercourse free from embarrassment, inhibitions, or self-consciousness.

There are many variations in normal vulvar anatomy, hence there is no such thing as a 'standard vulva' (Likes et al. 2008) and no definition for 'beauty.' Therefore, all patients require a thorough preoperative consultation exploring the issues motivating their desire for surgery; some countries have developed guidelines that outline recommendations for vulvar surgery. It is essential for the surgeon to clearly explain and document the extent and aims of surgery, with informed consent. If a presenting problem is likely to be a functional rather than physical as in cases of anorgasmia or lack of sexual pleasure, it is important to focus on addressing these issues with a specialist rather than performing surgery.

This chapter focuses on aesthetic vulvovaginal surgery but also covers some therapeutic techniques for dealing with scarring as a result of inflammatory disease such as lichen sclerosus.

AESTHETIC VULVOVAGINAL SURGERY

Labia minora labioplasty (labia minora reduction surgery)

This surgery is indicated when there is hypertrophy of the labia minora (**Figure 40.1 a** and **b**); however, the definition of hypertrophic labia is difficult since vulvar anatomy is highly variable (Likes et al. 2008). The average labia minora are asymmetrical, 20 mm (7–50 mm) in width and 60 mm (20–100 mm) in length (Lloyd et al. 2005). Some women with hypertrophic labia may complain of discomfort while doing exercise or physical activity such as riding a bicycle, having sexual intercourse, or even wearing tight clothes. The following procedures are generally performed in the outpatient setting under local anesthesia; however, general anesthesia may be preferred by some patients. These procedures generally take less than an hour. Postoperative advice includes avoiding intercourse and swimming for at least one month. There is currently no consensus regarding the best technique to employ.

Possible complications of these procedures include hematomas, wound dehiscence, infection, vulvar edema, necrosis, and most importantly sensory alterations and dyspareunia (**Table 40.1**).

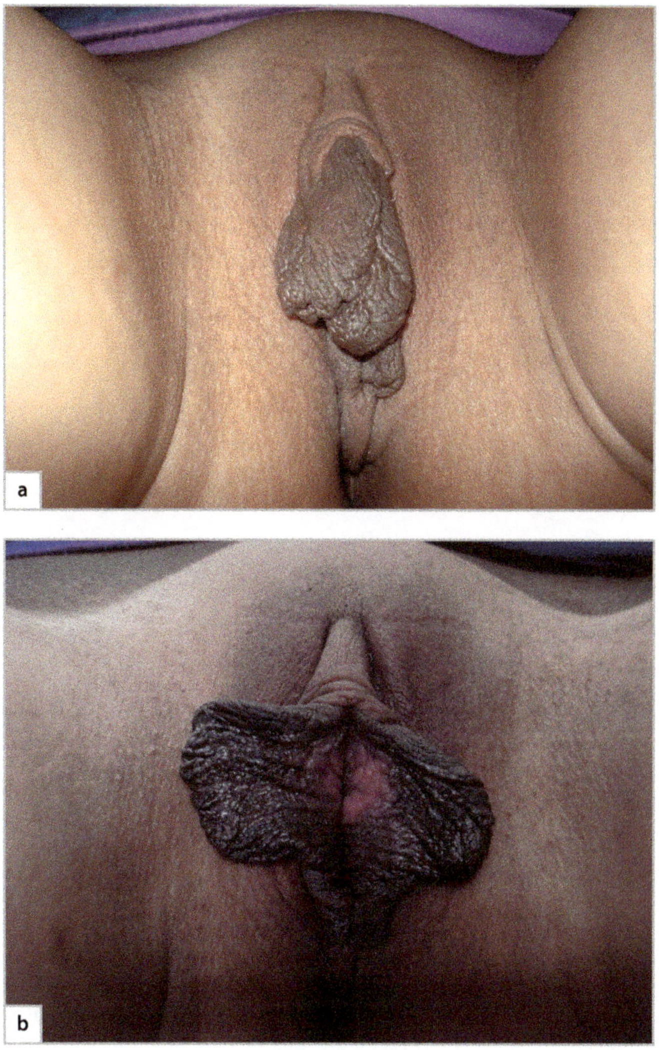

Figure 40.1 (a) A 33-year-old patient with hypertrophic labia minora. (b) A 27-year-old patient with hypertrophic labia minora.

Table 40.1 Labia minora reduction surgery: patients, follow-up, technique, and complications

Study	Number	Follow-up (months)	Technique	Complications				
				Necrosis	Infection	Dehiscence	Hematoma	Pain
Alter 1998	4	–	Central wedge resection	0	0	0	0	0
Maas & Hage 1998	13	72	Lateral W-resection	0	0	1(7,6)	1(7,6)	13(100)
Rouzier et al. 2000	163	30	Inferior V-resection	–	–	11(6,7)	–	104(64)
Choi & Kim 2000	6	–	Central de-epithelization	0	0	0	0	0
Giraldo et al. 2004	15	30	90° Z-plasty	0	0	2(13.3)	6(40)	0
Pardo et al. 2006	55	–	Laser labioplasty	0	0	3(5,4)	0	2(3,6)
Munhoz et al. 2006	21	46	Inferior wedge resection and reconstruction with superior pedicle	1(4,7)	1(4,7)	2(9,5)	1(4,7)	0
Marchitelli & Sluga 2010	42	19	Combined techniques	0	0	3 (7.4)	3(7.4)	–

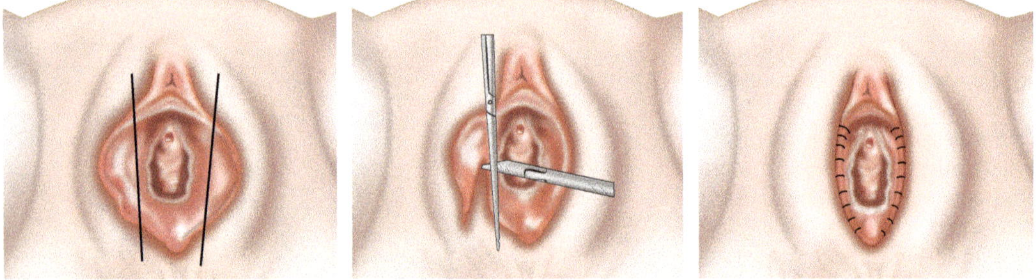

Figure 40.2 Free edge resection technique.

Free edge resection technique

The free edges of both labia minora are excised by an elliptical incision, always attempting to maintain and respect the vulvar anatomy. It is useful in those patients who do not wish to retain the hyperpigmented labial edge (**Figure 40.2** and **Figure 40.3**).

Wedge resection and reconstruction from remaining flaps is shown in **Figure 40.4.**

The original technique consists of a wedge-shaped resection of the inferior part of the labia and reconstruction with the remaining superior segment (Alter 1998). The aim of this technique is to hide the incisions and preserve the labium's natural pigmented border (**Figure 40.5**).

Inferior pedicle resection and reconstruction with superior pedicle flap

Rouzier et al. proposed a modified version of the previous technique describing a 'v' shaped resection of the inferior part of the labia (Rouzier et al. 2000). The color of the labia's free edge is preserved (**Figure 40.6**).

Central wedge resection technique with 90° Z-plasty

Two 90° Z-plasties are drawn facing each other on the internal and external surface of the labia minora (**Figure 40.7**). These 'Z's converge from the free edge of the midsection of the labia to a common origin at the base of each labia (pointing toward the ventral zone of the introital meatus). This outlines the irregular shape of the wedge, which is then removed. Finally, the edges of the resection are sutured directly with interrupted stitches with an absorbable suture, e.g. 4.0 Vicryl (Giraldo et al. 2004).

CO_2 laser technique

Any of the aforementioned techniques can be performed with a carbon dioxide laser. The laser must be set on scalpel mode allowing incision and coagulation simultaneously.

Complications

Possible complications of these procedures are listed in **Table 40.1**.

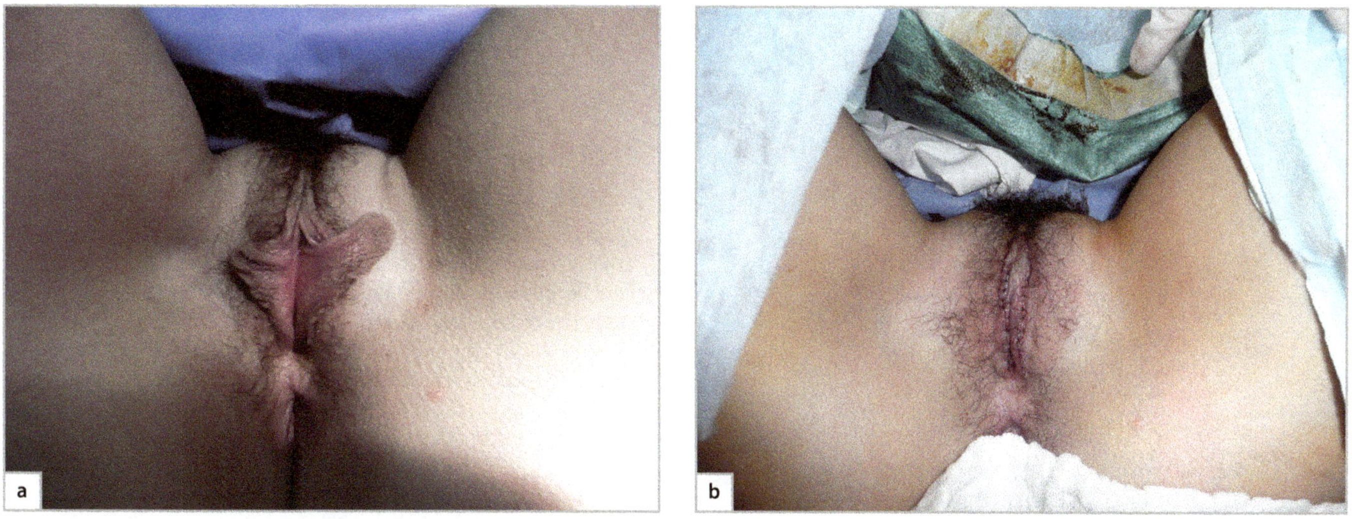

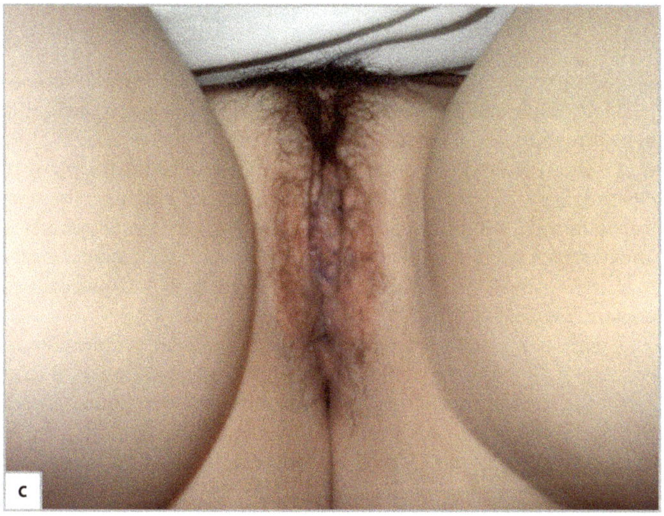

Figure 40.3 (a) Free edge resection technique before surgery. (b) Immediately postoperatively: resection of the free border. The longitudinal suture can be seen following the length of the labia minora. (c) 14 days postoperatively.

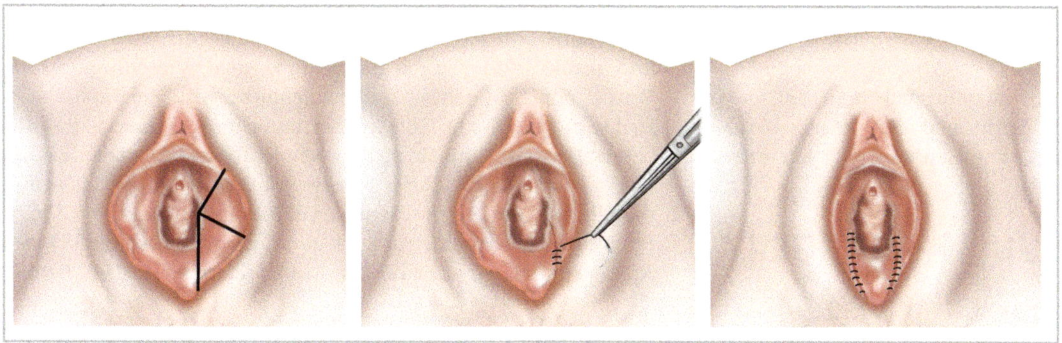

Figure 40.4 Wedge resection technique.

Labia majora labioplasty

The aim is to remove excess skin along with subjacent subcutaneous fatty tissue. It is indicated in cases of flaccidity of the labia majora, or in other diseases that affect the labial aesthetic, such as severe scarring from multiple sebaceous cysts or edematous hypertrophy of the labia associated with renal failure or ascites. Labia majora hypertrophy is usually asymptomatic and the surgery aims to improve the appearance. The most frequently employed technique is the elliptic excision of the skin and subcutaneous tissue, which is later repaired with absorbable sutures, with either a continuous intradermal stitch or interrupted stitches.

Reduction vaginoplasty

This procedure is sometimes referred to as 'vaginal rejuvenation.' The term 'reduction vaginoplasty' is preferred to 'colpoperineoplasty' when surgery involves reconstruction of the perineal body in the absence of pelvic organ prolapse or urinary incontinence.

Vaginal 'widening' may occur after childbirth and is often related to fetal size and the number of vaginal births. Other obstetric maneuvers, such as the use of forceps, may also affect vaginal width. Reduction vaginoplasty is only rarely indicated when an enlarged vagina results in painful sexual intercourse or incontinence of vaginal gas. In most cases, vaginal size does not interfere with female orgasm nor prevent

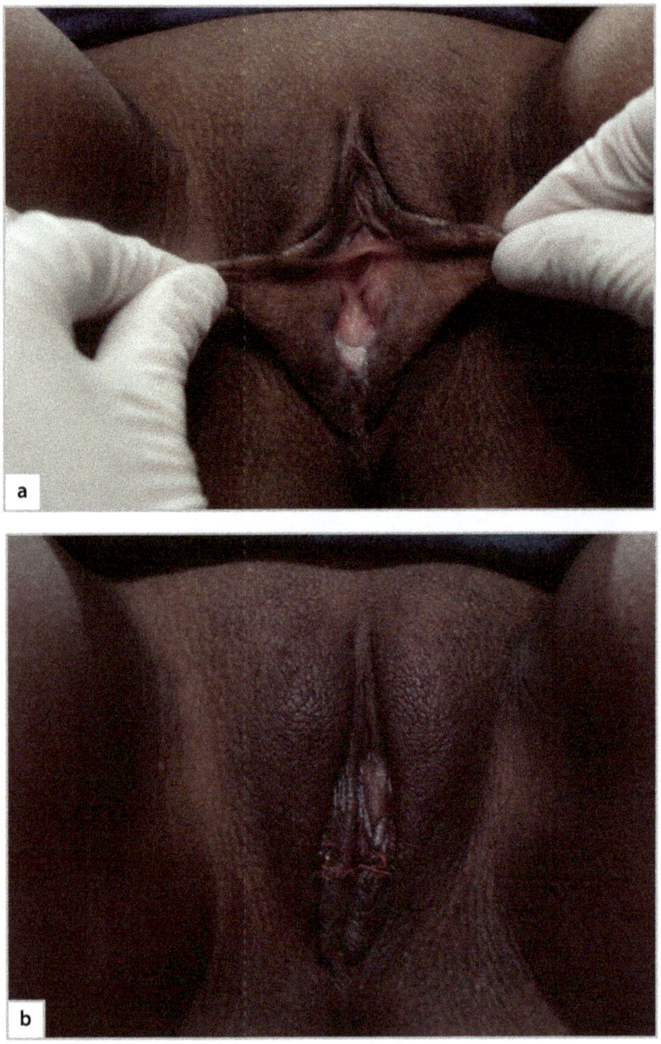

Figure 40.5 (a) Wedge resection technique before surgery. (b) Immediate postoperatively: the horizontal suture can be appreciated through the midsection of each labia, conserving the free edge.

a satisfactory sex life and is therefore not usually indicated. The patient must be fully informed and educated about female sexuality (Marchitelli et al. 2010). The main complications are dyspareunia and failure of vaginal penetration.

THERAPEUTIC VULVAR SURGERY

Fissures of the navicular fossa

These fissures arise in the midline between the hymen and the fourchette usually as a consequence of vaginal penetration. They may take several days to heal, tending to reoccur with every sexual relation. They are sometimes, but not always, associated with lichen sclerosus or lichen planus. The thin epithelium of this area may have been previously damaged by ablative or destructive treatments. Initial measures include advice to reduce the frequency of penetrative vaginal intercourse and use local estrogens and emollients. Contributing factors such as recurrent candidosis and vulvar eczema must be treated if necessary. If these measures fail, a surgical option should be considered.

The technique consists of excision of the fissure and vestibular mucosa that surrounds it, with dissection of the posterior vaginal wall for no less than 2 or 3 cm from the vestibule. This creates a free flap of vaginal wall, which fills the defect to allow tension-free closure (Paniel & Rouzier 2009).

Vulvoperineoplasty for lichen sclerosus

This surgery is indicated where there is stenosis of the vaginal introitus (Paniel & Rouzier 2009). The most frequent cause is advanced lichen sclerosus; however, lichen planus, Graft versus Host Disease, and rare genetic conditions may also result in narrowing. Previous aesthetic interventions, e.g. excessive reduction vaginoplasties may cause stenosis. Dyspareunia or apareunia are the most frequent symptoms.

Three-step procedure

1. Wide dissection and mobilization of the vaginal posterior wall
2. Shortening of the length of the perineal body
3. Eversion and advancement of the posterior vaginal wall

The first part of the procedure is the same as for a posterior colpoperineorrhaphy. A triangular flap of perineal skin is excised with the subcutaneous tissue, forming a triangular flap. The posterior vaginal wall is then dissected with scissors or a scalpel, allowing the plane of cleavage between the rectus and the vagina to be exposed. The next step is the medial incision of the perineal body, near the anal sphincter. The posterior vaginal wall is then advanced and exteriorized in order to fill the perineal defect. Absorbable 3.0 sutures provide a tension-free closure (**Figure 40.8a** and **b**).

This procedure allows maintenance of an adequate introitus diameter. Since the vaginal mucosa is typically not affected by lichen sclerosus, the success rate of this surgery is very high with improvement in dyspareunia in up to 90% and the quality of sexual intercourse in 86% (Rouzier et al. 2000). However, patients must continue treatment with local steroids for vulvar signs of lichen sclerosus.

Surgery for fourchette adhesions

Fourchette adhesions consist of synechiae that lead to fissures and cracks after vaginal penetration or a gynecologic exam. Postinflammatory adhesions due to lichen sclerosus are usually localized to the fourchette, labia minora, and clitoris (**Figure 40.9a**). The patients usually complain of dyspareunia. The treatment consists of a median perineotomy. This is usually performed by vertical incision of the adhesion, skin, vestibular mucosa, and vertex of the perineal body. By using transverse interrupted sutures, e.g. with absorbable Vicryl 3.0, closing of the mucosal edges can be performed (**Figure 40.9b**).

Surgery for labia minora adhesions

These adhesions usually occur in women with lichen sclerosus. In this case, the procedure is simply limited to incising and liberating the synechiae, the edges are then sutured with absorbable stitches. Postoperative continuous use of local steroids is essential aiming to prevent the development of new synechiae.

Surgery for clitoral adhesions

In patients with lichen sclerosus or mucosal lichen planus, there is frequent involvement of the clitoris. Although adhesions are usually asymptomatic and it is still possible to reach orgasm, many patients prefer the clitoris to be freed from adhesions for aesthetic reasons.

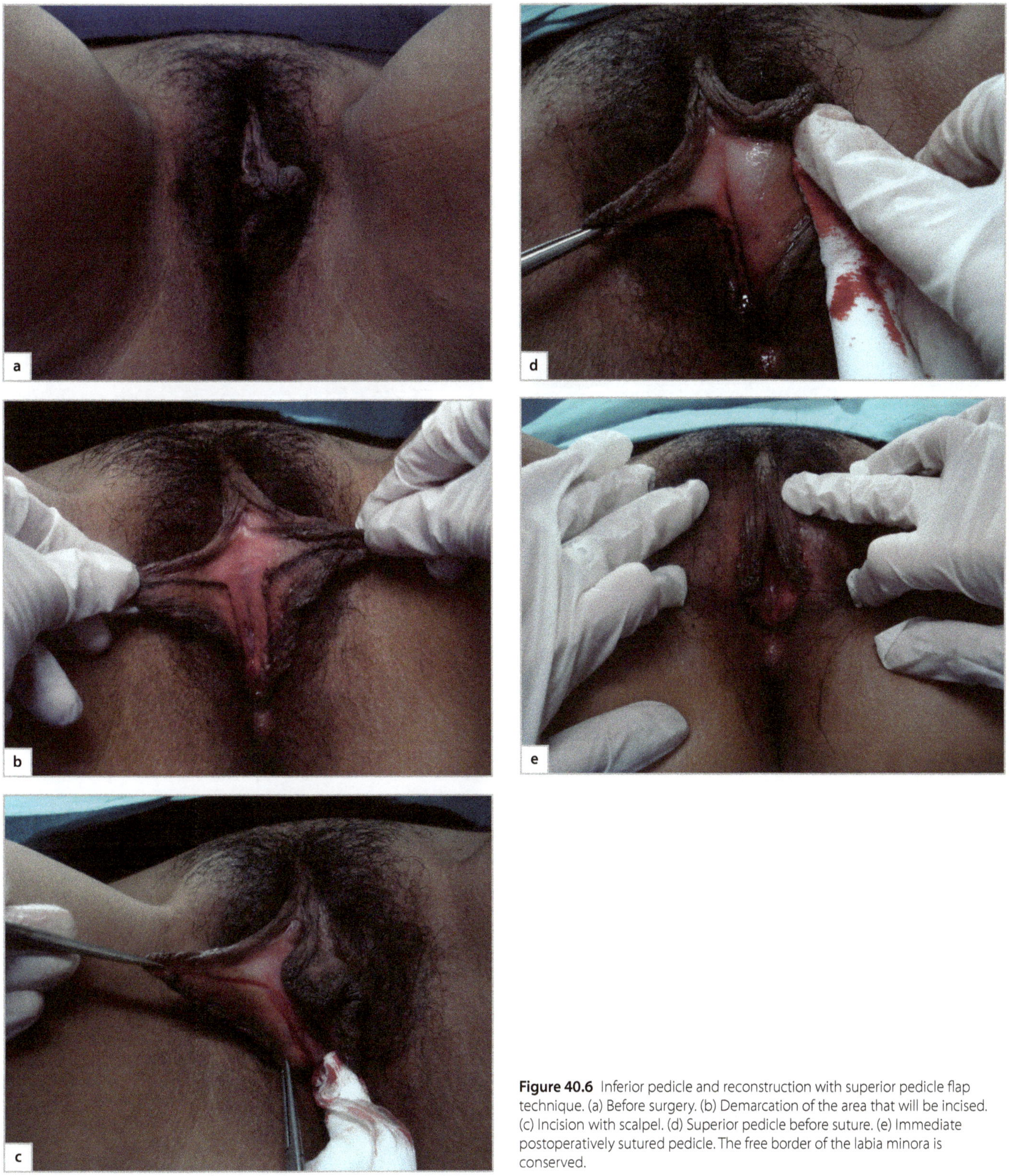

Figure 40.6 Inferior pedicle and reconstruction with superior pedicle flap technique. (a) Before surgery. (b) Demarcation of the area that will be incised. (c) Incision with scalpel. (d) Superior pedicle before suture. (e) Immediate postoperatively sutured pedicle. The free border of the labia minora is conserved.

In these cases, the adhesions are incised carefully and a small probe is used to release the hood of the clitoris from the glans (Paniel et al. 1984). In order to prevent readhesion, different techniques may be used, such as excision of the clitoral hood (circumcision) or partial resection of the hood with eversion of the free edge (**Figure 40.10**). However, it is possible to cause damage to sensory nerves, which may lead to difficulties achieving orgasm. In order to prevent recurrences, it is essential that the patient continues to use topical steroids.

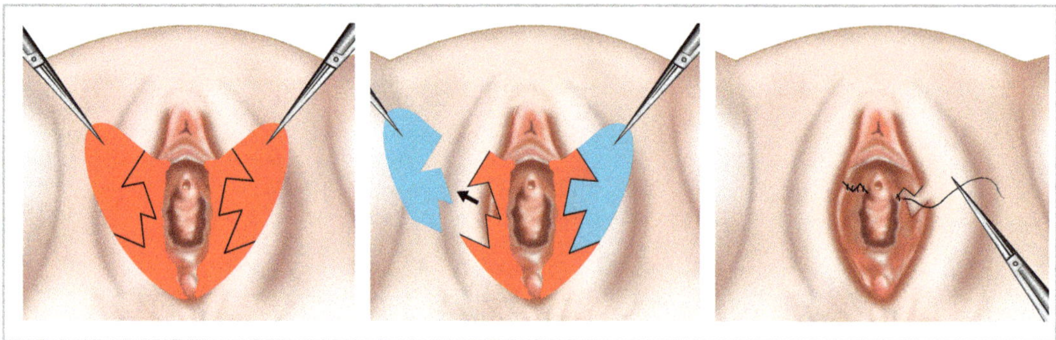

Figure 40.7 Ninety degrees Z-plasty technique.

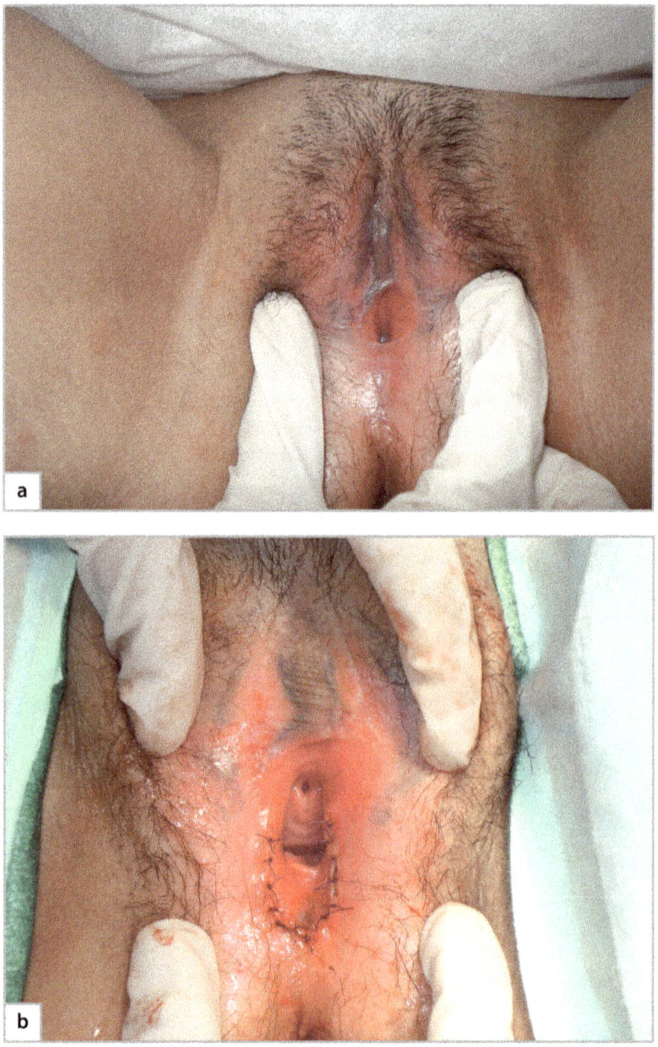

Figure 40.8 (a) A 35-year-old patient with lichen sclerosus and median fusion. (b) Immediately postoperatively: widening vaginoplasty in the same patient with lichen sclerosus.

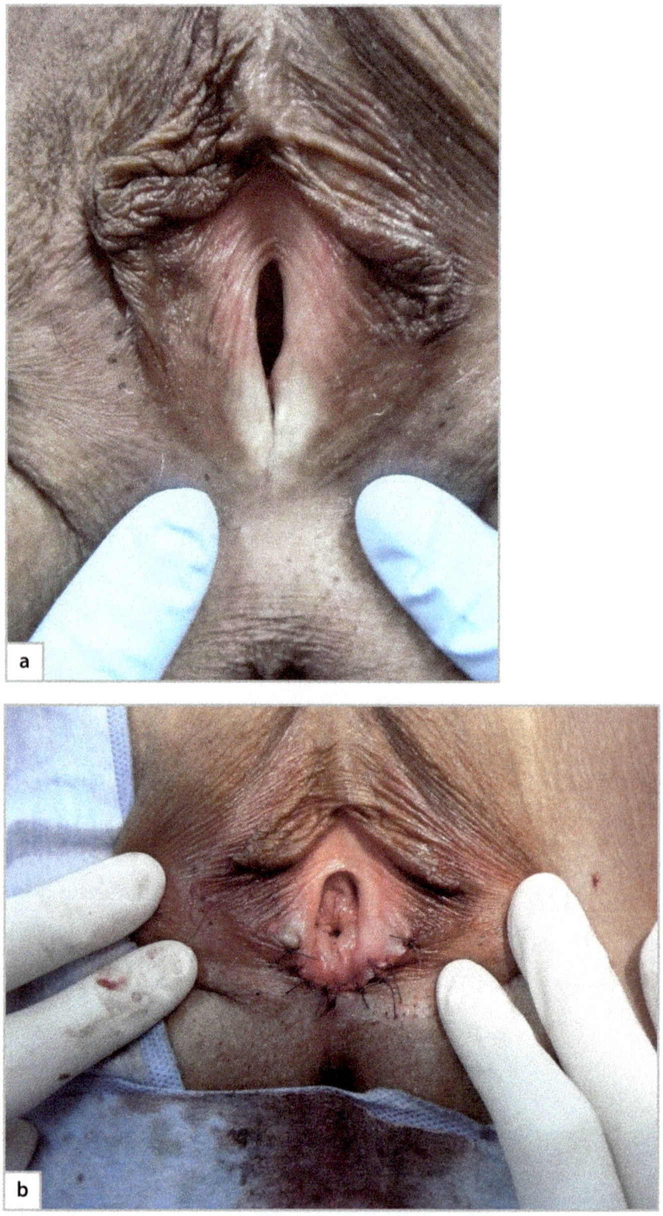

Figure 40.9 (a) Fourchette adhesions. (b) Immediate postoperative adhesion resection.

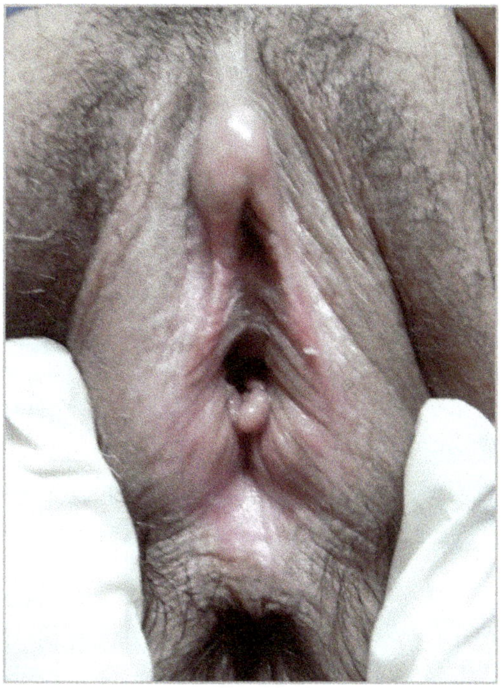

Figure 40.10 Clitoral adhesions in a patient with lichen sclerosus.

PRACTICES NOT RECOMMENDED DUE TO LACK OF EVIDENCE FOR THEIR EFFECTIVENESS

G-spot amplification

G-spot amplification with collagen, fatty tissue, or hyaluronic acid has become popular. However, the existence of the 'G-spot,' named after Dr Ernst Grafenberg who described it in 1944, is not proven. The technique and results of this surgery have not been published in the medical literature and thus experience is merely anecdotal. American Congress of Obstetricians and Gynecologists (ACOG) affirms that there is no evidence of increased sexual gratification following these procedures (ACOG Committee Opinion 2007).

Vulvar and/or anal bleaching

In vulvar and anal bleaching, the most common technique involves abrasion of the superficial layer of the epidermis with fractional laser or pulsed light. This stimulates the regeneration of epithelium, which in theory restores the vulva to its 'pink juvenile shade.' There are no studies to support this practice, and its use is discouraged because it can result in vulvodynia.

Reduction vaginoplasty

This is not recommended for patients consulting because of sexual issues (Marchitelli et al. 2010).

CONCLUSION

Performing aesthetic gynecological practices is ethically possible, by giving patients adequate information about a procedure, possible complications, and offering sexual counseling when necessary, based on ACOG recommendations (ACOG Committee Opinion 2007).

Cosmetic surgical procedures that potentially result in sexual problems, changes in function, or pain should not be performed, regardless of the patient's request. Work is needed to produce consensus opinions defining the indications and contraindications for these procedures and unethical practice must be eradicated. Patients must be informed about the lack of data regarding the efficacy and potential long-term complications of cosmetic surgery.

Prospective, randomized studies with long-term follow-up evaluating safety and efficacy of cosmetic procedures are clearly needed.

REFERENCES

ACOG Committee Opinion No.378. Vaginal rejuvenation and cosmetic vaginal procedures. Obstet Gynecol 2007; 110:737–738.

Alter GJ. A new technique for aesthetic labia minora reduction. Annals of Plast Surg 1998; 40:287–290.

Bramwell R, Morland C, Garder AS. Expectations and experience of labial reduction: a qualitative study. BJOG 2007; 114:1493–1499.

Choi HY, Kim KT. A New method for aesthetic reduction of labia minora (the deepithelialized reduction labioplasty). Plast Reconstr Surg 2000; 105:419–422.

Giraldo F, González C, de Haro F. Central Wedge Nymphectomy with a 90-Degree Z plasty for aesthetic reduction of the labia minora. Plast and Reconst Surg 2004; 113:1820–1825.

Likes WM, Sideri M, Haefner H, et al. Aesthetic Practice of Labial Reduction. J Low Genit Tract Dis 2008; 12:210–216.

Lloyd J, Crouch NS, Minto CL, Liao LM, Creighton SM. Female genital appearance: 'normality' unfolds. BJOG 2005; 112:643–646.

Maas SM, Hage JJ. Aesthetic labia minora reduction Ann Plast Surg 1998; 41:685.

Marchitelli CE, Sluga MC, Perrotta M, et al. Initial experience in a vulvovaginal aesthetic surgery unit within a general gynecology department. J Low Genit Tract Dis 2010; 14:295–300.

Munhoz AM, Filassi JR, Ricci, et al. Aesthetic labia minora reduction with inferior wedge resection and superior pedicle flap reconstruction. Plast Reconstr Surg 2006; 118:1237–1247.

Paniel BJ, Berville-Levy S, Moyal-Barracco M. La vulvopérinéoplastie. Journal de Gynécolgie. Obstétrique et Biologie de la Reproduction 1984; 31:91–99.

Paniel BJ, Rouzier R. Surgical procedures in benign vulvar disease. In: Neill S, Lewis F. Ridley's The Vulva 3rd edn. Oxford: Wiley-Blackwell, 2009.

Pardo J, Solà V, Ricci P, Guilloff E. Laser labioplasty of labia minora. Int J Gynaecol Obstet 2006; 93:38–43.

Renganathan A. Gynecological cosmetic surgery Expert Rev Obstet Gynecol 2009;4:101–104.

Rouzier R, Louis-Sylvestre C, Paniel B, et al. Hypertrophy of labia minora: Experience with 163 reductions. Am J Obst Gynecol 2000; 182:35–40.

Chapter 41 Vulvar body art

Christa De Cuyper

INTRODUCTION

Body-modifying practices, in particular tattooing and piercing, have become increasingly popular in the Western world in recent decades (De Cuyper et al. 2010, Stirn 2003). The aim of this chapter is to describe to physicians the procedures their patients may undergo, as most clinicians have little knowledge of these. In the genital area, piercing is the most popular procedure and is mainly used to enhance physical attraction and sexual pleasure (Angel 2014). However, according to the WHO classification genital piercings are categorised as type IV female genital mutilation. Some serious risks and complications are described. Body art practitioners are often unaware of the risks associated with such procedures. Complications include infections, allergies and permanent disfigurement.

PIERCING

Materials

Piercing materials

- Gold
- Titanium
- Surgical steel
- Plastics
- Polytetrafluoroethylene (PTFE) (inert thermoplastic polymer): non-stick properties, suitable for initial piercings, and difficult to heal piercings

Piercing retainers or 'sleepers'

- Silicone
- PTFE/Bioflex plastic

Piercings are available in a variety of materials and in different colors and designs. Common shapes are labret studs, captive bead rings or hoops, barbells, circular or curved barbells, and spirals (**Figures 41.1** and **41.2**). High-grade surgical steel is the most frequently used piercing material and is usually well tolerated. Since the introduction of the European Nickel Directive, a substantial decrease in the nickel content of most metal ornaments sold in Europe has resulted in a reduction in cases of nickel contact dermatitis (Lidén & Norberg 2005).

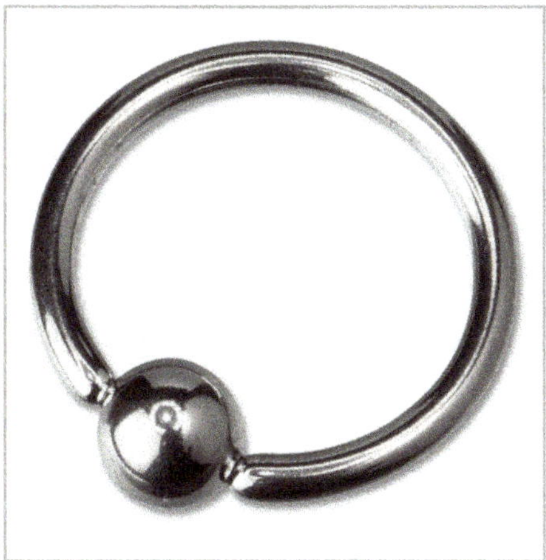

Figure 41.1 Ball closure ring.

Piercing retainers or 'sleepers'

Piercing retainers or 'sleepers' can be used to keep the 'tunnel' created by the piercing open, e.g. during medical interventions or X-ray procedures (**Figures 41.3** and **41.4**).

Bead closures

The captive bead ring or ball closure ring is circular and closed by the pressure present in the ring (**Figure 41.1**). To insert or remove the piercing, the hoop can be opened by internal or external pressure, thus widening the ring and loosening the ball. In a second type, the balls can be screwed on and off and replaced by a variety of designs and ornaments. Internally threaded balls and jewelry reduce the risk of tears in the skin and limit irritation (**Figures 41.5** and **41.6**). Many

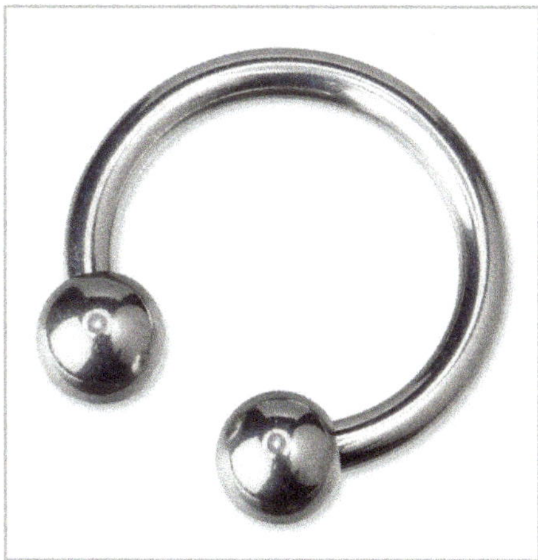

Figure 41.2 Circular barbell.

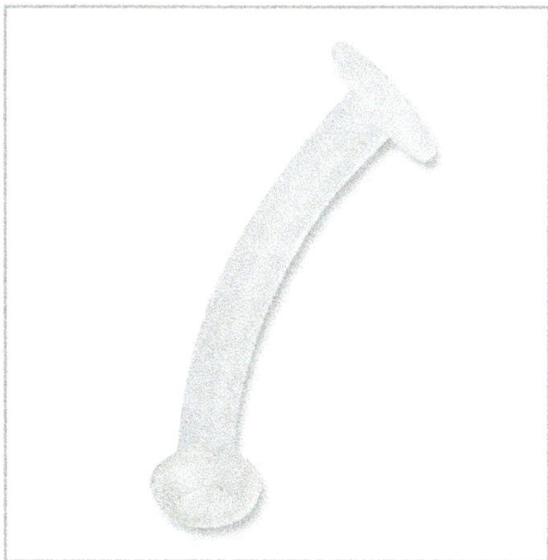

Figure 41.3 Bioplast banana retainer.

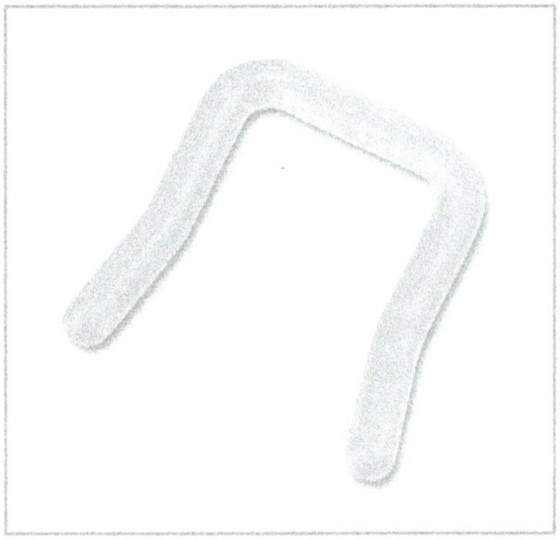

Figure 41.4 Bioplast septum retainer.

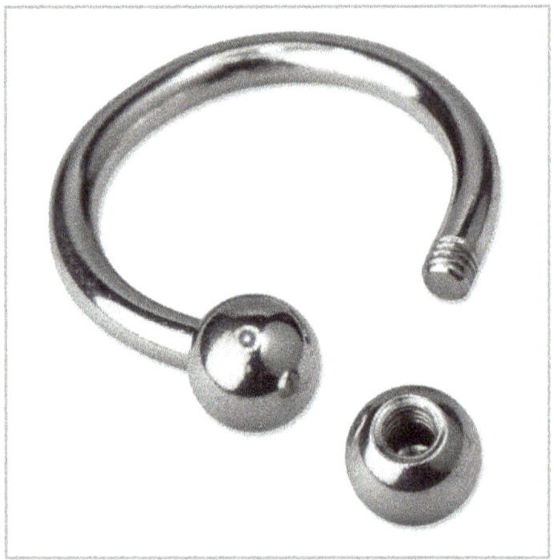

Figure 41.5 External thread circular barbell.

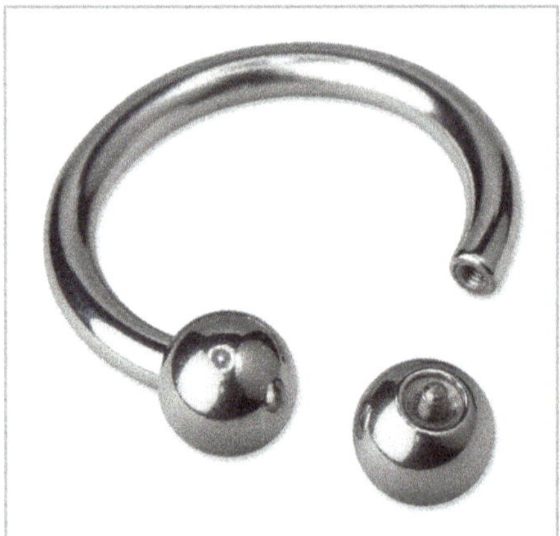

Figure 41.6 Internal thread circular barbell.

accessories can be bought online, including a wide variety of ornaments (De Cuyper 2010).

Procedure

Piercing is performed by perforating the skin, the mucosa and often the underlying cartilage, with a sharp tool followed by the insertion of an ornament or jewel. If this is performed by a trained professional there is little pain; painkillers containing acetyl salicylic acid should be avoided to reduce the risk of bleeding. In contemporary piercings, a temporary stainless steel bar or ring or a piercing retainer made of inert, biocompatible plastic is often used during the healing process. After epithelialization, an artificial 'tunnel' is created and the temporary piercing material can be replaced by another ornamental one.

Anatomical site and rationale for piercings

Almost every part of the body can be pierced for decorative purposes. In adults, more intimate sites are often pierced. Genital piercings are not only used to enhance physical attraction but are also associated with increased sexual pleasure.

Specific terminology is used in the body art world relating to anatomical site or historical associations (**Figure 41.7**). **Table 41.1** describes the anatomical sites and healing time of vulvar piercings.

Vertical and horizontal clitoral hood (VCH and HCH) piercings are perforations through the foreskin above the clitoris; they do not perforate the clitoris (**Figure 41.8**). They are intended to increase sexual desire and to stimulate orgasm. Long lasting complications may result from a VCH piercing in an anatomically unsuited vulva (Angel 2014). **Figure 41.9** demonstrates an incorrect placement of a VCH piercing: the cotton-stick is visible under the skin, indicating a piercing that is too close to the clitoris. Properly placed VCH piercings at the apex under the deepest part of the hood will provide clitoral stimulation. Triangle piercings are located underneath the shaft of the clitoris thereby stimulating the back of the clitoris. (**Figure 41.10**). Diana or Dukes piercings are similar to a VCH but located in an angle on the side of the clitoris. They may be placed singly, in pairs or in combination with a VCH piercing. The healing time varies from 4-8 weeks in this area. Inner labial piercings often heal much faster (4-6 weeks) in contrast to outer labial piercings that take 2-3 months. Outer labial piercings are often placed in pairs or ladders for aesthetic reasons (**Figure 41.11**). Not all women are anatomically suited for all types of genital piercings. A true clitoris piercing in a large exposed clitoris is rarely seen (**Figure 41.12**). Improperly placed VCH piercings that risk damaging the clitoral glans are quite common (**Figure 41.13**) and accidental piercing of the clitoral nerve bundle can be extremely painful (Angel 2014). A fourchette piercing is a vertical perineum piercing at the back edge of the vagina and only possible when there is sufficient tissue and a pinchable skin flap (**Figure 41.14**). This location is prone to infection due to the proximity of the anus: healing can take several months and requires attention to hygiene. To prevent infections, piercees must engage in safe and gentle sex during the healing process and avoid contact with partners' body fluids (even saliva). They should take showers; use of swimming pools, baths or jacuzzis should be avoided. Saline solution and mild fragrance free soaps can be used to keep the piercing clean (Angel 2014).

Side effects

Short-term side effects

Minor side effects are normal in the first days

- Mild bleeding
- Localized swelling
- Tenderness and bruising

Pain and swelling are immediate side effects, cooling may help. Itching and secretion of whitish or slightly coloured fluid can occur. Such side effects are under-reported, mostly transient and often dealt with by the piercers and customers. Trauma caused by the use of inappropriate jewels and/or vigorous sexual activity can cause bleeding (**Figure 41.15**).

Infections

The risk of infection largely depends on the hygienic conditions in which the procedure has been performed and of the pierced site.

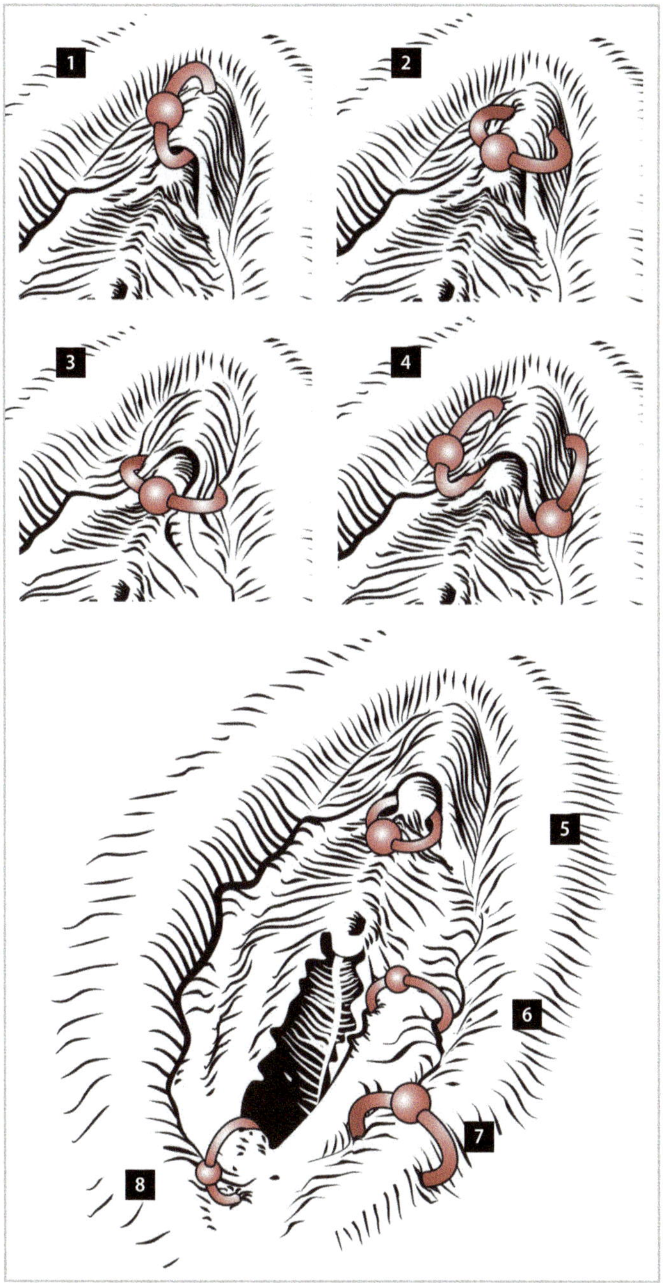

Figure 41.7 Anatomical site of vulvar piercings (numbers of anatomical sites correlate to numbers in the Table 41.1 below)

Table 41.1 Anatomical site of piercings and healing time (the numbers correspond to the numbers shown on Figure 41.7).

Anatomical site	Healing time
1. Vertical clitoral hood, above the clitoris	4–8 weeks
2. Horizontal clitoral hood	6–8 weeks
3. Triangle, underneath the shaft of the clitoris	2–3 months
4. Dukes or Diana	4–8 weeks
5. Clitoris	4–6 weeks
6. Inner labia	4–6 weeks
7. Outer labia	2–3 months
8. Fourchette	2–3 months

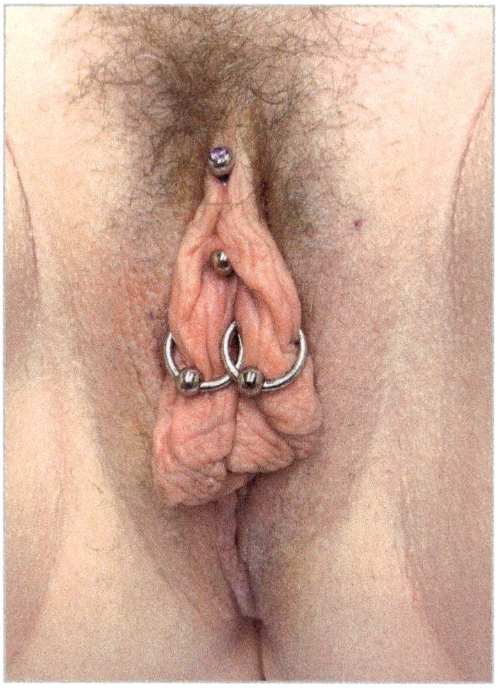

Figure 41.8 Correct vertical clitoral hood and inner labia piercings. By courtesy of Elayne Angel, Mérida, Mexico.

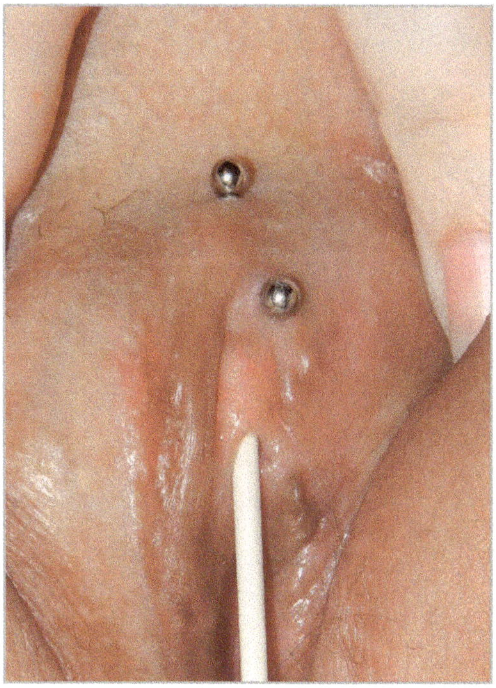

Figure 41.9 Swab test demonstrating the incorrect placement of a vertical clitoral hood piercing (too close to the edge). By courtesy of Elayne Angel, Mérida, Mexico.

Genital piercings often require a long healing time with an increased risk of infection. Most common are bacterial infections caused by *Streptococcus pyogenes* and *Staphylococcus aureus*, but Gram-negative microbial infections must also be considered. Evacuation of pus, inflammation with persistent or increasingly painful swelling can all be indications of infection. High-quality jewelry should be kept in position, allowing drainage of pus and helping to avoid abscess formation. If jewelry is removed, piercings may shrink and the opening will close rapidly. If the jewelry needs to be removed, non-metallic replacements are available. In localized bacterial

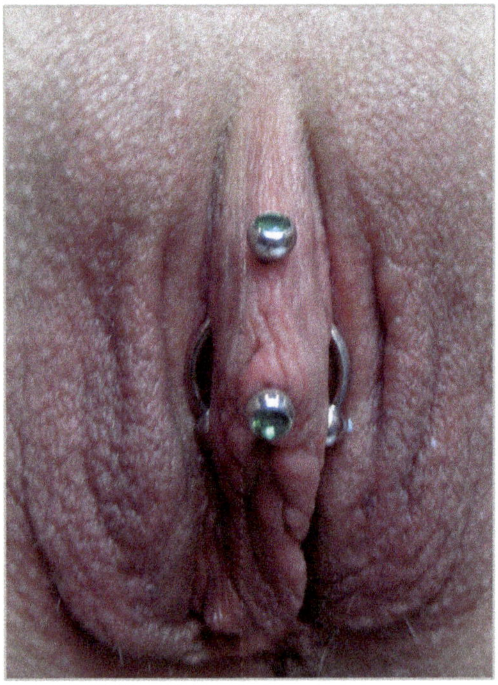

Figure 41.10 Correct vertical clitoral hood and triangle piercing. By courtesy of Elayne Angel, Mérida, Mexico.

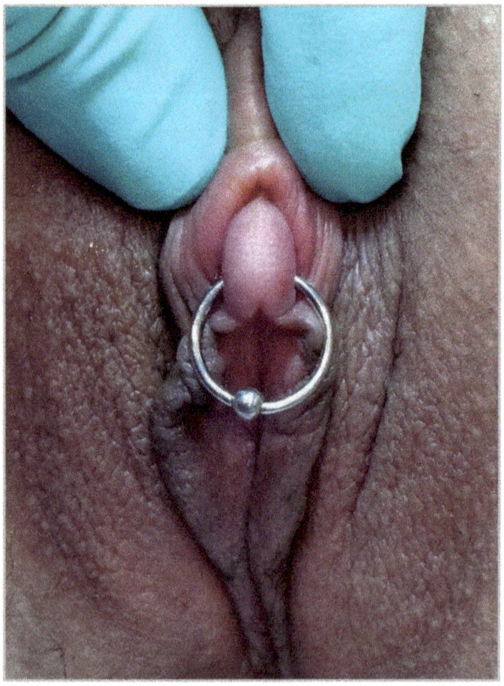

Figure 41.12 Clitoral piercing. By courtesy of Elayne Angel, Mérida, Mexico.

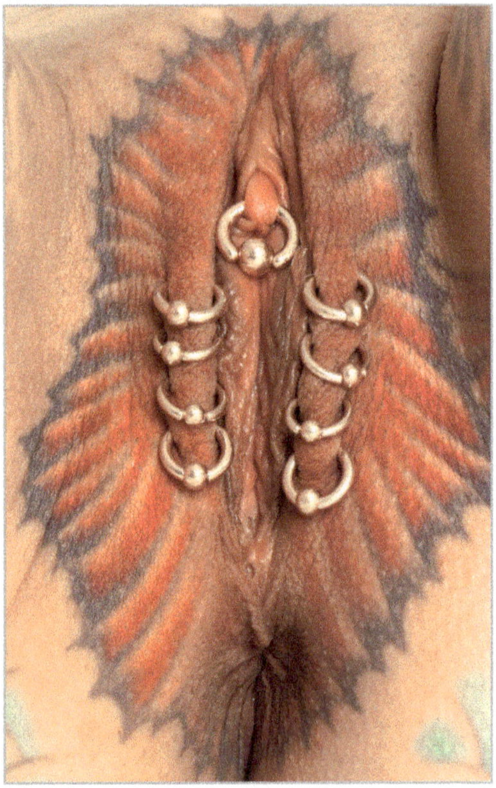

Figure 41.11 Vulvar tattoo, clitoral piercing, and outer labia piercings in ladder distribution. By courtesy of Elayne Angel, Mérida, Mexico.

infection, frequent rinsing with saline or mild soaps is advised. Mild disinfectants and topical antibiotics can also be used, but only for a short period because these products can cause irritation and induce contact dermatitis. Persistent and deep bacterial infections require treatment with systemic antibiotics. Herpes reactivation, common viral warts, and condylomata have all been reported after piercing. Blood-borne infections such as hepatitis B and C, but also human immunodeficiency virus, can be transmitted and should be ruled out serologically. Both the customer and the practitioner are at risk of acquiring a transfusion-transmitted disease. Preventive hepatitis B and tetanus vaccinations are recommended for all body art professionals. Blood donation is not accepted in many countries for 1 year after piercing or tattooing.

Long-term side effects

Trauma and scarring

Shallow VCH piercings or piercings located too close to the edge of the foreskin are at risk of damaging the mucosa (**Figure 41.16**) (Angel 2014). Chronic irritation can lead to granuloma formation and rejection (**Figures 41.17** and **41.18**). Misplacement of the piercings and the use of inappropriate jewelry often result in discomfort and disappointed customers. Figure 41.19 shows VCH piercing placing too cranially: it is too far away from the clitoris with a jewel that is much too short, retracting into the mucosa.

Atrophic scars are common after infections. Hypertrophic scars and keloid formation are observed predominantly in dark skinned individuals. Genital and urethral injuries may result in disfiguring scars and strictures. Infertility as a consequence of ascending infection has also been reported. Genital piercings may cause rupture of condoms during sexual intercourse.

Contact allergies

Contact dermatitis is mostly caused by nickel allergy. Therefore, only metal piercings made of high-grade stainless steel or an inert material should be used. Other compounds in the ornaments or materials used during the procedure and any products used for aftercare that contain additives, antiseptics, and topical antibiotics, can all be responsible for allergic reactions. Any material responsible or suspected to be responsible for allergic reactions must be removed. The use of topical steroids is helpful to reduce the itching and inflammation. In the case of protracted vulvitis, patch testing should be considered. Foreign body reactions, sarcoid-like granuloma, angiofibroma, and pseudolymphoma may be manifestations of unusual allergic reactions to piercings.

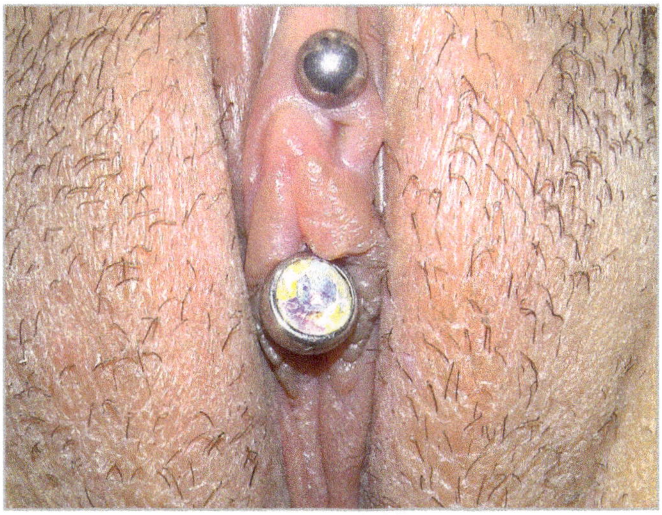

Figure 41.13 Incorrect vertical clitoral hood with accidental damage of the clitoris. By courtesy of Elayne Angel, Mérida, Mexico.

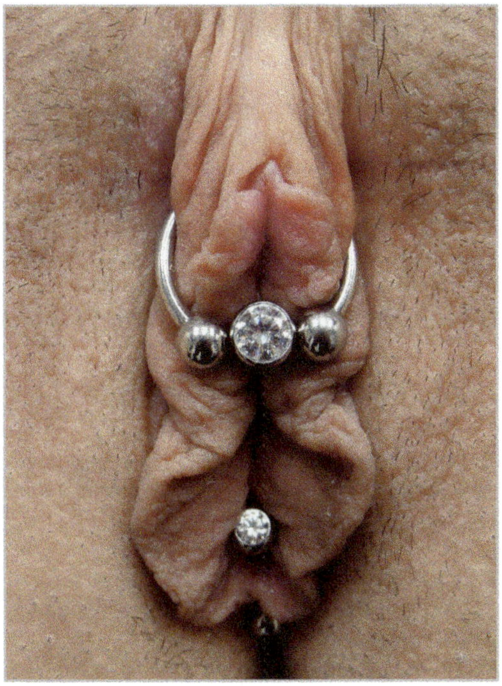

Figure 41.14 Triangle plus fourchette piercing. By courtesy of Elayne Angel, Mérida, Mexico.

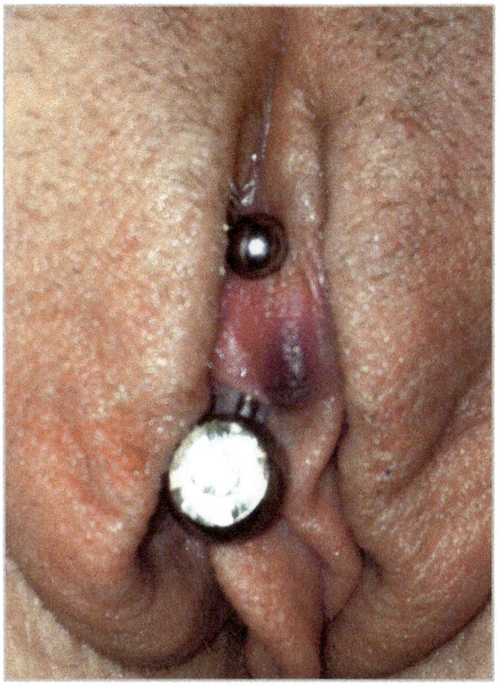

Figure 41.15 Bruising by too big jewelry. By courtesy of Elayne Angel, Mérida, Mexico.

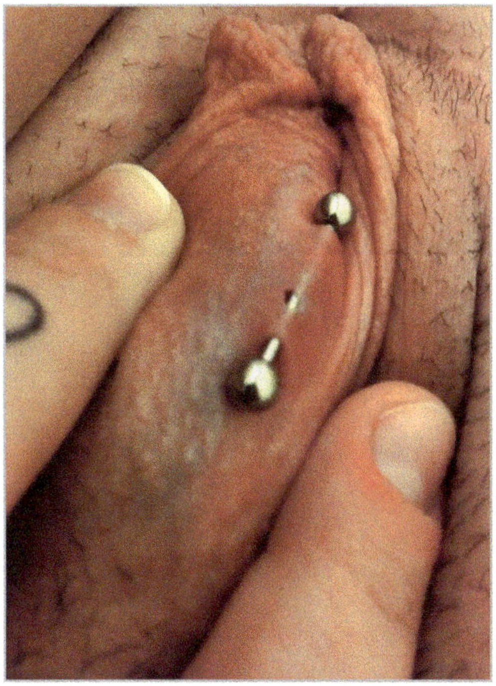

Figure 41.16 Shallow vertical clitoral hood straight barbell piercing with perforation of the foreskin. By courtesy of Elayne Angel, Mérida, Mexico.

Infections

Impetiginization can require antiseptic or antibiotic therapy. Concomitant candidosis must be considered in patients with persistent complaints.

Other complications

Improperly placed piercings may cause nerve damage, e.g. to the clitoral nerve bundle, with temporary or permanent pain or loss of sensation (Angel 2014).

Piercings and implants, in general, may interfere with diagnostic and therapeutic medical procedures. Imaging (ultrasound, radiology, magnetic resonance imaging) can be disturbed by the overlying material. Piercings can interfere with medical interventions, e.g. hindering the insertion of a urethral catheter in emergency situations. Skin burns may also occur if metal-containing piercings are not removed before electrocauterization. Health-care professionals, in particular in emergency and surgery units, should be familiar with the removal of piercings. Genital piercings should be removed before delivery to prevent trauma to the perineum or to the baby during delivery. Plastic 'sleepers' are useful in certain situations.

Documentation of piercings in a patient's medical notes, and discussion of any associated risks are recommended. It is also advisable to obtain the patient's informed consent before the removal of piercings if possible.

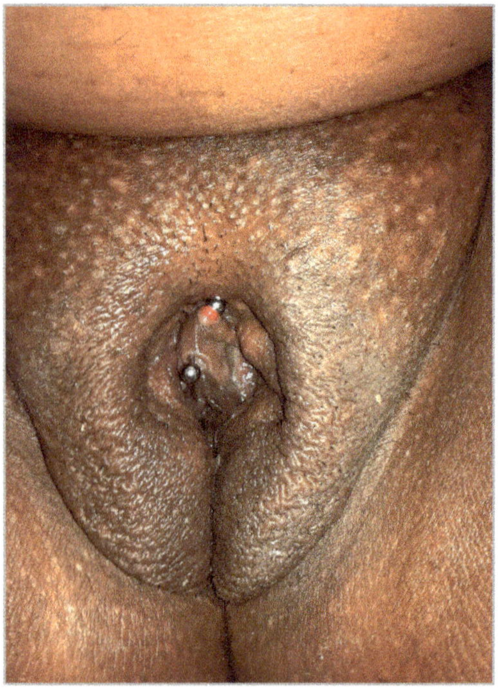

Figure 41.17 Vertical clitoral hood with granuloma. By courtesy of Elayne Angel, Mérida, Mexico.

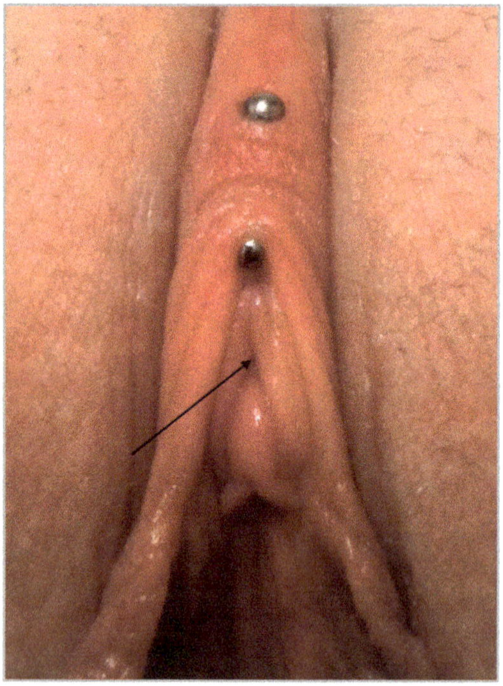

Figure 41.19 Improperly placed vertical clitoral hood piercing too high and too distal from the clitoris with a jewel that is much too short retracting into the mucosa. By courtesy of Elayne Angel, Mérida, Mexico.

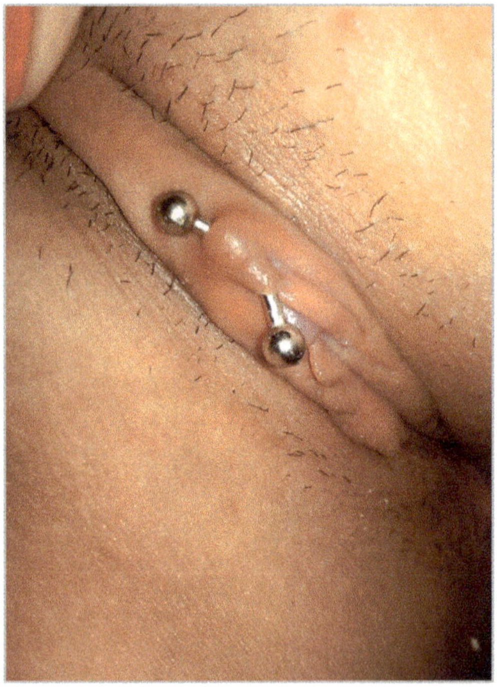

Figure 41.18 Incorrect placement of a curved bar or banana bell piercing with rejection. By courtesy of Elayne Angel, Mérida, Mexico.

TATTOOING

Procedure

The practice of tattooing involves the implantation of a colorant into the skin or the mucosa. The level of implantation depends on the skill of the performer, the purpose of the tattoo, and the type of device (Pérez-Cotapoz et al. 2010). For professionals, a wide range of electronic devices have been developed. Before the procedure, the skin is disinfected and a tattoo print is transferred to the skin. A fine layer of solid Vaseline is applied on the skin to avoid accidental staining of the surrounding skin by the pigments. After tattooing the area is cleaned using a mild soap or an antiseptic solution, then again more Vaseline is applied. However, the procedure will cause a localized inflammatory reaction leading to a relief-like appearance of the design in the first few weeks following the procedure. During the first few days after the procedure, a significant amount of pigment will extrude through the epidermis. After complete healing, the residual pigment will be stored within the macrophages in the dermis. Some pigment will also be transported to the draining lymph nodes.

Side effects

In general, the side effects of tattooing are very similar to the complications after piercings; however, infections are much more common in piercing (Pérez-Cotapoz et al. 2010).

Exacerbation of pre-existing conditions has been reported. Concomitant diseases such as psoriasis, lichen planus, and sarcoidosis can be triggered by tattooing. Psoriasis may occur as a Köbner phenomenon in the tattooed area.

Other complications as sequelae of tattooing include intolerance and allergic reactions to the pigments. This phenomenon occurs more frequently in colored (red/yellow) tattoos but has also been observed in black tattoos. The extent of the reaction is unpredictable, but fortunately often limited to the tattooed area. The mechanism of sensitization and causative allergen is unclear; patch testing is often inconclusive in suspected tattoo allergy: it is usually not positive to the inks used. The toxicological impact of tattooing on public health is still under research.

OTHER BODY-MODIFYING PROCEDURES

Scarring, scalping, branding, and cutting are extreme body-modifying procedures that can result in irreversible mutilation and functional impairment.

CONCLUSION

Body art has become increasingly popular in the Western world in recent decades, attracting in particular the younger generation. Body art practitioners and customers are often unaware of the risks associated with body art procedures. All procedures should be performed under hygienic conditions, with sterile equipment and by trained practitioners. Health-care professionals should be aware of the medical consequences of piercing and the implications for medical interventions.

ACKNOWLEDGMENTS

This chapter was realized with the advice and contribution of Elayne Angel who provided all clinical photos. Piercing material illustrations were provided by Davy D'hollander.

REFERENCES

De Cuyper C, Pérez-Cotapoz ML, Cossio L. Piercings. Techniques and complications. In: De Cuyper , Pérez-Cotapos ML (eds). Complications with body art: Tattoos, piercings and permanent make-up, 1st edition. Berlin: Springer Heidelberg 2010:43–52.

Elayne Angel. The Piercing Bible. The definitive guide to safe body piercing. Available from www.piercingbible.com/female-genital-piercings (accessed 24 November 2015)

Lidén C, Norberg K. Nickel on the Swedish market. Follow-up after implementation of the nickel directive. Contact Dermatitis 2005; 52:29–35.

Pérez-Cotapoz ML, De Cuyper C, Cossio L. Tattooing and scarring: techniques and complications. In: De Cuyper , Pérez-Cotapoz ML (eds), Complications with body art: tattoos, piercings and permanent make-up, 1st edition. Berlin: Springer Heidelberg 2010:29–41.

Stirn A. Body Piercing: medical consequences and psychological motivations. Review. Lancet 2003; 361:1205–1215.

Chapter 42 Vulvar disease in children

Ruth Murphy

INTRODUCTION

Vulvar skin conditions in children are relatively common. However, the lack of understanding from both health care professionals and carers presents a barrier to the optimum delivery of care. The common symptoms of itch, pain, and skin splitting may be frightening to children, making going to the toilet uncomfortable and leading to altered and disruptive behavior. Common skin problems such as irritant or atopic dermatitis can affect the vulva, but there are also more the specific vulvar dermatoses such as lichen sclerosus (LS). This chapter describes the commonest vulvar problems presenting in children, their signs, and symptoms and the best published evidence for how they are managed.

Conditions commonly seen in children

Fused labia	(see also Chapters 1)
Eczema/Dermatitis	(see also Chapters 16 and 17)
Psoriasis	(see also Chapter 22)
Lichen sclerosus	(see also Chapter 19)
Vulvar growths	(see also Chapters 33–35)
Congenital abnormalities	(see also Chapter 37)
Infectious diseases	(see also Chapters 29 and 30)

VULVA IN INFANCY AND CHILDHOOD

In girls, there is a lack of estrogen after the neonatal period and levels remain low until menarche. Without this hormonal influence, the vulvovaginal mucosa is thinner appearing redder than in adults and this can be easily mistaken by the unwary for inflammation. This thinner genital skin is also more easily damaged by common irritants used in bathing such as preservatives in soaps and bubble baths.

The inflammation makes the skin vulnerable to bacterial infection, especially in the presence of poor hygiene. Postmenarche, under the influence of estrogens, the skin becomes thicker and the pH is acidic favoring the colonization of lactobacilli species and supporting overgrowth with *Candida* species.

This is not so in the prepubertal vulva where the pH is between neutral and alkaline favoring the growth of common skin bacteria such as streptococcal and staphylococcal species. This explains why prior to menarche, vulvar infection with *Candida* is rare, although it is frequently but incorrectly attributed as to the cause of pruritus vulvae in children (Lewis & Neill 2009).

PRINCIPLES OF PEDIATRIC VULVAR CARE

Care of the pediatric vulva is essential in maintaining health and preservation of the skin barrier function will help support the fragile vulvar epithelium. This will make vulvar irritation more difficult that in turn minimizes skin damage. Key tips are avoiding cleansing with irritants such as bubble baths, perfumed or medicated cleaning wipes and soaps, and substituting with emollients as detailed in **Table 42.1** (Fischer 2010, Margesson 2004) [see also Chapter 3 (Vulvovaginal care) and Chapter 7 (General treatment considerations)].

FUSED LABIA

Synonym

Labial adhesions

This condition usually presents in young children and is nearly always an incidental finding by carers. Families need to be reassured that the vagina beyond the labia is normal. The cause of adhesion is either physiological and will resolve with time or 'stickiness' of the labia minora from low-grade inflammation resulting in fusion. The ensuing labial fusion or adhesion may occur anywhere from the clitoris to the posterior fourchette. Often there is complete fusion with loss of the vaginal opening (Fischer & Rogers 2000). General vulvar hygiene, as described in Table 42.1, prevents further inflammation of the labia and reduces the risk of recurrence of the adhesions. Most affected individuals or their carers have not been aware of any specific inflammatory condition that predisposes to fusion. It may rarely be an early sign of LS (Gibbon et al. 1999).

Treatment

The condition usually spontaneously resolves by the age of 6 years. However, if persistent, the labia may be teased apart by gentle surgery under a light general anesthesia.

DISCHARGE

Childhood vaginal discharge is a frequent reason for referral (**Figure 42.1**). The commonest cause of discharge in one case series was

Table 42.1 Recommendations for vulvar care in children

Washing	• Use an emollient instead of soap or a shower gel • Bath rather than shower, ensuring that the vulva is cleansed • Do not shampoo hair in the bath • Avoid bubble bath
Wiping	• Wipe front to back after defecation • Avoid commercial wipes with potential irritants and sensitizers
External irritants	• Avoid antifungal creams, perfumed products including herbal/natural creams
Clothing/nappies	• Avoid tight clothing, e.g. lycra ballet clothes or leotards • Wear only cotton or silk underwear • Change nappies regularly

Modified from Fischer (2010)

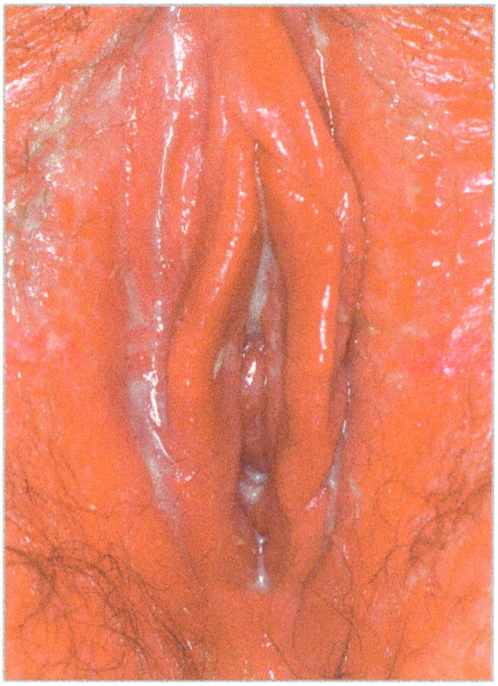

Figure 42.1 Discharge in a girl with *Candida* infection complicated by contact eczema. By courtesy of Prof. Dominique Parent, Belgium.

vulvovaginitis (82%) (McGreal & Wood 2013). Other important causes included suspected sexual abuse (5%), foreign body (3%), labial adhesions (3%), and vaginal agenesis (2%). Thirty-five percent of patients were admitted for vaginoscopy. In case of premenarcheal vaginal bleeding or bloody discharge, vaginoscopy under general anesthesia is recommended to exclude, e.g. foreign bodies or malignancies such as an embryonal rhabdomyosarcoma.

Treatment

Vulvovaginitis often responds to simple hygiene measures.

VULVAR DERMATITIS IN CHILDREN

Dermatitis

This is the most common cause of vulvar symptoms in prepubertal girls:

- **Irritant vulvitis:** due to irritation
- **Napkin dermatitis:** seen in very young children
- **Atopic vulvitis:** possibly part of an atopic diathesis
- **Allergic contact dermatitis:** rare in this age group

Irritant vulvitis

This is common, because, as previously described, the thin skin in the genital region is more prone to irritation. Any measures taken to reduce irritation, as suggested in **Table 42.1**, will help prevent this condition. The common symptom associated with irritant vulvitis is itch becoming painful when there is a superadded bacterial infection.

Napkin dermatitis

Napkin dermatitis is a subset of irritant dermatitis typically affecting children from 9 to 12 months of age. It has an estimated incidence of between 7% and 35% (Atherton 2004). Any gastrointestinal disturbance or neonatal malformation associated with increase of feces and/or urine trapped by the nappy or diaper against the skin will predispose to this condition.

Jacquet erosive dermatitis is a particularly unusual and potentially severe form of napkin dermatitis. It presents as skin-colored umbilicated papules or nodules with minimal erythema. With disposable nappies nowadays, this is relatively rare.

The risk of napkin dermatitis is reduced by frequent nappy changes, coupled with the use of agents to improve the skin barrier such as zinc oxide cream and petroleum jelly (Alonso et al. 2013) (see also Chapter 3 and 7 for vulvar care).

Atopic vulvitis

Atopic disease in the genital area ('atopic vulvitis') occurs more commonly in children with an atopic diathesis or family members affected with asthma, eczema, or hay-fever (see also Chapter 16 for atopic eczema). Atopic individuals are also more prone to irritant vulvitis (Fischer & Rogers 2000). A study from Australia found that 24% (9/38) of girls with 'vulvovaginitis' had clinical signs of atopic dermatitis on general skin examination (Fischer 2010) and in a larger case series of 130 girls, 33% (41/130) had atopic or irritant dermatitis (Fischer & Rogers 2000). Typical signs of atopic vulvitis are dry, red, itchy skin. If there is a secondary bacterial infection, there might be associated pain and vaginal discharge, sometimes with satellite pustular folliculitis. When children scratch, lichen simplex may ensue (**Figure 42.2**).

Treatment

The treatment principles are, as always, to optimize vulvar care as outlined in **Table 42.1** and to switch off the inflammation using a topical steroid of appropriate potency (NICE CG057 2007). Any secondary bacterial infection needs to be treated with antibiotics. It is important to stress that this is a relapsing and remitting condition and that while it is easy to treat, the regular use of emollients to restore barrier function is necessary with intermittent 'pulses' of moderately potent topical steroids.

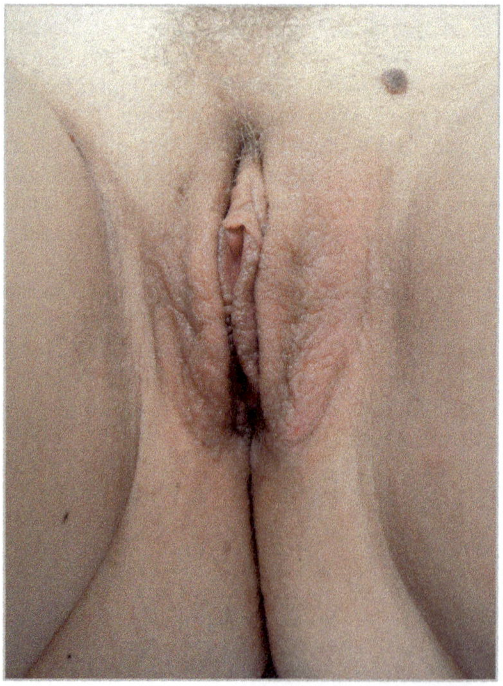

Figure 42.2 Lichen simplex in a teenager showing typical erythema, thickening of the skin, and lichenification. Patient had been scratching. By courtesy of Dr Karen Gibbon, Whipps Cross University Hospital, London, UK.

OTHER INFLAMMATORY DISEASES

Psoriasis

Vulvar psoriasis is a common cause of persistent vulvar problems, estimated to be 4% of cases of pediatric vulvitis (Kapila et al. 2012, Zamirska et al. 2008). Genital psoriasis appears as a well-demarcated erythematous plaque often extending to the inguinal folds and natal cleft (**Figures 42.3** and **42.4**). Flexural involvement means that there is a reduction in associated scale and the plaques may appear redder. Secondary bacterial and *Candida* infections are common and may be a cause of pain in the fissured skin (see also Chapter 22).

A family history of psoriasis (47%) and psoriasis elsewhere on the skin (78%) is usually reported (Kapila et al. 2012, Zamirska et al. 2008). Parents may not realize that an inflamed umbilicus or cracking behind the ears is psoriasis and this may result in under-reporting of the condition. Psoriasis in the vulvar region is both persistent and chronic.

Treatment and prognosis

It is important to manage the expectations around aspects of control rather than cure of the lesions.

To reduce the irritation and secondary infection, the vulvar hygiene techniques recommended in **Table 42.1** should be employed. The inflammation is reduced using a topical steroid of appropriate potency. The UK's National Institute for Health and Clinical Excellence (NICE) guidelines for psoriasis recommend short-term mild or moderate potency corticosteroids applied once or twice daily (for a maximum of 2 weeks) (NICE CG153 2012). Calcineurin inhibitors that are sometimes useful for treating genital psoriasis in adults are not licensed for use in the treatment of psoriasis in children.

Lichen sclerosus

Synonyms

Lichen sclerosus et atrophicus, kraurosis vulvae, lichen albus, hypoplastic dystrophy

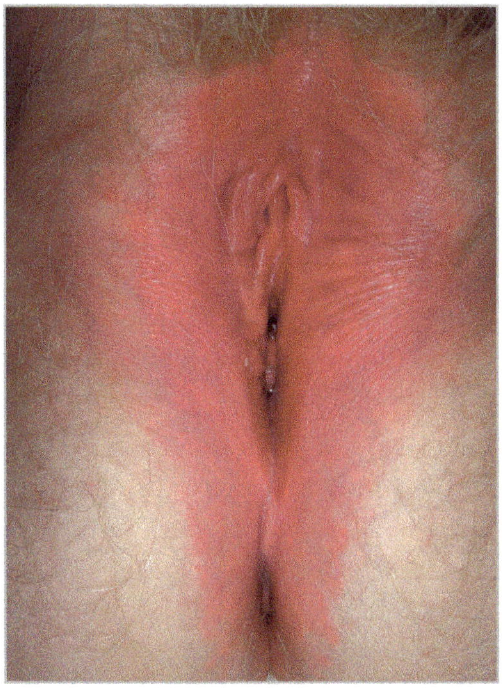

Figure 42.3 Vulvar psoriasis in a teenager showing the typical symmetrical, well-demarcated erythema with minimal scaling. By courtesy of Dr Karen Gibbon, Whipps Cross University Hospital, London, UK.

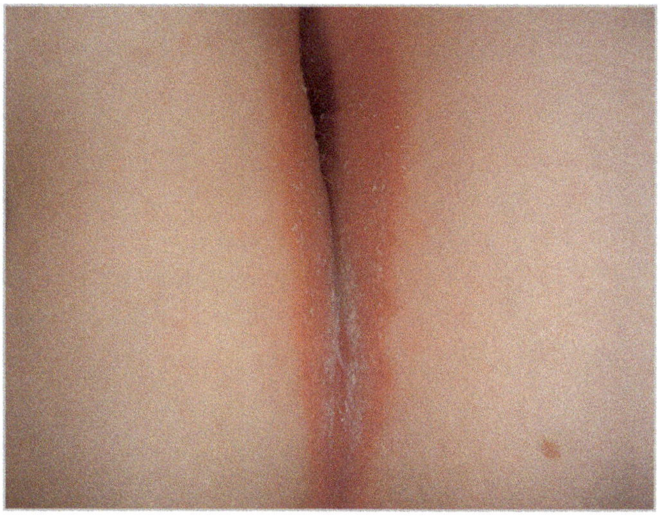

Figure 42.4 Vulvar psoriasis involving the natal cleft. This is a common site of involvement. By courtesy of Dr Karen Gibbon, Whipps Cross University Hospital, London, UK.

LS is predominantly a genital dermatosis, which can affect young girls as well as postmenopausal women (see also Chapter 19). It frequently presents with anogenital itch, splitting, and soreness. This leads to behavior changes such as 'grinding' often observed at school and pain and distress when going to the toilet due to dysuria and perianal skin splitting, which leads to constipation.

Vulvar examination will often show well-demarcated white plaques in a figure of eight distribution extending from the periclitoral skin to the anal margin (**Figure 42.5a** and **b**). In the early stages of inflammation, the affected skin appears to 'wrinkle' (**Figure 42.6a** and **b**). It is shiny and thinned, and easily bleeds when scratched producing characteristic dermal hemorrhage or ecchymoses (**Figure 42.7**). These distinct clinical features are usually diagnostic. However, if there is doubt, a biopsy should be carried out. There may be scarring with loss of the normal labia minora. The skin may fissure or erode (**Figure 42.8**).

Treatment

There are no random controlled trials for therapeutic interventions for the treatment of LS in children. Evidence is therefore largely collated from the clinical experience from reported case series. Superpotent topical steroids are more effective than moderate potency preparations to switch off the inflammation. They also appear to be well tolerated with very few side effects if used responsibly (Fischer & Rogers 2000, Powell & Wojnarowska 2001). To induce remission, there are two commonly used treatment regimens, each needing a reducing course of daily applied topical potent/superpotent topical steroid followed by a maintenance application usually of once weekly to fortnightly (Powell & Wojnarowska 2001). LS is very responsive to topical steroids and an apparent poor response or frequent relapse is generally due to parental fears about topical steroids and their side effects. Reassurance is essential in establishing adequate disease control. Second-line therapy with topical calcineurin inhibitors, e.g. pimecrolimus 1%, for resistant cases is reported in children but should not be used unless it is clearly established that disease resistance is driving the therapeutic escalation rather than parental fear and poor compliance with topical steroids (Boms et al. 2004, Kirtschig et al. 2015).

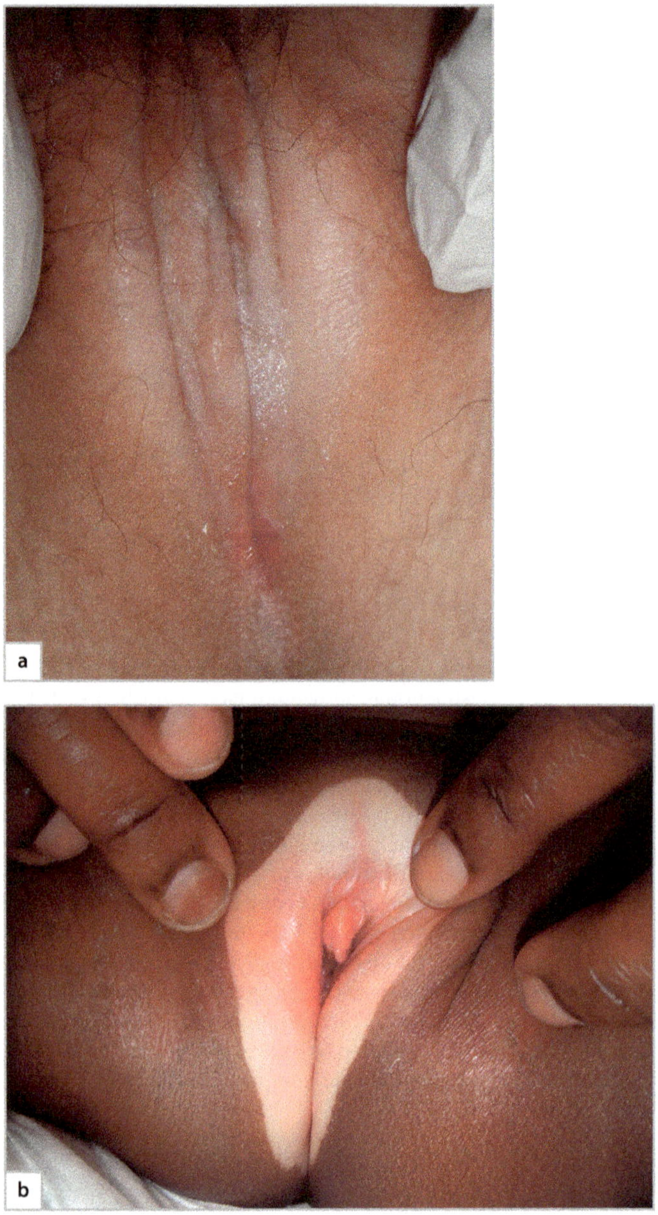

Figure 42.5a and b Lichen sclerosus in two girls showing pallor affecting the vulva and perianal area. By courtesy of Dr Karen Gibbon, Whipps Cross University Hospital, London, UK.

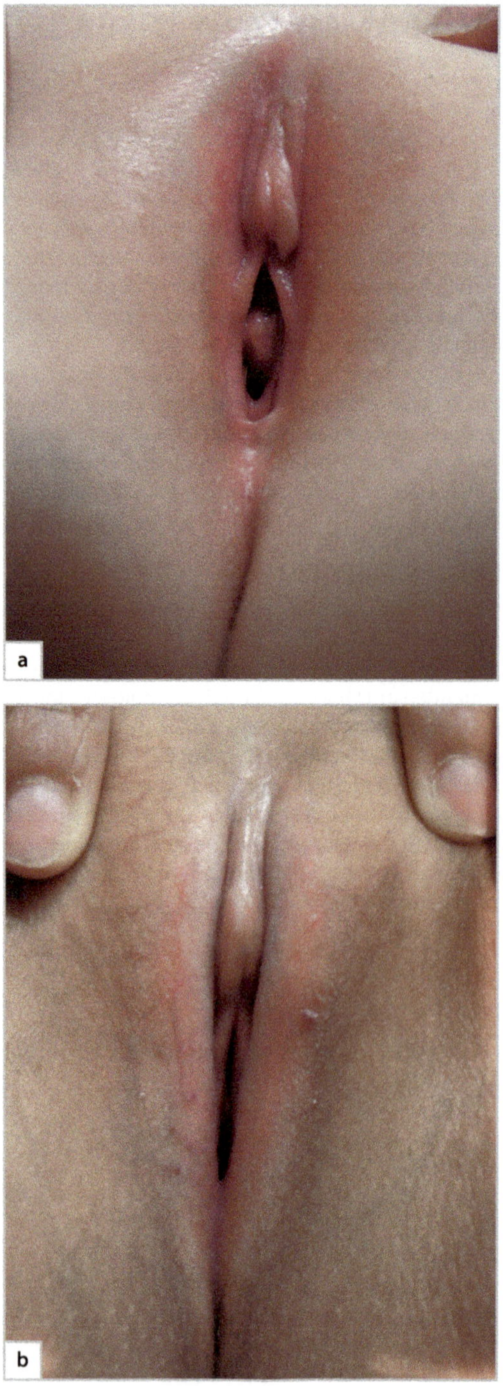

Figure 42.6 (a, b) Subtle pallor of lichen sclerosus. By courtesy of Dr Gudula Kirtschig, Tübingen, Germany.

Prognosis

Course after puberty

There is a risk of developing squamous cell carcinoma of the vulva in individuals affected with LS, and although some individuals developed the LS in childhood, it is not known whether early onset disease increases the likelihood of neoplastic transformation (Leibowitch et al. 1990). About one-third of cases may remit at puberty.

VULVAR GROWTHS

Benign growths in the vulvar region are relatively common accounting in one series for 12% (15/130) diagnoses (Fischer 2010). Moles or nevi mainly occur and melanoma, although rare, has been reported (see also Chapter 34). All nevi in this region should be assessed for malignancy similar to any other nevi on the skin, and the use of a dermatoscope is appropriate (Stricker et al. 2003). Hemangioma or 'strawberry marks' are relatively common in this region and are covered in Chapter 37.

COMMON VULVAR SKIN INFECTIONS IN CHILDREN

Candida infection

As previously described, prior to puberty, it is very unusual for girls to develop *Candida* infections in the genital region, unless they are

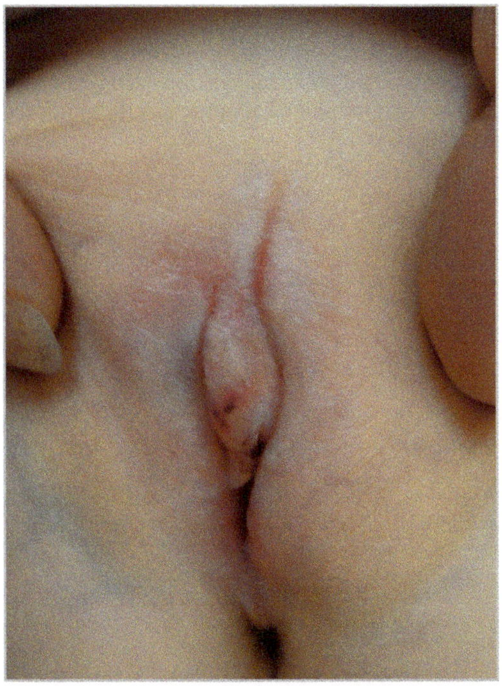

Figure 42.7 Lichen sclerosus in a young child showing pallor and ecchymoses. By courtesy of Dr Karen Gibbon, Whipps Cross University Hospital, London, UK.

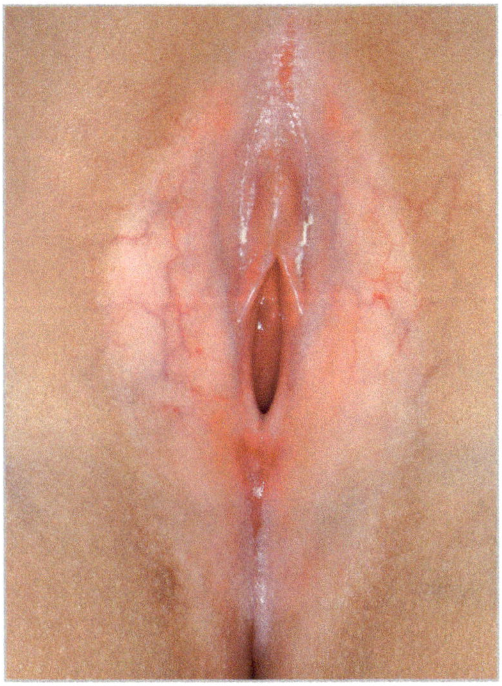

Figure 42.8 Lichen sclerosus showing postinflammatory hypopigmentation, fused labia minora above the clitoris and erosions. By courtesy of Dr Gudula Kirtschig Tübingen, Germany.

immunosuppressed (Fischer 2010) (see also Chapter 29). Despite this, vulvar 'thrush' is still commonly considered when children present with vulvovaginal irritation. This is evidenced by a study of swabs taken from 192 girls aged from 2 to 12 years who had symptoms of vulvovaginitis with the presumed diagnosis of *Candida* infection. Only two were found to have *Candida albicans* infection and in both of them it was considered to be secondary to psoriasis rather than a primary skin infection (Egan et al. 1997).

Bacterial infection

Infection of the genital region with streptococcal species is very common (see also Chapter 29). Streptococcal vulvitis commonly involves the perianal region followed by the perineum and genitalia. Studies of girls with vulvovaginal symptoms (i.e. erythema, discharge, and itch) aged 2–12 years found that 17/80 and 47/74 had swabs positive for β-haemolytic *Streptococcus* and *Streptococcus pyogenes*, respectively (Stricker et al. 2003). In a study of 23 girls with proven Group A streptococcal infection (Mogielnicki et al. 2000), symptoms in those with perianal infection ranged from perianal pruritus or tenderness to abdominal pain and rectal bleeding. In the same study, girls with vulvovaginitis complained of a variety of symptoms including dysuria, pruritus, tenderness, and discharge. There is usually a red swollen appearance to the vulva, sometimes with pustular lesions on the perineum and a thin greenish discharge. Treatment is with the antibiotics of appropriate sensitivity. In cases of recurrent infection, the possibility of a retained intravaginal foreign body should be considered.

Scabies

Scabies infection is caused by the mite *Sarcoptes scabiei* (see also Chapter 31). It is most common in children and young adults and is transmitted through close physical contact. The symptoms are of intense itch, often worse at night accompanied by the presence of burrows, vesicles, and pustules. In more advanced cases, nodules might be present in the genital region or elsewhere on the skin. While the head and neck are generally spared, in very young children this might not be the case.

Treatment

The Cochrane review group has recommended the use of Permethrin cream 5% as safe and effective in killing both the mites and their eggs (Strong & Johnstone 2007). Treatment should be used by the patient and close contacts and should be applied for at least 8 hours overnight from head-to-toe, and repeated 7 days later (see Chapter 31 for further advice).

Genital warts

Genital warts (condylomata acuminata), caused by human papilloma virus infection, are also relatively common in children and do not necessarily indicate sexual abuse (see also Chapter 30). Maternal transmission from the genital tract during birth is a well-recognized mode of infection of the virus. Consideration should always be given to the risk of sexual abuse. In general, older children presenting with genital warts are more likely to have acquired them sexually than younger children, with an increased likelihood over 11 years of age (for treatment recommendations, see Chapter 30).

Molluscum contagiosum

Molluscum contagiosum is one of the commonest skin infections in childhood (see also Chapter 30). It is caused by a poxvirus and has a peak incidence between 2 and 5 years of age (Kyriakis et al. 2007). The warm moist genital environment promotes spread and lesions commonly occur in this region. These lesions spontaneously resolve but can cause significant parental concern. A recently updated Cochrane systematic review found that many common treatments for molluscum, such as physical destruction techniques (e.g. with cryotherapy), have not been adequately evaluated and suggested that most infections be left to resolve naturally. However, this may take months or years in particular in patients with an atopic constitution.

CONCLUSION

Vulvar conditions in children are common. They often present with symptoms that may result in abnormal behavior at school or home. Carers are universally concerned and need reassurance. Due to generally poor understanding of these disorders, time is needed to fully explain the diagnosis, any necessary investigations, and management plan, including providing written instructions and information leaflets to affected young people and their families. Most conditions are treatable and carers should be reassured of this so that their children receive the best possible care.

REFERENCES

Alonso C, Larburu I, Bon E, et al. Efficacy of petrolatum jelly for the prevention of diaper rash: a randomized clinical trial. J Spec Pediatr Nurs 2013; 18:123–132.

Atherton DJ. A review of the pathophysiology, prevention and treatment of irritant diaper dermatitis. Curr Med Res Opin 2004; 20:645–649.

Boms S, Gambichler T, Freitag M, et al. Pimecrolimus 1% cream for anogenital lichen sclerosus in childhood. BMC Dermatol 2004; 4:14.

Egan CA, Bradley R, Logsdon VK, et al. Vulvar melanoma in childhood. Arch Dermatol 1997; 133:345–348.

Fischer G, Rogers M. Vulvar disease in children: a clinical audit of 130 cases. Pediatr Dermatol 2000; 17:1–6.

Fischer G. Chronic vulvitis in pre-pubertal girls. Australas J Dermatol 2010;51:118–123.

Gibbon KL, Bewley AP, Salisbury JA. Labial fusion in children: a presenting feature of genital lichen sclerosus? Pediatr Dermatol 1999; 16:388–391.

Kapila S, Bradford J, Fischer G. Vulvar psoriasis in adults and children: a clinical audit of 194 cases and review of the literature. J Low Genit Tract Dis 2012; 16:364–371.

Kirtschig G, Becker K, Günthert A, et al. Evidence-based (S3) Guideline on (anogenital) Lichen sclerosus. J Eur Acad Dermatol Venereol 2015 ;29:e1–e43.

Kyriakis KP, Palamaras I, Terzoudi S, et al. Case detection rates of molluscum contagiosum in childhood. Pediatr Dermatol 2007; 24:198–199.

Leibowitch M, Neill S, Pelisse M, et al. The epithelial changes associated with squamous cell carcinoma of the vulva: a review of the clinical, histological and viral findings in 78. women. Br J Obstet Gynaecol 1990; 97:1135–1139.

Lewis FM and Neill SM. Principles of examination, investigation and treatment. In: Neill SM, Lewis FM (eds), Ridley's The Vulva, Chichester, West Sussex: Wiley-Blackwell, 2009:34–43.

Margesson LJ. Contact dermatitis of the vulva. Dermatol Ther 2004; 17:20–27.

McGreal S and Wood P. Recurrent Vaginal Discharge in Children. J Pediatr Adolesc Gynecol 2013; 26: 205–208.

Mogielnicki NP, Schwartzman JD, Elliott JA. Perineal group A streptococcal disease in a pediatric practice. Pediatrics 2000; 106:276–281.

National Institute for Health and Clinical Excellence. Atopic eczema in children: management of atopic eczema in children from birth up to the age of 12 years. CG057. London: NICE, 2007.

National Institute for Health and Clinical Excellence. Chronic plaque psoriasis in adults and children. CG153. London: NICE, 2012.

Powell J, Wojnarowska F. Childhood vulvar lichen sclerosus: an increasingly common problem. J Am Acad Dermatol 2001; 44:803–806.

Stricker T, Navratil F, Sennhauser FH. Vulvovaginitis in prepubertal girls. Arch Dis Child 2003; 88:324–326.

Strong M, Johnstone P. Interventions for treating scabies. Cochrane Database Syst Rev 2007(3): CD000320.

Zamirska A, Reich A, Berny-Moreno J, et al. Vulvar pruritus and burning sensation in women with psoriasis. Acta Derm Venereol 2008; 88:132–135.

Index

Note: Page numbers in **bold** or *italic* refer to tables or figures respectively.

EU GSPR Authorised Reprsentative
Logos Europe, 9 rue Nicolas Poussin
1700, La Rochelle, France
Phone: +33 (0) 6 67 93 73 78
E-mail: contact@logoseurope.eu

www.ingramcontent.com/pod-product-compliance
Ingram Content Group UK Ltd.
Pitfield, Milton Keynes, MK11 3LW, UK
UKHW051912100926
8556IPUK00005B/855
9781909836013